Textbook of Microbiology for BSc Nursing

Textbook of Microbiology for BSc Nursing
SECOND EDITION

Surinder Kumar MD DNB MNAMS
Ex-Director Professor
Department of Microbiology
Maulana Azad Medical College
New Delhi, India

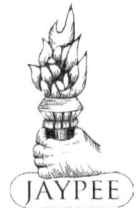

JAYPEE BROTHERS MEDICAL PUBLISHERS
The Health Sciences Publisher
New Delhi | London

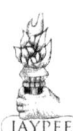 **Jaypee Brothers Medical Publishers (P) Ltd**

Headquarters
Jaypee Brothers Medical Publishers (P) Ltd
EMCA House
23/23-B, Ansari Road, Daryaganj
New Delhi - 110 002, India
Landline: +91-11-23272143, +91-11-23272703
+91-11-23282021, +91-11-23245672
Email: jaypee@jaypeebrothers.com

Corporate office
Jaypee Brothers Medical Publishers (P) Ltd
4838/24, Ansari Road, Daryaganj
New Delhi 110 002, India
Phone: +91-11-43574357
Fax: +91-11-43574314
Email: jaypee@jaypeebrothers.com

Overseas office
J.P. Medical Ltd
83 Victoria Street, London
SW1H 0HW (UK)
Phone: +44 20 3170 8910
Fax: +44 (0)20 3008 6180
Email: info@jpmedpub.com

Website: www.jaypeebrothers.com
Website: www.jaypeedigital.com

© 2022, Jaypee Brothers Medical Publishers

The views and opinions expressed in this book are solely those of the original contributor(s)/author(s) and do not necessarily represent those of editor(s) of the book.

All rights reserved. No part of this publication may be reproduced, stored or transmitted in any form or by any means, electronic, mechanical, photocopying, recording or otherwise, without the prior permission in writing of the publishers.

All brand names and product names used in this book are trade names, service marks, trademarks or registered trademarks of their respective owners. The publisher is not associated with any product or vendor mentioned in this book.

Medical knowledge and practice change constantly. This book is designed to provide accurate, authoritative information about the subject matter in question. However, readers are advised to check the most current information available on procedures included and check information from the manufacturer of each product to be administered, to verify the recommended dose, formula, method and duration of administration, adverse effects and contraindications. It is the responsibility of the practitioner to take all appropriate safety precautions. Neither the publisher nor the author(s)/editor(s) assume any liability for any injury and/or damage to persons or property arising from or related to use of material in this book.

This book is sold on the understanding that the publisher is not engaged in providing professional medical services. If such advice or services are required, the services of a competent medical professional should be sought.

Every effort has been made where necessary to contact holders of copyright to obtain permission to reproduce copyright material. If any have been inadvertently overlooked, the publisher will be pleased to make the necessary arrangements at the first opportunity.

Inquiries for bulk sales may be solicited at: jaypee@jaypeebrothers.com

Textbook of Microbiology for BSc Nursing

First Edition: 2015

Second Edition: **2022**

ISBN 978-93-5465-123-6

Dedicated to

My Father
Late Shri Lachhman Das,

Mother
Late Smt Bal Kaur,

Wife
Dr (Prof) Savita Kumari,

and
Sons
Dr Sourabh Kumar and Dr Sanchit Kumar

Whose love and energy make everything I do possible.

Preface to the Second Edition

This book, *Textbook of Microbiology for BSc Nursing* remains true to the goals of the first edition to provide a brief, accurate and up-to-date presentation with limited time and the latest syllabus for nursing students. These aims are achieved by using several different formats, which should make the book useful to students with varying study objectives and learning styles. It covers both applied microbiology and infection control including safety as per BSc Nursing syllabus.

After teaching medical microbiology for many years, I believe that students appreciate a book that presents the essential information in a readable, interesting, and varied format. I hope you find that the second edition of book meets these criterias. I shall be thankful for any comment or suggestions from students, teachers and all the readers of this book for further improvement.

I am thankful to Shri Jitendar P Vij (Group Chairman), Mr Ankit Vij (Managing Director), Mr MS Mani (Group President) of M/s Jaypee Brothers Medical Publishers (P) Ltd., New Delhi, India, for their support in this project.

The invaluable assistance of my wife Dr Savita Kumari, my sons Dr Sourabh Kumar and Dr Sanchit Kumar in making this book a reality is also gratefully acknowledged.

Surinder Kumar

Preface to the First Edition

Microbiology is an extremely diverse discipline and can be a bewildering field to the novice particularly for BSc Nursing students due to the limited syllabus. Nursing students are in a fix to take a particular book with limited time and syllabus. Traditional books are too long and detailed to be read by the typical nursing student who is trying to keep up with several classes of other nursing subjects simultaneously. The microbiology text presented here is written after 28 years of teaching of medical, dental and nursing students and searching for a book that was both readable and complete enough to meet the needs of nursing students. This *Textbook of Microbiology for BSc Nursing* contains all the information that is pertinent to students, who are studying microbiology, keeping in mind their examination. It also provides a solid background of microbiology while describing the organisms in a manner that is relevant to nursing practice.

The textbook is divided into eight sections, based on the major disciplines included within the syllabus of nursing microbiology—general bacteriology, immunology, systemic bacteriology, virology, medical mycology, medical parasitology, miscellaneous and diagnostic medical microbiology. To facilitate understanding of the subject matter, we have added tables, illustrated figures, and photographs throughout the text to help students understand and retain information. At the end of each chapter, the reader will find chapter summary as "Key Points" and "Important Questions" to reinforce comprehension and preparation for the examination. I hope, this book will be received with the enthusiasm and will fulfill the needs of nursing students. I shall be thankful for any comment or suggestions from students, teachers and all the readers of this book for further improvement.

Surinder Kumar

Acknowledgments

I am greatly indebted to a variety of mentors, friends and colleagues, especially who encouraged me and gave valuable suggestions for improving the text. I would like to thank my family for patiently enduring the writing of this book. Their support and encouragement at home are integral to my activities at work.

I am especially grateful to my wife Dr Savita Kumari, Professor, Department of Internal Medicine, Postgraduate Institute and Medical Research, Chandigarh, for her support and encouragement and to two special children, Dr Sourabh Kumar and Sanchit Kumar (medical student) who gave me their valuable moments without any complaint for completing this book so I could retain my sanity.

I am especially thankful to Dr Sanjeev R Saigal, my PhD student, and now Research Associate in Indian Council of Medical Research (ICMR), for his constant help for this book.

I am very grateful to the whole team of M/s Jaypee Brothers Medical Publishers (P) Ltd, New Delhi, India, who helped and guided me, especially Shri Jitendar P Vij (Group Chairman), Mr Ankit Vij (Managing Director), Mr MS Mani (Group President), Dr Madhu Choudhary (Publishing Head–Education), Ms Pooja Bhandari (Production Head), Ms Sunita Katla (Executive Assistant to Group Chairman and Publishing Manager), Ms Samina Khan (Executive Assistant to Publishing Head–Education), Ms Dolly Dominic (RN, MSN) (Development Editor), Mr Rajesh Sharma (Production Coordinator), Ms Seema Dogra (Cover Visualizer), Mr Laxmidhar Padhiary (Proofreader), Mr Jagvir Singh (Typesetter), Mr Pappu Kumar (Graphic Designer) and their team members, for all their support to work in this project and make it a success. Without their cooperation, I could not have completed this project.

Contents

SECTION 1: General Microbiology

1. **Historical Development of Microbiology** ... 3
   - Introduction and Scope ... 3
   - Importance and Relevance of Microorganisms ... 3
   - Importance of Microbiology in Nursing ... 4
   - The Discovery of Microorganisms ... 5
   - Scientific Development of Microbiology ... 5
   - Immunity and Immunization ... 6
   - Serotherapy and Chemotherapy ... 6
   - Branches of Microbiology ... 7
   - Nobel Prizes Awarded for Research in Microbiology ... 7

2. **Microscopy and Morphology of Bacteria** ... 11
   - Microscopy ... 11
   - Light Microscopy ... 11
   - Morphology of Bacteria ... 13
   - Naming and Classifying Microorganisms ... 13
   - Nomenclature ... 13
   - Comparison of Prokaryotic Cells and Eukaryotic Cells ... 13
   - Morphology of Bacteria ... 14
   - L-Forms of Bacteria (Cell-Wall-Defective Organisms) ... 20

3. **Physiology of Bacteria** ... 22
   - Principles of Bacterial Growth ... 22

4. **Culture Media and Culture Methods** ... 25
   - Classification of Media ... 25
   - Culture Methods ... 28

5. **Infection** ... 31
   - Sources of Infection ... 32
   - Modes of Transmission of Infection ... 32
   - Factors Predisposing to Microbial Pathogenicity ... 32

6. **Staining Methods** ... 36
   - Hanging Drop Preparation ... 36
   - Staining Methods ... 38

Gram Stain	39
Acid-fast Stain (Ziehl–Neelsen Staining of Acid-fast Bacilli)	41
Special Stains	43
Methods for Detection for Direct Microscopic Detection of Fungi in Clinical Specimens	43

SECTION 2: Immunology

7. Immunity — 47
- Definition — 47
- Classification — 47
- Types of Immunity — 48

8. Antigens — 51
- Types of Antigen — 51
- Antigenic Determinant or Epitome — 51
- Determinants of Antigenicity — 51

9. Antibodies (Immunoglobulins) — 53
- Antibody Structure — 53
- Immunoglobulin Classes — 54
- Role of Different Immunoglobulin Classes — 57

10. The Complement System — 58
- Complement System — 58

11. Antigen-Antibody Reactions — 62
- Uses — 62
- General Characteristics of Antigen-Antibody Reactions — 62
- Types of Antigen and Antibody Reactions — 63

12. Structure and Functions of the Immune System — 74
- Types of Immune Response — 74
- Organs and Tissues of the Immune System — 74
- Cells of the Lymphoreticular System — 75
- Major Histocompatibility Complex — 76

13. Immune Response — 78
- Definition — 78
- Type of Immune Response — 78
- Humoral Immunity — 78
- Monoclonal Antibodies — 79

Cell-mediated Immune Responses	80
Cytokines	80
Theories of Immune Response	80

14. Hypersensitivity Reactions — 82

Hypersensitivity	82
Classification of Hypersensitivity Reactions	82
Type I Hypersensitivity (IgE Dependent)	83
Type II Hypersensitivity: Cytolytic and Cytotoxic	84
Type III Hypersensitivity: Immune Complex-mediated	85
Type IV Hypersensitivity: Delayed Hypersensitivity	85
Type V Hypersensitivity (Stimulatory Type): Jones-Mote Reaction (or) Cutaneous Basophil Hypersensitivity	86

15. Autoimmunity — 88

Definition	88
Mechanisms of Autoimmunity	88
Classification of Autoimmune Diseases	88

SECTION 3: Systemic Bacteriology

16. Staphylococcus — 93

Staphylococcus aureus	93
Coagulase-Negative Staphylococci (CONS)	97

17. Streptococcus and Enterococcus — 100

Classification	100
Streptococcus pyogenes	101
Other Streptococci Pathogenic for Humans	104
Enterococcus	105
Viridans Streptococci	105

18. Pneumococcus — 107

Morphology	107
Cultural Characteristics	108
Biochemical Reactions	108
Resistance	108
Antigenic Structure	108
Pathogenesis	109
Laboratory Diagnosis	109
Treatment	110

19. Neisseria and Moraxella	**111**
Neisseria meningitidis	111
Neisseria gonorrhoeae (Gonococcus)	113
20. Corynebacterium	**117**
Corynebacterium diphtheriae	117
Schick Test	120
Diphtheroids	121
21. Bacillus	**123**
Bacillus anthracis	123
Anthracoid Bacilli	124
Bacillus cereus	125
22. Clostridium	**127**
Clostridium perfringens (Clostridium welchii)	127
Clostridium Tetani	129
Clostridium botulinum	131
Clostridium difficile	132
23. Nonsporing Anaerobes	**134**
Classification	134
Laboratory Diagnosis	134
24. Mycobacterium I: Mycobacterium Tuberculosis	**136**
Mycobacterium tuberculosis	136
25. Mycobacterium III: Mycobacterium Leprae	**141**
Mycobacterium leprae	141
26. Nontuberculous Mycobacteria	**144**
Classification	144
Pathogenesis	145
Laboratory Diagnosis	145
27. Actinomycetes: Actinomyces, Nocardia	**146**
Actinomyces	146
Nocardia	147
28. Enterobacteriaceae: Escherichia, Klebsiella, Proteus, and other Genera	**149**
Characteristics of the Family Enterobacteriaceae	149
Classification of Enterobacteriaceae	149
Escherichia coli	149
Edwardsville	152

Citrobacter	152
Klebsiella	152
Klebsiella pneumoniae	152
Enterobacter	153
Hafnia	153
Serratia	153
Tribe Proteae: *Proteus, Morganella,* and *Providencia*	153
Morganella	154
Providencia	154
Erwinia	154

29. Shigella — 156
Morphology — 156
Cultural Characteristics — 156
Antigenic Structure — 156
Classification — 156
Pathogenic Mechanisms — 157
Laboratory Diagnosis — 157
Treatment — 158

30. Enterobacteriaceae III: Salmonella — 159
Salmonella — 159
Vaccines Against Typhoid Fever — 162
Salmonella gastroenteritis — 163

31. Vibrio — 165
Vibrio cholerae — 165
Halophilic Vibrios — 169

32. Campylobacter and Helicobacter — 170
Campylobacter jejuni and *Campylobacter coli* — 170
Helicobacter — 171

33. *Pseudomonas, Stenotrophomonas,* and *Burkholderia* — 173
Pseudomonas aeruginosa — 173
Stenotrophomonas maltophilia — 174
Burkholderia cepacia — 174
Burkholderia mallei — 175
Burkholderia pseudomallei — 175

34. Legionella — 176
Legionella pneumophila — 176

35. Yersinia, Pasteurella and Francisella — 178
- Yersinia pestis — 178
- Yersinia pseudotuberculosis — 179
- Yersinia enterocolitica — 180

36. Haemophilus — 181
- Haemophilus influenzae — 181
- Haemophilus ducreyi — 183

37. Bordetella — 185
- Bordetella pertussis — 185

38. Brucella — 187

39. Spirochetes — 190
- Treponema — 190
- Borrelia — 195
- Borrelia vincentii (Treponema vincentii) — 196
- Leptospira — 197

40. Mycoplasma and Ureaplasma — 200
- Classification — 200
- Morphology — 200
- Cultural Characteristics — 200
- Pathogenicity — 201
- Laboratory Diagnosis — 201
- Treatment — 202

41. Miscellaneous Bacteria — 204
- Listeria monocytogenes — 204
- Erysipelothrix rhusiopathiae — 205
- Alcaligenes faecalis — 205
- Chromobacterium violaceum — 205
- Flavobacterium meningosepticum — 205
- Donovania Granulomatis (Calymmatobacterium granulomatis) or Klebsiella granulomatis — 205
- Acinetobacter (Mima polymorpha; Bacterium anitratum) — 206
- Rat Bite Fever (Streptobacillus moniliformis and Spirillum minus) — 206
- Gardnerella vaginalis — 206

42. Rickettsiaceae, Bartonellaceae, and Coxiella — 208
- Classification — 208
- Genus Rickettsia — 208

Genus *Orientia*	209
Genus *Ehrlichia*	210
Genus *Coxiella*: Q Fever	211
Bartonella	211
43. *Chlamydia* and *Chlamydophila*	**213**
Chlamydia	213
Chlamydia trachomatis	214
Chlamydophila psittaci	215

SECTION 4: Virology

44. General Properties of Viruses	**219**
Main Properties of Viruses	219
Morphology of Viruses	219
Structure and Chemical Composition of the Viruses	220
Cultivation of Viruses	220
Detection of Virus Growth in Cell Culture	222
Classification of Viruses	222
45. Laboratory Diagnosis, Prophylaxis, and Chemotherapy of Viral Diseases	**224**
Laboratory Diagnosis of Viral Infections	224
Immunoprophylaxis of Viral Diseases	224
Chemoprophylaxis and Chemotherapy of Virus Diseases	225
46. DNA Viruses	**226**
Poxviruses	226
Herpes Viruses	227
Varicella-Zoster Virus	229
Cytomegalovirus	230
Epstein–Barr Virus	230
Adenoviruses	231
Papovaviruses	232
Papillomaviruses	232
Polyomaviruses	232
Parvovirus	232
Hepatitis B Virus	232
47. Hepatitis Viruses	**234**
Type A Hepatitis (Infectious Hepatitis)	234

Hepatitis B Virus (Serum Hepatitis)	235
Hepatitis Type C	238
Type D (Delta) Hepatitis	238
Hepatitis E Virus	239
Hepatitis G Virus	239
Non-A, Non-B (NANB) Hepatitis	239

48. RNA Viruses — 241
- Picornaviruses — 241
- Poliovirus — 241
- Orthomyxovirus — 242
- Paramyxoviruses — 244
- Rhabdoviruses — 245
- Rabies Virus — 245
- Arboviruses — 247
- Alphavirus — 247
- Flavivirus — 247
- Rubella (German Measles) — 248
- Congenital Rubella — 248
- Rotaviruses — 248

49. Retroviruses: Human Immunodeficiency Virus — 251
- Human Immunodeficiency Virus — 251

SECTION 5: Medical Mycology

50. General Properties, Classification and Laboratory Diagnosis of Fungi — 259
- General Properties of Fungi — 259
- Classification of Fungi — 259
- Laboratory Diagnosis — 260
- Mycoses (Fungus Infections) — 260

51. Superficial, Cutaneous and Subcutaneous Mycoses — 262
- Superficial Mycoses — 262
- Cutaneous Mycoses — 262
- Subcutaneous Mycoses — 263

52. Systemic Mycoses — 266

53. Opportunistic Mycoses — 270
- Opportunistic Fungi — 270
- Yeast-like Fungi — 270

Cryptococcosis	272
Aspergillosis	273
Mucormycoses (Zygomycosis, Systemic Phycomycosis)	273
Penicilliosis	273
Pneumocystosis	274

SECTION 6: Medical Parasitology

54. Protozoology — 279
- Classification of Parasites — 279
- Protozoa — 279
- *Entamoeba histolytica* — 280
- *Entamoeba coli* — 283
- Flagellates — 283
- *Giardia lamblia (Giardia intestinalis)* — 284
- Trichomonas — 285
- *Trichomonas vaginalis* — 285
- Hemoflagellates — 286
- *Leishmania donovani* — 286
- Sporozoa — 288

55. Helminthology — 294
- **Cestodes** — 294
- *Taenia saginata* — 294
- *Taenia solium* — 295
- Genus *Echinococcus* — 298
- **Nematodes** — 301
- *Ascaris lumbricoides*—The Common Roundworm — 301
- *Ancylostoma duodenale* — 303
- *Necator americanus* — 305
- Visceral Larva Migrans — 306
- *Enterobius vermicularis* — 306
- *Wuchereria bancrofti* — 307
- Trematodes — 310

SECTION 7: Miscellaneous

56. Infective Syndrome* — 315
- Meningitis — 315
- Urinary Tract Infections — 317

Sore Throat	317
Diarrhea	317
Dysentery	318
Food Poisoning	318
Sexually Transmitted Diseases	319
Pyrexia of Unknown Origin	319

57. Laboratory Control of Antimicrobial Therapy — 321
- Antibiotic Sensitivity Tests — 321

58. Normal Microbial Flora of the Human Body — 324
- Normal Flora of the Skin — 324
- Normal Flora of the Conjunctiva — 324
- Normal Flora of the Nose, Nasopharynx and Accessory Sinuses — 324
- Normal Flora of the Mouth — 324
- Normal Flora of the Upper Respiratory Tract — 325
- Normal Flora of the Gastrointestinal Tract — 325
- Normal Flora of the Genitourinary Tract — 325

59. Antimicrobial Chemotherapy — 327
- Antibacterial Agents — 327
- Mechanisms of Action of Antibacterial Drugs — 327
- Resistance to Antimicrobial Drugs — 329

60. Immunoprophylaxis — 331
- Immunizing Agents — 331
- The Cold Chain — 332
- Immunization — 332

61. Vehicles, Vectors and Rodents — 337
- Vehicles and Vectors — 337
- Vehicle-Borne — 337
- Vector-Borne — 337
- Rodents — 338

62. Pathogenesis and Common Diseases — 340
- Common Diseases Caused by Different Microorganisms — 340
- Human Diseases Caused by Bacteria — 340

SECTION 8: Infection Control and Safety

63. Healthcare-associated Infections — 351
- Sources of Infections — 351

Routes of Transmission	351
Microorganisms Causing Healthcare-associated Infections (HAIs)	352
Types of Healthcare–associated Infections	352
Diagnosis and Control of Hospital Infection	353
Infection Control Policy	354
Prevention of Hospital-associated Infections	354

64. Isolation Precautions and use of Personal Protective Equipment — 358
- Isolation Technique — 358
- Standard Precautions in Health Care — 358
- Standard Precautions — 362
- Personal Protective Equipment — 364

65. Hand Hygiene — 368
- Hand Hygiene: Why, How and When? — 368
- Hand Wash — 369
- Hand Rub — 369
- Improving the Implementation of Hand Hygiene — 369
- Your 5 Moments for Hand Hygiene — 369

66. Sterilization and Disinfection — 376
- Methods of Sterilization and Disinfection — 376
- Cleaning — 385
- Asepsis — 386
- Spaulding's Classification — 386

67. Specimen Collection (Review) — 389
- Specimens — 389
- Universal Precautions — 389
- Collection of Specimens — 390
- Transport of Specimens — 392
- Health and Safety Precautions — 392

68. Biomedical Waste Management — 393
- Definition of Biomedical Waste — 393
- Categories of Biomedical Waste — 393
- Waste Segregation — 394
- Biomedical Waste Management in India — 399
- Laundry Management Process and Infection Control and Prevention — 399

69. Antibiotic Stewardship — 401
- Antimicrobial Stewardship — 401
- Goal of Antimicrobial Stewardship — 401

Need of Antimicrobial Stewardship	401
Implementing an Antimicrobial Stewardship Program	401
Monitoring of Antimicrobial Stewardship Program	402
Rational use of Antibiotics	403
Antimicrobial Resistance	404
Methicillin-resistant *Staphylococcus aureus*	405
Multidrug Resistant Organisms	406

70. Patient Safety Indicators — 409
Care of Vulnerable Patients	409
Prevention of Iatrogenic Injury	410
Care of Lines, Drains and Tubing's	411
Restraint Policy and Care: Physical and Chemical	411
Blood and Blood Transfusion Policy	412
Prevention of Intravenous Complications	413
Fall Prevention	414
Prevention of Deep Vein Thrombosis	414
Shifting and Transport of Patients	414
Surgical Safety	415
Care Coordination Event Related to Medication Reconciliation and Administration	415
Prevention of Communication Errors	415
Documentation	417

71. Incidents and Adverse Events — 419
Capturing of Incidents	419
Root Cause Analysis	420
Report Writing	421

72. International Patient Safety Goals — 423
Applications of International Patient Safety Goals in the Patient Care System	423

73. Safety Protocol — 426
High 5s Project	426
Radiation Safety	427
Laser Safety	427
Fire Safety	428
HAZMAT (Hazardous Materials) Safety	429
Spill	429
Material Safety Data Sheet or Safety Data Sheet	430

Environment, Health and Safety	430
Emergency Codes	432
Role of Nurse in Times of Disaster	433

74. Employee Safety Indicators — 436
Fall Prevention — 436
Annual Health Checkup — 437

75. Healthcare Worker Immunization and Management of Occupational Exposure — 439
Occupational Health and Safety Legislation in India — 439
Occupational Health Program — 439

Index — 445

General Microbiology

SECTION OUTLINE
1. Historical Development of Microbiology
2. Microscopy and Morphology of Bacteria
3. Physiology of Bacteria
4. Culture Media and Culture Methods
5. Infection
6. Staining Methods

Historical Development of Microbiology

LEARNING OBJECTIVES

After reading and studying this chapter, you should be able to:
1. Describe the following: (a) Contributions of Antony van Leeuwenhoek; (b) Contributions of Louis Pasteur; (c) Contributions of Robert Koch; (d) Koch's postulates; (e) Contributions of Paul Ehrlich.
2. Explain concepts and principles of microbiology and their importance in nursing.

INTRODUCTION AND SCOPE

Microbiology is the study of living organisms of microscopic size. **Medical microbiology** is the subdivision concerned with the causative agents of infectious disease of man, the response of the host to infection and various methods of diagnosis, treatment and prevention. The term microbe was first used by Sedillot in 1878, but now is commonly replaced by microorganisms. Microorganisms include a large and diverse group of microscopic organisms that exist as single cell or cell clusters (e.g., **bacteria, archaea, fungi, algae, protozoa and helminths**) and the **viruses,** which are microscopic but not cellular. Microorganisms are present everywhere on earth, which includes humans, animals, plants and other living creatures, soil, water, and atmosphere.

IMPORTANCE AND RELEVANCE OF MICROORGANISMS

Microorganisms are relevant to all of our lives in a multitude of ways. Sometimes, the influence of microorganisms on human life is beneficial, whereas at other times, it is detrimental.

Beneficial Influence

Examples:
1. **Production of important products:** Microorganisms are required for the production of **bread, cheese, yogurt, alcohol, wine, beer, antibiotics** (e.g., penicillin, streptomycin, and chloramphenicol), **vaccines, vitamins, enzymes** and many more important products.
2. **Contribution to public health:** Many products of microbes contribute to public health as aids to nutrition.
3. **Interruption of spread of disease:** Other products are used to interrupt the spread of disease.
4. **Improving the quality of life**: Still others hold promise for improving the quality of life in the year's ahead.
5. **Component of an ecosystem:** Microbes are also an important and essential component of an ecosystem. Molds and bacteria play key roles in the cycling of important nutrients in plant nutrition particularly those of carbon, nitrogen and sulfur. Bacteria referred to as **nitrogen fixers** live in the soil where they convert vast quantities of nitrogen in air into a form that plants can use.

6. **Energy production:** Microorganisms also play major roles in energy production. Natural gas (methane) is a product of bacterial activity, arising from the metabolism of methanogenic bacteria.
7. **Cleaning up pollution:** Microorganisms are also being used to clean up pollution caused by human activities, a process called **bioremediation (the introduction of microbes to restore stability to disturbed or polluted environments).** Bacteria and fungi have been used to consume spilled oil, solvents, pesticides and other environmentally toxic substances.

Harmful Influence

1. Microorganisms have also harmed humans and disrupted societies over the millennia. Microbial diseases undoubtedly played a major role in historical events, it was in the year 1347 when **plague** or **"black death"** struck Europe and within 4 years killed 25 million people, that is, one-third of the population.
2. Many common human diseases are caused by bacteria, fungi (molds and yeasts), protozoa, and helminths.

IMPORTANCE OF MICROBIOLOGY IN NURSING

Scope of Microbiology in Nursing

1. **To promote health:** Nursing care in the hospital and community is of paramount importance to promote health and it is considered to be the backbone of public health. To attain perfection in this profession, nurses should acquire sound knowledge of nursing microbiology, as nursing is an interdependent profession influenced by the recent scientific and technological advances of nursing sciences.

    Aseptic technique becomes almost second nature to the nurse, who practices it daily. However, the patient is less aware of the factors that promote the spread of infection or of the ways to prevent its transmission. A nurse will be obliged to educate patients about the nature of infection and the techniques to use in planning or controlling its spread.
2. **Diagnosis and treatment of infection:** The role of the laboratory in assisting clinicians in the diagnosis of infection is to provide the physician with information concerning the presence or absence of microorganisms that may be involved in the infectious disease process. These individuals and facilities also determine the susceptibility of microorganisms to antimicrobial agents. Application of knowledge of medical microbiology at the bedside of patients during nursing care will be possible due to nursing microbiology and nurses should acquire sound knowledge of nursing microbiology.
3. **Sterilization and disinfection:** Pathogenic microorganisms are infectious agents. Unwashed hands, wound dressings, soiled linen, and decaying teeth provide ideal areas for pathogenic growth. The strength of the microorganism, the number of microorganisms present, the effectiveness of a person's immune system, and the length of exposure to the microorganisms determine a pathogen's ability to produce disease. A nurse has a duty to provide a safe environment for a patient which can be accomplished by performing hand hygiene, donning gloves, disinfection (the use of a chemical that can be applied to objects to destroy microorganisms), using an antiseptic (a substance that tends to inhibit the growth and reproduction of microorganisms—may be used on humans), and sterilization.
4. **Prophylaxis:** In the final analysis the patient's well-being and health can benefit significantly from information provided by the clinical microbiology laboratory. Clinical microbiologists and clinical microbiology laboratories perform many services, all related to the identification and control of pathogens.
5. **Diagnosis and control of hospital infection—infection control team:** An infection control team of workers, headed by the **infection control doctor**. The *infection control nurse* is a key member of this team. The functions of this team include **surveillance**

and control of infection and monitoring of hygiene practices, advising the infection control committee on matters of policy relating to the prevention of infection and the education of all staff in the microbiologically safe performance of procedures.

THE DISCOVERY OF MICROORGANISMS

The First Observation of Microorganisms

As microbes are invisible to the unaided eye, direct observation of microorganisms had to await the development of the microscope.

Antony van Leeuwenhoek (1632–1723)

The credit for having first observed and reported bacteria belongs to Antony van Leeuwenhoek. Antony van Leeuwenhoek, the Dutchman, was a draper and haberdasher in Delft, Holland. He was the amateur microscopist and was the first person to observe microorganisms (1673) using a simple microscope. In 1683, he made accurate descriptions of various types of bacteria and communicated them to the Royal Society of London. Their importance in medicine and in other areas of biology came to be recognized two centuries later.

SCIENTIFIC DEVELOPMENT OF MICROBIOLOGY

The development of microbiology as a scientific discipline dates from Louis Pasteur, perfection on microbiological studies by Robert Koch, the introduction of antiseptic surgery by Lord Lister and contributions of Paul Ehrlich in chemotherapy.

Louis Pasteur (1822–1895)

Louis Pasteur (1822–1895) was born in the village of Dole, France on December 27, 1822 the son of humble parents. He was originally trained as a chemist, but his studies on fermentation led him to take interest in microorganisms.

Father of Microbiology: He is known as **"Father of Microbiology"** (Fig. 1.1).

Contributions of Louis Pasteur in Microbiology (Box 1.1)

Refer **Box 1.1.**

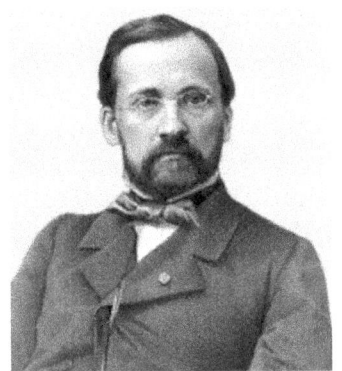

Fig. 1.1: Louis Pasteur.

> **Box 1.1: Contributions of Louis Pasteur in Microbiology.**
>
> 1. **Coined the term microbiology:** Pasteur coined the term microbiology for the study of living organisms of microscopic size.
> 2. **Proposed germ theory of disease:** He established that putrefaction and fermentation was the result of microbial activity and that different types of fermentations were associated with different types of microorganisms (1857).
> 3. **Disapproved theory of spontaneous generation:** He disapproved the theory of spontaneous generation in 1860–1861.
> 4. **Developed sterilization techniques:** He introduced sterilization techniques and developed the steam sterilizer, hot-air oven and autoclave in the course of these studies.
> 5. **Developed methods and techniques for cultivation of microorganisms.**
> 6. Studies on pebrine (silkworm disease), anthrax, chicken cholera and hydrophobia.
> 7. **Pasteurization:** He devised the process of destroying bacteria, known as pasteurization (1863–1865). This process (pasteurization) is employed to preserve milk and certain other perishable foods throughout the civilized world today.
> 8. **Coined the term vaccine.**
> 9. **Discovery of the process of attenuation and chicken cholera vaccine.**
> 10. **Developed live attenuated anthrax vaccine:** He attenuated cultures of the anthrax bacillus by incubation at high temperature (42–43°C) and proved that inoculation of such cultures in animals induced specific protection against **anthrax.**
> 11. **Developed rabies vaccine:** The crowning achievement of Pasteur was the successful application of the principle of vaccination to the prevention of rabies, or hydrophobia, in human beings and developed Pasteur rabies vaccine in 1885. He did not know that rabies was caused by a virus but he managed to develop a live attenuated vaccine for the disease.
> 12. **Noticed pneumococci.**

Joseph Lister (1827–1912)

Joseph Lister was a professor of Surgery in Glasgow Royal Infirmary. He was impressed with Pasteur's study on the involvement of microorganisms in fermentation and putrefaction.

- **Developed a system of antiseptic surgery:** He developed a system of antiseptic surgery designed to prevent microorganisms from entering wounds.
- **Father of modern surgery:** He established the guiding principle of antisepsis for good surgical practice and was milestone in the evolution of surgical practice from the era of "laudable pus" to modern aseptic techniques. For this work he is called the "**Father of modern surgery**".

Robert Koch (1843–1910)

Robert Koch (**Fig. 1.2**) was the German physician. Winner of the Nobel Prize in 1905, Robert Koch is known as "**Father of bacteriology**".

Contributions of Robert Koch

1. **Staining techniques:** He described **methods for the easy microscopic examination of bacteria**.
2. **Hanging drop method:** He was the first to use **hanging drop method** by studying bacterial motility.
3. He devised a **simple method for isolating pure cultures of bacteria** by plating out mixed material on a solid culture medium and to isolate pure cultures of pathogens.
4. **Discovered** the **causal agents of anthrax (1876), tuberculosis (1882), and cholera (1883)**.
5. **Koch's postulates:** Robert Koch proved that microorganisms cause disease. Koch used the criteria to establish the relationship between *Bacillus anthracis* and anthrax (**Fig. 1.3**). His criteria for proving the causal relationship between a microorganism and a specific disease are known as **Koch's postulates (1876) (Box 1.2)**.
6. **Koch's phenomenon:** Koch (1890) observed that a guinea pig already infected with the bacillus responded with an exaggerated response when injected with the tubercle bacillus or its protein. This hypersensitivity reaction is known as **Koch's phenomenon**.

Discovery of Viruses

As a science, virology evolved later than bacteriology.

IMMUNITY AND IMMUNIZATION

Edward Jenner (1749–1823)

The first scientific attempts at artificial immunizations in the late eighteenth century by **Edward Jenner (1749–1823)** from England. Edward Jenner is known as the "**Father of immunology**".

SEROTHERAPY AND CHEMOTHERAPY

Antisera: The work of **Behring and Kitasato** led to the successful use of antisera raised in animals for the treatment of patients with diphtheria, tetanus, pneumonia and other diseases. Antisera were the only specific therapeutic agents available for the management of infectious diseases till **Domagk (1935)** initiated scientific chemotherapy with the discovery of prontosil.

Magic bullet: Ehrlich (1909) discovered **salvarsan (arsphenamine),** sometimes called the "**magic bullet**" was capable of destroying the spirochete of syphilis with only moderate toxic effects.

Antibiotics-A Fortunate Accident: Sir Alexander Fleming (1881–1955) made accidental discovery that the fungus *Penicillium notatum* produces a substance which destroys staphylococci.

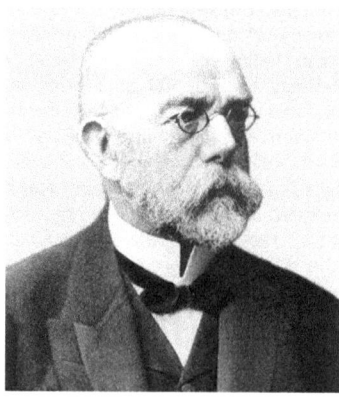

Fig. 1.2: Robert Koch.

Chapter 1: Historical Development of Microbiology

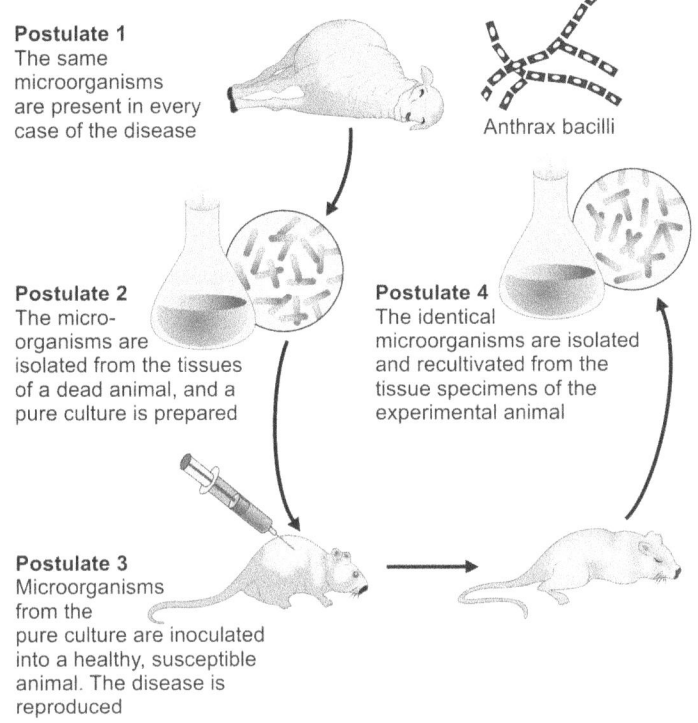

Fig. 1.3: Demonstration of Koch's postulates.

Box 1.2: Koch's postulates.

Koch's postulates are a series of guidelines for the experimental study of infectious disease. According to these, a microorganism can be accepted as the causative agent of an infectious disease only **(Fig. 1.3)** if the following conditions are satisfied:
Postulate 1: The organism should be regularly found in the lesions of the disease.
Postulate 2: It should be possible to isolate the organism in pure culture from the lesions.
Postulate 3: Inoculation of the pure culture into suitable laboratory animals should reproduce the lesion of the disease.
Postulate 4: It should be possible to reisolate the organism in pure culture from the lesions produced in the experimental animals.
  Subsequently, an additional fifth criterion introduced states that specific antibodies to the organism should be demonstrable in the serum of patients suffering from the disease.
Limitations of Koch's postulates: Even today Koch's postulates are considered whenever a new infectious disease arises. These criteria have proved invaluable in identifying pathogens, but they cannot always be met, for example, some organisms (including all viruses) cannot be grown on artificial media, and some are pathogenic only for man. *Mycobacterium leprae*, a causative agent of leprosy, has not been cultured on artificial medium so far and not fulfilling Koch's postulates.

BRANCHES OF MICROBIOLOGY

- **Bacteriology:** The study of bacteria
- **Mycology:** The study of fungi
- **Parasitology:** The study of parasites
- **Immunology:** The study of the immune system
- **Virology:** The study of viruses

NOBEL PRIZES AWARDED FOR RESEARCH IN MICROBIOLOGY

The number of Nobel laureates in medicine and physiology for their contribution in microbiology is evidence of the positive contribution made to human health by the science of microbiology. **(Table 1.1)**.

Section 1: General Microbiology

Table 1.1: Nobel laureates for research in microbiology.

Year	Nobel laureates	Contribution
1901	Emil A von Behring	Developed a diphtheria antitoxin
1902	Ronald Ross	Discovered how malaria is transmitted
1905	Robert Koch	Tuberculosis—discovery of causative agent
1907	CLA Laveron	Discovery of malaria parasite in an unstained preparation of fresh blood
1908	Paul Ehrlich and Elie Metchnikoff	Developed theories on immunity. Described phagocytosis, the intake of solid materials by cells
1913	Charles Richet	Anaphylaxis
1919	Jules Bordet	Discovered roles of complement and antibody in cytolysis, developed complement fixation test
1928	Charles Nicolle	Typhus exanthematicus
1930	Karl Landsteiner	Described ABO blood groups; solidified chemical basis for antigen-antibody reactions
1939	Gerhardt Domagk	Antibacterial effect of prontosil
1945	Alexander Fleming, Ernst Chain, and Howard Florey	Discovered penicillin
1951	Max Theiler	Yellow fever vaccine
1952	Selman A Waksman	Development of streptomycin. He coined the term "antibiotic"
1954	John F Enders, Thomas H Weller, and Frederick C Robbins	Cultured poliovirus in cell cultures
1960	Sir Macfarlane Burnet and Sir Peter Brian Medawar	Immunological tolerance, clonal selection theory
1962	James D Watson, Francis H C Crick, and Maurice AF Wilkins	Double helix structure of deoxyribonucleic acid (DNA)
1966	Francois Jacob, Andre Lwoff and Jacques Monod	Regulatory mechanisms in microbial genes (concept of "lac operon")
1966	Peyton Rous	Viral oncogenes (avian sarcoma)
1968	Robert Holley, Har Gobind Khorana, and Marshall W Nirenberg	Genetic code
1969	Max Delbruck, AD Hershey and Salvador Luria	Mechanism of virus infection in living cells
1972	Gerald M Edelman and Rodney R Porter	Described the nature and structure of antibodies
1975	David Baltimore, Renato Dulbecco and Howard M Temin	Interactions between tumor viruses and genetic material of the cells
1977	Rosalyn Yalow	Developed immunoassay
1980	Baruj Benacerraf, Jean Dausset and George Snell	HLA antigens
1984	César Milstein, Georges Köhler, Niels K Jerne	Developed hybridoma technology for production of monoclonal antibodies
1987	S Tonegawa	Described the genetics of antibody production
1989	J Michael Bishop and Harold E Varmus	Discovered cancer-causing genes called oncogenes
1990	Joseph E Murray and E Donnall Thomas	Performed the first successful organ transplants by using immunosuppressive agents

(Contd...)

Chapter 1: Historical Development of Microbiology

(Contd...)

Year	Nobel laureates	Contribution
1993	Kary B Mullis	Discovered the polymerase chain reaction (PCR) to amplify DNA
1996	Peter C Doherty and Rolf M Zinkernagel	Cell-mediated immune defenses
1997	Stanley B Prusiner	Prion discovery
2001	Leland H Hartwell, Paul M Nurse, and R Timothy Hunt	Discovered genes that encode proteins regulating cell division
2005	Barry J Marshall and J Robin Warren	*Helicobacter pylori* and its role in gastritis and peptic ulcer disease
2007	Mario R Capecchi, Oliver Smithies and Sir Martin J Evans	Creation of knockout mice for stem cell research
2008	Luc Montagnier and Francoise Barre-Sinoussi	Discovery of human immunodeficiency virus
	Harald zur Hausen	Human papillomaviruses causing cervical cancer
2011	Bruce A Beutler and Jules A Hoffmann	Discoveries concerning the activation of innate immunity
	Ralph M Steinman	Discovery of dendritic cell and its role in adaptive immunity
2012	Sir John B Gurdon and S Yamanaka	Discovery that mature cells can be programmed to become pluripotent
2015	William C Campbell and Satoshi Omura	For the discovery concerning a novel therapy against infections caused by roundworm parasites
	Youyou Tu	For the discovery concerning a novel therapy against malaria
2018	James P Allison and Tasuku Honjo	For the discovery of cancer by inhibition of negative immune regulation
2020	Harey J Alter, Michael Houghton and Charles M Rice	Discovery of hepatitis C virus

KEY POINTS

- Microbiology is the study of living organisms of microscopic size.
- Nursing care in the hospital and community is of paramount importance to promote health and it is considered to be the backbone of public health.
- Antony van Leeuwenhoek was the first person to describe microorganisms.
- **Louis Pasteur** is known as **"Father of Microbiology"**.
- **Robert Koch:**
  a. Koch developed the techniques required to grow bacteria on solid media and to isolate pure cultures of pathogens.
  b. Koch's postulates are used to prove a direct relationship between a suspected pathogen and a disease.

IMPORTANT QUESTIONS

1. Write short notes on:
   a. Contributions of Louis Pasteur
   b. Contributions of Robert Koch
   c. Koch's postulates
2. Write briefly on scope of microbiology in nursing.

MULTIPLE CHOICE QUESTIONS

1. Who was the first person to describe microorganisms?
   a. Louis Pasteur
   b. Robert Koch
   c. Paul Ehrlich
   d. Antony van Leeuwenhoek

Section 1: General Microbiology

2. Who is father of microbiology?
    a. Louis Pasteur
    b. Robert Koch
    c. Paul Ehrlich
    d. Joseph Lister
3. Who is father of bacteriology?
    a. Louis Pasteur
    b. Robert Koch
    c. Paul Ehrlich
    d. Joseph Lister
4. Who is father of immunology?
    a. Louis Pasteur
    b. Robert Koch
    c. Paul Ehrlich
    d. Edward Jenner

ANSWERS

1. d   2. a   3. b   4. d

CHAPTER 2

Microscopy and Morphology of Bacteria

LEARNING OBJECTIVES

After reading and studying this chapter, you should be able to:
- Discuss microscopic methods.
- Explain the principle and describe uses of the following:
  - Darkfield microscopy, phase-contrast microscopy
  - Fluorescent microscopy and electron microscopy
- Differentiate between prokaryotes and eukaryotes.
- Describe anatomy of bacterial cell.
- Describe cell envelope.
- Describe bacterial cell wall.
- Discuss capsule or bacterial capsule.
- Describe bacterial flagellae.
- Describe fimbriae or pili.
- Discuss bacterial spores or endospores.
- Explain L-forms of bacteria.

MICROSCOPY

Microscope is an optical instrument used to magnify (enlarge) minute objects or microorganisms which cannot be seen by naked eye. In general, microscopy is used in microbiology for two basic purposes: The initial detection of microbes and the preliminary or definitive identification of microbes.

LIGHT MICROSCOPY

Light microscopy refers to the use of any kind of microscope that uses visible light to observe specimens. Here we examine several types of light microscopy. A modern **compound light microscope (LM)** has a series of lenses and uses visible light as its source of illumination (**Fig. 2.1**).

Compound Light Microscopy

Parts of Microscope

An ordinary light microscope consists of different parts, such as the stand, the optical system, the body, the stage, the substage, and the mirror (**Fig. 2.1**).

1. **Stand:** The upright *stand* rests on a heavy *foot* and bears at its upper end an inclined binocular head with two *eye-pieces*, above, and a revolving *nose-piece* bearing several *objectives,* below. The stand rests on a heavy *foot* and the *limb* which bears the optical system.
2. **The optical system:** The stand bears at its upper end an inclined binocular head with two *eye-pieces*, above with (magnification x 5, x 6, or x 10), and a revolving *nose-piece* bearing several *objectives,* below with different magnifying powers. The three objectives most commonly used in microbiology are: (1) a low-power "dry" objective with magnification x 10, (2) a high-power "dry" objective with magnification x 40, and (3) an oil immersion objective with magnification x 100.
3. **The stage:** This is the platform on which material (i.e., the "object") is placed to be examined with a central hole over which the slide with specimen is held by clips. For focusing, the stage is racked upward or downward and the slide can be moved in two directions.

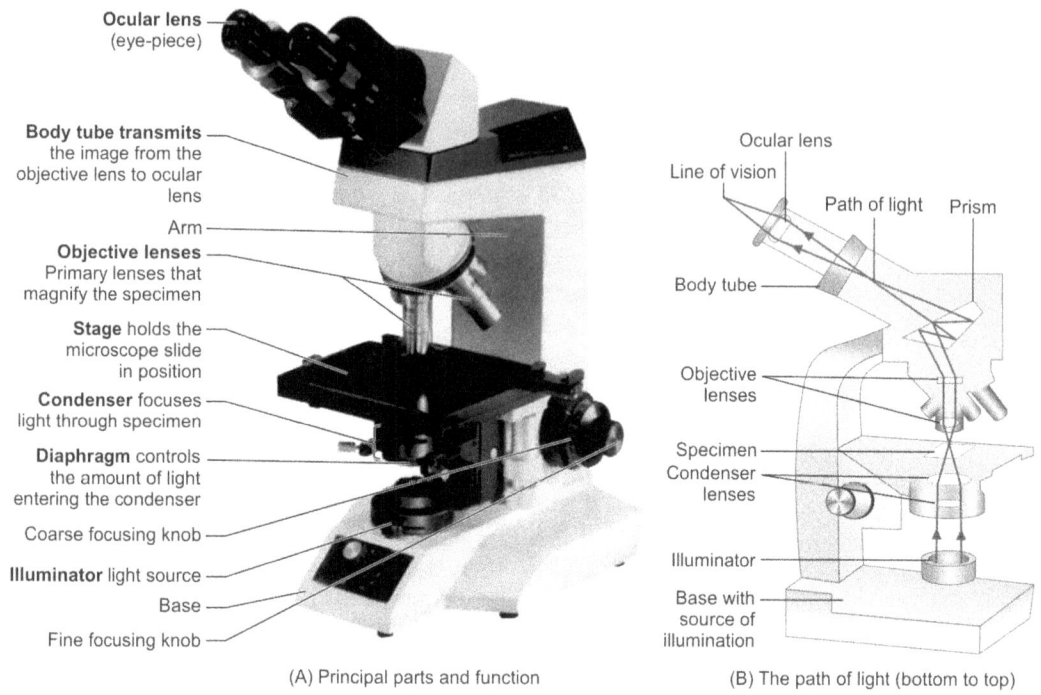

Fig. 2.1: The compound light microscope.

4. **The substage:** A built-in *lamp* in the foot of the microscope passes a beam of light upward through a *field diaphragm* (iris). The beam is focused on to the specimen by a *substage condenser* which is attached beneath the stage, centered by condenser centration adjustments and moved upward or downward by the turning of a *condenser focusing adjustment*. An *aperture diaphragm* (iris) with a lever for its control is incorporated in the condenser mounting.

Methods of Use of Light Microscope

1. Place the microscope at a convenient position on the bench
2. Check to ensure that the objectives and eye-pieces are free from dust and immersion oil
3. Rack up fully the substage condenser, i.e., until its top surface is within about 1 mm below the upper surface of the stage (undersurface of the slide)
4. Check that the filter carrier in the substage is in its correct position
5. Fully open the substage and lamp irises
6. Switch on the lamp at low intensity and then increase the intensity
7. Place the slide with the object on the stage, so that it is held by the stage clips
8. First view the specimen with a low power dry objective. Use the fine adjustment only to obtain and maintain exact focus
9. Adjust the distance between the eye-pieces so that a single field is seen
10. If continued examination with the **low power objective** is required, diffuse the light uniformly over the field by defocusing the condenser either by racking it down or swinging out its top lens
11. Before proceeding to use a **high-power objective**, check that the iris diaphragms are open, the condenser is focused
12. Before using an **oil-immersion objective**, place a moderately large drop of immersion oil on the middle of the specimen
    i. Rotate the nose-piece until the oil immersion lens is in position

ii. With the eye at the level of the stage, use the *coarse* focusing adjustment slowly to raise the stage until the oil on the slide makes contact with the objective
13. Apply the eyes to the eye-pieces and, while watching, slowly focus the objective *away* from the slide by lowering the stage with the coarse focusing adjustment
14. Wipe the oil from the objective with a clean tissue after use. Turn down the light intensity control to low and then switch off the light

MORPHOLOGY OF BACTERIA

Microorganisms are generally regarded as living forms that are microscopic in size and relatively simple, usually unicellular, in structure. The bacteria are single-celled organisms that reproduce by simple division, i.e., binary fission.

NAMING AND CLASSIFYING MICROORGANISMS

Microorganisms are a heterogeneous group of several distinct classes of living beings. Whittaker's system recognizes five-kingdoms of living things–**Monera (bacteria), Protista, Fungi, Plantae, and Animalia**. Five kingdoms have been modified further by the development of **three domains, or Superkingdoms** system—the **Bacteria,** the **Archaea** (meaning ancient), and the **Eukarya.**

NOMENCLATURE

The system of nomenclature (naming) for organisms in use today was established in 1735 by Carolus Linnaeus. Scientific names are latinized. Scientific nomenclature assigns each organism two names—the genus (plural: genera) is the first name and is always capitalized; the specific epithet (species name) follows and is not capitalized. The organism is referred to by both the genus and the specific epithet, and both names are underlined or italicized. With the initial of the genus followed by the specific epithet, e.g., *Staphylococcus aureus* (*Staphylococcus*-Genus; *aureus*-Species).

COMPARISON OF PROKARYOTIC CELLS EUKARYOTIC CELLS

All living organisms on earth are composed of one or the other of two types of cells *prokaryotic* cells and *eukaryotic* cells (**Table 2.1**).

Table 2.1: Principle differences between prokaryotic and eukaryotic cells.

Characteristic	Prokaryotic	Eukaryotic
Size (approximate)	0.5–3 µm	>5 µm
Nucleus		
• Nuclear membrane	Absent	Present
• Nucleolus	Absent	Present
• Chromosome	One (circular)	More than one (linear)
• Deoxyribonucleoprotein	Absent	Present
• Division	By binary fission	By mitosis
Cytoplasm		
• Cytoplasmic streaming	Absent	Present
• Mitochondria	Absent	Present
• Golgi apparatus	Absent	Present
• Lysosomes	Absent	Present
• Pinocytosis	Absent	Present
• Endoplasmic reticulum	Absent	Present
Chemical composition		
• Sterol	Absent	Present
• Muramic acid	Present	Absent
Examples	Eubacteria, Archaea All bacteria and blue-green algae	Fungi, slime molds, protozoa, higher plants, and animals including humans

1. **Prokaryotes—Bacteria and Archaea**: All bacteria and blue-green algae are prokaryotes.
2. **Eukaryotes—Eukarya**: Other algae (excluding blue-green algae), fungi, slime molds, protozoa, higher plants, and animals are eukaryotic **(Table 2.1)**.

Size of Bacteria

The unit of measurement in bacteriology is the micron or micrometer:
- 1 micron (μ) or micrometer (μm) = a millionth part of a meter or a thousandth of a millimeter.
- 1 millimicron (mμ) or nanometer (nm) = one thousandth of a micron or one millionth of a millimeter.
- 1 Angstrom unit (A) = one tenth of a nanometer

The diameter of the smallest body that can be resolved and seen clearly with naked eye is 200 μm. Bacteria of medical importance generally measure 0.2–1.5 μm in diameter and about 3–5 μm in length. To see bacteria a light microscope must be used. Following types of microscopes are used for examination of bacteria.

Study of Bacteria

Stained Preparations

Because most microorganisms appear almost colorless when viewed through a standard light microscope, we often must prepare them for observation. Staining simply means coloring the microorganisms with a dye that emphasizes certain structures.

Routine methods for staining of bacteria involve drying and fixing smears, procedures that kill them. Fixing simultaneously kills the microorganisms and attaches them to the slide. It also preserves various parts of microbes in their natural state with only minimal distortion. Various staining techniques are commonly used in bacteriology **(See Chapter 6)**.

MORPHOLOGY OF BACTERIA

Shape of Bacteria

Depending on their shape, bacteria are classified into several varieties **(Fig. 2.2)**:

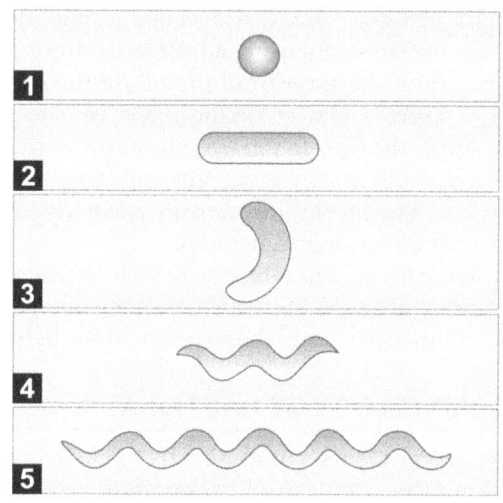

Fig. 2.2: Shape of bacteria: 1. coccus; 2. bacillus; 3. vibrio, 4. spirillum, 5. spirochete.

1. **Cocci:** Cocci (from kokkos meaning berry) are spherical, or nearly spherical
2. **Bacilli:** Bacilli (from baculus meaning rod) are relatively straight, rod shaped (cylindrical) cells. In some of the bacilli the length of the cells may be equal to width. Such bacillary forms are known as coccobacilli and have to be carefully differentiated from cocci
3. **Vibrios:** Vibrios are curved or comma-shaped rods
4. **Spirilla:** Spirilla are rigid spiral or helical forms
5. **Spirochetes:** Spirochetes (from speira meaning coil and chaite meaning hair) are flexuous spiral forms
6. **Mycoplasma:** Mycoplasma are cell wall deficient bacteria and hence do not possess a stable morphology

Arrangement of Bacterial Cells

Pathogenic bacterial species appear as sphere (cocci), rods (bacilli), and spirals. Bacteria sometimes show characteristic of cellular arrangement or grouping **(Figs. 2.3A and B)**.

Anatomy of the Bacterial Cell

The principal structures of the bacterial cell are shown in **Figure 2.4**.

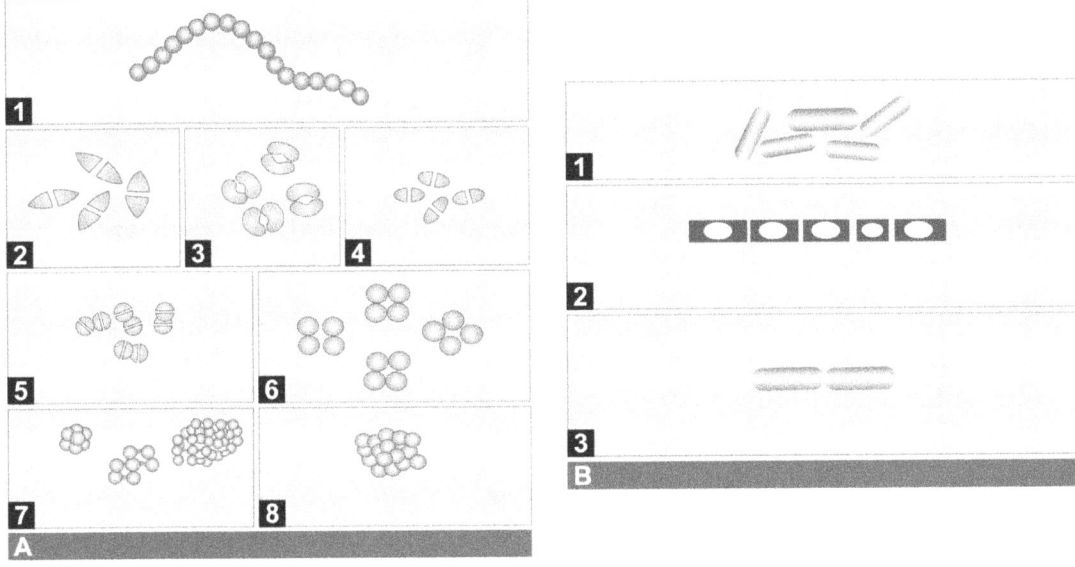

Figs. 2.3A and B: Arrangement of bacteria. (A) Cocci: 1. streptococci, 2. pneumococci, 3. gonococci, 4. meningococci, 5. *Neisseria catarrhalis*, 6. Gaffkya tetragena, 7. sarcina, 8. staphylococci. (B) Bacilli: 1. bacilli in cluster, 2. bacilli in chains (*Bacillus anthracis*) 3. diplobacilli (*K. pneumoniae*).

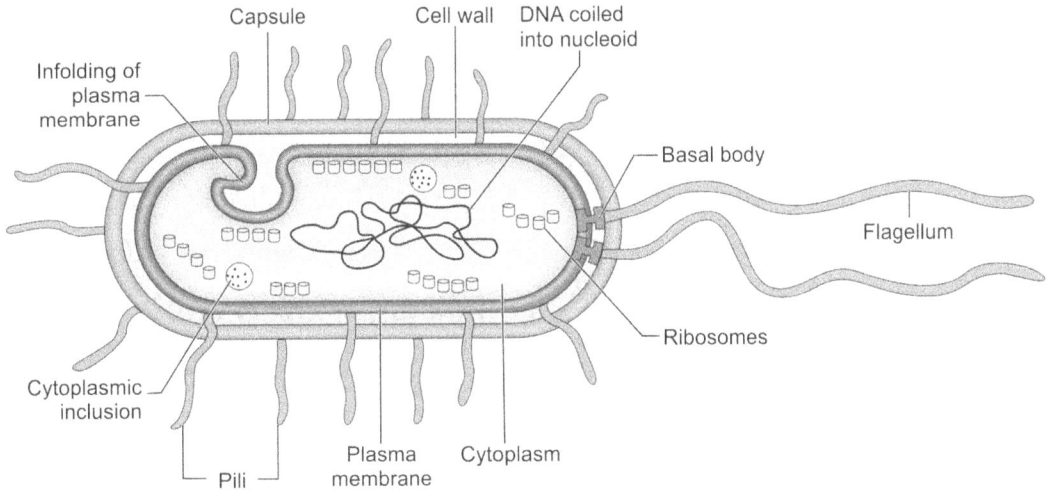

Fig. 2.4: Anatomy of a bacterial cell.

Bacterial Cell Components

It can be divided into:
A. Cell envelope and its appendages.
   a. **The outer layer or cell envelope** consists of two components:
      1. **Cell wall**
      2. **Cytoplasmic or plasma membrane**—beneath cell wall
   b. Cellular appendages—capsule, fimbriae, and flagella
B. **Cell interior:** Those structures and substances that are bounded by the cytoplasmic membrane compose the cell interior and include **cytoplasm, cytoplasmic inclusions, (mesosomes, ribosomes, inclusion granules, vacuoles) and a single circular**

chromosome of deoxyribonucleic acid (DNA).

Cell Envelope and Its Appendages
The Outer Layer or Cell Envelope
1. *Cell wall:* The cell wall is the layer that lies just outside the plasma membrane. It is thick, strong, and relatively rigid.

Gram-positive bacterial cell wall: In gram-positive bacteria, the cell wall consists mainly of peptidoglycan and teichoic acids **(Fig. 2.5)**.

- **Peptidoglycan**: It is thicker and stronger than those of gram-negative bacteria.
- **Teichoic acid:** In addition, the cell walls of gram-positive bacteria contain *teichoic acids.*

Gram-negative cell wall: The gram-negative cell wall is structurally quite different from that of gram-positive cells **(Fig. 2.6)**. It consists of **peptidoglycan and lipoprotein, outer membrane, and lipopolysaccharide.**

1. **Peptidoglycan layer:** It is bonded to lipoproteins covalently in the outer membrane and plasma membrane and is in the **periplasmic,** a gel-like fluid between the outer membrane and plasma membrane.

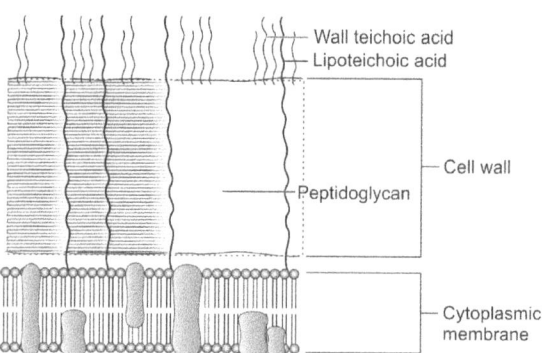

Fig. 2.5: Gram-positive cell wall.

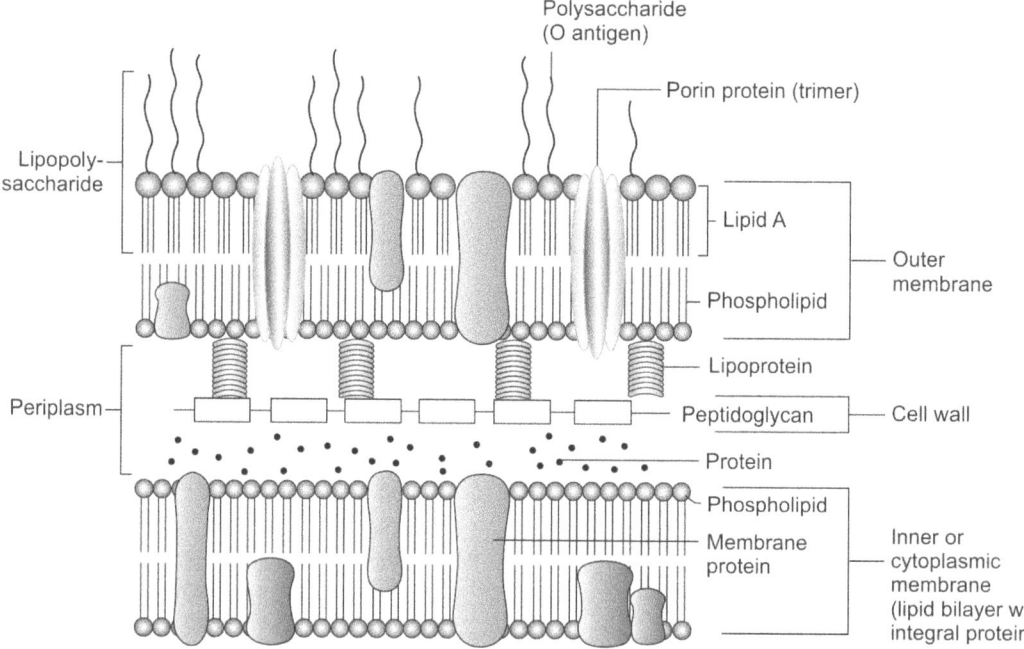

Fig. 2.6: Gram-negative cell wall.

2. **Lipopoprotein:** Lipopoprotein, or murein lipoproteins attach to the peptidoglycan, and to the outer membrane.
3. **Outer membrane:** External to the peptidoglycan and attached to it by lipoprotein is the outer membrane. It is bilayered structure. Its inner leaflet is composed of phospholipid and outer leaflet by lipopolysaccharide (LPS).
4. **Lipopolysaccharide (LPS):** Lipopolysaccharide (LPS) consists of three components:
   i. **Lipid A** is the lipid portion of LPS and is embedded in the top layer of the outer membrane. Lipid A functions as an **endotoxin**. All the toxicity of the endotoxin is due to lipid A, i.e., pyrogenicity, lethal effect, tissue necrosis, etc.
   ii. **The core polysaccharide** is attached to lipid A.
   iii. **O polysaccharide**: It is known as **O antigen**. Differences between cell wall of gram-positive and gram-negative bacteria are shown in **Table 2.2**.

2. *Cytoplasmic (plasma) membrane (Table 2.2)*
Structure: It is thin (5–10 nm thick), elastic and can only be seen with electron microscope.
Functions of cytoplasmic membrane:
   i. **Semipermeable membrane**
   ii. **Housing enzymes and proteins**
   iii. **Generation of chemical energy**
   iv. **Cell motility**
   v. **Mediation of chromosomal segregation during replication**

Cellular Appendages
Capsule or slime layer
Structure: Many bacteria synthesize large amount of extracellular polymer in their natural environments. When the polymer forms a condensed, well-defined layer closely surrounding the cell, it is called the capsule as in the pneumococcus. If the polymer is easily washed off and does not appear to be associated with the cell in any definite fashion, it is referred as a slime layer.

Composition of capsules and slime layers: Capsules and slime layers usually are composed of polysaccharide (e.g., *Pneumococcus*) or of polypeptide in some bacteria (e.g., *Bacillus anthracis* and *Yersinia pestis*).

Capsulated bacteria: *Streptococcus pneumoniae*, several groups of streptococci, *Neisseria meningitidis, Klebsiella, Haemophilus influenzae, Yersinia* and *Bacillus*.

Demonstration of capsule
   i. **Gram stain:** Slime has little affinity for basic dyes and is not visible in Gram stained smears.
   ii. **Special capsule staining techniques**: Usually, employing copper salts as mordants.
   iii. **India ink staining (negative staining):** The capsule appears as a clear halo around the bacterium, against a dark background in the film **(Fig. 2.7)**.
   iv. **Electron microscope**
   v. **Serological methods:** When a suspension of a capsulated bacterium is mixed with its specific anticapsular serum and examined under the microscope, the capsule becomes very prominent and appears "swollen" due to an increase in its refractivity. It is known as the **capsule-swelling reaction** or **Quellung reaction** (Quellung-*Ger; swelling*), described by Neufeld (1902).

Table 2.2: Comparison of cell walls of gram-positive and gram-negative bacteria.		
Characteristic	*Gram-positive*	*Gram-negative*
1. Thickness	Thicker	Thinner
2. Peptidoglycan	Thick layer (16–80 nm)	2 nm (thin layer)
3. Teichoic acid	Present	Absent
4. Variety of amino acids	Few	Several
5. Aromatic and sulfur-containing amino acids	Absent or scant	Present
6. Lipids	Absent or scant	Present
7. Porin proteins	Absent	Present
8. Periplasmic region	Absent	Present

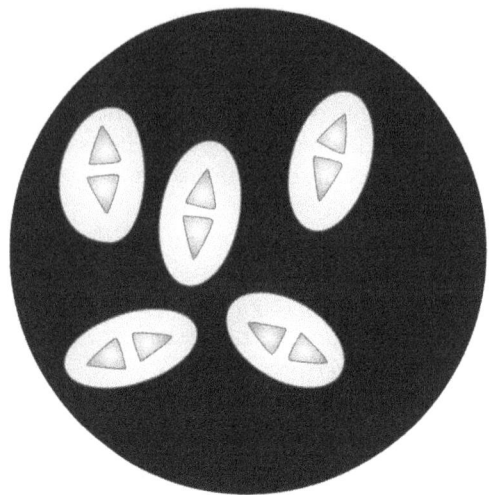

Fig. 2.7: Pneumococci negatively stained with India ink to show capsule.

Functions of capsule
i. **Virulence factor—by inhibiting phagocytosis**
ii. **Protection of the cell wall**
iii. **Identification and typing of bacteria**

Flagella
Motile bacteria possess one or more unbranched, long, sinuous filaments called **flagella**, which are the organs of locomotion.
Structure: They are 3–20 µm long and are of uniform diameter (0.01–0.013 µm) and terminate in a square tip. Flagella consists of largely or entirely of a protein, **flagellin**.

Parts and Composition
Each flagellum consists of three parts:
1. Filament
2. Hook
3. Basal body

Arrangement/Types (Fig. 2.8)
These are four types of flagella arrangement:
1. **Monotrichous**—single polar flagellum, e.g., cholera vibrio
2. **Amphitrichous**—single flagellum at both ends, e.g., *Alcaligenes faecalis*.
3. **Lophotrichous**—tuft of flagella at one or both ends, e.g., spirilla
4. **Peritrichous**—flagella surrounding the cell, e.g., typhoid bacilli

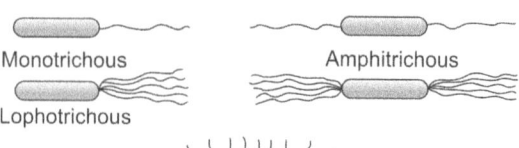
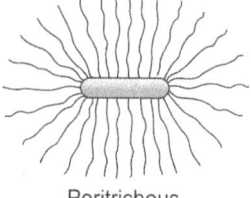

Fig. 2.8: Arrangement of flagella.

Demonstration of Flagella
Flagella are about 0.02 µm in thickness and hence beyond the resolution limit of the light microscope. The following methods are used for its demonstration:
i. **Dark ground illumination**
ii. **Special staining methods**: In which their thickness is increased by mordanting
iii. **Electron microscopy**
iv. **Indirect methods**: Indirect methods by which motility of bacteria can be seen or demonstrated.
   a. Microscopically in fluid suspensions (in a hanging drop or under a coverslip)
   b. **By spread of bacterial growth as a film over agar**, e.g., swarming growth of *Proteus* spp.
   c. **Turbidity spreading through semisolid agar**, e.g., Craigie tube method.

Fimbria or Pili
Structure and synthesis: Many gram-negative bacteria have short, fine, hair-like surface appendages which are called **fimbriae or pili**. They are shorter and thinner than flagella (0.1–1.5 µm in length and uniform width between 4 and 8 nm) and emerge from the cell wall. They originate in the **cytoplasmic membrane** and are composed of protein termed **pilins** like flagella.

Demonstration of Fimbriae
1. Electron microscopy
2. Hemagglutination

Functions of Pilli
Two classes can be distinguished on the basis of their function: **Ordinary (common) pili** and **sex pili**.

Cell Interior

1. **Cytoplasm:** The cytoplasm of the bacterial cell is a viscous watery solution or soft gel, containing a variety of organic or inorganic solutes, and numerous ribosomes and polysomes.
2. **Ribosomes:** The ribosomes are the location for all bacterial protein synthesis.
3. Mesosomes (Chondrioids)
   Structure: These are convoluted or multi-laminated membranous bodies formed as invaginations of the plasma membrane into the cytoplasm.
   Functions of mesosomes
   i. Compartmenting of DNA
   ii. Sites of the respiratory enzymes
4. **Intracytoplasmic inclusions:** These bodies are usually for storage. They consist of **volutin (polyphosphate), lipid, glycogen, starch or sulfur.**
5. **Bacterial nucleus:**
   Structure: The genetic material of a bacterial cell is contained in a single, long molecule of double-stranded deoxyribonucleic acid (DNA) which can be extracted in the form of a closed circular thread about 1 mm (1,000 µm) long, about 1,000 times the length of the cell. The bacterial chromosome is haploid and replicates by simple fission. Bacterial nucleus does not possess nuclear membrane.
   Plasmids: Bacteria may possess extranuclear genetic elements in the cytoplasm consisting of DNA termed *plasmids* or *episomes*.
   Function of plasmids: Plasmids are not essential for host growth and reproduction they inhabit, but may **confer on it certain properties**, such as drug resistance, enhanced pathogenicity, which may constitute a survival advantage.
6. **Bacterial spore:**
   A number of gram-positive bacteria, such as those of the genera *Clostridium* and *Bacillus* can form a special resistant dormant structure called an **endospore** or, simply, **spores.** Endospore develop when essential nutrients are depleted. Sporulation in bacteria, therefore, is not a method of reproduction but of preservation **(Fig. 2.9).**

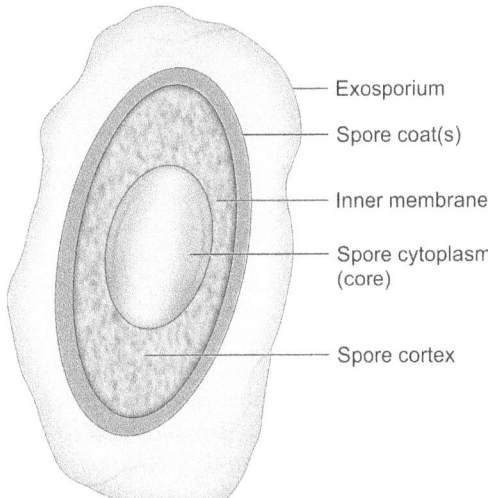

Fig. 2.9: Bacterial spore (cross-section).

Sporulation: Spore formation, sporogenesis or sporulation normally commences when growth ceases due to lack of nutrients, depletion of the nitrogen or carbon source (or both) being the most significant factor.
Stages: It is a complex process and may be divided into several stages.
- **Spore septum**
- **Forespore:** The spore septum becomes a **double-layered membrane** that surrounds the chromosome and cytoplasm. Structure, entirely enclosed within the original cell, is called a **forespore.**
- **Spore coat:** The forespore is subsequently completely encircled by dividing septum as a double layered membrane. The two spore membranes now engage in active synthesis of various layers of the spore. The inner layer becomes the **inner membrane.** Between the two layers there is laid **spore cortex** and outer layer is transformed into **spore coat** which consists of several layers. In some species **from** outer layer also develops **exosporium** which bears ridges and folds **(Fig. 2.9).**

Germination: Germination is the process of conversion of a spore into vegetative cells under suitable conditions.

Shape and position of spores
Spores may be central (equatorial), subterminal (close to one end), or terminal **(Fig. 2.10).**

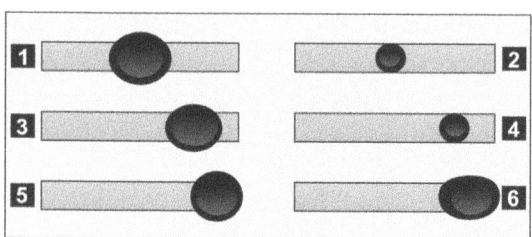

Fig. 2.10: Types of spores. 1. central, bulging, 2. central, not bulging, 3. subterminal, bulging, 4. subterminal, not bulging, 5. terminal, spherical, 6. terminal, oval.

The appearance may be spherical, ovoid or elongated, and being narrower that the cell, or broader and bulging it. The diameter of spore may be same or less than the width of bacteria (Bacillus), or may be wider than the bacillary body producing a distension or bulge in the cell (Clostridium).

Resistance
Bacterial spores constitute some of the most resistant forms of life. Spores of all medically important species are destroyed by autoclaving at 120°C for 15 minutes. Methods of sterilization and disinfection should ensure that spores also are destroyed. Sporulation helps bacteria survive for long periods under unfavorable environments.

Demonstration
i. **Gram stain:** Spores appear as an unstained refractile body within the cell.
ii. **Modified Ziehl–Neelsen (ZN) staining:** Spores are slightly acid-fast and may be stained differentially by a modification of the Ziehl–Neelsen method. Ziehl–Neelsen staining with 0.25–0.5% sulfuric acid (instead of 20% sulfuric acid as used in conventional method) as decoloring agent is used for spore staining.

Uses of spores
1. **Importance in food, industrial, and medical microbiology**
2. **Sterilization control:** For proper sterilization, spores of certain species of bacteria are employed as indicator, e.g., *Bacillus stearothermophilus* which is destroyed at a temperature of 121°C for 10–20 minutes (same temperature and time as used in autoclaving). Prior to its use, these spores may be kept in autoclave. Proper sterilization is indicated by the absence of the spores after autoclaving.
3. **Research**

L-FORMS OF BACTERIA (CELL-WALL-DEFECTIVE ORGANISMS)

Abnormal forms of the bacteria were named **L-forms** after the Lister Institute, London (hence, the "L").

Colonies of L-phase organisms on agar media are small and have a characteristic **"fried egg"** appearance.

L-forms are **nonpathogenic to laboratory animals.**

KEY POINTS

Microscopy: A simple microscope consists of one lens; a compound microscope has multiple lenses.

Anatomy of Bacterial Cell
A. Cell envelope and its appendages
B. Cell interior

Endospores are a dormant stage for survival during adverse environmental conditions.

IMPORTANT QUESTIONS

1. Name various microscopic instruments used in microbiology and describe the working principle of compound microscope.
2. Describe briefly the anatomy of bacterial cell.
3. Draw a labeled diagram of bacterial cell. Write briefly on cell wall of bacteria.
4. Write short notes on:
   a. Bacterial cell wall
   b. Capsule or bacterial capsule
   c. Bacterial flagella
   d. Bacterial spores or endospores

MULTIPLE CHOICE QUESTIONS

1. Which of the following is not a distinguishing characteristic of prokaryotic cells?
   a. They usually have a single, circular chromosome
   b. They lack membrane enclosed organelles
   c. They have cell walls containing peptidoglycan
   d. They lack a plasma membrane

Chapter 2: Microscopy and Morphology of Bacteria

2. Peptidoglycan layer of cell wall is thicker in:
   a. Gram-positive bacteria
   b. Gram-negative bacteria
   c. Fungi
   d. Parasites
3. All the following statements are true for lipopolysaccharide, *except*:
   a. It consists of three components: Lipid A, core polysaccharide and O polysaccharide.
   b. Lipid A functions as an endotoxin
   c. It is an integral part of the cell wall of the gram-positive bacteria
   d. Polysaccharide represents a major surface antigen of the bacterial cell
4. A tuft of flagella present at one or both ends of bacterial cell is known as:
   a. Monotrichous
   b. Amphitrichous
   c. Lophotrichous
   d. Peritrichous
5. Which of the following is not true about fimbriae?
   a. They originate in the cytoplasmic membrane.
   b. They are composed of protein.
   c. They may be used for attachment.
   d. They may be used for motility.
6. Which one of the following bacteria is cell wall deficient?
   a. Escherichia coli
   b. Streptococcus aureus
   c. Mycoplasma
   d. Treponema pallidum
7. All of the following are spore forming bacteria, *except*:
   a. Clostridium botulinum
   b. Bacillus anthracis
   c. Bacillus subtilis
   d. Vibrio cholerae

ANSWERS

1. d   2. a   3. c   4. c
5. d   6. c   7. d

CHAPTER 3: Physiology of Bacteria

LEARNING OBJECTIVES

After reading and studying this chapter, you should be able to:
- Explain generation time of bacteria.
- Describe and draw bacterial growth curve.
- Define the atmospheric requirement of microaerophilic bacteria and capnophilic bacteria.

PRINCIPLES OF BACTERIAL GROWTH

Bacterial Division

Bacteria divide by **binary fission** where individual cells enlarge and divide to yield two progeny of approximately equal size. Nuclear division precedes cell division. The cell division occurs by a constrictive or pinching process, or by the ingrowth of a transverse septum across the cell. The daughter cells may remain partially attached after division in some species.

Generation Time or Doubling Time

The interval of time between two cell divisions, or the time required for a bacterium to give rise to two daughter cells under optimum conditions, is known as the **generation time or doubling time**.
Examples: In coliform bacilli and many other medically important bacteria, it about 20 minutes, in tubercle bacilli, it is about 20 hours and in lepra bacilli, it is about 20 days.
Colonies: Bacteria growing on solid media form **colonies**.

Bacterial Count

Bacteria in a culture medium or clinical specimen can be counted by two methods:
1. **Total count:** This is total number of bacteria present in a specimen irrespective of whether they are living or dead.
2. **Viable count:** This measures only viable (living) cells.

Bacterial Growth Curve

If a suitable liquid medium is inoculated with bacterium and incubated, its growth follows a definitive course. Small samples are taken at regular intervals after inoculation and plotted in relation to time. A plotting of the data will yield a characteristic growth curve **(Fig. 3.1)**.

Phases of bacterial growth curve: The bacterial growth curve can be divided into four major phases: Lag phase, exponential or log

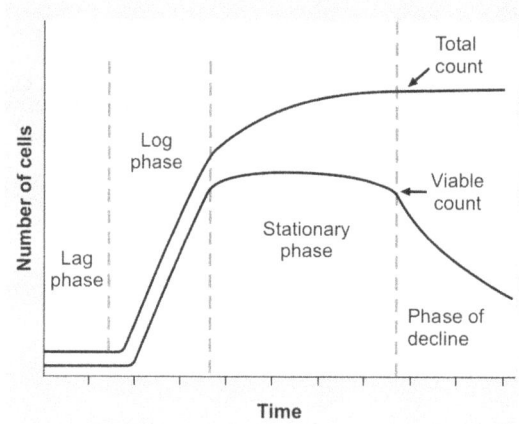

Fig. 3.1: Bacterial growth curve. The viable count shows lag, log, stationary and decline phases. In the total count, the phase of decline is not evident.

(logarithmic) phase, stationary phase, and decline phase.
1. **Lag phase:** When microorganisms are introduced into fresh culture medium, usually no immediate increase in cell number occurs, and therefore, this period is called the **lag phase.** After inoculation, there is an increase in cell size at a time when little are no cell division is occurring. This initial period is the time required for adaptation to the new environment, during which the necessary enzymes and metabolic intermediates are built up in adequate quantities for multiplication to proceed.
2. **Log (logarithmic) or exponential phase:** Following the lag phase, the cells start dividing and their numbers increase exponentially or by geometric progression with time. If the logarithm of the viable count is plotted against time, a straight line will be obtained.
3. **Stationary phase:** After a varying period of exponential growth, cell division stops due to depletion of nutrients and accumulation of toxic products. Eventually, growth slows down, and the total bacterial cell number reaches a maximum and stabilizes. The number of progeny cells formed is just enough to replace the number of cells that die. The growth curve becomes horizontal. The viable count remains stationary as an equilibrium exists between the dying cells and the newly formed cells.
4. **Decline or death phase:** The death phase is the period when the population decreases due to cell death. Eventually, the rate of death exceeds the rate of reproduction, and the number of viable cells declines. Like bacterial growth, death is exponential. Cell death may also be caused by autolysis besides nutrient deprivation and buildup of toxic wastes. Finally, after a variable period, all the cells die and culture becomes sterile.

Bacterial Nutrition

The minimum nutritional requirements for growth and multiplication of bacteria are water, a source of carbon, a source of nitrogen, and some inorganic salts. The water content of bacterial cells can vary from 75 to 90% of the total weight and is the vehicle for the entry of all cells and for the elimination of all waste products. It participates in the metabolic reactions and also forms an integral part of the protoplasm.

Categories of Requirements

The requirements for microbial growth can be divided into two main categories: Chemical and physical.
A. **Chemical requirements:** Chemical requirements include sources of carbon, nitrogen, sulfur, phosphorus, trace elements, oxygen, and organic growth factors.
B. Physical factors influencing microbial growth

1. Temperature

Optimum temperature: The temperature at which growth occur best is known as the **"optimum temperature"**. Thus, bacteria pathogenic for humans usually grow at 37°C (our body temperature).

2. Oxygen

Based on their O_2 requirements, prokaryotes can be separated into aerobes and anaerobes.
A. **Aerobic bacteria**—require oxygen for growth and may be:
   i. *Obligate aerobes*—have an absolute or obligate requirement for oxygen (O_2), like vibrio.
   ii. *Facultative anaerobes*—are ordinarily aerobic but can also grow in the absence of oxygen, though less abundantly.
   iii. *Microaerophilic organisms*—grow best at low oxygen tension.
B. **Anaerobic bacteria**—grow in absence of oxygen.
   Obligate anaerobes—may even die on exposure to oxygen. For example, *Clostridium tetani*.

3. Carbon Dioxide

All bacteria require small amount of carbon dioxide for growth.

4. Moisture and Drying
Moisture is very essential for the growth of the bacteria.

5. pH
Most bacteria can live and multiply within the range of pH 5 (acidic) to pH 8 (basic) and have a pH optimum near neutral (pH 7).

6. Light
Darkness provides a favorable condition for growth and viability of bacteria.

7. Osmotic Effect
Bacteria are more tolerant to osmotic variation.

8. Mechanical and Sonic Stresses
In spite of tough walls of bacteria, they may be ruptured by mechanical stress.

KEY POINTS
- **Bacterial growth curve:** The bacterial growth curve can be divided into four major phases: lag phase, exponential or log (logarithmic) phase, stationary phase, and decline phase.
- The requirements for microbial growth—chemical and physical.

IMPORTANT QUESTIONS
1. Draw a typical bacterial growth curve and describe it.
2. Write short notes on:
   a. Bacterial growth curve/growth phases of bacteria.
   b. Physical factors influencing microbial growth.

MULTIPLE CHOICE QUESTIONS

1. Generation time for *Mycobacterium tuberculosis* is:
   a. 20 seconds
   b. 20 minutes
   c. 20 hours
   d. 20 days
2. Bacteria which can grow at temperature between 20°C and 40°C are known as:
   a. Mesophiles
   b. Psychrophiles
   c. Thermophiles
   d. None of the above
3. The bacteria which require much higher level of carbon dioxide for their growth are known as:
   a. Microaerophilic bacteria
   b. Capnophilic bacteria
   c. Aerobic bacteria
   d. Phototrophs
4. Which one of the following acidophilic bacteria can grow in acidic conditions?
   a. *Escherichia coli*
   b. *Lactobacilli*
   c. *Pseudomonas aeruginosa*
   d. *Vibrio cholerae*
5. The enzyme catalase is present in:
   a. Aerobic bacteria
   b. Obligate anaerobic bacteria
   c. Aerobic and obligate anaerobic bacteria
   d. None of the above

ANSWERS
1. c 2. a 3. b 4. b
5. a

CHAPTER 4: Culture Media and Culture Methods

LEARNING OBJECTIVES

After reading and studying this chapter, you should be able to:
- Describe classification of media.
- Differentiate between the following: Enriched media and enrichment media; indicator media and differential media; selective media and differential media with suitable examples.
- Discuss liquid media and composition and uses.
- Discuss anaerobic culture methods.
- Explain the principle and describe uses of the following: McIntosh and Filde's anaerobic jar; cooked meat broth.

INTRODUCTION

Culture medium: A nutrient material prepared for the growth of microorganisms in a laboratory is called a **culture medium**.

CLASSIFICATION OF MEDIA

Media have been classified in many ways (**Table 4.1**).

A. Phases of Growth Media

Growth media are used in either of two phases: Liquid (broth) or solid (agar).

B. Based on Nutritional Factors

1. Simple Media (Basal Media)

Simple media are those which contain only basic nutrients, *e.g.*, peptone water, nutrient broth, and nutrient agar. These simple media are generally used as the basis of to prepare enriched media; hence, known as basal media.

2. Complex Media

Media that contain some ingredients of unknown chemical composition are called **complex media**.

Table 4.1: Classification of media.

A. Based on phases of growth media
  1. Liquid (broth) media
  2. Solid (agar) media
  3. Semisolid media

B. Based on nutritional factors
  1. Simple media (basal media)
  2. Complex media
  3. Synthetic or defined media

C. Special media
  1. Enriched media
  2. Enrichment media
  3. Selective media
  4. Indicator or differential media
  5. Transport media
  6. Sugar media

D. Reducing media
  Based on phases of growth media
  1. Liquid (broth) media
  2. Solid (agar) media
  3. Semisolid media

Nutrient Broth

A commonly used complex medium, **nutrient broth (in liquid form)**. It is a simple basal liquid medium, supports growth of many organisms.

Nutrient Agar (Table 4.2)

Nutrient agar is prepared by adding agar at a concentration of 2% to the nutrient broth.

Synthetic or Chemically Defined Media

They are prepared exclusively from pure chemical substances and their exact composition is known.

C. Special Media (Table 4.1)

1. Enriched Media (Table 4.2)

These are prepared to meet the nutritional requirements of more exacting bacteria by the addition of substances such as blood, serum or egg to a basal medium.

Examples:
i. **Blood agar:** Many medically important bacteria are fastidious, requiring a medium and commonly used in clinical laboratories is **blood agar**
ii. **Chocolate agar**
iii. **Loeffler's serum slope:** It is used for the isolation of *Corynebacterium diphtheriae*

2. Enrichment Media (Table 4.3)

When a substance is added to a liquid medium which inhibits the growth of unwanted bacteria and favors the growth of wanted bacteria is known as **enrichment medium**. This medium for an enrichment culture is **usually liquid**.

Usually, the nonpathogenic or commensal bacteria tend to overgrow the pathogenic ones, for example, *Salmonella* (*S*). Typhi being overgrown by *E. coli* in cultures from feces. In such situations, substances which have a stimulating effect on the bacteria to be grown or an inhibitory effect on those to be suppressed are incorporated in the medium.

Table 4.2: Representative types of agar media.		
Medium	**Composition**	**Characteristics**
A. Simple medium		
Nutrient agar	Nutrient broth, agar (2–3%)	Complex medium used for routine laboratory work
B. Enriched media		
i. Blood agar	Nutrient agar. Sheep blood (5–10%)	In addition to being enriched medium, it is an indicator medium showing the hemolytic properties of bacteria such as *Streptococcus pyogenes*
ii. Chocolate agar	Heated blood agar (55°C × 2 hours)	Culture fastidious of *Haemophilus influenzae*, *Neisseria* and *Pnemococcus*
iii. Loeffler's serum slope (LSS)	• Nutrient broth • Serum (of ox, sheep or horse) • Glucose	Culture of Corynebacterium diphtheriae
C. Indicator media		
MacConkey agar	• Peptone • Sodium taurocholate, • Agar • Neutral red • Lactose	Isolation and differentiation of lactose fermenting (LF) and nonlactose fermenting (NLF) enteric bacilli
D. Selective media		
Deoxycholate citrate agar (DCA)	• Nutrient agar • Sodium deoxycholate • Sodium citrate • Lactose • Neutral red	Suitable for the isolation of *Salmonella* and *Shigella*

Table 4.3: Representative types of liquid media.

Medium	Composition	Characteristics
1. Peptone water	• Peptone—10 g • Sodium chloride (Na Cl)—5 g • Water—1 liter (pH 7.4–7.5)	• Basis for carbohydrate fermentation media • For testing the formation of indole
2. Nutrient broth	• Peptone water • Meat extract	For routine culture
3. Glucose broth	Nutrient broth + glucose (1% most common)	• Blood culture • Promotes luxuriant growth of many organisms • Glucose acts as reducing agent
4. Enrichment media i. Tetrathionate broth	• Nutrient broth • Sodium thiosulphate • Calcium carbonate • Iodine solution • Phenol red	Enriches salmonellae and sometimes shigellae
ii. Selenite F broth	• Sodium selenite • Peptone • Lactose	It inhibits coliform bacilli while permitting salmonellae and many shigellae to grow
iii. Alkaline peptone water	• Peptone—10 g • Sodium chloride (NaCl)—10 g • Distilled water—1 liter	For enriching *V. cholerae* and other *Vibrio* species in a fecal specimen
5. Anaerobic media Robertson's cooked meat broth (RCM)	• Nutrient broth • Predigested cooked meat of ox heart	• Culture of anaerobic bacteria • Preservation of stock culture of aerobic bacteria

Examples:
a. **Tetrathionate broth:** Tetrathionate inhibits coliforms while allowing typhoid-paratyphoid bacilli to grow freely in fecal sample.
b. **Selenite F (F for Feces) broth:** It is used for dysentery bacilli.
c. **Alkaline peptone water:** It is used for (*Vibrio*) *V. cholerae* from feces.

3. Selective Media (Table 4.2)

When a substance is added to a solid medium which inhibits the growth of unwanted bacteria but favors the growth of wanted bacteria it is known as **selective media**. These media are used to isolate particular bacteria from specimens where mixed bacterial flora is expected.

Examples of Selective Media
a. **Deoxycholate citrate agar (DCA):** Addition of deoxycholate acts as a selective agent for dysentery bacilli (isolation of *Shigellae*)
b. **Lowenstein and Jensen medium:** Is used for *Mycobacterium tuberculosis*
c. **Potassium tellurite medium:** For the isolation of diphtheria bacilli

4. Indicator Media (Table 4.2)

These media contain an indicator which changes color when a bacterium grows in them.

Example:
a. **Mac Conkey agar:** Mac Conkey agar indicates fermenting properties. Lactose fermenter (LF) produce pink colonies and non-lactose fermenter (NLF) produce colorless colonies due to neutral red indicator.
b. **Wilson and Blair medium:** There is incorporation of sulfite in Wilson and Blair medium. *S. Typhi* reduces sulfite to sulfide in the presence of glucose and the colonies of *S. Typhi* have a black metallic sheen.

5. Differential Media

A medium which has substances incorporated in it, enabling it to bring out differing characteristics of bacteria and thus helping to distinguish between them, is called a **differential medium**.
Examples:
 a. **Blood agar**
 b. **MacConkey agar:** It is both differential and selective.

6. Sugar Media

For the identification of most of the organisms, sugar fermentation reactions are carried out.

7. Transport Media

A transport medium is a holding medium designed to preserve the viability of microorganisms in the specimen but not allow multiplication.

Delicate organisms (like gonococci) which may not survive the time taken for transporting the specimen to the laboratory or the normal flora may overgrow pathogenic flora *(Salmonella, Shigella* and *V. cholerae),* such special media are devised to maintain the viability of the pathogen termed as "transport media".

Example: *Stuart's transport medium* and *Amies transport medium* for gonococci.

D. Anaerobic Media (Table 4.3)

These media are used to grow anaerobic organisms, and contain reducing substances. These include:
 i. Thioglycolate broth
 ii. Cooked meat broth.

CULTURE METHODS

Methods of Bacterial Culture

The methods of bacterial culture used in the clinical laboratory include **streak culture, lawn culture, stroke culture, stab culture, pour-plate culture, shake culture, and liquid culture.** Special methods are employed for culturing **anaerobic bacteria.**

Streak Culture (Surface Plating)

This method is routinely employed for the isolation of bacteria in pure culture from clinical specimens. A platinum loop No. 23 SWG, 6.5 cm long, is charged with the specimen to be cultured. Owing to the high cost of platinum, loops for routine work are made of nichrome resistance wire, No. 24 SWG. The loop is flat, circular and completely closed with 2–4 mm internal diameter mounted on a handle.

One loopful of the specimen is smeared thoroughly over area A **(Fig. 4.1),** on the surface of a well dried plate, to give a **well-inoculum or "well"**. The loop is resterilized and drawn from the well in two or three parallel lines on to the fresh surface of the medium (B). This process is repeated as shown (C, D, E), care being taken to sterilize the loop, and cool it on unseeded medium, between each sequence. At each step the inoculum is derived from the most distal part of the immediately preceding strokes.

Plates are incubated in the inverted position with the lid underneath. On incubation, growth may be confluent at the site of original inoculation ("well"), but becomes progressively thinner, and well separated colonies are obtained over the final series of streaks.

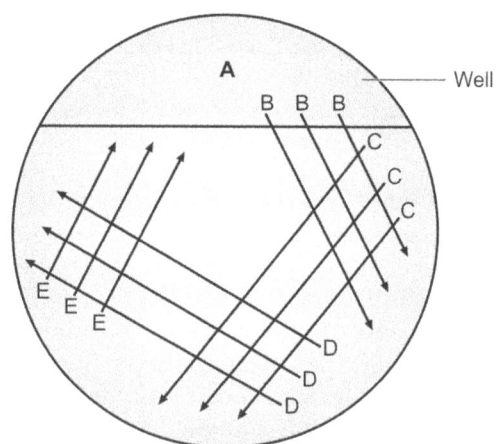

Fig. 4.1: Streak culture (streak plating) on solid media.

Lawn Culture or Carpet Culture

Lawn cultures are prepared by flooding the surface of the plate with a liquid culture or suspension of the bacterium, pipetting off the excess inoculum and incubating the plate. Alternatively, the surface of the plate may be inoculated by applying a swab soaked in the bacterial culture or suspension. After incubation, lawn culture provides a uniform growth of the bacterium.

Uses

i. **Antibiotic susceptibility testing**
ii. **Bacteriophage typing**
iii. **For preparation of bacterial antigens and vaccines**

Anaerobic Culture Methods

Anaerobic bacteria require incubation without oxygen and differ in their requirement and sensitivity to oxygen. Obligate anaerobes will not grow from small inocula unless oxygen is absent and the Eh of the medium is low.

Methods of Anaerobiosis

Anaerobiosis can be achieved by a number of methods.

McIntosh and Filde's anaerobic jar: Anaerobiosis obtained by **McIntosh and Filde's anaerobic jar (Fig. 4.2)** is the most dependable and widely used method.

The jar (20 × 12.5 cm) should be made of metal or robust plastic with a lid that can be clamped down on a gasket to make it airtight. The lid is furnished with two tubes with valves, one acting as gas inlet and the other as the outlet. The lid also has two terminals which can be connected to an electrical supply. On its undersurface it carries a gauze sachet carrying alumina pellets coated with palladium (palladinized alumina). It acts as a room temperature catalyst for the conversion of hydrogen and oxygen into water

Procedure: Inoculated culture plates are placed inside the jar with the medium uppermost and lid downward and the lid clamped tight. The outlet tube is connected to a vacuum pump and

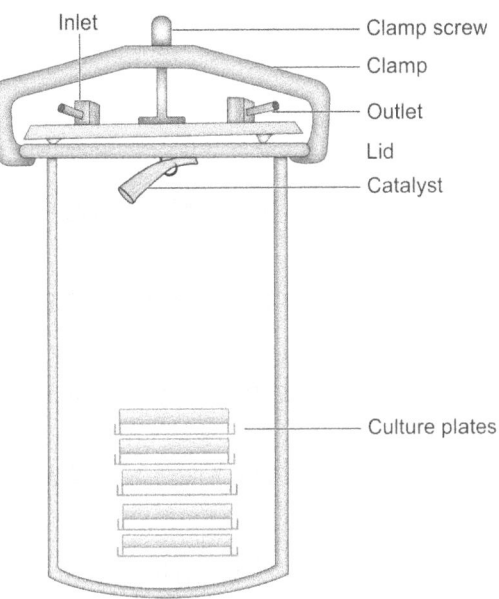

Fig. 4.2: McIntosh and Filde's anaerobic jar.

the air inside is evacuated. Approximately, 6/7 of the air is evacuated (pressure reduced to 100 mm Hg, i.e., 660 mm below atmospheric) and this is monitored on a vacuum gauge. The outlet tap is then closed and the inlet tube connected to a hydrogen supply. Hydrogen is drawn in rapidly.

Catalyst: After the jar is filled with hydrogen, the electrical terminals are connected to a current supply to heat the catalyst and if room temperature catalyst is used, heating is not required. The catalyst will help to combine hydrogen and residual oxygen to form water. The jar is then incubated at 37°C.

Indicator: Reduced methylene blue is generally used as indicator (mixture of NaOH, methylene blue, and glucose). It becomes colorless anaerobically but regains blue color on exposure to oxygen.

By Reducing Agents

Liquid media soon become aerobic unless a reducing agent is added such as glucose, ascorbic acid, cysteine sodium mercaptoacetate or thioglycollate, or the particles of meat in cooked meat broth.

KEY POINTS

A culture medium is any material prepared for the growth of bacteria in a laboratory.
- **Enriched media** are solid media supplemented with blood, serum, etc.
- **Enrichment media:** An enrichment culture is used to encourage the growth of a particular microorganism in a mixed culture and are the liquid media
- **Selective media:** By inhibiting unwanted organisms with salts, dyes, or other chemicals, selective media allow growth of only the desired microbes
- **Transport media** are used to maintain the viability of certain delicate organisms during their transport to the laboratory
- **Anaerobic jars:** Anaerobiosis obtained by **McIntosh and Filde's anaerobic jar** is the most dependable and widely used method

IMPORTANT QUESTIONS

1. What are culture media? Classify and discuss them briefly.
2. Distinguish between a selective medium and a differential medium.
3. Discuss in detail anaerobic culture methods.
4. Write short notes on:
   a. Enriched media.
   b. Enrichment media.
   c. Selective media.
   d. Indicator media.
   e. Differential media
   f. Transport media.
   g. Streak culture.
   h. Lawn culture.

MULTIPLE CHOICE QUESTIONS

1. The important source of nutrition for bacteria to grow is:
   a. Agar
   b. Electrolytes
   c. Inorganic salts
   d. Peptone
2. All of the following are examples of enriched media, *except*:
   a. Blood agar
   b. Chocolate agar
   c. Loeffler's serum slope
   d. Bile salt agar
3. All of the following are examples of selective media, *except*:
   a. Potassium tellurite medium
   b. Deoxycholate citrate agar
   c. Lowenstein and Jensen medium
   d. Nutrient agar
4. Which enrichment medium is preferred to grow *Vibrio cholerae*?
   a. Tetrathionate broth
   b. Selenite F broth
   c. Alkaline peptone water
   d. All of the above

ANSWERS

1. d   2. d   3. d   4. c

CHAPTER 5

Infection

LEARNING OBJECTIVES

After reading and studying this chapter, you should be able to:
- Define the terms saprophytes, parasite, commensal, and pathogen.
- Discuss modes of spread of infection giving suitable examples.
- List the differences between exotoxins and endotoxins.

INTRODUCTION

Infection and immunity involve interaction between the animal body (host) and the infecting microorganisms.

Microorganisms and Host

Based on their relationship to their host they can be divided into saprophytes and parasites.
A. **Saprophytes:** Saprophytes (from Greek *sapros*, decayed; and *phyton*, plant) are free-living microbes that live on dead or decaying organic matter.
B. **Parasites:** Parasites are microbes that can establish themselves and multiply in the hosts. Parasite microbes may be either pathogens or commensals:
   1. **Pathogens:** Pathogens (from Greek *pathos*, disease, and *gen*, to produce) are the microorganisms or agents, which are capable of producing disease in the host. Its ability to cause disease is called *pathogenicity*.
   Types of pathogens: They are of two types:
   a. **Primary (frank) pathogens**: Primary (frank) pathogens are the organisms, which are capable of producing disease in previously healthy individuals with intact immunological defenses.
   b. **Opportunist pathogens: Opportunist pathogens** rarely cause disease in individuals with intact immunological and anatomical defenses.
   2. **Commensals:** Commensals (organisms of normal flora) are the microorganisms that live in complete harmony with the host without causing any damage to it. Skin and mucous membranes are sterile at birth.

INFECTION

The lodgment and multiplication of a parasite in or on the tissues of a host constitute infection.

For a microorganism to be transported and be effective in continuing contamination, it follows a definite cycle or chain of events. The following six elements are necessary for infection to occur:
1. **The infectious agent**—a pathogen
2. **Reservoir**—where the pathogen can grow. Any natural habitat of a microorganism that promotes growth and reproduction is a **reservoir.**

    A **carrier,** or vector, is a person or animal who does not become ill but harbors and spreads an organism, causing disease in others.
3. **Exit route from reservoir—exit route:** A microorganism does not have the capacity to cause disease in another host without

finding a point of escape from the reservoir. Successful microbes must leave the body and then be transmitted to fresh hosts.

By performing hand hygiene, you have the capacity to prevent the spread of microorganisms, or cross contamination. Also, teach the patient to cover the nose and mouth when coughing or sneezing.

4. **Method or vehicle** of transportation, such as exudate, feces, air droplets, hands, and needles.
5. **Entrance through skin, mucous lining, or mouth**
6. **Host**—it is another person or animal where organism is nourished and harbored.

SOURCES OF INFECTION

A. **Human beings:** The most common source of infection for human beings is human beings themselves.
B. **Animals:**
   Reservoir hosts: Many pathogens are capable of causing infections in both human beings and animals. Therefore, animals may act as a source of infection of such organisms. These animals serve to maintain the parasite in nature and act as **reservoir** and they are, therefore, called **reservoir hosts**.
   Zoonosis: The diseases and infections, which are transmissible to man from animals are called **zoonosis**.
C. **Insects:** Blood-sucking insects, such as mosquitoes, ticks, mites, flies, and lice may transmit pathogens to human beings and diseases so caused are called *arthropod borne diseases*.
   Vectors: Insects that transmit infections are called *vectors*.
D. **Soil and water**
   i. **Soil**: Some pathogens can survive in the soil for long periods.
      Examples: a. Spores of tetanus and gas gangrene; b. Fungi and parasites
   ii. **Water**
E. **Food**: Contaminated food may act as source of infection of organisms causing food poisoning, gastroenteritis, diarrhea, and dysentery.

MODES OF TRANSMISSION OF INFECTION

These include:
1. **Contact:** Infection may be acquired by contact, which may be direct or indirect.
   a. **Direct contact**: Such as sexually transmitted diseases
   b. **Indirect contact**: Indirect contact may be through the agency of fomites, which are inanimate objects, such as clothing, pencils or toys which may be contaminated by a pathogen from one person and act as a vehicle for its transmission to another.
2. **Inhalation:** Respiratory infections, such as common cold, influenza, measles, mumps, tuberculosis and whooping cough are acquired by inhalation.
3. **Ingestion:** Intestinal infections are generally acquired by the ingestion of food or drink contaminated by pathogens.
4. **Inoculation:** The disease agent may be inoculated directly into the skin or mucosa, e.g., rabies virus deposited subcutaneously by dog bite.
5. **Insects**
6. **Congenital:** Some pathogens are able to cross the placental barrier and reach the fetus in utero. This is known as **vertical transmission**.
   Examples: So-called TORCH (Toxoplasma gondii, rubella virus, cytomegalovirus, and herpes virus) agents.
7. **Iatrogenic and laboratory infections:** If meticulous care in asepsis is not taken, infections, such as AIDS and hepatitis B may sometimes be transmitted during administration of injections, lumber puncture, and catheterization.

FACTORS PREDISPOSING TO MICROBIAL PATHOGENICITY

Pathogenicity and Virulence

Pathogenicity: Denotes the ability of a microbial species to cause disease. The term virulence (Latin *virulentia*, from *virus*, poison) denotes the ability of a strain of a species to produce disease.

Virulence: Provides a quantitative measure of pathogenicity, or the likelihood of causing disease.

Determinants of Virulence

1. **Transmissibility:** The first step of the infectious process is the entry of the microorganism into the host by one of several ports: the respiratory tract, gastrointestinal tract, urogenital tract, or through skin that has been cut, punctured, or burned.
2. **Adhesions:** The initial event in the pathogenesis is the attachment of the bacteria to body surfaces.
3. **Invasiveness:** Invasiveness signifies the ability of a pathogen to spread in the host tissues after establishing infection. Highly invasive pathogens characteristically produce spreading or generalized lesions (e.g., streptococcal septicemia following wound infection), while less invasive pathogens cause more localized lesions (e.g., staphylococcal abscess).
4. **Toxigenicity:** Some bacteria cause disease by producing toxins, of which there are two general types: the exotoxins and the endotoxins (**Table 5.1**).
    a. *Exotoxins:* These are soluble, heat-labile proteins inactivated at 60–80°C which are secreted by certain species of bacteria and diffuse readily into the surrounding medium.
    b. *Endotoxins:* These are heat-stable, lipopolysaccharide (LPS) components of the outer membranes of gram-negative but not gram-positive-bacteria. Their toxicity depends upon the component (lipid A). Intravenous injections of large doses of endotoxin and massive gram negative septicemias cause endotoxic shock (**Table 5.1**).

Table 5.1: Differences between exotoxins and endotoxins.

Exotoxins	Endotoxins
1. Proteins	1. Lipopolysaccharide on outer membrane. Lipid A portion is toxic
2. Heat-labile (inactivated at 60–80°C)	2. Heat-stable
3. Actively secreted by the cells; diffuse into the surrounding medium	3. Form integral part of the cell wall; do not diffuse into surrounding medium
4. Readily separable from cultures by physical means, such as filtration	4. Obtained only by cell lysis
5. Action often enzymic	5. No enzymic action
6. Specific pharmacological effect for each exotoxin	6. Nonspecific action of all endotoxins
7. Specific tissue affinities	7. No specific tissue affinities
8. Highly toxic and fatal in microgram quantities	8. Moderate toxicity. Active only in very large doses
9. Highly antigenic	9. Weakly antigenic
10. Action specifically neutralized by antibody	10. Neutralization by antibody ineffective
11. Usually, do not produce fever	11. Usually, produce fever by release of interleukin-1
12. Produced by both gram-positive bacteria and gram-negative bacteria	12. Produced by gram-negative bacteria only
13. Frequently controlled by extrachromosomal genes (e.g., plasmids)	13. Synthesized directly by chromosomal genes
14. Disease examples: Botulism diphtheria tetanus	14. Gram-negative infections, meningococcemia

5. **Avoidance of host defense mechanisms:** Bacteria also have evolved many mechanisms to evade host defenses. Several of these evasive mechanisms are such as **capsules**.
6. **Enzymes:** Many species of bacteria produce tissue-degrading enzymes that play important roles in the infection process.
   i. *Coagulase:* Coagulase is produced by S. aureus and prevents phagocytosis.
   ii. *Hyaluronidases:* Hyaluronidases facilitate the spread of infection along tissue spaces.
7. **Plasmids:** Plasmids are extrachromosomal DNA segments that carry genes for antibiotic resistance known as R-factors.
8. **Bacteriophages:** The classical example of phage directed virulence is seen in diphtheria.
9. **Communicability:** The ability of a microbe to spread from one host to another is known as communicability.
10. **Infecting dose:** Adequate number of bacteria is required for successful infections.
11. **Route of infection:** Certain bacteria are infective when introduced through optimal route.

Types of Infectious Diseases

Infectious diseases may be localized or generalized.
A. **Localized:** Localized infections may be superficial or deep seated
B. **Generalized:** Bacteremia, septicemia and pyemia.

KEY POINTS

- Parasites are microbes that can establish themselves and multiply in the hosts. Parasite microbes may be either pathogens or commensals:
- Sources of infection:
  A. Human beings
  B. **Animals**
  C. Insects
  D. Soil and water
  E. Food
- Modes of transmission of infection:
  1. **Contact**
  2. **Inhalation**
  3. **Ingestion**
  4. **Inoculation**
  5. **Insects**
  6. **Congenital**
  7. **Iatrogenic and laboratory infections**
- Pathogenicity denotes the ability of a microbial species to cause disease. The term virulence denotes the ability of a strain of a species to produce disease. Enhancement of virulence is known as *exaltation*. Reduction of virulence is known as *attenuation*.

IMPORTANT QUESTIONS

1. Describe in detail the sources of infections to human beings.
2. What are the various modes of spread of infection? Describe each in brief giving suitable examples.
3. Distinguish between exotoxins and endotoxins in a tabulated form.
4. Write short notes on:
   a. Modes of transmission of infection.
   b. Determinants of virulence.

MULTIPLE CHOICE QUESTIONS

1. The organisms can be transmitted vertically by all the following ways, *except*:
   a. Sexual contact
   b. Through the placenta
   c. Within the birth canal
   d. Through breast milk
2. Which of the following may cause teratogenic infections?
   a. Toxoplasma
   b. Rubella virus
   c. Cytomegalovirus
   d. All of the above
3. Which of the following statement is not true for exotoxins?
   a. They are proteins
   b. They are highly antigenic
   c. They are heat-labile
   d. They are obtained by cell lysis
4. Which of the statement is not true for endotoxins?
   a. These are lipopolysaccharides component of outer membrane of gram-negative bacteria
   b. These are heat-stable

c. They cannot be toxoided
d. They are highly antigenic
5. The disease that spreads rapidly, involving many persons in a particular area at the same time is known as:
   a. Sporadic
   b. Endemic
   c. Epidemic
   d. Pandemic

ANSWERS

1. a   2. d   3. d   4. d
5. c

CHAPTER 6

Staining Methods

LEARNING OBJECTIVES

After reading and studying this chapter, you should be able to:
- Describe common staining techniques.
- Describe the following: Simple stains; differential stains; Gram stain; acid-fast stain (Ziehl–Neelsen staining of acid-fast bacilli); Albert's stain.

INTRODUCTION

The morphological features of an organism can be studied by examining them under using unstained and stained preparations.

Examination of Living Bacteria in Unstained Preparations

The unstained preparations of living organisms can be studied by anyone of the following methods:
A. Wet coverslip preparation
B. Hanging drop preparation
C. Phase contrast microscope
D. Dark ground microscope

Wet Coverslip Preparation

"Wet" mounts, i.e., unstained preparations of fluid material, are widely used in looking at cells in urine, cerebrospinal fluid (CSF), feces, and vaginal secretions. They are ideal rapid methods (takes more than 5 or 10 minutes).

HANGING DROP PREPARATION

It is done to demonstrate motility and to study morphology of bacteria (**Fig. 6.1**).
- **Motility:** Motile or nonmotile.
- **Morphology:** Cocci, bacilli or coccobacilli

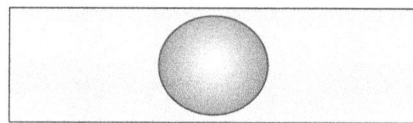
Step 1: Glass slide containing a plasticin ring

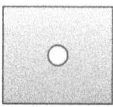
Step 2: Coverslip with a drop of culture medium

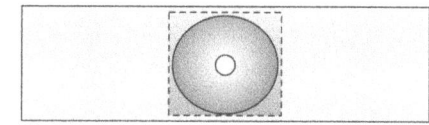
Step 3: Inverted glass slide from step 1 placed on to coverslip in step 2

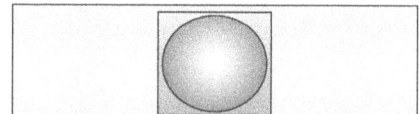
Step 4: Glass slide in step 3 is turned upside down

Fig. 6.1: Hanging drop preparation.

Requirements

1. A clean cavity (depression) slide
2. A clean coverslip
3. Young broth culture
4. Wire loop

5. Bunsen burner/spirit lamp
6. Microscope

Procedure
1. A "hollow ground" slide (a glass slide with a shallow, circular concavity in its center) is used for *hanging drop preparation.*
2. Encircle the concavity with a line streak of soft petroleum jelly applied with a glass rod to the surface of the slide just outside the concavity.
3. Place drop of culture using the sterile wire loop on the center of the coverslip.
4. Invert the cavity slide over the coverslip so that the drop of the culture is in the center of the cavity; press it lightly, so that the coverslip adheres to the vaseline ring.
5. Then quickly turn round the slide so that the coverslip is uppermost. The drop will then be hanging from the coverslip in the center of the concavity, that is why it is called *hanging drop.*
6. Proceed to examine first with a **low-power objective** and then with a **high-power one**.
7. First focus the edge of a hanging drop preparation under **low-power objective (X10)** of microscope, after reducing the light intensity (by partial closing of iris diaphragm) so that the edge of the drop is exactly in the center of the microscopic field.
8. Turn high-power objective (X40) into position and focus the edge of the hanging drop and observe for the motility and morphology of bacteria. Their shape, approximate size, and general structure can be observed **(Fig. 6.2)**.

Note: Instead of slide with a shallow, circular concavity, in many institutions, plasticine is provided to students. Make a ring of plasticine and place it in the center of a clean glass slide. Invert the glass slide containing the plasticine ring and place it on the coverslip. Rest procedure is the same.

Reasons for Focusing the Edge of the Drop
The edge of the drop is focused to observe the motility and morphology for the following reasons:
- The concentration of the organism is more at the edge because:
  - Aerobic organisms tend to move toward the edge.
  - Surface tension is less at the edge, hence the concentration of organisms is more.
- Density is less at the edge of the drop, hence the contrast is better so that the organisms are clearly visible. The differences in refractive index of light rays that pass through glass slide and liquid gives a better contrast at the edge.

Important Points for Observing Motility of Organisms
When examining living organisms for the property of active locomotion, it is essential to distinguish **true motility**, whereby the organisms move in different directions and change their positions in the field, from either:
1. **Passive drifting** of the organisms in the same direction in a convectional current in the fluid or

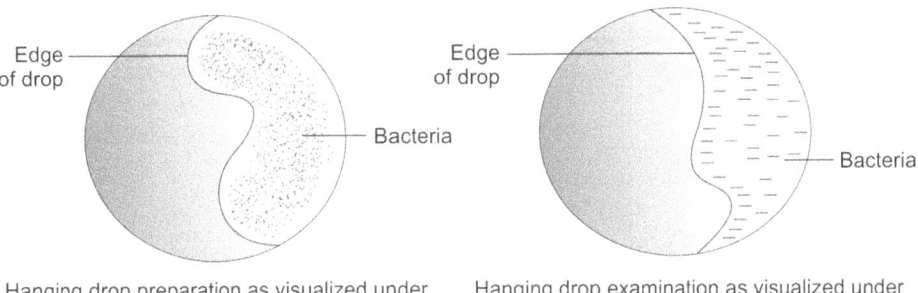

Hanging drop preparation as visualized under X10 objective

Hanging drop examination as visualized under preparation X40 objective

Fig. 6.2: Examination of hanging drop preparation under the microscope.

2. **Brownian movement**, which is an oscillatory movement about a nearly fixed point possessed by all small bodies suspended in fluid and due to irregularities in their bombardment by molecules of water.

Motile Gram Negative Bacilli
- *Escherichia coli*
- *Proteus*
- *Salmonella* sp.
- *Enterobacter*
- *Citrobacter*
- *Hafnia*
- *Serratia* sp.
- *Morganella morganii*
- *Providencia stuartii, rettgeri*
- *Chromobacterium violaceum*
- *Peudomonas aeruginosa*
- *Burkholderia cepacia*
- *Burkholderia pseudomallei*
- *Vibrio cholerae*
- *Campylobacter*
- *Helicobacter*
- *Clostridium tetani*

Nonmotile Gram Negative Bacteria
- *Klebsiella pnemoniae*
- *Shigella* spp.
- *Burkholderia mallei*
- *Streptococcus moniliformis*
- *Gardnerella vaginalis*
- *Flavobacterium menigosepticum*
- Anaerobes:
  - *Bacteroides fragilis*
  - *Fusobacterium* sp.
  - *Leptotrichia buccalis*
  - *Prevotella* spp.
  - *Porphyromonas* sp.

STAINING METHODS

Because most microorganisms appear almost colorless when viewed through a standard light microscope, we often must prepare them for observation. Live bacteria do not show much structural detail under the light microscope due to lack of contrast. Hence, it is customary to use staining techniques to produce color contrast.

Preparing Film or Smear for Staining

Slides
Film preparations are made either on coverslips or on 3 × 1 in glass slides, usually the latter. It is essential that the coverslips or slides be perfectly clean and free from grease.

Smear preparation: A thin film of material containing the microorganisms is spread over the surface of the slide. This film, called a **smear**, is allowed to air dry.

Fixation: Before the microorganisms can be stained, however, they must be fixed (attached) to the microscope slide. In most staining procedures the slide is fixed by passing it through the flame of a Bunsen burner several times, smear side up. Air drying and flaming fix the microorganisms to the slide. Fixing simultaneously kills the microorganisms and attaches them to the slide. It also preserves various parts of microbes in their natural state with only minimal distortion.

Staining: Stain is applied and then washed off with water; then the slide is blotted with absorbent paper. Without fixing, the stain might wash the microbes off the slide. The stained microorganisms are now ready for microscopic examination.

Types of Stain

Basic dyes: Dyes, which include crystal violet, methylene blue, malachite green, and safranin are more commonly used than acidic dyes.

Acidic dyes: These are **eosin, acid fuchsin, and nigrosin.**

Negative staining: Preparing colorless bacteria against a colored background is called **negative staining**. It is valuable in the observation of overall cell shapes, sizes, and capsules.

Stained Preparations

Staining simply means coloring the microorganisms with a dye that emphasizes certain structures. Routine methods for staining of bacteria involve drying and fixing smears, procedures.

Common Staining Techniques
- Simple stains
- Differential stains
  - Gram stain
  - Acid-fast stain (Ziehl-Neelsen staining of acid-fast bacilli)
- Special stains
  - Negative staining
  - Impregnation methods:

Simple Stains
Some of the simple stains commonly used in the laboratory are **methylene blue, carbol fuchsin, crystal violet, and safranin.**

Differential Stains
Gram stain and the **acid-fast stain** are two most widely used differential stains.

GRAM STAIN
It was first devised by the histologist Hans Christian Gram (1884) as a method of staining bacteria in tissues. It is one of the most useful staining procedures because it classifies bacteria into two large groups: gram-positive and gram-negative.

Reagents
- **Violet dye:** Crystal violet or methyl violet is used at concentrations of 0.5–2%. Solution is facilitated if the dye is first dissolved in alcohol and then added to the water.
  - Crystal violet or methyl violet 6B—10 g
  - Absolute alcohol (100% ethanol)—100 mL
  - Distilled water—1 L
- **Gram's iodine**
  - Iodine—10 g
  - Potassium iodide—20 g
  - Distilled water—1 L
- **Decolorizer**
  - Acetone
  - Absolute alcohol (100% ethanol)
  - Acetone-alcohol: This is a mixture of 1 volume of acetone with 1 volume of 95% ethanol. It requires application for about 10 seconds.
- **Safranin counterstain:** Safranin 0.5% in distilled water.

Procedure
1. Heat-fixed smear is covered with a basic purple dye, usually **crystal violet (primary stain)** for **1 minute**.
2. Wash the smear thoroughly with water.
3. Cover the smear with Gram's iodine for **1 minute**.
4. Wash again with water.
5. Decolorize the smear with acetone for **10 seconds or less** taking care not to over-decolorize (alcohol can be substituted for acetone).
6. Immediately wash with water to remove the decolorizer.
7. Cover the slide with dye safranin (counterstain) for **1 minute**.
8. Wash off the smear with water, blot and dry.
9. Examine the stained smear under the 100 X (oil) immersion objective of the microscope **(Fig. 6.1)**.

Interpretation of Gram Stain (Figs. 6.3A and B and Table 6.1)
Two broad groups:
1. **Gram-positive:** Gram-positive bacteria are those that resist decolorization and retain the primary stain, appearing violet.
2. **Gram-negative:** Gram-negative bacteria are decolorized by organic solvents (acetone/alcohol) and, therefore, take the counterstain, appearing red.

Gram Staining Mechanism
The exact mechanism is not understood. It may, however, be attributed to following:
1. **Protoplasm:** There is a more **acidic protoplasm in the gram-positive cells,** which is responsible for retaining the basic dye more strongly than the gram-negative bacteria.
2. **Cell wall structure:** Different kinds of bacteria react differently to the gram stain, because of structural differences in their cell walls.

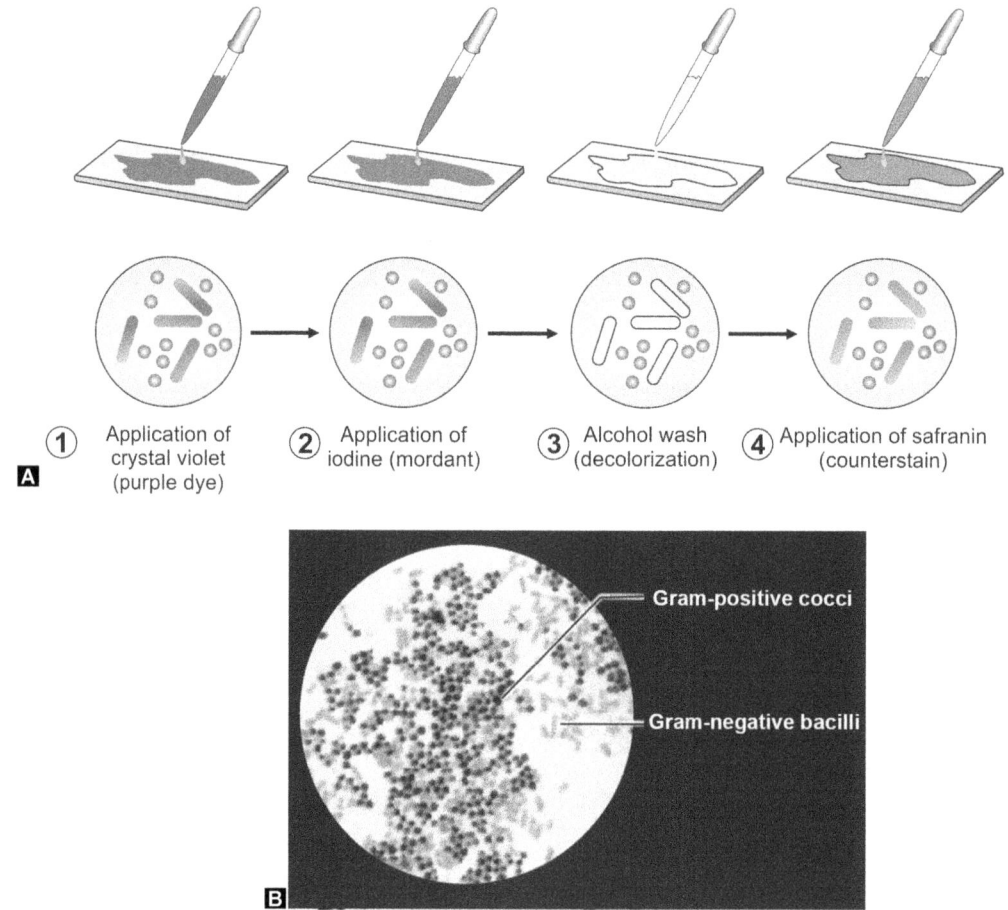

Figs. 6.3A and B: Gram Stain: (A) Steps in the Gram Stain procedure; (B) Results of a Gram Stain. The gram-positive cells (purple) are *Staphylococcus aureus*; the gram-negative cells (reddish-pink) are *Escherichia coli*.

Gram-positive cells: Gram-positive bacteria have a **thicker peptidoglycan cell wall** than gram-negative bacteria. The complex **crystal violet-iodine (CV-I) complex** is larger than the crystal violet molecule that entered the cells, and, because of its size, it cannot be washed out of the intact peptidoglycan layer of gram-positive cells by **acetone/alcohol.** Consequently, gram-positive cells retain the color of the crystal violet dye.

Gram-negative: Gram-negative bacterial cell walls are **thinner,** have a **smaller amount of peptidoglycan** and contain a high percentage of lipids. There is a layer of lipopolysaccharide as part of their cell wall. They dissolve during treatment with acetone alcohol, forming **larger pores** in the cell wall**,** and the **CV-I complex** is washed out through the thin layer of peptidoglycan. Causing outflow of dye-iodine complex and take up counter stain, thus appearing red/pink (Gram-negative).

Cell wall integrity: It has been found that gram-positivity depends on the integrity of cell wall and presence of specific magnesium-ribonucleate-protein complex. The gram-positive bacteria become gram-negative when cell wall is damaged.

Table 6.1: Gram-positive and negative bacteria.	
Gram-positive bacteria	**Gram-negative bacteria**
Cocci • Staphylococcus • Streptococcus • Enterococcus Gram-positive diplococci- Streptococcus pnemoniae	Cocci Bacillu Neisseria

Bacilli
• Corynebacterium
• Bacillus
• Clostridium
• Lactobacillus
• Mycobacterium
• (Some, *Mycobacteria*, including *Mycobacterium tuberculosis* are stained only faintly or not at all by Gram's method)
➤ Actinomyces
➤ Nocardia
	Bacilli
	• Enterobacteria
	  ➤ *Escherichia coli*
	  ➤ *Klebsiella*
	  ➤ *Salmonella*
	  ➤ *Shigella*
	  ➤ *Proteus*
	  ➤ *Yersinia*
	• *Vibrio*
	• *Pseudomonas*
	• *Parvobacteria*
	  ➤ *Haemophilus*
	  ➤ *Bordetella*
	  ➤ *Brucella*
	• *Bacteroides*

ACID-FAST STAIN (ZIEHL–NEELSEN STAINING OF ACID-FAST BACILLI)

Acid-fast stain was discovered by Ehrlich (1882), who found that after staining with aniline dyes, tubercle bacilli resist decolorization with acids. The method, as modified by Ziehl and Neelsen, is in common use now.

Principle

Some bacteria, such as mycobacteria are resistant to aniline dyes and do not readily penetrate the substance of the tubercle bacillus and are therefore unsuitable for staining it. The dye can be made to penetrate the bacillus by the use of a powerful staining solution that contains **phenol**, and the **application of heat**. Once stained the tubercle bacillus cannot be decolorized even with powerful decolorizing agents for a considerable time and thus still retains the stain when everything else in the microscopic preparation has been decolorized. Hence, they are called **acid-fast bacilli (AFB)**.

The stain used consists of **basic fuchsin**, with **phenol** (acts as a mordant) added. The dye is basic and its combination with a mineral acid used as decolorizer produces a compound that is **yellowish brown in color** which is readily dissolved out of all structures except acid-fast bacteria. Any strong acid can be used as a decolorizing agent, but 20% sulfuric acid (by volume) is usually employed. In order to show structures and cells, including nonacid-fast bacteria, that have been decolorized, and to form a contrast with the red-stained bacilli, the preparation is counterstained with **methylene blue or malachite green (Fig. 6.4)**.

Acid fastness has been ascribed to the high content and variety of lipids, fatty acids, and higher alcohols found in tubercle bacilli. A lipid peculiar to acid fast bacilli, a high molecular weight hydroxy acid wax containing carboxyl groups **(mycolic acid)** is acid fast in the free state. Acid-fastness depends also on the **integrity of the cell wall** besides lipid contents.

Make a smear on a numbered slide, dry and fix by flaming by passing the *dried* slide, film downward, three times slowly through the flame, or by heating through the glass slide (the slide is held, film upward) in the top of the Bunsen flame for a few seconds so' that the slide becomes hot.

Procedure

1. The slide containing fixed smear is covered with carbol fuchsin. The carbol fuchsin is left on the slide for **5–10 minutes** with intermittent heating during that period. Heat the slide until the steam rises, but without boiling. (Do not allow the stain to dry, to counteract

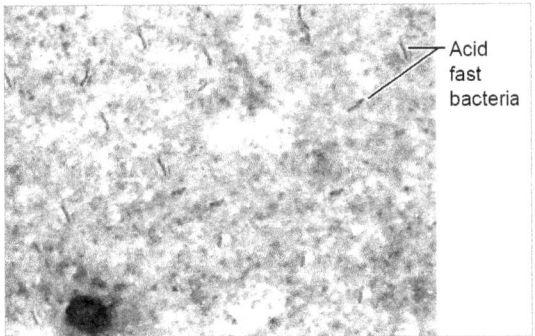

Fig. 6.4: Ziehl–Neelsen stain (100X).

drying more solution of stain is added to the slide and the slide reheated).
2. Wash in tap water.
3. The stained smear is decolorized with **20% sulfuric acid.** The red color of the preparation is changed to **yellow brown**. After about 1 minute in the acid, wash the slide with water, and pour on fresh acid. Repeat this procedure several times. When it is complete, the film, after washing, is only very faintly pink.
4. The smear is counterstained with a contrasting dye such as methylene blue for **1–2 minutes**. Malachite green can also be used as counterstain instead of methylene blue.
5. Wash with water, blot with clean paper, dry and mount.
6. Examine under oil immersion (X100) objective.

Important Points in Observation

Acid-fast bacilli such as *Mycobacterium tuberculosis* appear red while other organisms, tissue cells and debris are stained blue or green according to the counterstain used **(Fig. 6.2)**.

Acid-fast Organisms

1. All mycobacteria are acid-fast, *e.g., Mycobacterium tuberculosis, Mycobacterium bovis, Mycobacterium leprae,* atypical mycobacteria.
2. *Nocardia asteroides, Nocardia braziliensis*
3. *Cryptosporidium*—a protozoan coccidian parasite, which causes opportunistic infections in AIDS is acid-fast.
4. Bacterial spores are weakly acid-fast.

Ziehl–Neelsen (ZN) Reagents

1. **Ziehl–Neelsen (ZN) carbol fuchsin**
   - Basic fuchsin (powder)—5 g
   - Phenol (crystalline)—25 g
   - Alcohol (95% or 100% ethanol)—50 mL
   - Distilled water—500 mL
2. **Sulfuric acid (20%) decolorizer**
   - Concentrated sulfuric acid—250 mL (98%, 1.835 g/mL)
   - Distilled water—1 L

3. **Alcohol 95%:** Ethanol 95 mL plus water to 100 mL, *or* industrial methylated spirit
4. **Acid-alcohol decolorizer**
   - Concentrated hydrochloric acid—75 mL
   - Industrial methylated spirit—2,425 mL
5. **Methylene blue counterstain**
   - Loeffler's methylene blue (see above)
6. **Saturated solution**
   - Methylene blue in alcohol—300 mL
   - KOH, 0.01% in water—1 L

Staining of Volutin Containing Organisms

Well-developed granules of volutin (polyphosphate) may be seen in unstained wet preparations as round refractile bodies within the bacterial cytoplasm. They tend to stain more strongly than the rest of the bacterium with **basic dyes,** and with **toluidine blue or methylene blue** they stain metachromatically, a **reddish-purple color.** They are demonstrated most clearly by special methods, such as Albert's and Neisser's, which stain them dark purple but the remainder of the bacterium with a contrasting counterstain. For routine use the following method is recommended:

Albert's stain

A fixed smear is provided for Albert's staining. If the smear is unfixed, it is fixed by passing the *dried* slide, film downward, three times slowly through the flame, or by heating through the glass slide (the slide is held, film upward) in the top of the Bunsen flame for a few seconds so that the slide becomes hot.

Procedure

1. Make film, dry in air, and fix by heat
2. Cover slide with Albert's stain (Albert's solution A) and allow to act for **3–5 minutes**
3. Wash in water and blot dry
4. Cover slide with Albert's iodine (Albert's solution B) for **1 minute**
5. Wash with water and blot dry. Observe under the oil-immersion objective (X100)

The metachromatic (volutin) granules of *Corynebacterium diphtheriae* stain **bluish black**, and the bacterial protoplasm **green** and other organisms mostly **light green (Fig. 6.5)**.

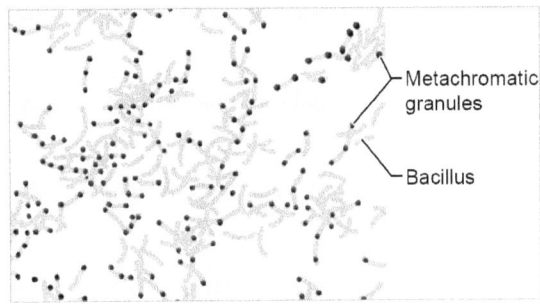

Fig. 6.5: Albert's stain (100X).

Important points in observation
1. In case of *Corynebacterium diphtheriae*, green colored bacilli with bluish black metachromatic (volutin) granules are observed.
2. Bacilli are arranged in *Chinese letter* or *cuneiform arrangement* (**Fig. 6.5**).
3. Show your observations to the examiner by focusing a good stained field of your smear as such and by drawing a well-labeled diagram using colored pencils.

SPECIAL STAINS

Special stains are used to stain specific structures inside or outside of a cell color and isolate specific parts of microorganisms, such as capsule stain, endospore stain, and flagella stain.

Staining of Capsules

India ink Preparation Procedure
1. Carefully wipe a microscopic slide free from particles of dust or dirt.
2. Place a large loopful of undiluted India ink on the slide.
3. Emulsify a very small portion of solid material culture or a small loopful of liquid culture in the ink.
4. Place a clean coverslip on the ink drop and press it down through a sheet of blotting paper to make the film very thin and thus pale in color.
5. Examine under **× 100 to × 1,000 magnification.**
6. The highly refractile outline of the bacterium is seen. Between this refractive surface membrane and the clear background of the particles there is a clear space which represents the capsule. **The capsule appears as a clear halo around the yeast cell.**
   Uses: The India ink method is useful for demonstrating the presence of a capsule **especially *Cryptococcus neoformans*** in clinical specimens, particularly cerebrospinal fluid. **Species.**

Staining of Spores
- **Gram stain:** The body of the bacillus is deeply colored, whereas the spore is unstained and appears as a clear halo in the organism.
- **Malachite green stain for spores:**
  - Place the slide over a beaker of boiling water, resting it on the rim with the bacterial film uppermost.
  - When, within several seconds, large droplets have condensed on the underside of the slide, flood it with 5% aqueous solution of malachite green and leave to act for 1 minute while the water continues to boil.
  - Wash in cold water.
  - Treat with 0.5% safranin or 0.05% basic fuchsin for 30 seconds.
  - Wash and dry.
  - Examine under oil immersion (X100) objective.
  - Spore-colors green; vegetative bacilli-red

METHODS FOR DETECTION FOR DIRECT MICROSCOPIC DETECTION OF FUNGI IN CLINICAL SPECIMENS

Potassium Hydroxide (KOH) Preparation
1. A drop of the KOH (10–20%) preparation is added to a slide.
2. An aliquot of specimen (nail scrapings, hair, skin scales, or thin slices of tissue) are added to the drop, and a coverslip is added.
3. The slide is held at room temperature for 5–30 minutes after the addition of KOH,

depending on the specimen type, to allow digestion to occur. Digestive capabilities can be enhanced with gentle heating or the addition of 40% dimethyl sulfoxide.
4. Hyaline molds and yeasts appear transparent, while dematiaceous molds may display golden visible brown hyphae. It can be used in combination with calcofluor hydroxide of specimen to make for fluorescence microscopy (KOH) fungi more readily.

Lactophenol Cotton (Aniline) Blue (LPCB) Stain

Needle-mount Method

1. Place a drop of 95% alcohol on the slide. Gently tease out a fragment of the culture in the alcohol with needles or straight wires. When it is satisfactorily spread, let most of the alcohol evaporate and then a drop of stain.
2. Apply a coverslip.
3. Remove any excess stain round the coverslip with the edge of a piece of blotting paper.
4. Examine at ×100 to ×400 magnification.
   Uses: It is commonly used for the microscopic examination of fungal cultures by tease or tape preparation. The addition of 10% polyvinyl alcohol (LPCB-PVA) makes an excellent permanent stain or fixative for mounting slide culture preparations.

KEY POINTS

- Hanging drop preparation: It is done to demonstrate motility and to study morphology of bacteria.
- The Gram stain procedure uses a purple stain (crystal violet), iodine as a mordant, an alcohol decolorizer, and a red counterstain. Gram-positive bacteria stain purple and gram-negative bacteria stain pink.
- The acid-fast stain is used to stain organisms, such as *Mycobacteria*; acid-fast organisms stain pink and all other organisms stain blue.

IMPORTANT QUESTIONS

1. Describe in detail the Gram's stain. Describe Gram staining mechanism.
2. Give an account of differential stains.
3. Write short notes on:
   a. Simple staining.
   b. Acid-fast stain or Ziehl–Neelsen's stain.

MULTIPLE CHOICE QUESTIONS

1. All include basic dyes, *except*:
   a. Crystal violet
   b. Methylene blue
   c. Malachite green
   d. Nigrosin
2. Special stains are used to color and isolate various structures, such as:
   a. Capsule
   b. Endospore
   c. Flagella
   d. All of the above

ANSWERS
1. d   2. d

Immunology

SECTION OUTLINE
7. Immunity
8. Antigens
9. Antibodies (Immunoglobulins)
10. The Complement System
11. Antigen–Antibody Reactions
12. Structure and Functions of the Immune System
13. Immune Response
14. Hypersensitivity Reactions
15. Autoimmunity

Immunity

LEARNING OBJECTIVES

After reading and studying this chapter, you should be able to:
- Describe innate immunity, artificial active immunity, natural passive immunity, and herd immunity.
- Differentiate between active and passive immunity.

DEFINITION

Immunity refers to the resistance exhibited by the host toward injury caused by microorganisms and their products.

The complex reaction a host animal undergoes after contact with microorganisms can be grouped under the broadly defined heading of **resistance.**

CLASSIFICATION

Immunity against infectious diseases is of different types. The discrimination between self and nonself, and the subsequent destruction and removal of foreign material, is accomplished by two arms of immune system, the **innate** (or "**natural**") **immune system,** and the **adaptive** (or "**acquired**"), **specific immune system.**

IMMUNITY

Innate or Natural Immunity

It is the resistance to infections which an individual possesses by virtue of his genetic or constitutional make up. Repeated exposure to a pathogen does not enhance the innate immune system.

Nonspecific and Specific Immunity

It may be **nonspecific**, when it indicates a degree of resistance to infections in general, or **specific** where resistance to a particular pathogen is concerned. Innate immunity may be considered at the level of **species, race or individual.**

Mechanisms of Innate Immunity

1. **Mechanical barriers and surface secretions:**
   A. **Skin:** The intact skin and the mucous membranes provide mechanical barriers. Secretions from the sebaceous glands contain both saturated and unsaturated fatty acids that kill many bacteria and fungi.
   B. **Mucous membrane:**
      General protective mechanisms: A major protective component of mucous membranes is the **mucus** itself.
      Specific protective characteristics:
      i. **Mouth or oral cavity:** The mouth or oral cavity is protected by the flow of saliva that physically carries microorganisms away from the cell surfaces and also contains the lysozyme, which destroys bacterial cell walls, and antibodies.
      ii. **Gastrointestinal tract:** The low pH and proteolytic enzymes of the stomach help to keep the numbers of microorganisms low. In the **small intestine**, protection is provided by the presence of bile salts.
      iii. **Upper respiratory tract:** Cough reflex is an important defense mechanism

of the respiratory tract. Nasal and respiratory secretions contain **mucopolysaccharide** capable of combining with influenza and certain other viruses.
   iv. **Genitourinary tract:**
      a. **Normal flow of urine:** The normal flow of urine flushes the urinary system.
      b. **Spermine and zinc:** Spermine and zinc present in the semen carry out antibacterial activity.
      c. **Acidity of the adult vagina:** The low pH (acidity) of the adult vagina provides an inhospitable environment for colonization by pathogens.
   v. **Conjunctiva:** Conjunctiva is continually being assaulted by microbe-laden dust and is kept moist by the continuous flushing action of tears (lachrymal fluid). Tears contain the antibacterial substance lysozyme.
2. **Antibacterial substances in blood and tissues:** Many microbial substances are present in the tissue and body fluids. These are nonspecific:
   - Complement system
   - Other substances.
3. **Microbial antagonisms:** The skin and mucous surfaces have resident bacterial flora which prevent colonization by pathogens.
4. **Cellular factors in innate immunity:** Natural defense against the invasion of blood and tissues by microorganisms and other foreign particles is mediated to a large extent by phagocytic cells which ingest and destroy them.
5. **Inflammation:** If the surface chemical and physiologic defenses of the body are breached by a pathogen, inflammation can result, which is an important, nonspecific defense mechanism.
6. **Fever:** Following infection a rise of temperature is a natural defense mechanism.
7. **Acute phase proteins:** A sudden increase in the plasma concentration of certain proteins, collectively termed **"acute phase proteins"** occurs as a result of infection or tissue injury.

TYPES OF IMMUNITY

Acquired Immunity

Acquired immunity refers to the resistance that an individual acquires during his lifetime. Acquired immunity is of two types: active immunity, and passive immunity **(Table 7.1)**.

A. Active Immunity

Active immunity is induced after contact with foreign antigens.

Immune response:
A. **The primary response:** Active immunity sets in only after a **latent period.** There is often a **negative phase.** Once developed, the active immunity is **long lasting.**
B. **Secondary response:** If an individual who has been actively immunized against an antigen, experiences the same antigen

Table 7.1: Comparison of active and passive immunity.	
Active immunity	**Passive immunity**
• Produced actively by host's immune system	• Received passively. No active host participation
• Induced by infection or by immunogens	• Readymade antibody transferred
• Durable effective protection	• Transient, less effective
• Immunity effective only after lag periode, i.e., time required for generation of antibodies and immunocompetent cells	• Immediate immunity
• Immunological memory present	• No memory
• Booster effect on subsequent dose	• Subsequent dose less effective
• "Negative phase" may occur	• No negative phase
• Not applicable in the immunodeficient	• Applicable in immunodeficient

subsequently, the immune response occurs more quickly and abundantly than during the first encounter. This is known as **secondary response**.

Types of active immunity:
1. **Natural active immunity:** Natural active immunity results from either a clinical or an inapparent infection by a microbe. Such immunity is usually **long lasting**. The immunity is **life-long** following many viral diseases such as chickenpox or measles.
2. **Artificial active immunity:** Artificial active immunity is the resistance induced by vaccines. **Vaccines** are preparations of live or killed microorganisms or their products used for immunization. Vaccines are made with either (1) live, attenuated microorganisms; (2) killed microorganisms; (3) microbial extract; (4) vaccine conjugates; or (5) inactivated toxoids. Both bacterial and viral pathogens are targeted by these diverse means.

Examples of Vaccines
1. **Bacterial vaccines**
   a. Live (BCG vaccine for tuberculosis)
   b. Killed (Cholera vaccine)
   c. Subunit (Typhoid Vi antigen)
   d. Bacterial products (Tetanus toxoid)
2. **Viral vaccines**
   a. *Live*
      - Oral polio vaccine—Sabin
      - 17D vaccine for yellow fever
      - MMR vaccine for measles, mumps, rubella
   b. *Killed:* Injectable polio vaccine—Salk
      - Neural and nonneural vaccines for rabies
      - Hepatitis B vaccine
   c. *Subunit:* Hepatitis B vaccine

B. Passive Immunity

The immunity that is transferred to a recipient in a "readymade" form is known as **passive immunity**.

Main advantage of passive immunity:
i. The prompt availability of large amount of antibody.
ii. It is employed where **instant immunity** is required because of its immediate action.

1. Natural Passive Immunity

This is the resistance passively transferred from mother to baby through the placenta. After birth, immunoglobulins are passed to the newborn through the **breast milk**. The **human colostrum**, is rich in IgA antibodies which gives protection to the neonate up to 3 months of age.

2. Artificial Passive Immunity

Artificial passive immunity is the resistance passively transferred to a recipient by the administration of antibodies. The agents used for this purpose are pooled human gamma globulin, hyperimmune sera of animal or human origin and convalescent sera. These are used for prophylaxis and therapy.

Indications of passive immunization:
1. **To provide immediate protection**—to a nonimmune host exposed to an infection and lack active immunity to that pathogen and when there is insufficient time for active immunization to take effect.
2. **Treatment of some infections.**
3. **For the suppression of active immunity**—when it may be injurious, e.g., administration of anti-Rh (D) IgG to Rh-negative mother, bearing Rh-positive baby at the time of delivery to prevent isoimmunization.
4. **Immunocompromised or immunodeficient individuals,** e.g., children with hypogammaglobulinemia, individuals with AIDS, patients receiving chemotherapy, organ transplant recipients receiving immunosuppressive therapy.

Combined Immunization

Combined immunization is a combination of active and passive methods of immunization which is sometimes employed. For example, it is often undertaken in some diseases such as tetanus, diphtheria, and rabies. Passive immunity provides the protection necessary till the active immunity becomes effective.

Local Immunity

Local immunity is conferred by secretory immunoglobulin A (*secretory IgA*) produced locally by plasma cells present on mucosal surfaces or in secretory glands. There appears to be a selective transport of such antibodies between the various mucosal surfaces and secretory glands.

Examples
1. **Poliomyelitis immunization**
2. **Influenza immunization**

Herd Immunity

It is the level of resistance of a community or a group of people to a particular disease and is relevant in the control of epidemic diseases.

High level of herd immunity: Eradication of communicable diseases depends on the development of a high level of herd immunity rather than on the development of a high level of immunity in individuals.

KEY POINTS

- Innate or natural immunity—is the resistance to infections which an individual possesses by virtue of his genetic or constitutional make up.
- Acquired immunity refers to the resistance that an individual acquires during his lifetime.
- Artificial active immunity is the resistance induced by vaccines.

IMPORTANT QUESTIONS

1. Tabulate the differences between active and passive immunity.
2. Write short notes on:
   a. Innate immunity
   b. Active immunity
   c. Passive immunity

MULTIPLE CHOICE QUESTIONS

1. All are acute phase proteins, *except*:
   a. C-reactive protein
   b. Mannose binding protein
   c. Serum amyloid P component
   d. Antibody
2. Clinical or inapparent infection leads to:
   a. Natural active immunity
   b. Artificial active immunity
   c. Natural passive immunity
   d. Artificial passive immunity
3. Vaccine induces:
   a. Active natural immunity
   b. Active artificial immunity
   c. Passive natural immunity
   d. Passive artificial immunity
4. All the following statements are true for artificial passive immunity, *except*:
   a. Artificial passive immunity is the resistance passively transferred to a recipient by the administration of antibodies
   b. It is short lived and lasts only a few weeks to a few months
   c. This type of immunity is immediate
   d. This immunity may be induced by maternal antibodies
5. All of the following are live vaccines, *except*:
   a. BCG
   b. MMR
   c. Sabin vaccine
   d. TAB vaccine
6. All of the following are killed vaccines, *except*:
   a. Salk vaccine
   b. Nonneural vaccines for rabies
   c. Hepatitis B vaccine
   d. BCG

ANSWERS

1. d   2. a   3. b   4. d
5. d   6. d

CHAPTER 8

Antigens

LEARNING OBJECTIVES

After reading and studying this chapter, you should be able to:
- Describe haptens, heterophile antigens, and super antigens.

INTRODUCTION

Antigens (**antibody generator**) are the substances that can stimulate an immune response and, given the opportunity, react specifically by binding with the effector molecules (antibodies) and effector cells (lymphocytes).

TYPES OF ANTIGEN

1. **Complete antigen:** Complete antigen is able to induce antibody formation and produce a specific and observable reaction with antibody so produced.
2. **Haptens (incomplete immunogen);** Haptens (Latin *haptein*, to grasp) **are** low-molecular-weight molecules which cannot induce an immune response when injected by themselves but can do so when covalently coupled to a large protein molecule, called the *carrier* molecule. Haptens may be simple or complex.

ANTIGENIC DETERMINANT OR EPITOME

The smallest unit of antigenicity is known as the *antigenic determinant* or *epitope*. Each antigen can have several **antigenic determinant sites** or **epitopes.** The combining area on the antibody molecule, corresponding to the epitope, is called the *paratope*.

DETERMINANTS OF ANTIGENICITY

A number of properties have been identified which make a substance antigenic but the exact basis of antigenicity is still not clear.
1. **Size—molecular weight:** Very large molecules are very powerful antigens. Some low-molecular weight chemical substances may be antigenic.
2. **Chemical nature:** In general, proteins are the best immunogens and carbohydrates are weaker immunogens.
3. **Foreignness:** Only antigens which are "**foreign**" to the individual (**nonself**) induce an immune response.
4. **Susceptibility to tissue enzymes:** Only those substances which can be metabolized and susceptibility to the tissue enzymes behave as antigens.
5. **Antigenic specificity:** Foreignness of a substance to an animal can depend on the presence of chemical groupings that are not normally found in the animal's body.
6. **Species specificities:** Tissues of all individuals in a species possess species specific antigens.
7. **Isospecificities:** Isoantigens or alloantigens are antigens found in some but not all members of a species. On the basis of isoantigens a species may be divided into different groups, e.g., **human erythrocytes antigens.**

8. **Autospecificity—sequestrated antigens:** Certain self-antigens are present in closed system and are not accessible to the immune apparatus and these are known as **sequestrated antigens,** e.g., lens protein and sperm.
9. **Organ specificity:** Some organs, such as brain, kidney and lens protein of different species, share the same antigens. These antigens are known as organ-specific antigens, characteristic of an organ or tissue and are found in different species.
10. **Heterogenetic (heterophile) specificity:** Same or closely related antigens occurring in different biological species, classes and kingdoms are known as **heterogenetic or heterophile antigens**.

Biological Classes of Antigens

Depending on their ability to induce antibody formation, antigens are classified as **T cell dependent (TD)** and **T cell independent (TI) antigens.**

KEY POINTS

- Antigens are the substances that can stimulate an immune response and, given the opportunity, react specifically by binding with the effector molecules (antibodies) and effector cells (lymphocytes).
- Types of antigen are: (1) Complete antigen; (2) Haptens (incomplete immunogen).
- Determinants of antigenicity are: (1) Size; (2) Chemical nature; (3) Foreignness; (4) Susceptibility to tissue enzymes; (5) Antigenic specificity; (6) Species; specificities; Isospecifities; (8) Autospecificity; (9) Organ specificity; (10) Heterogenetic (heterophile) specificity.

IMPORTANT QUESTIONS

1. What is an antigen? Discuss briefly various determinants of antigenicity.
2. Write short notes on:
    a. Haptens
    b. Heterophile antigens

MULTIPLE CHOICE QUESTION

1. The substances that are least immunogenic are:
    a. Proteins
    b. Polysaccharides
    c. Nucleic acids
    d. None of the above

ANSWER

1. c

CHAPTER 9

Antibodies (Immunoglobulins)

LEARNING OBJECTIVES

After reading and studying this chapter, you should be able to:
- Define antibody and draw labeled diagram of immunoglobulin.
- Describe structure and functions of IgG, IgA, and IgM.
- Discuss properties of IgM, IgG, IgA, IgD, and IgE.
- Draw labeled diagram of IgG, IgM, and IgA.

INTRODUCTION

Antibody or immunoglobulin (Ig): An **antibody or immunoglobulin (Ig)** is a glycoprotein that is made in response to an antigen, and can recognize and bind to the antigen that caused its production.

All antibodies are immunoglobulins, but all immunoglobulins may not be antibodies.

Physicochemical and antigenic structure: On the basis of physicochemical and antigenic structure Igs can be divided into five distinct classes or isotypes namely IgG, IgA, IgM, IgD, and IgE.

ANTIBODY STRUCTURE

All immunoglobulins are composed of the same basic units consisting of four chains: **Two identical "light" (L) chains** and **two identical heavy chains**. The L chain is attached to the H chain by a disulfide bond. The two H chains are joined together by 1-5 S-S bonds, depending on the class of immunoglobulins **(Fig. 9.1)**. The smaller chains are called **"light" (L)** chains and the larger ones **"heavy" (H)** chains. The variable region contains the **antigen-binding site**; the **constant region** encompasses the entire fragment crystallizable (Fc) region as well as part of the fragment antigen-binding (Fab) regions.

Classes of L Chains

The L chains are similar in all classes of immunoglobulins. There are two classes of L chains, designated kappa (κ) and lambda (λ).

Classes of H Chains

The H chains are structurally and antigenically distinct for each class and are designated by the Greek letter corresponding to the immunoglobulin class. In humans there are five classes of heavy chains designated by lowercase Greek letters: gamma (γ), alpha (α), mu (μ), delta (δ), and epsilon (ε).

Constant and Variable Regions

All immunoglobulin chains possess a **constant ("C") region** and a **variable ("V") region**. Both light and heavy chains contain two different regions. L chain has **constant regions (C_L) and variable region (V_L)**.

The H chain also has **constant regions (C_H)** and **variable regions (V_H)**.

Fc Fragment

The Fc fragment is composed of the carboxy terminal portion of the H chains. It can be crystallized, and is therefore called **fragment-crystallizable (Fc)**.

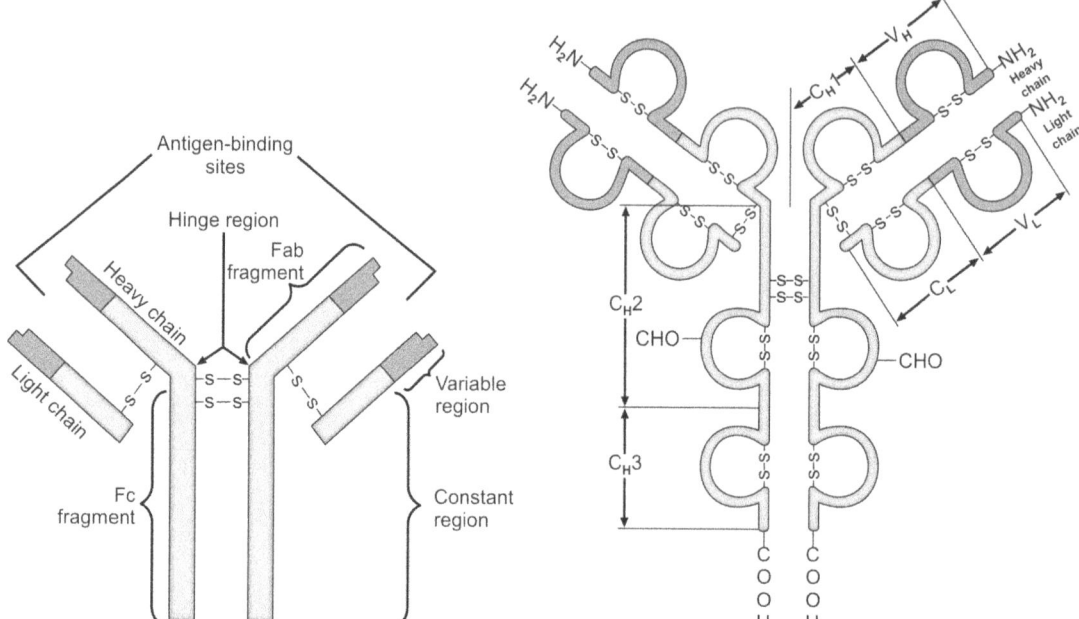

Fig. 9.1: The four-peptide chain structure of the IgG molecule composed of two identical heavy (H) and two identical light (L) chains linked by interchains **disulfide** bonds. Loops formed by intrachain disulfide bonds are domains (shown stippled). Each chain has one domain in the variable region (VH and VL). Each light chain has one domain in the constant region (CL) while each heavy chain has three domains in the constant region (CHl, CH2 and CH3). Between CH1 and CH2 is the hinge region.

IMMUNOGLOBULIN CLASSES

Human serum contain five classes of immunoglobulins—IgG, IgA, IgM, IgD, and IgE in the descending order of the concentration. **Table 9.1** shows their differentiating features.

Immunoglobulin G (IgG)

1. This is the **major immunoglobulin** in human serum, accounting for about 80% of the total immunoglobulin pool.
2. It has a sedimentation coefficient of **7S** and a molecular weight of **150,000**.
3. It contains less carbohydrate than other immunoglobulins.
4. The normal serum concentration of IgG is about **8–16 mg/mL**.
5. IgG is distributed nearly equally between extra- and intravascular spaces.

Functions of IgG

1. **Transfer from mother to fetus:** IgG is the only class of Igs that can cross the placenta and is responsible for the protection of the infant during first few months of life.
2. **Opsonization**
3. **Fixing to guinea pig skin**
4. **Immunological reactions:** IgG participates in complement fixation, precipitation and neutralization of toxins and viruses.

Immunoglobulin A (IgA) (Fig. 9.2)

1. It is the second most abundant class, constituting about 10–13% of serum immunoglobulins.
2. The normal serum level is 0.6–4.2 mg per mL.
3. IgA is the primary immunoglobulin found in external secretions, such as mucus, tears, saliva, gastric fluid, colostrum, and sweat.

Chapter 9: Antibodies (Immunoglobulins)

Table 9.1: Physical, physiologic, and biologic properties of human serum immunoglobulins.

Property	IgG	IgA*	IgM	IgD	IgE
A. Physical properties					
1. Sedimentation coefficient (S)	7	7	19	7	8
2. Molecular weight in kilodaltons	150,000	160,000	900,000	180,000	190,000
3. Carbohydrate (%)	3	8	12	13	12
4. Number of four-chain units per molecule	1	1–3	5–6	1	1
B. Physiologic properties					
1. Normal adult serum concentration (mg/mL)	12	2	1.2	0.03	0.00004
2. Half-life (in days)	23	6	5	2–8	1–5
3. Daily production (mg/kg)	34	24	3.3	0.4	0.0023
4. Intravascular distribution (%)	45	42	80	75	50
C. Biologic properties					
1. Complement-fixation					
Classical	++	–	+++	–	–
Alternative	–	+	–	–	–
2. Placental transport to fetus	+	–	–	–	–
3. Present in milk	+	+	–	–	–
4. Selective selection by submucous glands	–	+	–	–	–
5. Anaphylactic hypersensitivity	–	–	–	–	++++
6. Heat stability	+	+	+	+	–
D. Major characteristics	Most abundant Ig; Longest half-life: Crosses placenta; Opsonizes antigen	Protects mucosal surfaces	Very efficient against bacteremia	Mainly lymphocyte receptor; major surface components of B cells	Initiates inflammation; raised in helminthic infections; causes allergy symptoms

*IgA may occur in 7S, 9S, and 11S forms

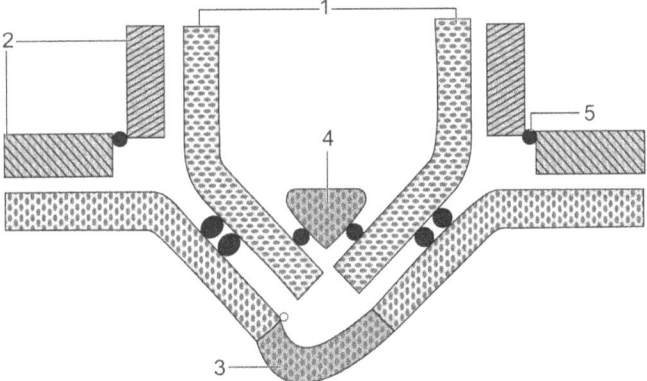

Fig. 9.2: Secretory IgA: 1. Heavy chain, 2. Light chain, 3. J-chain, 4. Secretory component, 5. **Disulfide** bond.

It exists in different forms in these various solutions.
4. IgA occurs in two forms.
   i. **Serum IgA:** Serum IgA is monomeric (one four-chain unit) 7S molecule (MW about 160,000).
   ii. **Secretory IgA (SIgA):** In contrast, IgA found on mucosal surfaces and in secretions is a dimer formed by two monomer units joined together at their carboxy terminals by a glycopeptide termed the **J chain (J for joining).** This dimeric form is more important form, known as **secretory IgA (SIgA).**

Functions of IgA
1. **Local immunity**—plays an important role in local immunity against respiratory and intestinal pathogens.
2. **Prevention of organisms entry into body tissues**
3. **Newborn protection**
4. **Agglutination**
5. **Alternative pathways activation**
6. **Phagocytosis and intracellular killing**

Immunoglobulin M (IgM)
1. It is a heavy molecule (19S; MW 900,000–1,000,000 daltons, hence called "**millionaire molecule**")
2. The normal serum level of IgM is 1.2 mg/mL.
3. IgM is the first immunoglobulin to appear after exposure to an antigen.
4. In the circulation, IgM exists as a pentamer of five four-chain units. The five identical IgM monomers are connected to each other by a polypeptide **joining (J) chain (Fig. 9.3).**
5. Most of IgM (80%) is intravascular in distribution.
6. They are relatively short-lived hence their demonstration in the serum indicates recent infection.
7. IgM agglutinates bacteria, activates complement by the classical pathway, and enhances the ingestion of pathogens by phagocytic cells. IgM is normally restricted

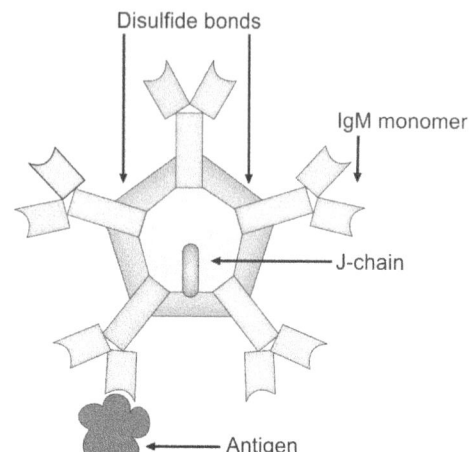

Fig. 9.3: Pentameric IgM molecule, composed of five identical monomers.

to the intravascular space because of its high molecular weight.

Immunoglobulin D (IgD)
1. IgD has a monomer structure similar to IgG.
2. Its molecular weight is 180,000 daltons.
3. IgD is found in trace amounts in the blood serum (0.03 mg/mL).

Immunoglobulin E (IgE)
1. It resembles IgG structurally and also known as reagin antibody.
2. IgE is an 8S molecules (MW 19,000).
3. It exhibits unique properties, such as **heat lability**.
4. It does not pass the placental barrier.
5. IgE does not activate complement nor agglutinate antigens.
6. **Allergic reactions:** IgE molecules bind tightly to receptors on mast cells and basophils, specialized cells that participate in allergic reactions. IgE may be elevated in allergic (atopic) individuals, and is responsible for many of the symptoms of allergies, bronchial asthma, and even systemic anaphylaxis. Allergy mediated by IgE is termed as type I hypersensitivity response.
7. **Immunity against helminthic parasites.**

8. **Extravascular:** It is mostly found **extravascularly**.

ROLE OF DIFFERENT IMMUNOGLOBULIN CLASSES

- IgG: Protects the body fluids
- IgA: Protects the body surfaces
- IgM: Protects the blood stream
- IgE: Mediates type I hypersensitivity
- IgD: Role not known

KEY POINTS

- An antibody or immunoglobulin (Ig) is a glycoprotein that is made in response to an antigen, and can recognize and bind to the antigen that caused its production.
- There are five major antibody classes, IgM, IgG, 1gA, IgD, and IgE, and each has distinct functions.

IMPORTANT QUESTIONS

1. Name various classes of immunoglobulins and describe structure and functions of IgG.
2. Write short notes on:
   a. Immunoglobulin G (IgG)
   b. Immunoglobulin M (IgM)
   c. Immunoglobulin A (IgA)

MULTIPLE CHOICE QUESTIONS

1. The immunoglobulin that crosses the placenta is:
   a. IgG
   b. IgM
   c. IgA
   d. IgE

2. The J chain is present in the immunoglobulin:
   a. IgG
   b. IgM
   c. IgA
   d. IgE

3. All the following immunoglobulins are heat stable, *except*:
   a. IgG
   b. IgM
   c. IgA
   d. IgE

4. Which is the earliest immunoglobulin to be synthesized by the fetus?
   a. IgG
   b. IgM
   c. IgA
   d. IgE

5. The immunoglobulin that mediates type I hypersensitivity reaction is:
   a. IgG
   b. IgM
   c. IgA
   d. IgE

6. Antibodies that are bound to mast cells and involve in allergic reactions are:
   a. IgG
   b. IgM
   c. IgA
   d. IgE

7. The first antibodies synthesized, especially against microorganisms:
   a. IgG
   b. IgM
   c. IgA
   d. IgE

ANSWERS

1. a   2. b   3. d   4. b
5. d   6. d   7. b

CHAPTER 10

The Complement System

LEARNING OBJECTIVES

After reading and studying this chapter, you should be able to:
- Describe sequence of events when the classical pathway and the alternative pathway of the complement system is activated.

The term **"complement" (C)** refers to a system of factors which occur in normal serum and are' activated characteristically by antigen–antibody interaction and subsequently mediate a number of biologically significant consequences.

COMPLEMENT SYSTEM

The **complement system** is an alarm and a weapon against infection, especially bacterial infection. The complement system includes serum and membrane-bound proteins that function in both acquired and constitutive (natural) host defense system.

Components of Complement

Complement is a complex of nine different fractions called C1–C9. The component C1 is made up of three protein subunits named C1q, C1r, and C1s.

Complement is normally present in circulation in inactive form, but when its activity is induced by antigen-antibody reaction or other stimuli, complement components react in a specific sequence as a cascade either through the classical or alternative pathway. Both the pathways have same result, i.e., lysis or damage of target cell.

A. **Classical complement pathway:** The chain of events in which C components react in a specific sequence following activation of C1 and typically culminate in immune cytolysis is known as the classical pathway (**Fig. 10.1**). It consists of the following steps:

1. **Antigen–antibody binding:** The first step is the binding of C1 to the antigen-antibody complex. The recognition unit of C1 is C1q, which reacts with the Fc piece of bound IgM or IgG. C1q binding in the presence of calcium ions leads to sequential activation of C1r and s.

2. **Production of C3 convertase:** Activated C1s is an esterase (C1s esterase), one molecule of which can cleave several molecules of C4—an instance of amplification. Activated C1 cleaves C4 into two pieces C4a and C4b (C4 → C4a + C4b). C4a is an anaphylatoxin and C4b which binds to cell membrane along with C1.
C14b in the presence of magnesium ions cleaves C2 into two pieces (C2 → C2a + C2b). C2a remains linked to cell bound C4b, and C2b which is released into fluid phase. The pieces recombine, forming C4b2a has enzymatic activity and is referred to as the classical pathway C3 *convertase*.

3. **Production of C5 convertase**: C3 convertase cleaves C3 into two fragments (C3 → C3a + C3b). C3a is soluble, and is an anahylotoxin, and C3b which remains

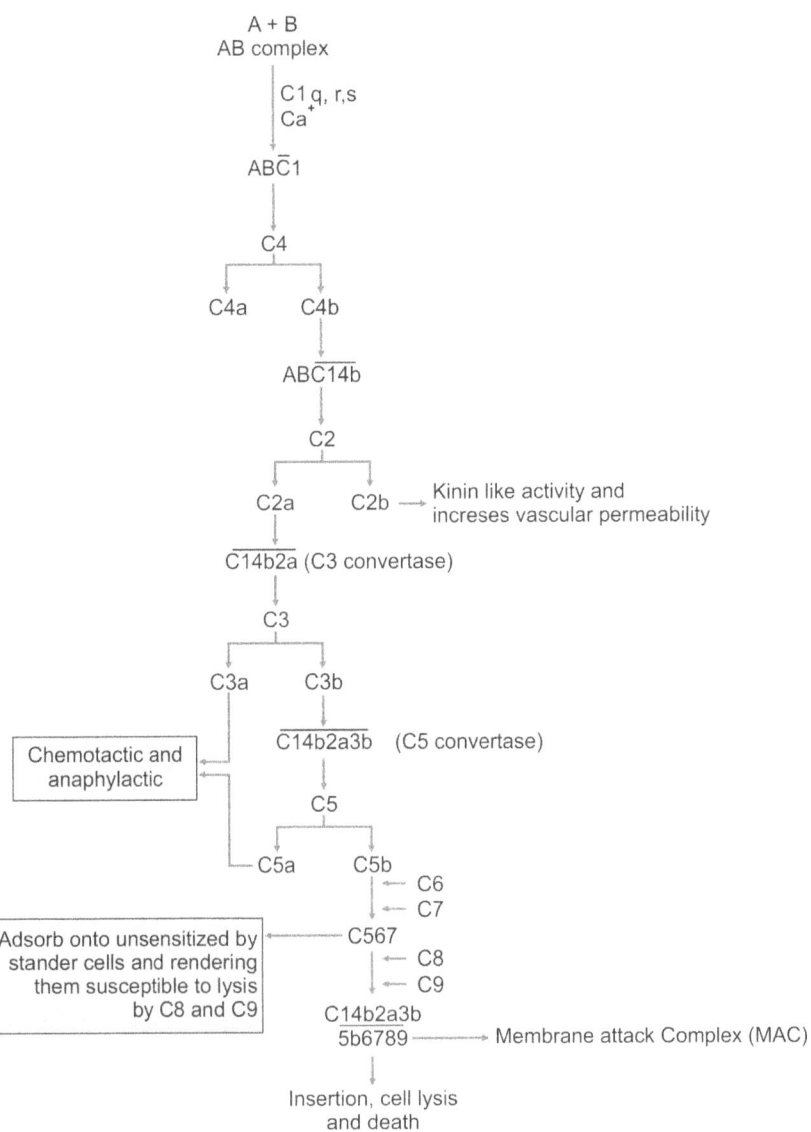

Fig. 10.1: Complement cascade—the classical pathway.

cell-bound along with C4b2a to form a trimolecular complex C4b2a3b which has enzymatic activity and is called **C5 convertase** of the classic pathway.

4. **Formation of the membrane attack complex (MAC):** The terminal stage of the classic pathway involves creation of **membrane attack complex (MAC),** which is also called **the lytic unit.**

Initiation of **membrane attack complex (MAC)** assembly begins with cleavage of C5 by C5 convertase into C5a and C5b fragments (C5 → C5a + C5b). The C5a the most potent anaphylatoxin in the body and C5b, which continues with the cascade. C6 and C7 then join together. A heat stable trimolecular complex **C567** is formed part of which binds to the cell membrane and prepares it for lysis by C8 and C9 which join the reaction subsequently. This complex (C5b67) inserts itself into the plasma membrane of the target cell. Most of C567 escape and serve to amplify the reaction by adsorbing onto unsensitized "bystander cells" and rendering them susceptible to lysis by C8 and C9.

The unbound C567 has chemotactic activity, though the effect is transient due to its rapid inactivation. C8 and C9 then bind, forming the **membrane attack complex** (C5b6789) that creates a pore in the plasma membrane of the target cell. The mechanism of complement-mediated cytolysis is the production of "holes", approximately 100 A in diameter on the cell membrane. This disrupts the osmotic integrity of the membrane, leading to the release of the cell contents.

B. **Alternative complement pathway:** In the complement cascade the central process is the activation of C3, which is the major component of C. In the classical pathway, activation of C3 is achieved by C42 (classical C3 convertase). The activation of C3 without prior participation of C142 is known as the "alternative pathway".

The alternate pathway of complement activation (the *properdin pathway*) does not require the formation of antigen–antibody complexes for activation. These activators include bacterial endotoxins, IgA and D, the cobra venom factor and the nephritic factor (a protein present in the serum of glomerulonephritis patients).

1. **Production of alternative pathway C3 convertase:** The binding of C3b to an activator is the first step in the alternative pathway. Although, C3b is present in the circulation but in the free state it is rapidly inactivated by the serum protein factors H and I. However, bound C3b is protected from such inactivation. The bound C3b, in the presence of Mg++, interacts with plasma protein factor B forming C3bB which is also known as "C3 pro activator convertase" to form a magnesium-dependent complex

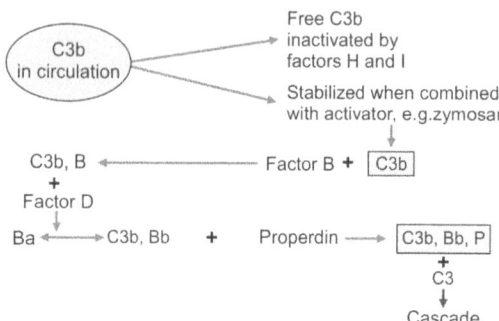

Fig. 10.2: Complement cascade—the alternative pathway.

"C3b, B". Factor B in the complex is cleaved by serum factor D (also called "C3 pro activator convertase") into two fragments— Ba and Bb. Fragment Ba is released into the medium. Fragment Bb remains bound to C3b producing C3bBb. C3bBb acts as the alternate pathway C3 convertase, capable of producing more C3b. This enzyme C3bBb is extremely labile. The function of properdin (also called Factor P) a serum protein, is to stabilize the C3 convertase, which hydrolyses C3, leading to further steps in the cascade, as in the classical pathway **(Fig. 10.2)**.

2. **Production of alternative pathway C5 convertase and MAC:** C3b produced by C3 convertase binds to C3bBb, producing the alternative *C5 convertase* (C3bBb3b). C5 convertase may or may not still have factor P attached. Properdin enters the reaction sequence and binds both C3 and C5 convertase.

Once the C5 convertase is formed, C5 is cleaved to form C5a and C5b, and the spontaneous formation of the attack complex (C5b-9) quickly follows. C5b is necessary for formation of the membrane attack complex and cell lysis. The formation of this attack complex proceeds in the same manner as it does in the classic pathway **(Fig. 10.1)**.

Biological Effects of Complement (C)

1. **Bacteriolysis and Cytolysis**
2. **Virus neutralization**
3. **Anaphylatoxins**

4. **Immune adherence and opsonization**
5. **Chemotaxis**
6. **Hypersensitivity reaction**
7. **Autoimmune diseases**
8. **Endotoxic shock**

KEY POINTS

- Complement activation occurs by the classical, alternative, or lectin pathways, each of which is initiated differently.
- The classical pathway is activated with the formation of soluble antigen–antibody complexes (immune complexes) or the binding of antibody to antigen on a suitable target, such as a bacterial cell. Reactions of IgM and certain IgG subclasses activate this pathway.
- Activation of the alternative pathway is antibody-independent.

IMPORTANT QUESTIONS

1. Define complement. What is the sequence of events when the classical pathway of the complement system is activated?
2. Write short notes on:
   a. Alternative pathway of complement.
   b. Biological effects of complement.

MULTIPLE CHOICE QUESTIONS

1. The activation of complement takes place through either of the following pathways, *except*:
   a. The classical pathway
   b. The lectin pathway
   c. The alternative pathway
   d. The lipid pathway

2. Classical pathway of the complement is activated by:
   a. Antigen
   b. Antibody
   c. Antigen–antibody complex
   d. None of the above

3. The alternative pathway of the complement is initiated by:
   a. Endotoxins
   b. Lipopolysaccharides
   c. Yeast cell walls
   d. All of the above

ANSWERS

1. d   2. c   3. d

CHAPTER 11: Antigen-Antibody Reactions

LEARNING OBJECTIVES

After reading and studying this chapter, you should be able to:
- Differentiate between precipitation and agglutination.
- Describe prozone phenomenon.
- Discuss mechanism and applications of precipitation reactions giving suitable examples.
- Describe types of precipitation reactions.
- Describe principle and applications of immunoelectrophoresis, radial immunodiffusion, counterimmunoelectrophoresis (CIE), rocket electrophoresis.
- Describe applications of agglutination reactions and their uses.
- Discuss principle and applications of agglutination reactions.
- Describe principle of complement fixation test.
- Discuss principle and clinical applications of immunofluorescence technique.
- Discuss principle, various types and clinical applications of ELISA technique.

INTRODUCTION

The antigen-antibody interaction is a bimolecular association that exhibits exquisite specificity. It is similar to an enzyme-substrate interaction, with an important distinction.

USES

1. In vivo or in the body
   i. **Protection:** Protecting the animal against the continuous onslaught of viruses, microorganisms and their products, certain macromolecules, and cancer cells.
   ii. **Basis of antibody-mediated immunity**
2. In vitro or in the laboratory
   i. Use **to detect the presence of either antibody or antigen**
   ii. **Vital roles in diagnosing diseases.**
   iii. **Identifying molecules of biological or medical interest.**

GENERAL CHARACTERISTICS OF ANTIGEN-ANTIBODY REACTIONS

1. **Highly specific**
2. **Lock and key arrangement:** Both antigens and antibodies participate in the formation of agglutinates or precipitates. The molecules are held together in lock and key arrangement.
3. **No denaturation**
4. **Surface antigens:** During combination only surface antigens participate.
5. **Entire molecules react**
6. **Combination is firm and reversible.**
7. **Combination in varying proportions.**

Serological reactions: The study of antigen-antibody reactions in vitro is called *serology*. Antigen-antibody reactions in vitro are known as serological reactions.

TYPES OF ANTIGEN AND ANTIBODY REACTIONS

A. **Precipitation reactions**
B. Agglutination reactions
C. Complement fixation test (CFT)
D. Neutralization tests
E. Opsonization
F. Immunofluorescence
G. Radioimmunoassay (RIA)
H. Enzyme-linked immunosorbent assay (ELISA)
I. Immunoelectroblot techniques
J. Immunochromatographic tests
K. Immunoelectronmicroscopic tests

A. Precipitation Reactions

Precipitation: When a soluble antigen combines with its antibody in the presence of electrolytes (NaCl) at a suitable temperature and pH, the antigen-antibody complex forms an insoluble **precipitate** and is called **precipitation**.

Flocculation: When instead of sedimenting, the precipitate remains suspended as floccules, the reaction is known as **flocculation**.

Zone phenomenon: A quantitative precipitation reaction can be performed by placing a constant amount of antibody in a series of tubes and adding increasing amounts of antigen to the tubes. This plot of the amount of antibody precipitated versus increasing antigen concentration (at constant total antibody) reveals three zones **(Fig. 11.1)**. This is called **zone phenomenon**. Zoning occurs in agglutination and some other serological reactions.

Three Zones

1. **Zone of antibody excess or prozone (ascending part)**
   Importance of prozone: The prozone is of importance in clinical serology, as sera rich in antibody or may sometimes give a false negative precipitation or agglutination result, unless several dilutions are tested.
2. **Equivalence zone (peak)**
3. **Zone of antigen excess or postzone (descending part)**

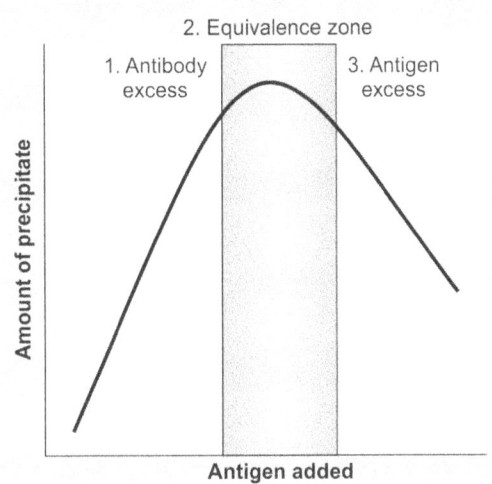

Fig. 11.1: A quantitative precipitation test showing: 1. prozone (zone of antibody excess); 2. zone of equivalence; 3. zone of antigen excess.

Mechanism of Precipitation

The **lattice hypothesis** was proposed by Marrack (1934) to explain the mechanism of precipitation. According to this concept, multivalent antigens combine with bivalent antibodies in varying proportions, depending on the antigen-antibody ratio in the reacting mixture. Precipitation results when a large lattice is formed consisting of alternating antigen and antibody molecules. This is possible only in the **zone of equivalence**. In the zones of antigen or antibody excess, as the valencies of the antibody and the antigen, respectively are fully satisfied and extensive lattices cannot be formed and precipitation is inhibited **(Figs. 11.2A to C)**. The lattice hypothesis holds good for agglutination also.

Applications of Precipitation Reaction

1. Forensic application in the identification of blood and seminal stains.
2. In testing for food adulterants.
3. To standardize toxins and antitoxins.

Types of Precipitation and Flocculation Tests

A. **Ring test:** This consists of layering the antigen solution over a column of antiserum in a narrow tube. A precipitate forms at the

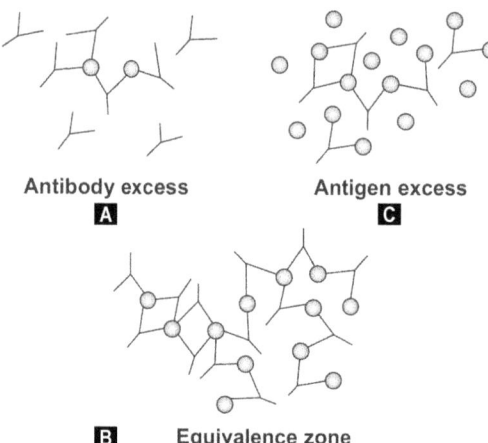

Figs. 11.2 A to C: Mechanism of precipitation by lattice formation. In A (antibody excess) and C (antigen excess), lattice formation does not occur. In B (zone of equivalence, lattice formation, and precipitation occur optimally).

junction of the two liquids. Ring tests have only a few clinical applications now.
Examples:
i. Ascoli's thermoprecipitin test.
ii. The grouping of streptococci by the Lancefield technique.
B. **Slide test (slide flocculation test):** When a drop each of the antigen and antiserum are placed on a slide and mixed by shaking, floccules appear.
Example: The venereal disease research laboratory (VDRL) test for syphilis.
C. Tube test (tube flocculation test):
i. **The Kahn test for syphilis** is an example of a tube flocculation test.
ii. **Standardization of toxins and toxoids**
D. **Immunodiffusion (precipitation reactions in gels):** Immunodiffusion refers to a precipitation reaction that occurs between an antibody and antigen in an agar gel medium. Immunodiffusion is usually performed in a soft (1%) agar gel.

Types of Immunodiffusion Tests
1. **Single diffusion in one dimension (Oudin procedure):** Antibody is incorporated in agar gel in a test tube. Antigen solution is then layered over it. The antigen diffuses downward through the agar gel and wherever it reaches in optimum concentration with antibody a line of precipitation is formed (Fig. 11.3A).
2. **Double diffusion in one dimension (Oakley-Fulthorpe procedure):** Here, the antibody is incorporated in gel in a test tube, above which is placed a column of plain agar and antigen is layered on surface of this. Antigen and antibody diffuse (double diffusion) toward each other (in one dimension) through the intervening column of plain agar and forms a band of precipitate where they meet at optimum proportion (Fig. 11.3B).

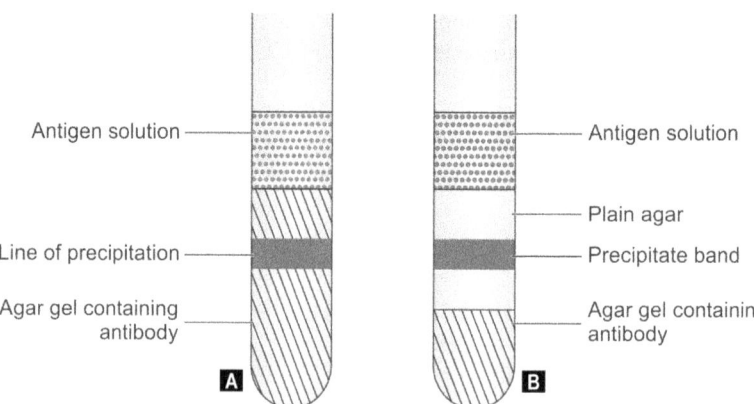

Figs. 11.3A and B: (A) Single diffusion in one dimension (Oudin procedure); (B) Double diffusion in one dimension (Oakley–Fulthorpe procedure).

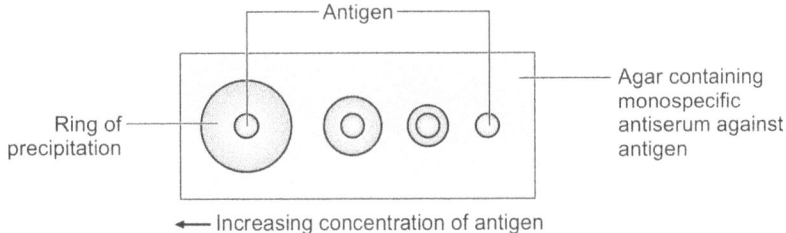

Fig. 11.4: Single diffusion in two dimensions (Radial immunodiffusion: Mancini method).

3. **Single diffusion in two dimensions (radial immunodiffusion—mancini method):** The assay is carried out by incorporating monospecific antiserum into melted agar and allowing the agar to solidify on a glass plate in a thin layer. Wells then are punched into the agar, and different dilutions of the antigen are placed into the various wells. As the antigen diffuses into the agar, and a ring of precipitation forms around the well **(Fig. 11.4)**. The area of the precipitin ring is proportional to the concentration of antigen.
   Uses
   i. To quantitate serum immunoglobulins, complement proteins.
   ii. For screening sera for antibodies to influenza viruses, among others.
4. **Double diffusion in two dimensions (Ouchterlony technique):** When soluble antigen and soluble antibody are placed in separate small wells punched into agar that has solidified on a slide or glass plate, the antigen and the antibody will diffuse through the agar and will interact to form a line of precipitate in the area in which they are in optimal proportions **(Fig. 11.5)**.

   The visible line of precipitation permits a comparison of antigens for identity (same antigenic determinants), partial identity (cross-reactivity), or nonidentity against a given selected antibody, e.g., **Elek test for toxigenicity in diphtheria bacilli**.
5. **Immunoelectrophoresis:** Immunoelectrophoresis is a procedure that combines electrophoresis and double diffusion in gels. In this procedure antigens are separated by electrophoresis in an agar gel. A small drop of solution containing the antigens is placed into a small well punched out of solidified agar on a small glass plate. The plate then is placed in an electric field to allow for the electrophoretic migration of the antigens. A trough is then cut next to the wells and filled with antibody and diffusion allowed to proceed for 18–24 hours. The antibody and the antigens diffuse toward each other, resulting in the formation of precipitin bands or arcs wherever they are in optimal proportions **(Fig. 11.6)**.
   Uses
   i. To separate many antigens
   ii. To separate the major blood proteins in serum.

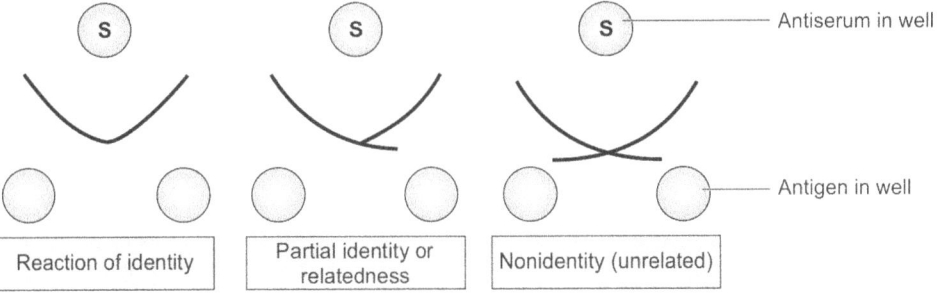

Fig. 11.5: Double diffusion in two dimensions (Ouchterlony technique).

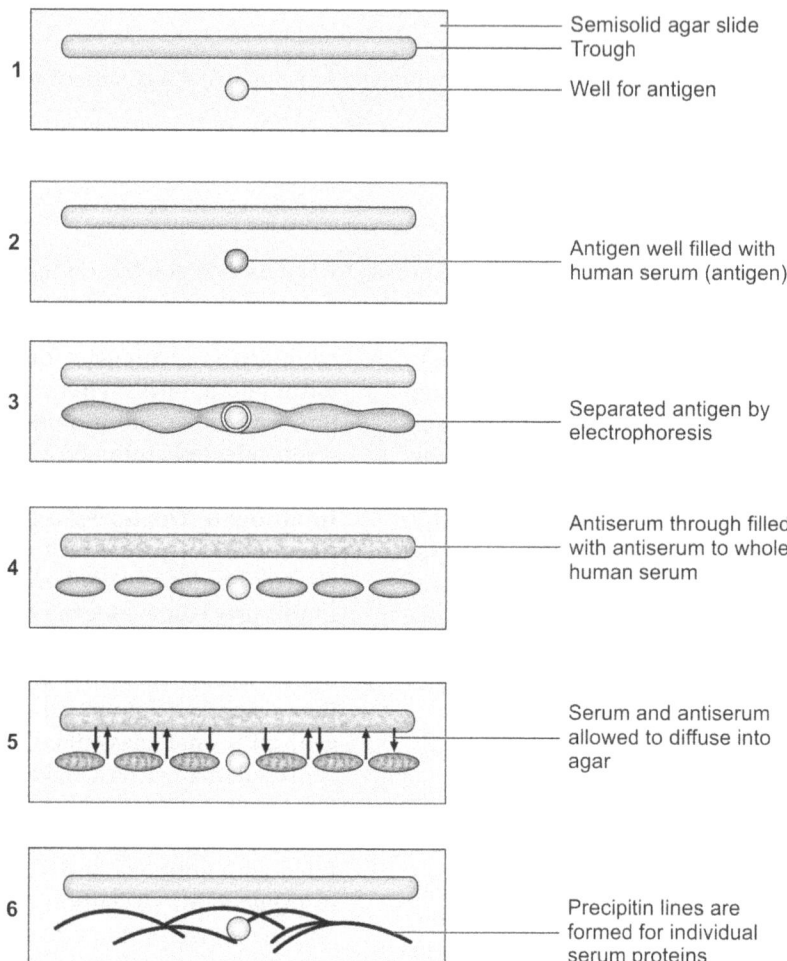

Fig. 11.6: Immunoelectrophoresis.

iii. For testing for normal and abnormal proteins in serum and urine.
6. **Electroimmunodiffusion:** Immunodiffusion is a slow process. The development of precipitin lines can be speeded up by electrically driving the antigen and antibody in a gel. Various methods have been described combining electrophoresis with diffusion such as one dimensional double electroimmunodiffusion (counterimmunoelectrophoresis).

Counterimmunoelectrophoresis (CIE) or Countercurrentelectrophoresis (CIEP)
Counterimmunoelectrophoresis can be used only for antigens and antibody that migrate in opposite directions in the electric field. Two wells are punched about in an agar slab on a glass plate. The antigen and antibody solutions are placed in these wells and that when the electric field is applied across the plate, the antigen will migrate toward the antibody, and the antibody will migrate toward the antigen resulting in precipitation at a point between them **(Fig. 11.7)**.

Clinical Applications
i. **For detection of various antigens:** Such as hepatitis B surface antigen (HBs antigen) and alpha-fetoprotein in serum and meningococcal and cryptococcal antigens in cerebrospinal fluid (CSF).

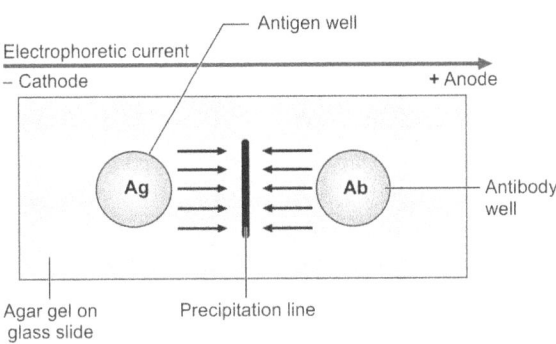

Fig. 11.7: Counterimmunoelectrophoresis (CIE).

ii. **To detect the presence of anti-DNA antibody in the serum of patients with several autoimmune disorders.**

B. Agglutination Reactions

When a particulate antigen is mixed with its antibody in the presence of electrolytes at a suitable temperature and pH, the particles are **clumped or agglutinated**. This reaction is analogous to the precipitin reaction, in that antibody acts as a bridge to form a lattice network of antibody and cells. Agglutination occurs optimally when antigen and antibodies react in equivalent proportion.

Prozone phenomenon: The zone phenomenon may be seen when either an antibody or an antigen is in excess.

Applications of Agglutination Reaction

1. Slide agglutination
2. Tube agglutination
3. Antiglobulin (Coombs') test
4. Passive (indirect) agglutination test

1. Slide Agglutination

A drop of sterile saline is placed on one of the divisions of the slide or plate and is emulsified in it, bacterial culture. With a small loop the diagnostic serum is taken and is placed on the slide and is then mixed it into the latter. Distinct clumping within 60 seconds is a positive result.
Uses:
  i. **For the identification of unknown bacterial cultures**—such as *Salmonella* and *Shigella*.
  ii. **Very rapid**

iii. **Also, the method for blood grouping and cross matching.**

2. Tube Agglutination

Serum from a patient thought to be infected with a given bacterium is serially diluted in a series of tubes to which the bacteria is added. The last tube showing visible agglutination will reflect the serum antibody **titer** of the patient. The reciprocal of the greatest serum dilution that elicits a positive agglutination is known as the agglutinin titer.

Uses of Tube Agglutination

Tube agglutination is routinely employed for the serological diagnosis of typhoid, brucellosis and typhus fever.

3. Antiglobulin (Coombs') Test

Principle of the antiglobulin test: When sera containing incomplete anti-Rh antibodies are mixed with Rh positive red cells, the antibody coats the surface of the erythrocytes but they are not agglutinated. When such antibody-coated erythrocytes are washed to free all unattached protein and are treated with a rabbit antihuman antiserum against human gamma globulin (antiglobulin or Coombs' serum) the cells are agglutinated. This is the principle of the antiglobulin test.

Types of Coombs' test: Coombs' test is of two types: direct and indirect.

4. Passive (indirect) Agglutination Test

A precipitation reaction can be converted into agglutination reaction by coating soluble antigen on to the surface of **carrier particles,** such as red cells, latex particles or bentonite. Such test is more convenient and more sensitive for detection of antibodies. Such tests are known as passive agglutination tests.

Reversed passive agglutination: When instead of antigen, the antibody is adsorbed to carrier particles in tests for estimation of antigens, the technique is known as **reversed passive agglutination.**

Examples of Passive Agglutination
  i. **Hemagglutination test**
      a. **Rose–Waaler test**
      b. ***Treponema pallidum* hemagglutination (TPHA):** Serological diagnosis of treponemal infection.
  ii. **Latex agglutination test**: Polystyrene latex, as it can adsorb several types of antigens. Latex agglutination tests (latex fixation tests) are widely employed in clinical laboratory for the detection of antistreptolysin O (ASO), C reactive protein (CRP), RA factor, human chorionic gonadotropin (hCG), and many other antigens.
  iii. **Coagglutination**

Principle: Certain strains of *Staphylococcus aureus* (the Cowan strain, ATCC 12498) have a high content of surface protein A. Protein A on the *Staph. aureus* cell wall binds the Fc portion of the immunoglobulin molecule, leaving the Fab portion free to bind antigen. When the corresponding antigen is mixed with these coated cells, Fab terminal binds to antigen resulting in agglutination. Visible agglutination of the staphylococcal cells serves as a positive test to indicate antigen-antibody binding **(Fig. 11.8).**

Uses
  i. For detecting the presence of antigens in serum, urine, and CSF.
  ii. Identification of antigens of various streptococcal groups, *Streptococcus pneumoniae; Neisseria meningitidis; N. gonorrhoeae;* and *Haemophilus influenzae* types A to F grown in culture.

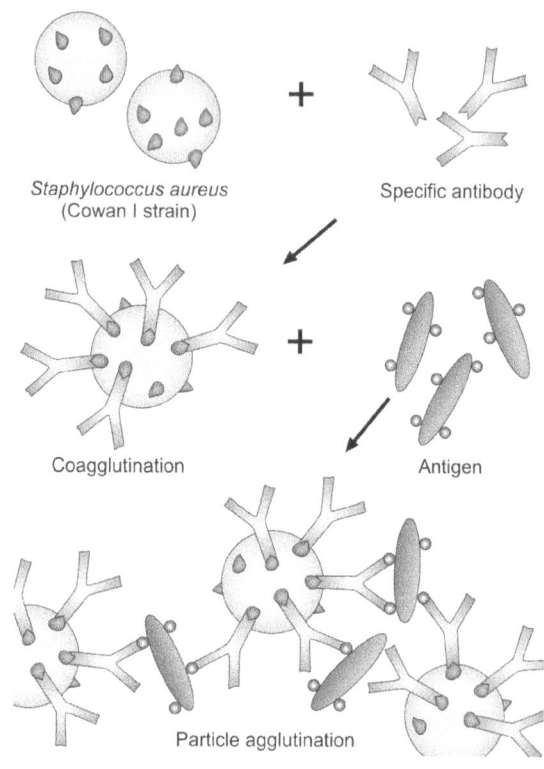

Fig. 11.8: Coagglutination.

C. Complement Fixation Test (CFT)

When complement binds to an antigen-antibody complex. It becomes "fixed" and "used up."

This test consists **of two separate systems and** these two systems are tested in sequence **(Fig. 11.9).**

Procedure

A. **Test system:** Consists of—(i) **Antigen:** Suspected of causing the patient's disease; (ii) **Patient's serum (antibody);** (iii) **Complement.**

B. **Indicator system:** Consists of **sheep red cells (antigen) coated with antisheep-red cell antibody and complement.**

Interpretation

Positive CF test: Absence of lysis

Negative CF test: Lysis of the indicator cells

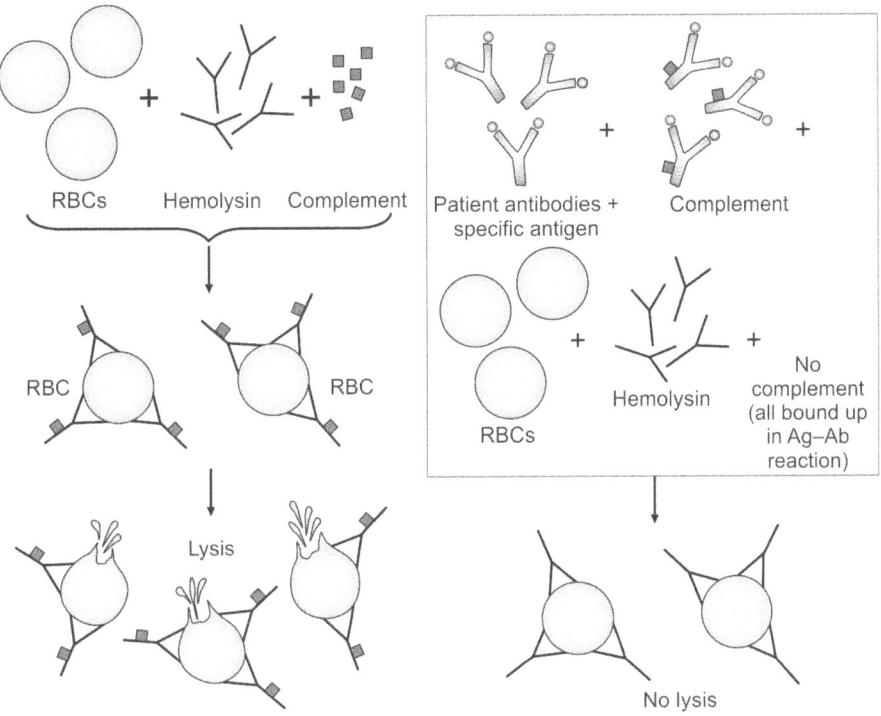

Fig. 11.9: Complement fixation text.
(RBC: red blood cell)

Lysis of the indicator cells indicates lack of antibody and a negative CF test. Lysis of the indicator cells **(Fig. 11.9)** results if immune complexes do not form in part of the test because the antibodies are not present in the test serum, complement remains and lyses the indicator cells.

D. Neutralization Tests
These are of two types:
1. Viral neutralization tests
2. Toxin neutralization tests

E. Opsonization
Opsonization is the process in which microorganisms or other particles are coated by antibody and/or complement, and thus prepared for "recognition" and ingestion by phagocytic cells.

F. Immunofluorescence
Immunofluorescence is a process in which dyes called fluorochromes are exposed to UV, violet, or blue light to make them fluoresce or emit visible light. Fluorescent molecules absorb light of one wavelength (excitation) and emit light of another wavelength (emission).

Fluorescent dyes: Rhodamine B or **fluorescein isothiocyanate (FITC)**—most commonly used fluorescent dyes. **Fluorescein** emits an intense yellow-green fluorescence. **Rhodamine** emits a deep red fluorescence.

Types of Immunofluorescence
There are two main kinds of fluorescent antibody assays: Direct and indirect **(Figs. 11.10A and B)**.
1. **Direct immunofluorescence**: In **direct staining** the specific antibody (the primary antibody) is directly conjugated with fluorescein. It involves fixing the specimen (cell or microorganism) containing the antigen of interest onto a slide. Fluorescein-labeled antibodies are then added to the slide and examined with the fluorescence microscope for fluorescence.

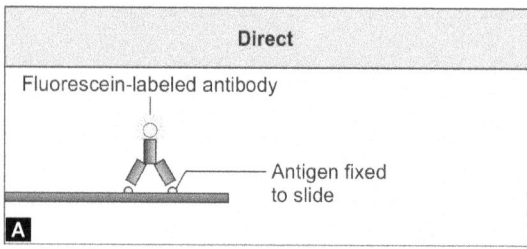

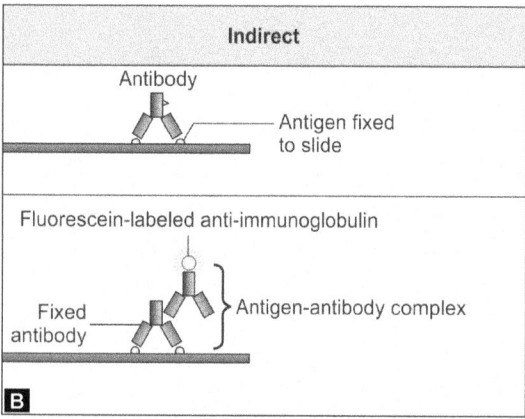

Figs. 11.10A and B: Direct and indirect immunofluorescence: (A) In the direct fluorescent-antibody (FA) technique, the specimen containing antigen is fixed to a slide. Fluorescenated antibodies that recognize the antigen are then added, and the specimen is examined under a UV microscope for yellow-green fluorescence; (B) Indirect fluorescent-antibody technique (IFA). The antigen on a slide reacts with an antibody directed against it. The antigen-antibody complex is located with a fluorescent antibody that recognizes immunoglobulins.

Uses
i. It is used to identify antigens group A streptococci.
ii. To diagnose bacteria, virus and other antigens.
iii. To diagnose rabies virus.

2. **Indirect immunofluorescence:** Indirect immunofluorescence is used to detect the presence of antibodies in serum following an individual's exposure to microorganisms. In this technique a known antigen is fixed onto a slide. The test antiserum is then added, and if the specific antibody is present, it reacts with antigen to form a complex. When fluorescein-labeled anti-immunoglobulin is added, it reacts with the fixed antibody. The slide is examined with the fluorescence microscope. The occurrence of fluorescence shows that antibody specific to the test antigen is present in the serum.

Uses
Diagnosis of Syphilis

G. Radioimmunoassay (RIA)

One of the most sensitive techniques for detecting antigen or antibody is RIA.

Principle of RIA

The principle of RIA is based on competitive binding of radiolabeled antigen, e.g., ^{125}I and unlabeled antigen to a high-affinity antibody. The labeled and unlabeled (test) antigens compete for the limited binding sites on the antibody. This competition is determined by the level of the unlabeled (test) antigen present in reacting system.

H. Enzyme-linked Immunosorbent Assay

Enzyme-linked immunosorbent assay, commonly (ELISA), is similar in principle to RIA but the radioactive tag used in RIA techniques can be replaced with an enzyme. When this enzyme is linked to an antibody and used to detect and measure other antibodies or antigens, the assay is called the enzyme-linked immunosorbent assay (ELISA). An enzyme conjugated with antibody reacts with a colorless substrate to generate a colored reaction product. Such a substrate is called a chromogenic substrate.

The test is usually done using microtiter plates (96-well) suitable for automation.

Types of ELISA (Figs. 11.11A to C)

1. Indirect ELISA

The indirect immunosorbent assay **detects antibodies** rather than antigens. Serum or other sample containing primary antibody is added to antigen-coated microtiter well. Any free antibody is washed away and the presence of antibody bound to the antigen is detected by adding an enzyme-conjugated secondary

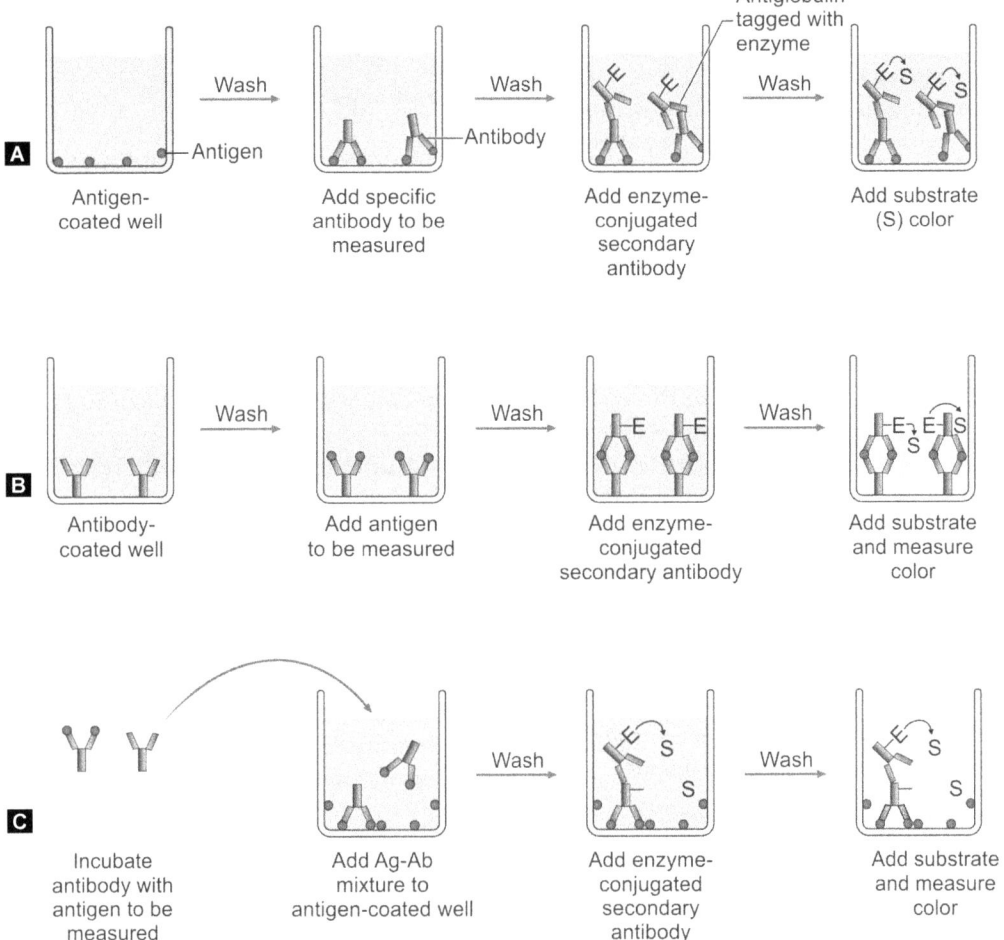

Figs. 11.11A to C: Types of enzyme-linked immunosorbent assay (ELISA).
(A) Indidect ELISA; (B) Sandwich ELISA; (C) Competitive ELISA.

anti-isotype antibody (Antibody 2), which binds to the primary antibody. Any free antibody-2 then is washed away, and a substrate for the enzyme is added. The amount of colored reaction product that forms is measured by specialized spectrophotometric plate readers, which can measure the absorbance of all of the wells of a 96-well plate in less than a few seconds.

2. Sandwich ELISA

The most frequently used ELISA for **detecting microbial antigen** is the sandwich solid-phase ELISA. It is of two types:

i. **Single antibody or direct sandwich ELISA:** In this technique, the antibody (rather than the antigen) is immobilized on a microtiter well. The test sample is then exposed to the solid-phase antibody, to which the antigen, if present, will bind. After the well is washed, a second enzyme-linked antibody specific for test antigen is added and allowed to react with the bound antigen. The conjugated antibody will react with the antigen held to the solid-phase by the first antibody, forming an **antibody-antigen-antibody sandwich** on the solid phase. After any free second antibody is removed by washing, substrate is added, and the colored reaction product is measured.

If the antigen has reacted with the absorbed antibodies in the first step, the ELISA test is positive. If the antigen is not recognized by the absorbed antibody, the ELISA test is negative.

3. Competitive ELISA

In this technique, antibody is first incubated in solution with a sample containing antigen. The antigen-antibody mixture is then added to an antigen coated microtiter well. The more antigen present in the sample, the less free antibody will be available to bind to the antigen-coated well. Addition of an enzyme-conjugated, secondary antibody specific for the isotype of the primary antibody can be used to determine the amount of primary antibody bound to the well as in an indirect ELISA. In the competitive assay, however, the higher the concentration of antigen in the original sample, the lower the absorbance.

Illustration: The principle of this test too can be illustrated by outlining its application for detection of anti-HIV antibodies in the patient serum.

Uses of ELISA

ELISA has been used to detect antigens and antibodies of various microorganisms.

Examples

Parasites
- *Entamoeba histolytica* antigens in feces
- *Toxoplasma* antigens in the patient serum

Bacteria
- *Haemophilus influenzae* antigens in spinal fluid.
- β-hemolytic streptococcal antigen in spinal fluid.
- Labile enterotoxin of *E. coli* in stools.

To detect antibody specific for:
- Mycoplasmas
- Chlamydiae
- *Borrelia burgdorferi*

Viruses
To detect antibody specific for:
- Hepatitis virus antigens
- Herpes simplex viruses 1 and 2
- Respiratory syncytial virus (RSV)
- Cytomegalovirus
- Human immunodeficiency virus (HIV)
- Rubella virus (both IgG and IgM)
- Adenovirus antigens—in nasopharyngeal specimens

I. Immunoelectroblot Techniques

Western blotting (immunoblotting): Identification of a specific protein in a complex mixture of proteins can be accomplished by a technique known as Western blotting, named for its similarity to Southern blotting, which detects DNA fragments, and Northern blotting which detects mRNAs. It is a variation of an ELISA.

J. Immunochromatographic Tests

A one-step qualitative immunochromatographic technique has found wide application in serodiagnosis due to its simplicity, economy, and reliability.

K. Immunoelectronmicroscopic Tests

1. **Immunoelectronmicroscopy**
2. **Immunoferritin test**
3. **Immunoenzyme test**

KEY POINTS

- The antigen-antibody reaction is a bimolecular association that exquisite specificity.
- There are many types of antigen-antibody reactions.
- The enzyme-linked immunosorbent assay (ELISA) depends on an enzyme-substrate reaction that generates a colored reaction product.

IMPORTANT QUESTIONS

1. Name various antigen-antibody reactions. Describe the principle and applications of precipitation reactions giving suitable examples.
2. Define agglutination reaction. Discuss the principle and applications of agglutination reactions giving suitable examples.
3. Write short notes on:
    a. Immunodiffusion (or) gel diffusion.
    b. Counterimmunoelectrophoresis (CIE).
    c. Coagglutination.

Chapter 11: Antigen-Antibody Reactions

D. Latex agglutination test complement fixation test (CFT).
e. Immunofluorescence tests.
f. Enzyme-linked immunosorbent assay (ELISA)—its principle and application.

MULTIPLE CHOICE QUESTIONS

1. The prozone phenomenon is:
   a. Zone of antibody excess
   b. Zone of antigen excess
   c. Zone of equivalence of antigens and antibody
   d. None of the above
2. Which immunoglobulin class is the most efficient to produce agglutination reaction?
   a. IgG
   b. IgM
   c. IgA
   d. IgE
3. Which immunoglobulin class is the most efficient to produce precipitation reaction?
   a. IgG
   b. IgM
   c. IgD
   d. IgE
4. Ring test is used for:
   a. C-reactive protein test
   b. Streptococcal grouping of Lancefield technique
   c. Both of the above
   d. None of the above
5. VDRL test is an example of:
   a. Agglutination test
   b. Flocculation test
   c. Immunofluorescence
   d. All of the above
6. Radial immunodiffusion can be used to estimate the following immunoglobulin classes:
   a. IgG
   b. IgM
   c. IgA
   d. All of the above
7. Counterimmunoelectrophoresis is used for detecting:
   a. Hepatitis B antigens
   b. Cryptococcal antigens
   c. *Neisseria meningitidis*
   d. All of the above
8. Tube agglutination test is used for serological diagnosis of:
   a. Enteric fever
   b. Infectious mononucleosis
   c. Typhus fever
   d. All of the above
9. Which of the following is/are example/s of heterophile agglutination test?
   a. Weil–Felix reaction
   b. Paul–Bunnel test
   c. *Streptococcus* MG agglutination test
   d. All of the above
10. Which of the following is/are example/s of passive agglutination test?
    a. Latex agglutination test
    b. Hemagglutination test
    c. Coagglutination
    d. All of the above
11. Which of the following is/are example/s of neutralization test?
    a. Schick test
    b. Antistreptolysin "O" test
    c. Nagler reaction
    d. All of the above
12. Direct immunofluorescence test may be used for detection of:
    a. Rabies virus antigens
    b. Antibodies in syphilis
    c. Both of the above
    d. None of the above
13. Indirect immunofluorescence test may be used for detection of:
    a. Rabies virus antigens
    b. Antibodies in syphilis
    c. Both of the above
    d. None of the above
14. ELISA can be used for detection of antigens and for antibodies in:
    a. HIV
    b. Rotavirus
    c. Hepatitis B virus
    d. All of the above
15. The technique of immunoblotting to analyze RNA is named as:
    a. Southern blot
    b. Northern blot
    c. Western blot
    d. None of the above

ANSWERS

1. a   2. b   3. a   4. c
5. b   6. d   7. d   8. d
9. d   10. d   11. d   12. a
13. b   14. d   15. b

Structure and Functions of the Immune System

LEARNING OBJECTIVES

After reading and studying this chapter, you should be able to:
- Differentiate between T and B cells in a tabulated form.
- Describe cluster of differentiation (CD).
- Discuss the following: Natural killer cells or NK cells; killer cells or K cells or ADCC cells; human leukocyte antigen (HLA).

INTRODUCTION

The lymphoreticular system is a complex organization of cells of diverse morphology distributed widely in different organs and tissues of the body responsible for immunity. **Lymphoreticular cells** consist of lymphoid and reticuloendothelial components. The lymphoid cells (lymphocytes and plasma cells) are primarily concerned with the specific immune response. The phagocytic cells (polymorphonuclear leukocytes and macrophages), forming part of the reticuloendothelial system, are primarily concerned with the "scavenger" functions of eliminating effete cells and foreign particles, thus contributing to nonspecific immunity by removing microorganisms from blood and tissues. They also play a role in specific immunity, both in the afferent and efferent limbs of the immune response.

TYPES OF IMMUNE RESPONSE

The immune response to an antigen, whatever its nature, can be of two broad type:
1. **Humoral or antibody mediated immunity (HMI or AMI):** Humoral immunity is mediated by antibodies produced by plasma cells.
2. **Cellular or cell-mediated immunity (CMI):** Cellular immunity is mediated directly by sensitized lymphocytes.

ORGANS AND TISSUES OF THE IMMUNE SYSTEM

Based on function, the organs and tissues of the immune system can be divided into primary or secondary lymphoid organs or tissues.
A. **Primary (central) organs or tissues**
   - Thymus
   - Bone marrow—the primary lymphoid tissue
B. **Secondary (peripheral) organs and tissues**
   - Lymph nodes
   - Spleen
   - Various mucosal-associated lymphoid tissues (MALT)—such as gut-associated lymphoid tissue (GALT), SALT (skin-associated lymphoid tissues)

Central (Primary) Lymphoid Organs

The place where immature lymphocytes mature and differentiate into antigen-sensitive mature B and T cells are called primary organs or tissues. The thymus and bone marrow are the primary (or central) lymphoid organs, where maturation of lymphocytes takes place. The thymus is the primary lymphoid organ and bone marrow is the primary lymphoid tissue.

CELLS OF THE LYMPHORETICULAR SYSTEM

Lymphoid cells: Cells of the immune system—the cells responsible for both nonspecific and specific immunity are the white blood cells called **leukocytes.**

Lymphocytes: Lymphocytes constitute 20–40% of the body's white blood cells and 99% of the cells in the lymph. Lymphocytes are now recognized as the major cellular elements responsible for immunological responses. Lymphocytes are mainly T cells and B cells.

i. T Lymphocytes

On the basis of functions these can be of the following types:

Regulatory T cells
1. **Helper/inducer cell (TH):** Helper/inducer cell (TH) generally stimulate and promote the growth of T cells and macrophages. They help B cells make antibody in response to antigenic challenge; stimulate cell-mediated immunity. Helper cells constitute about 65% and suppressor cells about 35% of circulating T lymphocytes.
2. **Suppressor T cells (T_S cells):** These have cluster of differentiation 8 (CD8) surface marker and major histocompatibility complex (MHC) class I restriction. They can suppress B-cell and T-cell response.

Effector Cells
1. **Delayed type-hypersensitivity T cells (Td cells):** They are involved in delayed hypersensitivity and cell-mediated immune response.
2. **Cytotoxic T cells (T_C cells):** They are also called CD8⁺ cells with CD8 surface marker and MHC class I restriction. They can kill and lyse target cells carrying new or foreign antigens, including tumor, allograft and virus infected cells.

ii. B Cells and Plasma Cells

B Cell Maturation

The B lymphocyte derived its letter designation from its site of maturation, in the bursa of Fabricius in birds; and the bone marrow of mammals.

Mature B cell undergoes **clonal proliferation** on contact with its appropriate antigen. In this process, the B cell divides repeatedly and differentiates, generating a population of **plasma cells** and **memory cells**. Memory cells circulate until activated by specific antigen.

Plasma Cell

Plasma cells are fully differentiated antibody-secreting effector cells of the B-cell lineage. Plasma cells are factories of antibody production.

Null Cells

A small proportion of lymphocytes that lack distinguishing phenotypic markers characteristic of T or B lymphocytes are called null cells. Because of their morphology, they are also known as *large granular lymphocytes* (LGL). The member of this group is the:
a. Natural killer (NK) cells: The most important member
b. Antibody dependent cellular cytotoxic (ADCC) cells
c. Lymphokine activated killer (LAK) cells

The term NK cell is sometimes used as a common name for all null cells.

a. **Natural killer (NK) cells:** Natural killer (NK) cells are derived from large granular lymphocytes (LGL). They differ from K cells in being independent of antibody. NK activity is "natural" or "nonimmune" as it does not require sensitization by prior antigenic contact.
   Function: They are important in natural defense against virus infected and malignant mutant cells.
b. **Antibody-dependent cell-mediated cytotoxicity (ADCC):** They are capable of lysing or killing target cells sensitized with IgG antibodies.

c. **Lymphokine activated killer (LAK) cells:** These NK lymphocytes are cytotoxic to a wide range of tumor cells without affecting normal cells.

Phagocytic Cells

Phagocytic cells are the **mononuclear macrophages** (of blood and tissues) and the **polymorphonuclear microphages**.

Mononuclear cells: The mononuclear phagocytic system consists of monocytes circulating in the blood and macrophages in the tissues, macrophages (histiocytes) spread throughout the animal body and take up residence in specific tissues where they are given special names, e.g., alveolar macrophages in the lung, Kupffer cells in the liver.

Functions of Macrophages
1. **Phagocytosis:** The primary function of macrophages is phagocytosis
2. Antigen presentation to T cells to initiate immune responses
3. Secretion of cytokines to activate and promote innate immune response
   Macrophages secrete interleukin-1, interleukin-6, tumor necrosis factor, and interleukin-12 in response to bacterial interaction, which stimulate immune and inflammatory responses, including fever.

Polymorphonuclear Microphages
Microphages are the **polymorphonuclear leukocytes or PMNs** of the blood: basophils, eosinophils, and neutrophils.
a. **Neutrophils:** Neutrophils are actively phagocytic, nonspecific and form the predominant cell type in acute inflammation.
b. **Eosinophils:** Eosinophils possess phagocytic activity to a limited degree. They are found in large numbers in allergic inflammation, parasitic infections and around antigen-antibody complexes.
c. **Basophils:** Basophil leukocytes are found in the blood and tissues (**mast cells**). Degranulation of mast cells, with release of pharmacologically active agents, constitutes the effector mechanism in anaphylactic and atopic allergy.

MAJOR HISTOCOMPATIBILITY COMPLEX

The major histocompatibility complex (MHC) is a remarkable cluster of genes that control T cell recognition of self and nonself. In humans, the MHC is called the **human leukocyte antigen (HLA) complex**.

Human Leukocyte Antigen (HLA) Complex

The major antigens determining histocompatibility in human beings are alloantigens, characteristically found on the surface of leukocytes. Human MHC antigens are therefore synonymous with human leukocyte antigens (HLA), and the MHC of genes with the HLA complex.

The HLA complex of genes is located on the short arm of chromosome 6 (**Fig. 12.1**). It consists of three separate clusters of genes:
1. **HLA class I comprising A, B and C loci:** HLA class I comprising A, B and C loci. HLA class I antigens (A, B and C) are found on the surface of virtually all nucleated cells.

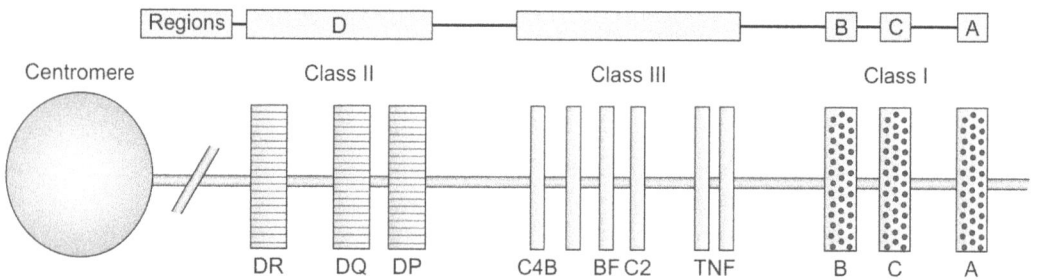

Fig. 12.1: Human leukocyte antigen complex loci on chromosome. (TNF: tumor necrosis factor)

They are the principal antigens involved in graft rejection and cell mediated cytolysis.

2. **Class II or the D region consisting of DR, DQ and DP loci:** Class II consists of three main sets: the DP, DQ and DR encoded molecules. HLA class II antigens are more restricted in distribution, being found only on cells of the immune system—macrophages, dendritic cells, activated T cells, and particularly on B cells. They are involved in graft rejection and in the regulation of immune response.

3. **Class III or the complement region:** Class III or the complement region containing genes for complement components C2 and C4 of the classical pathway, as well as properdin factor B of the alternative pathway, heat shock proteins and tumor necrosis factors alpha and beta.

KEY POINTS

- The lymphoid organs, based on their function, are classified into **primary (central) and secondary (peripheral) lymphoid organs**.
- There are three types of lymphocytes: B cells, T cells, and natural killer cells (NK cells).
- The MHC in humans is known as HLA complex.

IMPORTANT QUESTIONS

1. Give an account of lymphocytes.
2. Describe major histocompatibility complex (MHC).
3. Write short notes on:
   a. T lymphocytes
   b. B lymphocytes
   c. Null cells (or) large granular lymphocytes (LGL)
   d. Human leukocyte antigen (HLA)

MULTIPLE CHOICE QUESTIONS

1. All the following are examples of secondary-lymphoid organs, *except*:
   a. Lymph nodes
   b. Thymus
   c. Spleen
   d. Mucosa-associated lymphoid tissues

2. The CD4$^+$ T cells that recruit and activate phagocytic cells acting against intracellular microbes are called:
   a. Th-0 cells
   b. Th-1 cells
   c. Th-2 cells
   d. Antigen-presenting cells

3. The molecule expressed on surface of the mature T cells is:
   a. CD 19
   b. CD 8
   c. CD 3
   d. CD 1d

4. All the following statements are true for helper T cells, *except* that they:
   a. Carry CD4 marker
   b. Help or induce immune responses
   c. Kill intracellular microorganisms by secreting cytokines
   d. Recognize antigen in association with class I MHC

5. Class II MHC antigens are present on:
   a. Macrophages
   b. Monocytes
   c. Activated T lymphocytes (CD4)
   d. All of the above

6. Class I proteins are encoded by:
   a. HLA-A, -B, and -C loci
   b. HLA-DR, HLA-DQ, and HLA-DP loci
   c. Complement loci that encode C2 and C4
   d. Complement loci that encode factor B

7. Which of the following HLA types is associated with ankylosing spondylitis?
   a. HLA-B27
   b. HLA-DR4
   c. HLA-DP
   d. None of the above

8. Which of the following HLA types is associated with rheumatoid arthritis?
   a. HLA-B27
   b. HLA-DR4
   c. HLA-Al
   d. None of the above

ANSWERS

1. b 2. c 3. c 4. d
5. d 6. a 7. b 8. b

Chapter 13: Immune Response

LEARNING OBJECTIVES

After reading and studying this chapter, you should be able to:
- Differentiate between primary and secondary humoral immune responses.
- Describe the following: Monoclonal antibodies, cytokines.

DEFINITION

The immune response is the specific reactivity induced in a host by an antigenic stimulus.

TYPE OF IMMUNE RESPONSE

The immune response can be divided into two types—the humoral (antibody mediated) and the cellular (cell mediated) types.

1. **Antibody-mediated immunity (AMI)**
   - Provides primary defense against most extracellular bacterial pathogens
   - Helps in defense against viruses that infect through the respiratory or intestinal tracts
   - Prevents recurrence of virus infections
   - It also participates in the pathogenesis of immediate (types 1, 2, and 3) hypersensitivity and certain autoimmune diseases.
2. **Cell-mediated immunity (CMI)**
   - Protects against fungi, viruses and facultative intracellular bacterial pathogens such as *Mycobacterium tuberculosis, Mycobacterium leprae, Brucella* and *Salmonella,* and parasites such as *Leishmania* and *trypanosomes.*
   - It also participates in the rejection of homografts and graft-versus-host reaction.
   - It mediates the pathogenesis of delayed (type 4) hypersensitivity and certain autoimmune diseases.
   - It provides immunological surveillance and immunity against cancer

HUMORAL IMMUNITY

Synthesis of Antibody

On exposure to antigen, antibody production follows a characteristic pattern (**Fig. 13.1**). The production of antibodies consists of four steps:
1. **Lag phase:** A lag phase, the immediate stage following antigenic stimulus during which no antibody is detectable in circulation.
2. **Log phase:** A log phase in which there is steady rise in the titer of antibodies.

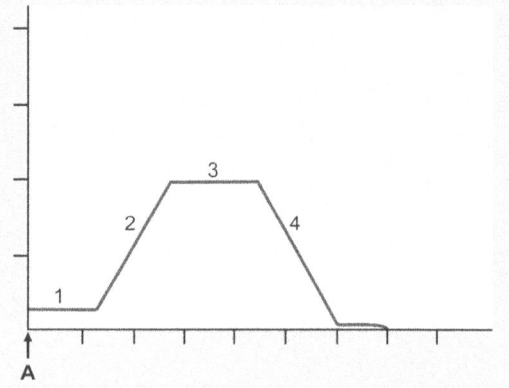

Fig. 13.1: Primary immune response. An antigenic stimulus: 1. Latent period; 2. Log phase (rise in titer of serum antibody); 3. Steady state of antibody titer; 4. Decline of antibody titer.

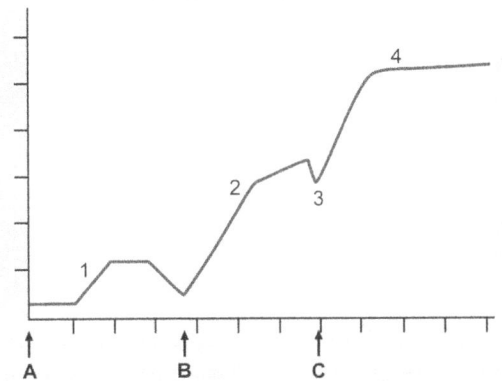

Fig. 13.2: Effect of repeated antigenic stimulus. A, B, C antigenic stimuli. 1. Primary immune response; 2. Secondary immune response; 3. Negative phase; 4. High level of antibody following booster injection.

3. **A plateau or steady state:** There is equilibrium between antibody synthesis and catabolism.
4. **The phase of decline:** The catabolism exceeds the production and the titer falls (Fig. 13.2).

Primary and Secondary Responses

a. Primary Humoral Response

The first contact of an exogenous antigen with an individual generates a primary humoral response, characterized by the production of antibody-secreting plasma cells and memory B cells.

b. Secondary Humoral Response

The secondary response has a shorter lag period, reaches a greater magnitude, lasts longer and is also characterized by secretion of antibody with a higher affinity for the antigen, and isotypes other than IgM predominate.

Priming dose and booster doses: The first injection is known as the **'priming' dose** and subsequent injections as **'booster' doses**.

Production of Antibodies

Immune response to an antigen is brought about by three types of cells—antigen processing cells (APC) principally macrophages and dendritic cells, T cells and B cells. Antibody production frequently requires T cell help.

Antigen Processing and Presentation

Antigen-presenting cell (APC) can ingest antigen, degrade it and present it to T cells.

T Cell Activation

Cytotoxic T (CD8/Tc) cells: Cytotoxic T (CD8/Tc) cells are activated when they contact antigens presented along with major histocompatibility complex (MHC) class I molecules. On contact with a target cell carrying the antigen on its surface, the activated Tc cells release **cytotoxins** that destroy the target, which may be virus infected or tumor cells. Some Tc cells also become memory cells.

B Cell Activation

The activated T-helper (H) cell forms interleukin-2 and other cytokines required for B cell activation and activate B cells and differentiate into antibody-secreting **plasma cells**. A small proportion of activated B cells, instead of being transformed into plasma cells, become long lived **memory cells** producing a secondary type of response to subsequent contact with the antigen.

Class Switching

Under the direction of cytokines produced by effector T-helper cells, some B cells become programmed to produce antibodies other than IgM. Terminal differentiation leads to production of plasma cell.

MONOCLONAL ANTIBODIES

Monoclonal antibodies: When a clone of lymphocytes or plasma cells undergoes selective proliferation, as in multiple myeloma, antibodies with a single antigenic specificity accumulate. Such antibodies produced by a single clone and directed against a single antigenic determinant are called **monoclonal antibodies,** e.g., plasma cell tumor (myeloma).

By laboratory manipulation, Köhler and Milstein (1975) prepared a hybrid cell line (hybridoma) by fusion of a mouse myeloma cell with an antibody producing lymphocyte from spleen or lymph node of the same inbred strain of mouse. Such hybrid cells can produce virtually unlimited quantities of monoclonal antibody of any required specificity indefinitely in cell culture conditions.

Uses of Monoclonal Antibody

1. In the typing of tissue
2. Identification and epidemiological study of infectious microorganisms
3. Identification of tumor and other surface antigens
4. In the classification of leukemias
5. In identification of functional populations of different types of T cells

CELL-MEDIATED IMMUNE RESPONSES

The term "cell mediated immunity" (CMI) refers to the specific immune responses which involves T-lymphocyte-mediated functions that do not involve antibodies. This form of immunity can be transferred from donor to recipient with intact lymphocytes, but not with antisera, hence it is called **cell-mediated immune reaction**.

Scope of Cell-mediated Immunity (CMI)

Cell-mediated immunity (CMI) participates in the following immunological functions:
1. Delayed hypersensitivity (Type IV hypersensitivity)
2. Immunity in infectious diseases caused by obligate and facultative intracellular parasites
3. Transplantation immunity and graft-versus-host reaction
4. Immunological surveillance and immunity against cancer
5. Pathogenesis of certain autoimmune diseases (for example, thyroiditis, encephalomyelitis)

Induction of Cell-mediated Immunity

Antigen-specific cell-mediated immunity is mediated by T lymphocytes. A second, smaller population of cells includes natural killer (NK) and killer (K) cells. As in case of antibody-mediated immune response, cell-mediated immune response can also be divided into primary and secondary cell-mediated immune responses.

CYTOKINES

Cytokines are biologically active substances produced by cells that influence other cells. Biologically active substances released by activated T lymphocytes are called **lymphokines**. When released from mononuclear phagocytes, these proteins are called **monokines**.

The term **interleukin** was introduced for those products of leukocytes which exert a regulatory influence on other cells; and if their effect is to stimulate the growth and differentiation of immature leukocytes in the bone marrow, they are called **colony-stimulating factors (CSFs)**.

Interferons, growth factors, and others were found to have similar effects. Therefore, all of them have been grouped under the term **cytokines**.

Immunological Tolerance

Immunologic tolerance is defined as the absence of a specific immune response resulting from a previous exposure to the inducing antigen. This nonreactivity is specific to the particular antigen, immune reactivity to other antigens being unaffected.

THEORIES OF IMMUNE RESPONSE

Theories of immunity fall into two categories: instructive and selective.
1. Instructive theories
   - Direct template theories
   - Indirect template theory

2. Selective theories
   - Side chain theory
   - Natural selection theory
   - Clonal selection theory

KEY POINTS

- The immune response can be divided into two types—the humoral (antibody mediated) and the cellular (cell mediated) types.
- **Cytokines:** Cytokines are biologically active substances produced by cells that influence other cells.

IMPORTANT QUESTIONS

1. Discuss primary and secondary humoral immune responses.
2. Write briefly on:
   a. Production of antibodies
   b. Humoral immunity
   c. Cell-mediated immunity (CMI)
   d. Monoclonal antibodies—production and applications.
   e. Cytokines

MULTIPLE CHOICE QUESTIONS

1. The synthesis and production of antibodies typically is dependent on complex interaction of all the following cells, *except*:
   a. Macrophages
   b. Helper T cells
   c. Cytotoxic T cells
   d. B cells

2. Which animal is used for monoclonal antibodies production:
   a. Guinea pig
   b. Mouse
   c. Rabbit
   d. None of the above

3. Interleukin-I is a protein produced mainly by:
   a. Macrophages and monocytes
   b. Polymorphonuclear leukocytes
   c. Lymphocytes
   d. Stem cells

4. Development of cell-mediated immunity can be detected by:
   a. Skin test for delayed hypersensitivity
   b. Lymphocyte transformation test
   c. Migration inhibiting factor test
   d. All of the above

5. Transfer factor shows all the following features, *except*:
   a. It is an extract from the leukocytes from the immunized host
   b. Transfers humoral immunity
   c. Transfers CMI
   d. Transferred immunity is systemic

6. Clonal selection theory was postulated by:
   a. Breinl and Haurowitz
   b. Burnet and Fenner
   c. Ehrlich
   d. Burnet

ANSWERS

1. c   2. b   3. a   4. d
5. b   6. d

CHAPTER 14

Hypersensitivity Reactions

LEARNING OBJECTIVES

After reading and studying this chapter, you should be able to:
- Compare major types of hypersensitivity reactions.
- Differentiate between immediate and delayed hypersensitivity.
- Discuss type I, type II, type-III, and type IV hypersensitivity reactions—mechanism and examples.

HYPERSENSITIVITY

Hypersensitivity is an exaggerated immune response that results in tissue damage and is manifested in the individual on second or subsequent contact with an antigen.

Immune responses to foreign antigens are, for the most part, beneficial to the responding individual. Nevertheless, at times the response to a seemingly innocuous antigen can result in tissue damage and even death. This inappropriate immune response is termed hypersensitivity or allergy.

CLASSIFICATION OF HYPERSENSITIVITY REACTIONS

Hypersensitivity reactions have been classified traditionally into "immediate" and "delayed" types, based on the time required for a sensitized host to develop clinical reactions on re-exposure to the antigen.

The major differences between the immediate and delayed types of hypersensitivity reactions are shown in **Table 14.1**.

Gell and Coombs Classification

The Gell-Coombs classification system divides hypersensitivity into four types: I, II, III, and IV.
Type I (Anaphylactic, IgE or reagin dependent)
Type II (Cytotoxic or cell stimulating)
Type III (Immune complex or toxic complex disease)
Type IV (Delayed or cell-mediated hypersensitivity)

The classification and some of the features of hypersensitivity reactions are shown in **Table 14.2**.

Table 14.1: Distinguishing features of immediate and delayed types of hypersensitivity.		
Characteristic	*Immediate hypersensitivity*	*Delayed hypersensitivity*
1. Time of reaction after challenge with antigen	1. Reaction appears and recedes rapidly	1. Appears slowly, lasts longer
2. Induction	2. Antigens or haptens	2. Antigen or hapten intradermally or with by any route
3. Immune response	3. "Antibody-mediated" reaction	3. "Cell-mediated" reaction
4. Transfer of hypersensitivity	4. Passive transfer possible with serum	4. Cannot be transferred with serum; but possible with T cells or transfer factor
5. Desensitization	5. Easy, but short-lived	5. Difficult, but long-lasting

Chapter 14: Hypersensitivity Reactions

Table 14.2: Comparison of major types of hypersensitivity reactions.

Type of reaction	Time required for manifestation	Mediators	Clinical syndrome
Type 1: IgE type	Minutes	IgE: Histamine and other pharmacological agents	1. Anaphylaxis 2. Atopy
Type II: Cytolytic and cytotoxic	Variable: Hours to days	IgG: IgM, complement	1. Transfusion reactions 2. Rh incompatibility
Type III: Immune complex	Variable: Hours to days	IgG: IgM, C, leukocytes	1. Arthus reaction 2. Serum sickness
Type IV: Delayed hypersensitivity	Hours to days	T cells: lymphokines; macrophages	1. Tuberculin test 2. Contact dermatitis 3. Graft rejection 4. Tumor immunity

TYPE 1 HYPERSENSITIVITY (IgE DEPENDENT)

A type I hypersensitive reaction is induced by certain types of antigens referred to as **allergens**.

Anaphylaxis

Anaphylaxis is an inclusive term for the reactions caused when certain antigens combine with IgE antibodies. Anaphylactic responses can be:

A. **Systemic reactions:** Systemic reactions produce shock and breathing difficulties and are sometimes fatal.

B. **Localized reactions:** Localized reactions is chronic or recurrent, nonfatal, typically localized form called **atopy**.

A. Systemic Anaphylaxis (or Anaphylactic Shock)

Systemic anaphylaxis is a generalized response that occurs when an individual sensitized to an allergen receives a subsequent exposure to it. Systemic anaphylaxis is a shock-like and often fatal state whose onset occurs within minutes of a type I hypersensitive reaction.

Antigens: A wide range of antigens have been shown to trigger this reaction in susceptible humans, including the venom from bee, wasp, hornet, and ant stings; drugs, such as penicillin, insulin, and antitoxins; and seafood and nuts. If not treated quickly, these reactions can be fatal.

Mechanism of anaphylaxis: *The immunologic basis for hypersensitivity is cytotropic IgE antibody.*

After an initial contact with an antigen, the individual produces IgE antibodies. IgE molecules are bound to surface receptors on mast cells and basophils. These cells carry large numbers of such receptors. IgE molecules attach to these receptors by their Fc end, leaving two antigen-binding sites free. Mast cells and basophils coated by IgE are said to be sensitized, making the individual allergic to the allergen **(Fig. 14.1)**.

Following exposure to the shocking dose, the antigen molecules combine with the cell bound IgE, bridging the gap between adjacent antibody molecules. This cross-linking increases the permeability of the cells to calcium ions and leads to degranulation, with release of biologically active substances contained in the granules. The pharmacologically active

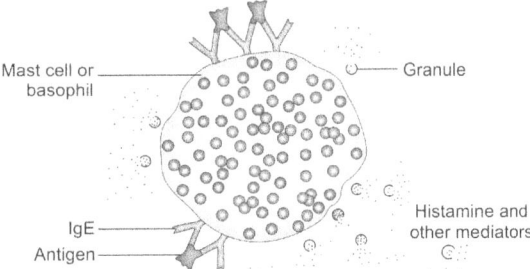

Fig. 14.1: Antigen-induced mediator release from mast cell.

mediators released from the granules act on the surrounding tissues. The manifestations of anaphylaxis are due to pharmacological mediators, which can be classified as two types either **primary or secondary.**

Primary mediators of anaphylaxis: The primary mediators are produced before degranulation and are stored in the granules.

1. **Histamine:** Histamine induces smooth muscle contraction in diverse tissues and organs, including vasculature, intestines, uterus, and especially the bronchioles.
2. **Heparin:** It contributes to anaphylaxis in dogs, but apparently not in human beings.
3. **Serotinin:** It induces contraction of smooth muscle, increased vascular permeability, and capillary dilatation.
4. **Chemotactic factors:**
   i. **Eosinophil chemotactic factor (ECF-A):** These probably contribute to the eosinophilia.
   ii. **Neutrophil chemotactic factors (NCF):** Attracts neutrophils (NCF).
5. **Proteases**: Result in increased permeability to a variety of cell types.

Secondary mediators of anaphylaxis:
1. **Platelet activating factor (PAF):** It induces a rapid wheal and flare reaction when injected into human skin.
2. **Leukotrienes and prostaglandin**—are bronchoconstrictors.
3. **Cytokines**: These cytokines leading to the recruitment of inflammatory cells.

B. Localized Anaphylaxis (Atopy)

The term "atopy" (literally meaning out of place or strangeness) refers to naturally occurring familial hypersensitivities of human beings. It was introduced by Coca (1923) and typified by hay fever and asthma. The antigens commonly involved in atopy are **inhalants contact allergens**, to which the skin and conjunctiva may be exposed.

Predisposition to atopy is genetically determined, genotypes. Atopy therefore runs in families.

Mechanism of Atopy

The mechanism of development of atopy is essentially the same as that of systemic anaphylaxis. The symptoms of atopy are caused by the release of pharmacologically active substances following the combination of the antigen and the cell fixed IgE.

Atopic sensitivity is due to an overproduction of IgE antibodies.

Clinical Expression of Atopic Reactions

The clinical expression of atopic reactions is usually determined by the portal of entry of the antigen-conjunctivitis, rhinitis, gastrointestinal symptoms and dermatitis following exposure through the eyes, respiratory tract, intestine or skin, respectively.

TYPE II HYPERSENSITIVITY: CYTOLYTIC AND CYTOTOXIC

These reactions involve a combination of **IgG (or IgM) antibodies** with an antigenic determinants on the surface of cells. Antibody can activate the **complement** system, creating pores in the membrane of a foreign cell, or it can mediate cell destruction by **antibody dependent cell-mediated cytotoxicity (ADCC).** Type II hypersensitivity is generally called **cytolytic or cytotoxic reactions** because it results in the destruction of host cells, either by lysis or toxic mediators (**Fig. 14.2**).

Examples:
1. **Transfusion reactions:** A **transfusion reaction** can occur if a patient receives erythrocytes differing antigenically from his or her own during blood transfusion.
2. **Hemolytic disease of the newborn**: If the child is Rh+ and mother Rh− will cross the placenta and destroy fetal RBCs.
3. **Drug-induced cytotoxic reactions:** Blood platelets (thrombocytes) that are destroyed by drug-induced cytotoxic reactions in the disease called **thrombocytopenic purpura** (quinine is a familiar example). Immune-caused destruction of granulocytic white

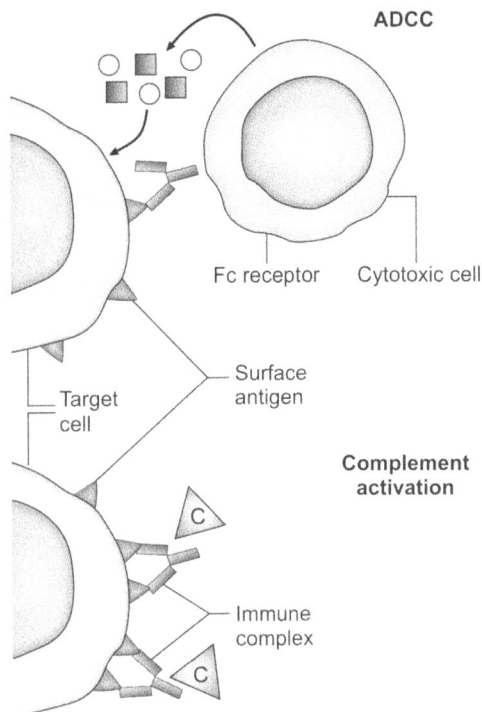

Fig. 14.2: Hypersensitivity.
(ADCC: antibody-dependent cell-mediated cytotoxicity)

cells is called **agranulocytosis.** When RBCs are destroyed in the same manner, the condition is termed **hemolytic anemia.**
4. Anemia due to infectious diseases.

TYPE III HYPERSENSITIVITY: IMMUNE COMPLEX-MEDIATED

Type III reactions involve antibodies against soluble antigens circulating in the serum. The antigen-antibody complexes are deposited in organs and cause inflammatory damage. The tissue damage that results from the deposition of immune complexes is caused by the activation of complement, platelets and phagocytes; in essence, an acute inflammatory response.

Models of Immune Complex-mediated Disease

Two basic models of immune complex-mediated disease have been well characterized: **The Arthus reaction** and **serum sickness.**

Arthus Reaction (Local Immune Complex Disease)

A localized form of experimental immune complex mediated vasculitis is called **Arthus reaction**. This is a local manifestation of generalized hypersensitivity.

Serum Sickness (Systemic Immune Complex Disease)

This is a systemic form of type III hypersensitivity. When large amounts of antigen enter the bloodstream and bind to antibody, circulating immune complexes can form. If antigen is in excess, small complexes form, they can cause tissue damaging type III reactions at various sites. This appears 7–12 days following a single injection of a high concentration of foreign serum such as the diphtheria antitoxin.

Pathogenesis: The pathogenesis is the formation of immune complexes (consisting of the foreign serum and antibody to it that reaches high enough titers by 7–12 days) and the circulating immune complexes deposit in the blood vessel walls and tissues, leading to increased vascular permeability and thus to inflammatory diseases such as glomerulonephritis and arthritis. Antigen–antibody aggregates can fix **complement** leading to **inflammation** and tissue damage.

Diseases Associated with Immune Complexes

- Systemic lupus erythematosus
- Rheumatoid arthritis
- Poststreptococcal glomerulonephritis
- Dengue hemorrhagic fever

TYPE IV HYPERSENSITIVITY: DELAYED HYPERSENSITIVITY

Type IV hypersensitivity reactions (delayed hypersensitivity) constitute one aspect of cell-mediated immune response and are caused mainly by T cells. These are typically provoked by intracellular microbial infections or haptens and consist of a mixed cellular reaction involving

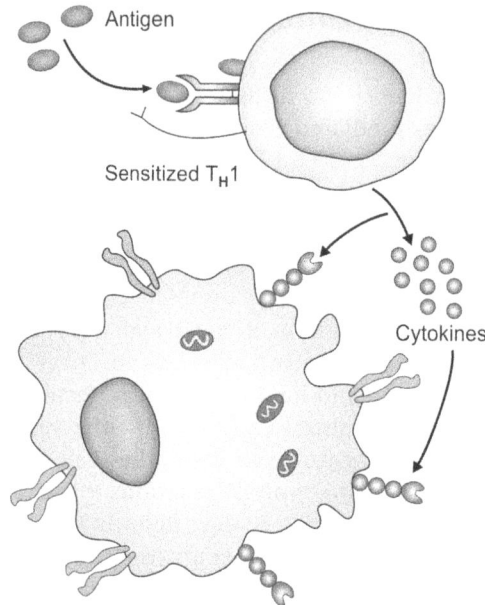

Fig. 14.3: Type IV (delayed or cell-mediated hypersensitivity).

lymphocytes and macrophages in particular. It is named delayed hypersensitivity because it appears in 24–48 hours after the presensitized host encounters the antigen, while immediate hypersensitivity reactions develop in 0.5–12 hours (**Fig. 14.3**).

Delayed hypersensitivity cannot be passively transferred by serum but can be transferred by lymphocytes or the transfer factor.

Types of Delayed Hypersensitivity

Two types of delayed hypersensitivity are recognized: The tuberculin (infection) type and the contact dermatitis type.

1. *Tuberculin (infection) type*
In tuberculin hypersensitivity, tuberculin or purified protein derivative (PPD) is injected into the skin of the forearm. Intradermally, in an individual sensitized to tuberculoprotein by prior infection or immunization. An indurated (firm and hard) inflammatory reaction, 10 mm or more in diameter, develops at the site of injection within 48–72 hours. It is characterized by erythema due to increased blood flow to the damaged area and the infiltration with a large number of mononuclear cells, mainly T lymphocytes and about 10–20% macrophages into the injection site are responsible for the induration.

The tuberculin test; therefore, provides useful indication of the state of delayed hypersensitivity (cell-mediated immunity) to the bacilli. Tuberculin type hypersensitivity develops in many infections with bacteria, fungi, viruses and parasites.

2. *Contact dermatitis type*
Allergic contact dermatitis is caused by haptens that combine with proteins in the skin to form the allergen that elicits the immune response.

Examples: Examples of these haptens include cosmetics, plant materials topical chemotherapeutic agents, metals (nickel and chromium), and chemicals.

TYPE V HYPERSENSITIVITY (STIMULATORY TYPE): JONES-MOTE REACTION (OR) CUTANEOUS BASOPHIL HYPERSENSITIVITY

This is an antibody-mediated hypersensitivity and is a modification of Type II hypersensitivity reaction.

Shwartzman Reaction

This is not an immune reaction but rather a perturbation in factors affecting intravascular coagulation.

KEY POINTS

Hypersensitivity is an exaggerated immune response that results in tissue damage and is manifested in the individual on second or subsequent contact with an antigen. Hypersensitivity reactions are of five types: Types I, II, III, IV, and V.

IMPORTANT QUESTIONS

1. What is hypersensitivity? How do you classify various types of hypersensitivity reactions? Describe type I hypersensitivity reactions.

2. Write short notes on:
   a. Anaphylaxis
   b. Atopy
   c. Type III hypersensitivity (or) immune complex diseases
   d. Arthus reaction
   e. Serum sickness
   f. Type IV hypersensitivity (or) delayed hypersensitivity (DTH)

MULTIPLE CHOICE QUESTIONS

1. All the following statements are true for type I hypersensitivity reaction, *except*:
   a. It is called immediate hypersensitivity reaction
   b. It always involves IgE-mediated degranulation of basophils or mast cells
   c. This reaction is always rapid
   d. Atopy is one of the manifestation
2. All are primary mediators of anaphylaxis, *except*:
   a. Histamine
   b. Proteases
   c. Eosinophil chemotactic factors of anaphylaxis
   d. Platelet activating factor
3. Schultz-Dale phenomenon is an example of:
   a. Type I hypersensitivity reaction
   b. Type II hypersensitivity reaction
   c. Type III hypersensitivity reaction
   d. Type IV hypersensitivity reaction
4. All the followings diseases are true for Arthus reaction, *except*:
   a. It is a local manifestation of generalized hypersensitivity
   b. The tissue damage is due to formation of local precipitating immune complexes
   c. This is systemic form of type II hypersensitivity
   d. It manifests after a single injection of a high concentration of foreign serum
5. All the followings diseases are true for serum sickness, *except*:
   a. It manifests after a single injection of a high concentration of foreign serum
   b. Disease is self-limited
   c. This is systemic form of type II hypersensitivity
   d. It is a localized inflammatory reaction due to deposition of immune complexes
6. Delayed hypersensitivity reaction is mediated by:
   a. T lymphocytes
   b. B lymphocytes
   c. Macrophages
   d. Basophils
7. Shwartzman reaction is an example of:
   a. Type I hypersensitivity reaction
   b. Type II hypersensitivity reaction
   c. Type III hypersensitivity reaction
   d. None of the above

ANSWERS

1. b   2. d   3. c   4. d
5. d   6. a   7. d

Autoimmunity

CHAPTER 15

LEARNING OBJECTIVES

After reading and studying this chapter, you should be able to:
- Describe the mechanisms of autoimmunity.
- Classify autoimmune diseases.
- List autoimmune diseases.

INTRODUCTION

One of the classically accepted features of the immune system is the capacity to distinguish self from nonself. Normally, a person is tolerized to self-antigens during the development of the immune system as a fetus and later in life by other mechanisms (e.g., oral tolerization).

DEFINITION

Autoimmunity is a condition in which structural or functional damage is produced by the action of immunologically competent cells or antibodies against the normal components of the body. Autoimmunity is due to copious production of autoantibodies and autoreactive T cells.

MECHANISMS OF AUTOIMMUNITY

A variety of mechanisms have been proposed for induction of autoimmunity.
1. **Forbidden clones:** During embryonic life, clones of cells that have immunological reactivity with self-antigens are eliminated. Such clones are called **forbidden clones**. Their persistence or development in later life by somatic mutation can lead to autoimmunity.
2. **Neoantigens or altered antigens:** Cells or tissues may undergo antigenic alteration as a result of physical, chemical or biological influences. Such altered or "neoantigens" may elicit an immune response.
3. **Molecular mimicry:** The fortuitous similarity between some foreign and self-antigens is the basis of the "cross reacting antigens" theory of autoimmunity.
4. **Polyclonal B-cell activation**
5. **Activity of helper and suppressor T-cells**
6. **Sequestered antigens:** Certain self-antigens are present in closed systems and are not accessible to the immune apparatus. These are known as **sequestered antigens**, e.g., (i) Lens antigen of the eye; (ii) Sperm antigens; (iii) Heart muscle antigens.
7. **Defects in the idiotype-anti-idiotype network**
8. **Genetic factors**

CLASSIFICATION OF AUTOIMMUNE DISEASES

Based on the site of involvement and nature of lesions, autoimmune diseases may be classified as:
A. Localized (or organ specific), e.g., Hashimoto's thyroiditis (self-antigen is thyroid proteins and cell; immune response autoantibodies).
B. Systemic (or nonorgan specific), e.g., rheumatoid arthritis (self-antigen is

connective tissue, IgG; immune response is autoantibodies, immune complexes).

KEY POINT

Autoimmunity is a condition in which structural or functional damage is produced by the action of immunologically competent cells or antibodies against the normal components of the body.

IMPORTANT QUESTIONS

1. What is autoimmunity? What are the mechanisms of autoimmune diseases giving suitable examples?
2. Write briefly on:
   a. Autoimmunity
   b. Mechanisms of autoimmune diseases

MULTIPLE CHOICE QUESTIONS

1. Lens protein of eye is an example of:
   a. Sequestered antigen
   b. Neoantigen
   c. Cross reacting antigen
   d. Molecular mimicry
2. **All of the following diseases are examples of organ-specific autoimmune diseases, *except*:**
   a. Goodpasture's syndrome
   b. Graves' disease
   c. Insulin-dependent diabetes mellitus
   d. Systemic lupus erythematosus

ANSWERS

1. a   2. d

Section 3

Systemic Bacteriology

SECTION OUTLINE

16. *Staphylococcus*
17. *Streptococcus* and *Enterococcus*
18. *Pneumococcus*
19. *Neisseria* and *Moraxella*
20. *Corynebacterium*
21. *Bacillus*
22. *Clostridium*
23. Nonsporing Anaerobes
24. *Mycobacterium I: Mycobacterium tuberculosis*
25. *Mycobacterium III: Mycobacterium leprae*
26. Nontuberculous Mycobacteria
27. Actinomycetes: *Actinomyces, Norcardia*
28. Enterobacteriaceae: *Escherichia, Klebsiella, Proteus*, and other Genera
29. *Shigella*
30. Enterobacteriaceae III: *Salmonella*
31. *Vibrio*
32. *Campylobacter* and *Helicobacter*
33. *Pseudomonas, Stenotrophomonas*, and *Burkholderia*
34. *Legionella*
35. *Yersinia, Pasteurella* and *Francisella*
36. *Haemophilus*
37. *Bordetella*
38. *Brucella*
39. Spirochaetes
40. *Mycoplasma* and *Ureaplasma*
41. Miscellaneous Bacteria
42. Rickettsiaceae, Bartonellaceae, and *Coxiella*
43. *Chlamydia* and *Chlamydophila*

CHAPTER 16

Staphylococcus

LEARNING OBJECTIVES

After reading and studying this chapter, you should be able to:
- Describe species of *Staphylococcus*.
- Describe morphology and culture characteristics of *Staphylococcus aureus*.
- List characteristics of *S. aureus* strains.
- Explain coagulase test.
- List and describe toxins and enzymes of *S. aureus*.
- Describe staphylococcal diseases.
- Discuss laboratory diagnosis of infections caused by *S. aureus*.
- Explain methicillin-resistant staphylococci and its clinical problem.
- Describe the following: coagulase-negative staphylococci (CNS); Micrococci.
- Distinguish characteristics of *S. aureus, S. epidermidis,* and *S. saprophyticus*.

INTRODUCTION

Staphylococci are gram-positive cocci that occur in grape-like clusters. They are ubiquitous and the most common cause of localized suppurative lesions in human beings.

Species: Species of staphylococci are classified by the coagulase test into two groups: the **coagulase-positive** (*Staphylococcus aureus*) and **coagulase-negative staphylococci (CNS)**, e.g., *S. epidermidis* and *S. saprophyticus*.

STAPHYLOCOCCUS AUREUS

Morphology

They are spherical cocci, approximately 1 μm in diameter, arranged characteristically in grape-like clusters (**Fig. 16.1**). Cluster formation is due to cell division occurring in three planes, with daughter cells tending to remain in close proximity. They stain readily with aniline dyes and are uniformly gram positive.

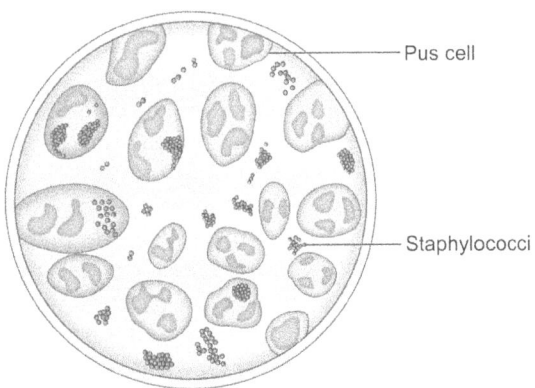

Fig. 16.1: *Staphylococcus* in a smear of pus.

Cultural Characteristics

They are aerobes and facultative anaerobes. Optimum temperature for growth is 37°C (range being 12–44°C). Optimum pH is 7.5. They can grow readily on ordinary media.

1. **Nutrient agar:** After aerobic incubation for 24 hours at 37°C, colonies are 2–4 mm in diameter and have a smooth glistening

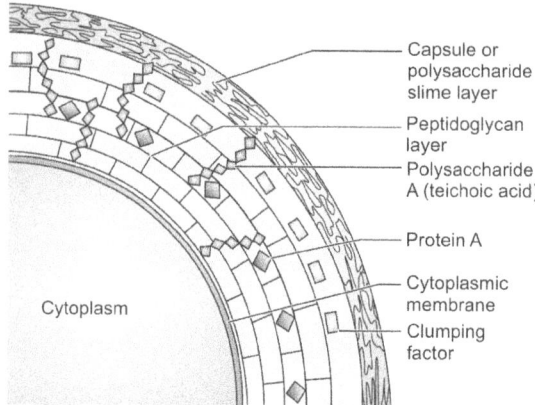

Fig. 16.2: Structure of staphylococcal cell wall.

Table 16.1: Characteristics of *Staphylococcus aureus* strains.
1. Beta hemolysis-produce clear hemolysis on blood agar
2. Golden yellow pigment
3. Coagulase positive
4. Greater biochemical activity, ferment mannite
5. Liquefy gelatin
6. Produce phosphatase
7. Black colonies on potassium tellurite blood agar
8. Produce thermostable nucleases, which can be demonstrated by the ability of boiled cultures to degrade DNA in an agar diffusion test.

surface, an entire edge, a soft butyrous consistency and an opaque, pigmented appearance. Most strains produce golden-yellow *(aureus)* pigment. The pigment is believed to be lipoprotein allied to carotene.
2. **Blood agar:** The colonies have the same appearances as on nutrient agar, but may be surrounded by a zone of β-**hemolysis (Fig. 16.2)**.
3. **MacConkey agar:** Colonies are smaller and are pink due to lactose fermentation.
4. **Milk agar:** On this medium, the colonies of *S. aureus* are larger than those on nutrient agar and pigmentation is well developed.
5. **Phenolphthalein phosphate agar:** This is an indicator medium and assists in the identification of *S. aureus* in mixed cultures.
6. **Selective salt media:** For selective medium **7–10%** of sodium chloride may be added to **nutrient agar (salt agar)** or **milk agar (salt milk agar), mannitol salt agar,** and **Ludlam's medium,** and salt-cooked meat broth.

Biochemical Reactions

1. **Sugar fermentation:** *S. aureus* ferments a range of sugar-producing acid but no gas.
2. **Catalase:** Catalase positive.
3. **Lipolytic**
4. **Phosphatase test:** This is a useful screening procedure for differentiating *S. aureus* from *S. epidermidis* in mixed cultures.
5. **Deoxyribonulease (DNAase) test:** It is positive.

Table 16.1 shows characteristics of *S. aureus*.

Resistance

Staphylococcus aureus and the other micrococcaceae are among the hardest of the nonsporing bacteria. They have been isolated from dried pus after 2–3 months. It withstands moist heat at 60°C for 30 minutes but is killed after 60 minutes.

Antigenic Structure of *Staphylococcus aureus*

The antigenic structure of *S. aureus* (**Fig. 16.2**) is complex. It is as follows:

A. Cell-associated Polymers

1. **Capsule:** Capsular polysaccharide surrounding the cell wall inhibits opsonization.
2. **Peptidoglycan: The cell wall polysaccharide peptidoglycan** confers rigidity and structural integrity to the bacterial cell.
3. **Teichoic acids:** Teichoic acid, an antigenic component of the cell wall.

B. Cell Surface Proteins

1. **Protein A:** Protein A is a group-specific antigen unique to *S. aureus* strains.
2. **Cytoplasmic membrane**
3. **Clumping factor (bound coagulase):** The component, on the cell wall of *S. aureus* that results in the clumping of whole

staphylococci in the presence of plasma, is referred to as the clumping factor (also called **bound coagulase**).

Toxins and Enzymes

Staphylococcus aureus forms a number of toxins and enzymes. They are important virulence factors for producing a disease in the host including:
1. Cytolytic or membrane-damaging toxins [alpha, beta, delta, gamma, and Panton-Valentine (P-V) leukocidin]
2. Enterotoxins (A-E, G-I)
3. Exfoliative toxins
4. Toxic shock syndrome toxin-l (TSST-1)

A. Toxins

1. Cytolytic Toxins
At least five cytolytic or membrane-damaging toxins (alpha, beta, delta, gamma, and P-V) leukocidin are produced by *S. aureus*.

2. Enterotoxins
This toxin is responsible for the manifestations of staphylococcal food poisoning.

3. Toxic Shock Syndrome Toxin-I (TSST-1)
Staphylococcus aureus is associated with toxic shock syndrome (TSS), a severe and often fatal disorder characterized by multiple organ dysfunctions.

4. Epidermolytic Toxins (Exfoliative Toxins)
This toxin, also known as ET or "exfoliatin" is responsible for the "staphylococcal scalded skin syndrome (SSSS)".

B. Enzymes

Staphylococcus aureus produces a number of enzymes, such as coagulase catalase, hyaluronidase, fibrinolysin, lipases, nucleases, and penicillinase.

Coagulase: *S. aureus* produces an extracellular enzyme called **coagulase,** which brings about clotting of human or rabbit plasma. It acts along with a **'coagulase reacting factor' (CRF)** present in plasma, binding to prothrombin and converting fibrinogen to fibrin. Coagulase test is the standard criterion for the identification of *S. aureus* isolates.

Coagulase and clumping factor ('bound coagulase') differ in many respects.

Coagulase test: Coagulase test is done by two methods—slide and tube coagulase test. The slide or tube coagulase test is performed to distinguish *S. aureus* from coagulase-negative species.

a. **Slide coagulase test:** The slide test detects bound coagulase. It can be detected by emulsifying a few colonies of the bacteria in a drop of normal saline on a clean glass slide and mixing it with a drop of rabbit plasma. Prompt clumping of the organisms indicates the presence of clumping factor (bound coagulase). Positive and negative controls also are set up.

b. **Tube coagulase test:** The tube coagulase test detects free coagulase. Place 1 mL volume in small test tubes of a 1- in-6 dilution of the human or rabbit plasma in saline. Emulsify a colony of the *Staphylococcus* under test in a tube of the diluted plasma. Alternatively, 0.1 mL of an overnight broth culture is added to 0.5 mL of undiluted plasma. The mixture is incubated in a water bath at 37°C for up to 4 hours. Examine at 1, 2, and 4 hours for clot formation. If positive, the plasma clots and does not flow when the tube is tilted or inverted.

False positive reaction: Citrated plasma should not be used because contaminating gram-negative bacilli (e.g., *Pseudomonas*) may utilize the citrate and produce false positive reaction. Oxalate, EDTA, or heparin, are suitable anticoagulants.

Pathogenesis

Staphylococcal infections are characteristically localized pyogenic lesions, in contrast to the spreading nature of streptococcal infections. *S. aureus* causes disease through the direct invasion and destruction of tissue or through the production of toxin.
   A. **Cutaneous infections:** These include: wound and burn infection, pustules, furuncles

or boils, carbuncles, styes, impetigo, and pemphigus neonatorum.
B. **Deep infections:** These include: osteomyelitis, periostitis, tonsillitis, pharyngitis, sinusitis, bronchopneumonia, empyema, septicemia, meningitis, endocarditis, breast abscess, renal abscess, and abscesses in the other organs.
C. **Toxin-mediated diseases**
  i. **Food poisoning:** Staphylococcal food poisoning may follow 2-6 hours after the ingestion of food in which *S. aureus* has multiplied and formed enterotoxin.
  ii. **Toxic shock syndrome (TSS):** Toxin-producing strains of *S. aureus* have been implicated in most cases of TSS, a multisystem disease that primarily afflicts young women. Most cases occur in menstruating women who use tampons. However, nonmenstruating women, children, and men with boils or staphylococcal infections of wounds can also have TSS.
  iii. **Exfoliative diseases:** These lesions are produced by the strains of S. *aureus,* which produce epidermolytic toxins. This toxin is responsible for **the SSSS,** exfoliative skin diseases in which the outer layer of epidermis gets separated from the underlying tissues. The severe form of SSSS is known as **Ritter's disease** in the newborn and **toxic epidermal necrolysis** in older patients. Milder forms are **pemphigus neonatorum** and **bullous impetigo**. Bullous impetigo is a localized form of SSSS.

Bacteriophage Typing

Staphylococci may be typed, based on their susceptibility to bacteriophages. An internationally recognized set of 23 standard typing phages is used for epidemiological studies and tracing the source of infection. Staphylococci can seldom be characterized by lysis by a single phage, but many different patterns of lysis are obtained with a set of phages. The strength of the method is more to demonstrate differences between strains than to confirm relatedness.

Staphylococcal phage typing is done by a pattern method. The strain to be typed is inoculated on a plate of nutrient agar to form a lawn culture. After drying, the phages are applied over marked squares in a fixed dose (routine test dose). After overnight incubation the culture will he observed to be lysed by some phages but not by others.

Virulent phages cause lysis of staphylococci that they can infect, and thus produce a clearing in the lawn of growth. The phage type of a strain is expressed by designation of the phages that lyse it, and there is international agreement on the interpretation of results. Thus, if a strain is lysed only by phages 3C, 55, and 71, it is called phage type 3C/55/71.

The reference center for staphylococcal phage typing in India is located in the Department of Microbiology, Maulana Azad Medical College, New Delhi.

Laboratory Diagnosis

1. **Specimens:** The specimens to be collected depend on the type of lesion, e.g., pus from suppurative lesions; Sputum from respiratory infections; food remains and vomit from cases of food poisoning; nasal and perineal swabs from suspected carriers.
2. **Direct microscopy:** Direct microscopy with Gram-stained smears is useful in the case of pus, where cocci in clusters may be seen. This is of no value for specimens like sputum where mixed bacterial flora is normally present.
3. **Culture:** The specimens are cultured on a **blood agar plate.** Specimens, where staphylococci are expected to be outnumbered by other bacteria, are inoculated on selective media like **Ludlam's or salt-milk agar or Robertson's cooked meat medium** containing 10% sodium. The inoculated media are incubated at 37°C for 18-24 hours. On blood agar plate, look for hemolysis around the colonies. The plates are inspected for golden-yellow or white colonies. Smears are examined from the culture and coagulase test done when staphylococci are isolated.

4. **Identification:** Relatively simple biochemical tests [e.g., positive reactions for coagulase (clumping factor), heat-stable nuclease, alkaline phosphatase, and mannitol fermentation] can be used to differentiate *S. aureus* and the other staphylococci.
   Coagulase test: Coagulase test is done by two methods—slide and tube coagulase test.
5. **Antibiotic sensitivity tests:** As a guide to treatment antibiotic sensitivity tests should be performed appropriate to the clinical situation.
6. **Bacteriophage typing:** Bacteriophage typing may be done, if the information is desired for epidemiological purposes.
7. **Serological tests:** Serological tests may sometimes be of help in the diagnosis of hidden deep infections.

Treatment

Benzyl penicillin is the most effective antibiotic, if the strain is sensitive. Patients allergic to penicillins may be given erythromycin, vancomycin or first-generation cephalosporins. Cloxacillin, oxacillin, flucloxacillin and methicillin are penicillinase-resistant penicillin.

Methicillin-resistant *Staphylococcus aureus* (MRSA) are also resistant to other penicillins and cephalosporins. Glycopeptides (vancomycin or teicoplanin) are the agents of choice in the treatment of MRSA infection.

For cutaneous infections, oral therapy with semisynthetic penicillin, such as cloxacillin or dicloxacillin, is usually efficacious. For **mild superficial lesions**, applications of drugs, as bacitracin, chlorhexidine or mupirocin may be sufficient.

COAGULASE-NEGATIVE STAPHYLOCOCCI (CoNS)

Staphylococcus epidermidis

Staphylococcus epidermidis is invariably present on normal human skin. It is nonpathogenic ordinarily but can cause disease when the host defenses are breached. *S. epidermidis* has a distinct predilection for foreign bodies, such as artificial heart valves, indwelling intravascular catheters, central nervous system shunts, and hip prostheses. Their etiological role is proved by repeated isolation.

Clinical Infection

1. Stitch abscesses; *Endocarditis Bacteremia*
2. Osteomyelitis
3. Wound infections
4. Prosthetic joint infections

Staphylococcus Saprophyticus

Staphylococcus saprophyticus occurs on the normal skin and in the periurethral and urethral flora. It is a common cause of urinary tract infections in sexually active young women. It may also cause urethritis in men and women, catheter-associated urinary tract infections, prostatitis in elderly men, and rarely bacteremia, sepsis, and endocarditis.

Table 16.2 lists the features useful for distinguishing the major species of staphylococci.

Sensitivity to Antibiotics

Before the introduction of penicillin, most of the strains of *S. aureus* were sensitive to this antibiotic. Staphylococci quickly developed drug resistance after penicillin was introduced. Penicillin resistance is of three types:

1. **Production of beta lactamase (penicillinase)** which inactivates penicillin by splitting the beta lactam ring. Penicillinase is an inducible enzyme and its production is usually controlled by plasmids, which are transmitted by' transduction or conjugation.
2. **Changes in bacterial surface receptors** reduce binding of beta-lactam antibiotics to cells.
3. **Development of tolerance** to penicillin, by which the bacterium is only inhibited but not killed.

Methicillin-resistant *Staphylococcus aureus* (MRSA)

Methicillin was the first compound developed to combat resistance due to penicillinase

Section 3: Systemic Bacteriology

Table 16.2: Characteristics distinguishing three species of the genus *Staphylococcus*.

Character	S. aureus	S. epidermis	S. saprophyticus
Anaerobic growth and fermentation of glucose	+	+	-
Mannitol			
Acid aerobically	+	V	V
Acid anaerobically	+	-	-
Coagulase	+	-	-
DNAase	+	-	-
Phosphatase	+	-/weak+	-
α –Toxin	+	-	-
Protein A in cell wall	+	-	-
Novobiocin sensitivity	Sensitive	Sensitive	Resistant

Table 16.3: Differentiation between Staphylococci and Micrococci.

Property	Staphylococcus	Micrococcus
Gram staining	Gram positive Grape-like clusters Uniform staining	Gram positive, darkly stained in groups of four (tetrad) or eight Often staining is not uniform
Colony characters	Colonies are golden yellow Size 1 mm	Colonies are white in color generally Size larger than staphylococcus
Anaerobic acid production from glucose	+	-
Aerobic acid production form glycerol in the presence of erythromycin	+	-
Modified oxidase	-	+
Resistance to bacitracin (0.04 unit disc)	Resistant	Sensitive
Lysosome (50 µg disk)	Resistant	Sensitive
Lysostaphin test	Sensitive	Resistance

(beta lactamase) production by staphylococci. But **methicillin-resistant S. aureus (MRSA)** became common, which were resisant not merely to penicillin, but also to all other beta lactam antibiotics and many others besides. **Glycopeptides (vancomycin or teicoplanin)** are the agents of choice in the treatment of MRSA infection.

Micrococci

Micrococci are catalase-positive, gram-positive, coagulase-negative, and usually oxidase-positive. They may occasionally colonize the skin or mucous membrane of humans, but they are only rarely associated with infections.

Only two species, *Micrococcus luteus* and *Micrococcus lylae*, remain in the genus. **Table 16.3** gives some differentiating features of *Staphylococcus* and *Micrococcus*.

KEY POINTS

Staphylococcus aureus
- *Staphylococcus* is gram-positive cocci arranged in clusters.
- **Coagulase test:** The slide or tube coagulase test is performed to distinguish *S. aureus* from coagulase-negative species.
- **Coagulase-negative Staphylococci (CoNS):** Coagulase-negative staphylococci are opportunistic pathogens that cause infection in

Chapter 16: Staphylococcus

debilitated or compromised patients, e.g., *S. epidermidis* and *S. saprophyticus*.

IMPORTANT QUESTIONS

1. Classify staphylococci. Discuss pathogenicity and laboratory diagnosis of *Staphylococcus aureus*.
2. Write short notes on:
   a. Antigenic structure of *Staphylococcus aureus*
   b. Coagulase or staphylocoagulase
   c. Toxins and enzymes of *Staphylococcus aureus*
   d. Coagulase-negative staphylococci
   e. Micrococci

MULTIPLE CHOICE QUESTIONS

1. *Staphylococcus aureus* shows the following characters, *except*:
   a. It produces golden-brown pigment on the blood agar
   b. It ferments mannitol
   c. It is novobiocin sensitive
   d. It has protein A
2. Protein A is a cell wall components of:
   a. *Staphylococcus aureus*
   b. *Staphylococcus epidermidis*
   c. All of the above
   d. None of the above
3. The enzyme coagulase shows all of the following features, *except*:
   a. It has eight serotypes
   b. It is extracellular
   c. It is detected by tube coagulase test
   d. Undiluted serum is used in the test
4. Scalded skin syndrome is caused by the following toxin of *Staphylococcus aureus*:
   a. Enterotoxins
   b. Toxin shock syndrome
   c. Exfoliative toxin
   d. Leukocidin
5. Which of the following *Staphylococcus* is novobiocin resistant?
   a. *Staphylococcus aureus*
   b. *Staphylococcus epidermidis*
   c. *Staphylococcus saprophyticus*
   d. None of the above
6. The most common cause of cystitis in a young healthy sexually active women is:
   a. *Staphylococcus aureus*
   b. *Staphylococcus epidermidis*
   c. *Staphylococcus saprophyticus*
   d. *Staphylococcus saccharolyticus*
7. All are coagulase negative staphylococci, *except*:
   a. *Staphylococcus epidermidis*
   b. *Staphylococcus saprophyticus*
   c. *Staphylococcus haemolyticus*
   d. *Staphylococcus aureus*

ANSWERS

1. a   2. a   3. d   4. c
5. c   6. c   7. d

Streptococcus and Enterococcus

LEARNING OBJECTIVES

After reading and studying this chapter, you should be able to:
- Classify streptococci.
- Describe antigenic structure of *Streptococcus pyogenes*.
- List and describe toxins and enzymes of *Streptococcus pyogenes*.
- Discuss pathogenicity of streptococci.
- List and describe toxins and enzymes of *Streptococcus pyogenes*.
- Describe nonsuppurative complications of *S. pyogenes* infections.
- Discuss laboratory diagnosis of streptococcal infections.
- Discuss group B streptococci, group D streptococci, and viridans group.

INTRODUCTION

The genus *Streptococcus* comprises of gram-positive cocci that grow in pairs or chains (**Fig. 17.1**). They are normal flora of humans and animals.

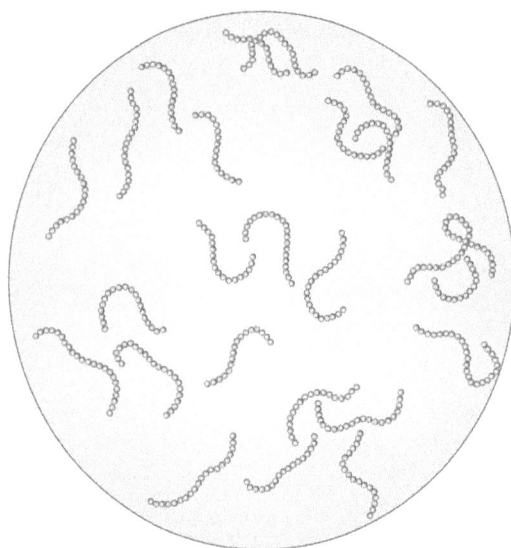

Fig. 17.1: Streptococci.

CLASSIFICATION

Streptococci are first divided into obligate anaerobe and facultative anaerobes. Obligate anaerobes are designated as peptostreptococci (**Flowchart 17.1**).

Three different schemes are used to classify the organism, as follows:
- A. **Hemolytic patterns**: Complete (β) hemolysis, incomplete (α) hemolysis, and no (γ) hemolysis.
- B. **Serologic properties**: Lancefield groupings A to H, K to M, and O to V.
- C. **Biochemical (physiologic) properties**.

A. Hemolytic Activity

1. Alpha-hemolytic (α) Streptococci

They produce a zone of partial hemolysis with a greenish discoloration around the colonies on blood agar. The zone of lysis is small (1–2 mm wide) with indefinite margin, with in this zone unlyzed erythrocytes can be made out microscopically. The streptococci producing α-hemolysis are also known as viridans streptococci (from 'virdis' meaning green).

Flowchart 17.1: Classification of streptococci.

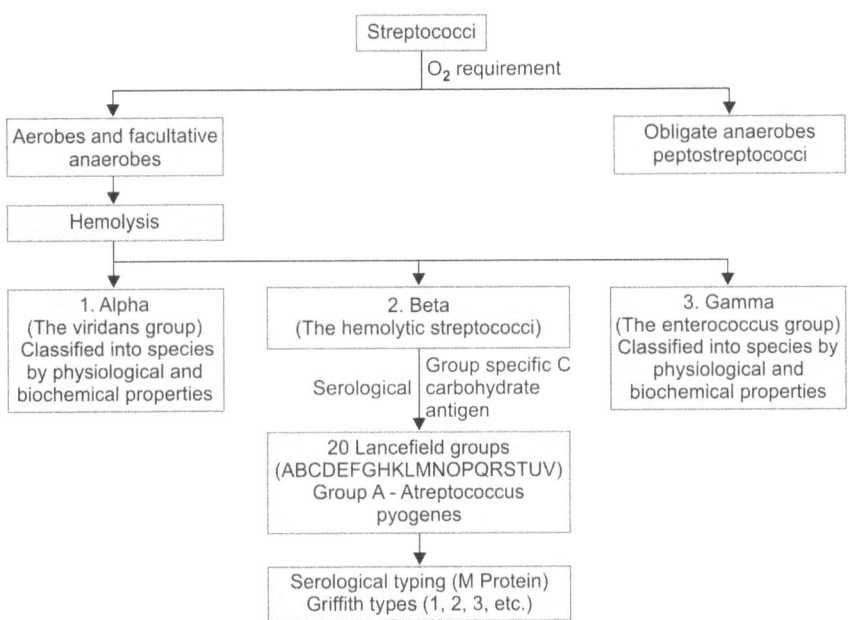

2. Beta (β) Hemolytic Streptococci

They produce a sharply defined, clear, colorless zone of hemolysis (2-4 mm wide) around the colony, caused by complete lysis of red blood cells in the agar medium induced by bacterial hemolysins. No red blood cell is visible on microscopic examination in clear zone of complete hemolysis.

3. Gamma (γ) or Nonhemolytic Streptococci

They produce no hemolysis on blood agar.

B. Serological Properties

1. **Lancefield grouping:** On the basis of group-specific carbohydrate (C) antigens in the cell wall, β-hemolytic streptococci are divided into 21 serological groups from A to W (without I and J). These are known as **Lancefield groups**.
2. **Griffith typing:** Hemolytic streptococci of group A are known as *S. pyogenes*. These are further divided into **types** based on the protein (M, T, and R) antigens present on the cell surface **(Griffith typing)**. About 80 types of *S. pyogenes* have been recognized so far (types 1, 2, 3, and so on).

C. Biochemical (Physiologic) Properties

Biochemical and other criteria are also used in defining various species within a single serogroup, and some species contain strains of more than one serogroup.

STREPTOCOCCUS PYOGENES

Morphology

Streptococcus pyogenes are gram-positive, spherical to ovoid organisms 0.5-1.0 mm in diameter. The organism grows in short or moderately long chains. Chain formation is due to the cocci dividing in one plane only and the daughter cells failing to separate completely.

Streptococci are nonmotile and nonsporing.

Cultural Characteristics

They are aerobe and facultative anaerobes, growing best at a temperature of 37°C (range 22-42°C). The optimal pH for growth is 7.4-7.6.

It is exacting in nutritive requirements, growth occurring only in media containing fermentable carbohydrates or enriched with blood or serum.

On **blood agar,** *S. pyogenes* colonies are small (0.5–1 mm in diameter), circular, semitransparent, low convex disks surrounded by a wide zone of β-hemolysis, several times greater than the diameter of the colony after incubation for 24 hours. An enhancement of growth and hemolysis are promoted by 10% CO_2.

Crystal violet blood agar and **PNF medium** (blood agar containing polymyxin-B, neomycin and fusidic acid) are selective for beta hemolytic streptococci.

In **liquid media,** such as glucose or serum broth, growth occurs as a granular turbidity with a powdery deposit. No pellicle is formed.

Biochemical Reactions

i. *S. pyogenes* is **catalase negative**.
ii. Insoluble in 10% bile unlike *S. pneumoniae*.
iii. It ferments several sugars producing acid and no gas.
iv. **Hydrolysis of pyrrolidonyl naphthylamine (PYR test)** is positive.

Antigenic Structure

Cell wall of *S. pyogenes* (**Fig. 17.2**) consists of:
1. **Capsule:** The capsule when present is composed of hyaluronic acid and inhibits phagocytosis.
2. **Group-specific polysaccharide antigen:** The cell well is composed of an outer protein (fimbria-containing protein) and lipoteichoic acid, a middle layer of group-specific carbohydrate, and inner layer of peptidoglycan.
   Serologic classification of β-hemolytic streptococci is based on their cell wall polysaccharide antigen.
3. **Type specific antigens:** Several proteins antigens have been identified in the outer layer of the cell wall. *S. pyogenes* can be typed, based on the surface proteins M, T, and R.

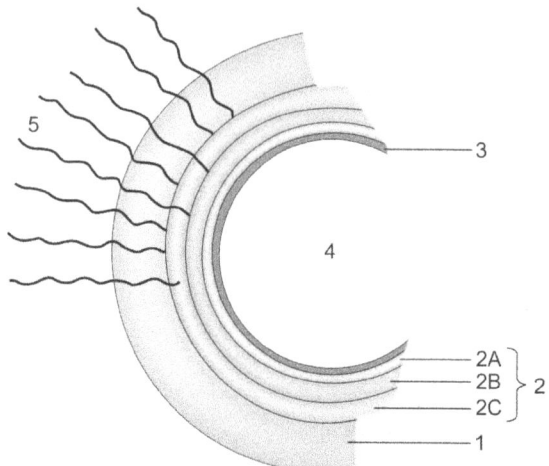

Fig. 17.2: Antigenic structure of *S. pyogenes*. (1. Hyaluronic acid capsule; 2. Cell wall comprising 2A. peptidoglycan; 2B, group specific carbohydrate; and 2C. Protein lipoteichoic acid fimbria; 3. Cytoplasmic membrane; 4. Cytoplasm; 5. Pili covered with lipoteichoic acid).

Toxins and Enzymes

1. **Hemolysins:** Two hemolytic and cytolytic toxins—streptolysin O (SLO) and streptolysin S (SLS)—are produced by most strains of group A streptococci and many strains of groups C and G.
   i. **Streptolysin O (SLO):** SLO is so called because it is oxygen-labile hemolysin. SLO is heat-labile protein, cytolytic, and capable of lysing erythrocytes, leukocytes, platelets, and cultured cells.
   ASO test: SLO is strongly antigenic and anti-streptolysin O (ASO) antibodies appears in sera following streptococcal infection. Estimation of this antibody is useful for documenting recent group A streptococcal infection (ASO test).
   ii. **Streptolysin S:** SLS is an **oxygen-stable** and causes the hemolysis around the colonies on aerobic blood culture.
2. **Pyrogenic exotoxins (erythrogenic dick, scarlatinal toxin):** The primary effect of the toxin is induction of fever and so it was renamed **Streptococcal pyrogenic exotoxin (SPE)**. This toxin was originally

called **'erythrogenic' toxins** because its intradermal injection into susceptible individuals produced an erythematous reaction (Dick test, 1924). Antitoxin injected into the skin of a patient with scarlet fever causes localized blanching as a result of neutralization of erythrogenic toxin **(Schultz–Charlton reaction).** The Dick test and Schultz Charlton reaction are now only of historical value as scarlet fever is no longer a common or serious disease.

3. **Deoxyribonucleases (Streptodornase DNAase):** There are four antigenically distinct nucleases (A, B, C, and D), of which B is the most antigenic in human beings.
4. **Streptokinase (fibrinolysin):** Streptokinase, plays a role in streptococcal infections by breaking down the fibrin barrier around the lesions and facilitates the spread of infection.
5. **Hyaluronidase:** Hyaluronidase splits hyaluronic acid, and favors the spread of infection along the intercellular spaces.
6. **Proteinase:** It destroys several proteins.
7. **Serum opacity factor (SOF):** It is produced mainly by strains causing skin infections.
8. **Nicotinamideadenine dinucleotidase (NADase):** It is believed to be leucotoxic.
9. **Other enzymes**: Many strains of streptococci also produce ATPase, phosphatase, esterases, amylase, N-acetylglucosaminidase, neuraminidase, and other toxins or enzymes.

Pathogenesis

Acute diseases associated with *Streptococcus pyogenes* occur chiefly in the **respiratory tract, bloodstream,** or the **skin**. Two post streptococcal sequelae (rheumatic fever following respiratory infection and glomerulonephritis following respiratory or skin infection), occur in 1–3% of untreated infections.

A. Suppurative Streptococcal Disease

I. Respiratory Infections

1. **Sore throat** is the most common of streptococcal disease.
2. **Suppurative complications:** The infection may spread to the surrounding tissues from the throat which may cause **suppurative complications** of streptococcal pharyngitis.

II. Skin and Soft Tissue Infections

The two typical streptococcal skin infections are erysipelas and impetigo. The main causes leading to acute glomerulonephritis in children in the tropics are impetigo and streptococcal infection of scabies lesions. It also causes cellulites, ***necrotizing fasciitis* (streptococcal gangrene) and streptococcal toxic shock syndrome.**

III. Other Suppurative Infections

1. **Puerperal sepsis:** Streptococcal puerperal sepsis used to take a heavy toll of life before antibiotics became available.
2. **Abscesses in internal organs, such as the brain, lungs, liver, and kidneys**
3. **Septicemia and pyemia**

B. Nonsuppurative Sequelae

Streptococcus pyogenes infections lead to two important nonsuppurative sequelae: acute rheumatic fever (ARF) and acute glomerulonephritis (AGN). Both are caused by immune reactions induced by the streptococcal infection. These complications ensue 1–5 weeks after the acute infection, so that the organism may not be detectable when sequelae set in.

1. Acute Rheumatic Fever

Rheumatic fever is a nonsuppurative inflammatory reaction. Typically, rheumatic fever follows persistent or repeated streptococcal throat infection with a strong antibody response.

2. Acute Poststreptococcal Glomerulonephritis

Acute glomerulonephritis (AGH) may be seen after either a pharyngeal or a cutaneous infection. AGN is most often seen in children.

Laboratory Diagnosis

1. Acute Suppurative Infections

A. **Specimens:** Throat and nose swabs, high vaginal swabs, pus or pus swabs are the usual specimens collected. Serum is obtained for antibody demonstration.

B. **Microscopy:** Presumptive information may be obtained by an examination of Gram stained films from pus and CSF. The observation of typical gram-positive cocci in chains may indicate the likelihood of the presence of streptococcal infection. In contrast, smears are of no value in infections of throat or genitalia, where streptococci may form part of the resident flora and has a poor predictive value.

C. **Culture:** The specimen is plated on blood agar and incubated at 37°C anaerobically or under 5–10% CO_2, as hemolysis develops better under these conditions. **Crystal violet blood agar** and **PNF medium** are selective media.

D. **Identification: Colonies** of *S. pyogenes* on sheep blood agar (SBA) are small, transparent, and smooth with a well-defined area of β-hemolysis. A **Gram stain** will reveal gram-positive cocci with some short chains. Hemolytic streptococci are grouped by the **Lancefield technique** using serologic methods, or biochemical tests can be performed. **The fluorescent antibody technique** has been employed for the rapid identification of group A streptococci. A key test that should be done is **bacitracin susceptibility** or **PYR hydrolysis.**
Typing of *S. pyogenes* is required for epidemiological in specialized reference laboratories.

E. **Antigen detection:** Enzyme immunoassay (EIA) or agglutination tests are used to demonstrate the presence of the antigen.

2. Nonsuppurative Complications

Serological tests: Detection of antibodies against antigens of *S. pyogenes* is an important means of establishing the diagnosis of poststreptococcal rheumatic fever and glomerulonephritis.

Anti-streptolysin O (ASO) test is used most frequently. ASO titers higher than 200 Todd units/mL are indicative of prior streptococcal infection. High levels are usually found in ARF but in glomerulonephritis, titers are often low.

Anti-deoxyribonuclease B (antiDNase B) estimation is also commonly employed. Titers higher than 300 or 350 are taken as significant. **AntiDNase B** and **anti-hyaluronidase (ASH) tests** are very useful for the retrospective diagnosis of streptococcal pyoderma.

Treatment

Streptococcal pyogenes is very sensitive to penicillin. Erythromycin or an oral cephalosporin can be used in patients with a history of penicillin allergy.

OTHER STREPTOCOCCI PATHOGENIC FOR HUMANS

Group B Streptococci: *Streptococcus agalactiae*

Streptococcus agalactiae Previously, *Streptococcus agalactiae* was recognized primarily as a cause of bovine mastitis (*agalactia*, want of milk). However, since 1960 it has become the leading cause of **neonatal infections** in industrialized countries and is also an important cause of morbidity among peripartum women and nonpregnant adults with chronic medical conditions.

S. agalactiae is found in the vaginocervical tract of female carriers, and the urethral mucus membranes of male carriers, as well as in the gastrointestinal (GI) tract, especially the rectum.

Clinical Diseases

1. **Infection in the neonate:** Two forms of neonatal disease: early-onset and late-onset; these diseases are characterized by meningitis, pneumonia, and bacteremia. **Other group B infections in neonates are** osteomyelitis, conjunctivitis, sinusitis, otitis media, endocarditis, and peritonitis may also occur.
2. **Infections in the adult:** Puerperal sepsis, pneumonia, endometritis, urinary tract infection, wound infection, and bacteremia.

Diagnosis

Identification: Presumptive identification method is based on their ability to hydrolyze

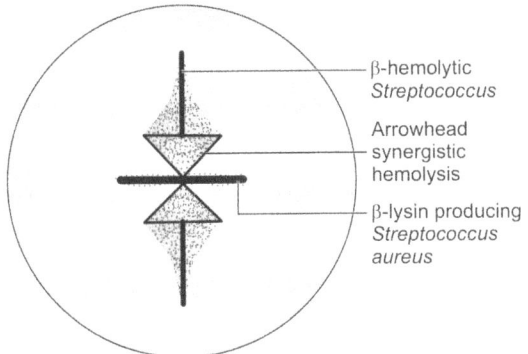

Fig. 17.3: CAMP reaction.

hippurate. They may be identified by the CAMP reaction (Christie, Atkins, and Munch–Peterson), which can be demonstrated as an accentuated zone of hemolysis (arrowhead-shaped area of enhanced hemolysis) when *S. agalactiae* is inoculated perpendicular to a streak of *S. aureus* grown on blood agar (**Fig. 17.3**).

Group D streptococci

Until the mid-1980s, the group D streptococci were divided into the two groups:
1. Enterococcus group (enterococci or fecal streptococci), which have been reclassified as a separate genus called *Enterococcus*
2. Nonenterococcal group, e.g., *S. bovis, S. equinus.*

ENTEROCOCCUS

The enterococci are gram-positive cocci typically arranged in pairs and short chains.

Species
- *Enterococcus fecalis* ("pertaining to feces").
- *Enterococcus fecium* ("of feces").

Distinctive Features of Enterococci

1. The enterococci grow in the presence of:
   - 6.5% NaCl
   - 40% bile
   - at pH 9.6
   - at 45°C
   - in 0.1% methylene blue
2. It survives heating at 60°C for 30 minutes, and also grows within a wider range of temperatures (10–45°C).
3. On MacConkey medium they produce deep pink colonies.
4. Enterococci are PYRase test positive. They do not hydrolyze hippurate.

Identification

The identification of enterococcus species is made on biochemical characteristics.

Clinical Infections

The enterococci inhabit the gastrointestinal tract and the genitourinary tract in humans and other animals. Enterococci are frequent causes of nosocomial infections and may cause **urinary tract infection, bacteremia, infective endocarditis, biliary tract infection, intra-abdominal abscess complicating diverticulitis, peritonitis, and wound infection.**

VIRIDANS STREPTOCOCCI

The viridans streptococci are commensals of mouth and upper respiratory tract. The viridans groups of streptococci are heterogeneous collection of α-hemolytic and nonhemolytic streptococci. The term *viridis* means "green" (Latin for "green") because many of these bacteria produce a greenish discoloration (α-hemolysis) on blood agar media. Some of them may be nonlytic. This group contains many species, such as *S. anginosus, S. sanguis, S. mitis, S. mutans, S. salivarius,* etc.

Clinical Infections

They are ordinarily nonpathogenic but can on occasion cause disease. Two clinically important phenomena are associated with viridans streptococci **dental caries** and **subacute endocarditis**. *Streptococcus anginosus* is responsible for causing **pyogenic infections**. They have also been implicated in meningitis, abscesses, osteomyelitis, and empyema.

Dental Caries

S. mutans is the principal cause of **dental caries (tooth decay).**

KEY POINTS

- *Streptococcus pyogenes.*
- Gram-positive cocci arranged in long chains.
  1. Suppurative streptococcal disease
     Diseases:
     A. Respiratory infection
     B. Pyogenic cutaneous infections.
     C. *Streptococcal toxic shock syndrome.*
  2. Nonsuppurtive sequelae: Rheumatic fever and acute glomerulonephritis

IMPORTANT QUESTIONS

1. Classify streptococci. Describe the laboratory diagnosis of streptococcal sore throat.
2. Write short notes on:
   a. Antigenic structure of *S. pyogenes*
   b. Lancefield grouping.
   c. Toxins and enzymes of *Streptococcus pyogenes*
   d. Pathogenicity of streptococci
   e. Nonsuppurative complications of *S. pyogenes* infections
3. Write briefly about:
   a. Group B streptococci
   b. CAMP reaction
   c. Group D streptococci
   d. Enterococci (or) fecal streptococci
   e. Viridans streptococci

MULTIPLE CHOICE QUESTIONS

1. Which type of hemolysis is produced by *Streptococcus pyogenes on* blood agar?
   a. Alpha hemolysis
   b. Beta hemolysis
   c. Gamma hemolysis
   d. None of the above
2. Group-specific antigen extraction of *Streptococcus pyogenes* by treating with hydrochloric acid method is known as:
   a. Lancefield's method
   b. Fuller's method
   c. Maxted's method
   d. Randall's method
3. Erythrogenic toxin is responsible for:
   a. Pyoderma
   b. Schultz–Charlton reaction
   c. Necrotizing fasciitis
   d. All of the above
4. Which of the following is selective medium for *Streptococcus pyogenes*?
   a. Blood agar
   b. Crystal violet blood agar
   c. Potassium tellurite blood agar
   d. Chocolate agar
5. Susceptibility to *bacitracin* can be used to identify:
   a. *Streptococcus pyogenes*
   b. *Streptococcus viridans*
   c. *Streptococcus mitis*
   d. *Streptococcus agalactiae*

ANSWERS

1. b   2. a   3. b   4. b
5. a

CHAPTER 18

Pneumococcus

LEARNING OBJECTIVES

After reading and studying this chapter, you should be able to:
- Describe morphology and cultural characters of pneumococci.
- Describe quellung reaction.
- Discuss laboratory diagnosis of pneumococcal infections.
- Differentiate between *Streptococcus pneumoniae* and *Streptococcus viridans*.

INTRODUCTION

Pneumococcus, a gram-positive lanceolate *Diplococcus*, formerly classified as *Diplococcus pneumomiae*, has been reclassified as *Streptococcus pneumoniae* because of its genetic relatedness to *Streptococcus*. Pneumococcus differs from other streptococci chiefly in its morphology, bile solubility, optochin sensitivity and possession of a specific polysaccharide capsule.

MORPHOLOGY

Pneumococci are gram-positive cocci in pairs (diplococci). The cocci are about 1 µm slightly elongated cocci, with one end broad or rounded and the other pointed, presenting a **flame-shaped or lanceolate appearance**. They may occur singly, in pairs, or in short chains but most often are seen as pairs (diplococci), with the broad ends in apposition, the long axis of the coccus parallel to the line joining the two cocci in a pair. They are nonmotile and nonsporing.

All freshly isolated strains are **capsulate (Fig. 18.1)**. The capsule encloses each pair. The capsule may be demonstrated as a clear halo in Indian ink preparations or may be stained directly by special techniques or by use of homologous type-specific antibody in the quellung reaction (**Fig. 18.2**).

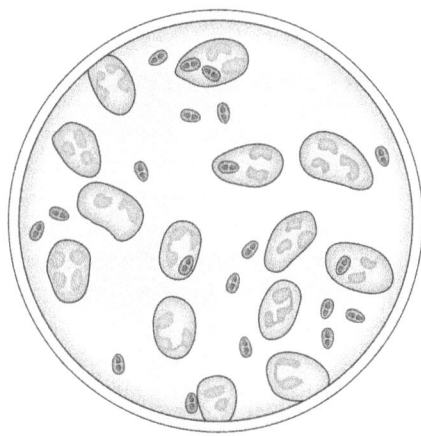

Fig. 18.1: *Streptococcus pneumoniae* in pus.

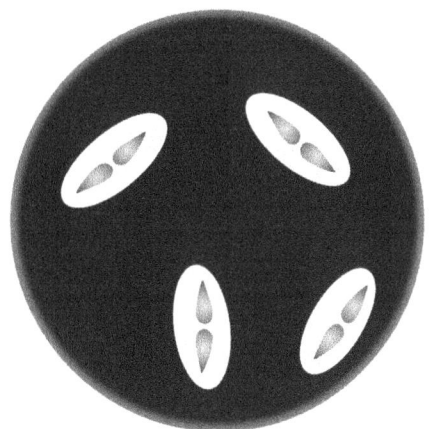

Fig. 18.2: Pneumococci. Indian ink preparation to show capsules.

CULTURAL CHARACTERISTICS

They are aerobes and facultative anaerobes. It grows best in air or hydrogen with 5-10% CO_2, for which some strains have a strict requirement. Optimum temperature being 37°C (range 25-40°C) and pH 7.8 (range 6.5-8.3).

On **blood agar**, after incubation for 18 hours, the colonies are small (0.5-1 mm), dome-shaped and glistening, with an area of green discoloration (alpha hemolysis) around them. On further incubation, the colonies become flat with raised edges and depressed centrally, so that concentric rings are seen on the surface when viewed from above **(draughtsman or carrom coin appearance)**, which is due to autolysis of bacteria within the flat pneumococcal colonies.

In **liquid media** such as glucose broth, growth occurs as uniform turbidity.

BIOCHEMICAL REACTIONS

1. **Inulin fermentation:** Pneumococci ferment several sugars with the production of acid and no gas. Fermentation is tested in Hiss's serum water or serum agar slopes. Fermentation of inulin by *Pneumococci* is a useful tests for differentiating them from streptococci as the latter do not ferment it.
2. **Bile solubility test:** For bile solubility test, grow the isolate to be tested in serum, digest broth or infusion broth, and add 10% sodium deoxycholate solution. Pneumococci are lysed and the initially turbid culture becomes clear and transparent. Pneumococci are soluble in bile; viridans and other streptococci are not.
   Alternatively, a rapid presumptive test may be made on the primary plate culture. Touch a suspected pneumococcal colony with a loopful of 2% sodium deoxycholate solution. Colonies of pneumococcus disappear leaving an area of α-hemolysis on the blood agar. Bile solubility is an important diagnostic test to differentiate *Pneumococcus* from viridans and other streptococci.
3. **Pneumococci are catalase and oxidase negative.**

RESISTANCE

Pneumococci are delicate organisms and are killed by moist heat at 55°C in 10 minute, and readily by most disinfectants.

Optochin sensitivity: Pneumococci are highly sensitive to killing by optochin (ethyl hydrocuprein hydrochloride), in a concentration of 1/50,000 and is useful in distinguishing them from *Viridans streptococci*. For testing, place a paper disc containing 5 μg of optochin on an area of a blood agar plate inoculated with *Pneumococcus*-like colonies from the primary diagnostic plate. A growth of *Pneumococcus* will be inhibited in a zone extending radially for at least 5 mm from the margin of the disk on incubation. *Viridans streptococci* will grow right up to the disk.

ANTIGENIC STRUCTURE

A. Capsular Antigens

The most important antigen of the *Pneumococcus* is the type specific capsular polysaccharide. It is also called the **"specific soluble substance (SSS)"** as this polysaccharide diffuses into the culture medium or infective exudates and tissues. These polysaccharides are antigenic and form the basis for the separation of pneumococci into different serotypes. A total of 90 different capsular serotypes have been identified. The serotypes are designated by numbers, and those that are structurally related are grouped together (1, 2, 3. 4, 5, 6A, 68, etc.).

The type of a *Pneumococcus* is determined by its reactions with type-specific antisera. The tests may be done by:

1. Agglutination of washed capsulate cocci.
2. Precipitation of SSS from culture supernates.
3. **Quellung reaction or capsule swelling reaction**

   It was described by Neufeld (1902). In the capsule swelling or 'quellung' reaction (quellung = swelling), a suspension of pneumococci is mixed on a slide with a drop of the type specific antiserum and a loopful of methylene blue solution and then examined using the oil-immersion objective. The capsule becomes apparently swollen, sharply delineated and refractile in the presence of the homologous antiserum.

B. Somatic Antigen

a. **C polysaccharide:** The cell wall of *S. pneumoniae* contains a species-specific carbohydrate antigen, referred to as **C substance**. A β-globulin in human serum, called the ***C-reactive protein (CRP)***, reacts with C substance to form a precipitate. CRP is an abnormal protein (beta globulin) that precipitates with the somatic 'C' antigen of pneumococci. It appears in acute phase sera of cases of pneumonia but disappears during convalescence. It is known as CRP. It is an 'acute phase' substance, produced in hepatocytes. Its production is stimulated by bacterial infections, inflammation, malignancies, and tissue destruction.
b. **F antigen**
c. **M protein**

PATHOGENESIS

1. **Pneumonia:** Pneumococci are one of the most common bacteria causing pneumonia, both **lobar and bronchopneumonia.** They also cause **acute tracheobronchitis** and **empyema.**
2. **Acute exacerbations in chronic bronchitis**
3. **Meningitis:** *S. pneumoniae* is among the leading causes of bacterial meningitis.
4. **Bacteremia**
5. **Other infections:** Pneumococci may also produce suppurative lesions in other parts of the body—empyema, pericarditis, otitis media, sinusitis, conjunctivitis, suppurative arthritis and peritonitis, usually as complications of pneumonia.

LABORATORY DIAGNOSIS

A. **Specimens:** Sputum, lung aspirate, pleural fluid, cerebrospinal fluid, urine, or blood are collected according to the site of lesion. Blood culture is useful in pneumococcal septicemia.
B. **Collection and transport:** All the specimens should be collected in sterile containers under all aseptic conditions. They should be processed immediately. CSF specimen should never be refrigerated in case of delay and should be kept at 37°C *(H. influenzae,* another causative agent of pyogenic meningitis may die at cold temperature).
C. **Microscopy and antigen detection:** Gram stain of sputum specimens is a rapid way to diagnose pneumococcal disease. If the smears are positive for gram-positive lancet-shaped diplococci, a presumptive diagnosis of pneumococcal pneumonia may be made. A centrifuged deposit of the CSF should be examined immediately in a Gram film in case of meningitis and presumptive diagnosis may be made by finding gram-positive diplococci both inside the polymorphs and extracellularly.
Pneumococcal antigen is often detectable by coagglutination (COA), latex agglutination (LA) or counterimmunoelectrophoresis (CIE), and ELISA.
D. **Capsule swelling tests:** For the identification of pneumococci by direct examination is the quellung reaction.
E. **Culture:** Specimen is inoculated on the plates of blood agar and heated-blood agar incubated in air with 5-10% CO_2 for 18-24 hours. Typical colonies develop with α-hemolysis. The colonies are small (0.5-1 mm), dome-shaped, and glistening, with an area of green discoloration (alpha hemolysis) around them. On further incubation, the colonies have **draughtsman or carrom-coin appearance.**
F. **Identification:** Procedures commonly used to distinguish *S. pneumoniae* from the *Viridans streptococci* are optochin susceptibility, bile solubility, and the quellung reaction. *S. pneumoniae* is susceptible to optochin, whereas other α-hemolytic species are resistant (**Table 18.1**).
G. **Intraperitoneal injection into mice:** Isolation may be obtained by intraperitoneal

Table 18.1: Differential characters of pneumococci and viridans streptococci.

Character	Pneumococcus	Viridans streptococci
Morphology	Ovoid or lanceolate diplococci; some short chains	Short or long chains of rounded cocci
Capsule	Present	Usually absent
Colonies	Become flattened or draughtsman	Convex
Effect on blood agar	Narrow zones of α-hemolysis	Wide or narrow zone of α-hemolysis
Optochin sensitivity	Sensitive	Resistant
Bile solubility	+	–
Inulin fermentation	+	–
Virulence in mice	+	–

inoculation in mice from specimens where pneumococci are expected to be scanty. Inoculated mice die in 1–3 days, and pneumococci may be demonstrated in the peritoneal exudate and heart blood.

H. **Blood culture:** In the acute stage of pneumonia, the organism may be obtained from blood culture in glucose broth.

I. **Antibiotic sensitivity test:** It is especially useful in strains which are resistant.

TREATMENT

Penicillin is the drug of choice for susceptible strains. Cephalosporin, erythromycin, chloramphenicol, or vancomycin are used for patients allergic to penicillin or for treatment of penicillin-resistant strains.

- Diseases—pneumonia, meningitis, sinusitis and otitis media, and a variety of systemic infections, including bacteremia and endocarditis.

IMPORTANT QUESTIONS

1. Describe the laboratory diagnosis of pneumococcal infections.
2. Differentiate between S. pneumoniae and S. viridans in a tabulated form.

MULTIPLE CHOICE QUESTIONS

1. Which of the following bacteria produce alpha hemolysis on blood agar?
   a. Staphylococcus aureus
   b. Streptococcus pyogenes
   c. Streptococcus pneumoniae
   d. All of the above
2. Draughtsman appearance colony is a characteristic feature of:
   a. Streptococcus pyogenes
   b. Streptococcus pneumoniae
   c. Enterococcus jacecalis
   d. Viridans streptococci
3. Streptococcus pneumoniae causes following infections, *except*:
   a. Otitis media
   b. Urinary tract infections
   c. Meningitis
   d. Sinusitis
4. Streptococcus pneumoniae shows following characteristics, *except*:
   a. Optochin sensitivity test positive
   b. Bile solubility test positive
   c. Inulin fermentation test positive
   d. Bacitracin test positive
5. Pneumococcal 23-valent polysaccharide is given to the following persons, *except*:
   a. Child younger than 2 years
   b. Persons older than 65 years
   c. Persons with HIV infections
   d. Persons with diabetes mellitus

KEY POINTS

- **Streptococcus pneumoniae** are **elongated or "lancet-shaped"**, gram-positive cocci arranged in pairs (diplococci). They are **capsulated.**

ANSWERS

1. c 2. b 3. b 4. d
5. b

CHAPTER 19

Neisseria and Moraxella

LEARNING OBJECTIVES

After reading and studying this chapter, you should be able to:
- Describe morphology, culture characteristics, biochemical reactions, and antigenic structure of *Neisseria meningitidis*.
- Discuss pathogenicity and laboratory diagnosis of meningococcal meningitis.
- Describe morphology, culture characteristics, biochemical reactions of *Neisseria gonorrheae*.
- Discuss pathogenicity of *N. gonorrhoeae*.
- Discuss laboratory diagnosis of gonorrhea.

INTRODUCTION

Members of the genus *Neisseria* are aerobic, gram-negative cocci typically arranged in pairs (diplococci) with adjacent sides flattened together (resembling coffee beans). All species are oxidase-positive, and most produce catalase-properties.

Species: Important species of the genus *Neisseria* are: *N. meningitidis, N. gonorrheae, N. flavescens, N. subflava, N. sicca, N. mucosa, N. lactamica,* and *N. polysaccharaeae*. *N gonorrheae* is always pathogenic, but *N. meningitidis* may be found as a commensal inhabitant of the upper respiratory tract of carriers. Other *Neisseria* species occur as commensals in the upper respiratory tract.

NEISSERIA MENINGITIDIS

(Meningococcus; Diplococcus intracellularis meningitidis)

Morphology

Meningococci are **gram-negative** oval or spherical **cocci** (0.6–0.8 µm in size), typically arranged in pairs, with the adjacent sides flattened or concave opposing edges and the long axes parallel. They are typically seen in large numbers inside polymorphonuclear leukocytes **(Fig. 19.1)**. Most fresh isolates are capsulated. They are nonsporing and nonmotile.

Cultural Characteristics

They are strict aerobes, no growth occurring anaerobically. The optimum temperature for growth is 35–36°C. No growth takes place below 30°C. Optimum pH is 7.0–7.4. Growth is facilitated

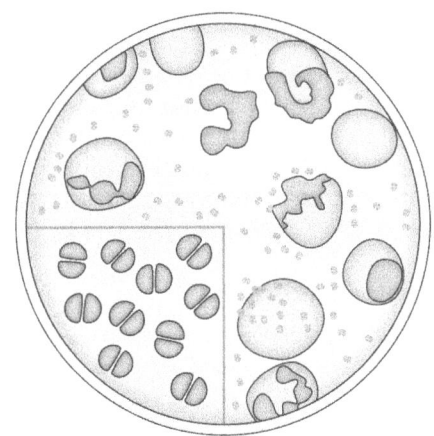

Fig. 19.1: *N. meningitidis* in cerebrospinal fluid. Inset—enlarged view showing flat adjacent sides of cocci.

by 5–10% CO_2 and high humidity. Meningococci have exacting growth requirements and do not grow on ordinary media. Growth occurs on media enriched with blood, serum or ascitic fluid. Blood agar, chocolate agar, and Mueller-Hinton starch casein hydrolysate agar are the media commonly used for culturing meningococci. Modified Thayer-Martin (with vancomycin, colistin and nystatin) is a useful selective medium.

On **blood agar** after 24 hours incubation, colonies are 1–2 mm in diameter, round, convex, gray, translucent, and nonhemolytic.

Heated blood (chocolate) agar—colonies are slightly larger on heated blood (chocolate) agar than on ordinary blood agar. Growth is poor in liquid media, producing a granular turbidity with little or no surface growth.

Biochemical Reactions

1. They are **catalase and oxidase positive**.
   Oxidase test: The oxidase test is a key test for identifying them. When 1% solution of oxidase reagent (tetramethylparaphenylene-diamine-dihydrochloride) is poured on culture media, *Neisseria* colonies quickly turn deep-purple. This prompt oxidase reaction helps in the identification of meningococci and gonococci in mixed cultures.
   The test may also be performed by rubbing a little of the growth with a loop on a strip of filter paper moistened with the oxidase reagent (Kovacs' method). A deep purple color appears immediately.
2. **Sugar fermentation:** Meningococci ferment glucose and maltose with the production of acid but no gas but not lactose or sucrose (gonococci ferment glucose but not maltose).
3. **Indole and hydrogen sulfide** are not produced and **nitrates** are not reduced.

Antigenic Classification

Based on their capsular polysaccharide antigens, meningococci are classified into at least 13 serogroups: A, B, C, X, Y, Z, Zl (29E) and W135. Further serogroups H, I, K, and L have also been described. Groups A, B, and C are the most important. Serogroups are further classified into **serotypes** and **subtypes**.

Resistance

Meningococci are very delicate organisms, being highly susceptible to heat, desiccation, alterations in pH and to disinfectants. They die within a few days at room temperature. They are killed by heating at 55°C in 5 minutes.

Pathogenicity

Meningococci are strict human parasites inhabiting the nasopharynx. Infection is usually asymptomatic. In some, local inflammation ensues, with rhinitis and pharyngitis. Dissemination occurs only in a small proportion.

Stages of Meningococcal Infections

There are three stages of meningococcal infection.
1. **First stage: Nasopharyngeal infection**
2. **Second stage: Meningococcal septicemia**—in a small percentage of cases the meningococci enter the bloodstream. This stage, called **meningococcemia.** The organisms may also cause lesions in the joints and lungs and rarely cause massive bilateral hemorrhages in the adrenals **(Waterhouse-Friderichsen syndrome).** It is an overwhelming and usually fatal condition, characterized by shock, **disseminated intravascular coagulation (DIC),** and **multisystem failure**.
3. **Third stage: Meningitis**

Laboratory Diagnosis

1. **Specimens**
   i. Cerebrospinal fluid (CSF)
   ii. Blood for culture
   iii. Aspirate from skin lesions or pus from an infected joint
   vi. Throat or nasopharyngeal swabs
   Swabs should be transported in Stuart's transport medium. All specimens where meningococcal infection is suspected must be submitted to the laboratory immediately.
2. **Examination of CSF:** If meningitis is suspected, a lumbar puncture should be performed.
   i. **Perform a cell count.** The exudate in meningococcal meningitis is typically polymorphonuclear.

ii. **Centrifuge the remaining CSF.** Make a smear of the centrifuged deposit and stain with Gram stain. CSF from a typical case of meningococcal meningitis will show gram-negative diplococci inside a limited proportion of the pus cells; many are extracellular.
Stain a second film with methylene blue to determine the cell type; occasionally, diplococci may be seen more easily with this stain.
If fluorescein isothiocyanate-coupled antiserum is available, a smear of the deposits may be examined for the direct identification of the meningococcal serogroup responsible for infection.
iii. **Divide the supernatant CSF into two aliquots:** One to be kept if necessary for **biochemical examination**, the other to be examined for the presence of **meningococcal polysaccharide antigen** by counterimmunoelectrophoresis, latex agglutination or coagglutination using meningococcal antisera.
iv. **Culture:** Plate out the centrifuged deposit on both blood and heated blood agar (chocolate agar) and incubate at 37°C in 5–10% CO_2. Colonies appear after 18–24 hours, which may be identified by morphology and biochemical reactions.
Subculture: Add Robertson's cooked meat broth to the remaining deposit, incubate overnight and subculture in the same way.
v. **Sugar utilization tests** or commercial kits are used to identify any gram-negative diplococci. The oxidase test is performed on colonies on solid medium.
vi. Set up antibiotic sensitivity tests.
vii. **Serogrouping** is performed by slide agglutination with hyper immune sera.
3. **Blood cultures:** Blood culture is often positive in meningococcemia and in early cases of meningitis. Cultures should be incubated for 4–7 days. Subculture to blood agar and heated blood agar, incubate cultures in 5–10% CO_2 for 24 hours and examine oxidase-positive colonies of gram-negative diplococci as above.
4. **Pus, aspirates, and swabs:** In addition to blood agar and heated blood agar, Thayer-Martin selective medium is used for the culture of materials.
5. **Petechial lesions:** For microscopy and culture
6. **Serological diagnosis:** Hemagglutination test, ELISA tests
7. **Polymerase chain reaction** (PCR)

Treatment

Penicillin is currently the antibiotic of choice, either chloramphenicol or a third generation cephalosporin such as cefotaxime or ceftriaxone is used in persons allergic to penicillin allergy.

Prophylaxis

1. **Chemoprophylaxis: Minocycline** and **rifampin** have been used effectively for antibiotic-mediated chemoprophylaxis. **Ciprofloxacin** is widely used as a prophylactic for adolescents and adults as a single, oral dose.
2. **Immunoprophylaxis:** A polyvalent vaccine effective against serogroups A, C, Y, and W135, which can be administered to children older than 2 years, has been developed. There is no Group B vaccine available at present.

NEISSERIA GONORRHOEAE (GONOCOCCUS)

Neisseria gonorrhoeae causes the venereal disease gonorrhea.

Morphology

In smears from the urethral discharge in acute gonorrhea, the organism appears as a diplococcus with the adjacent sides concave, being typically kidney shaped. It is found predominantly within the polymorphs, some cells containing as many as a hundred cocci (**Fig. 19.2**).

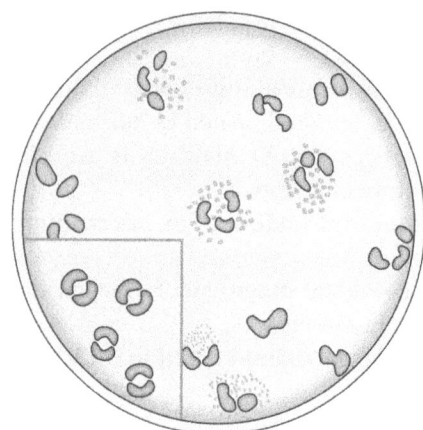

Fig. 19.2: *N. gonorrheae* in urethal pus. Inset—enlarged view showing diplococci with adjacent surfaces concave.

Cultural Characters

Gonococci are more difficult to grow than meningococci. They are aerobic but may grow anaerobically also. Growth occurs best at pH 7.0–7.4 and at a temperature of 35–36°C. It is essential to provide 5–10% CO_2.

They grow well on **chocolate agar** and **Mueller–Hinton agar.** A popular selective medium is the **Thayer–Martin medium (chocolate agar containing vancomycin, colistin, and nystatin),** which inhibits most contaminants including nonpathogenic neisseria. Colonies are small, round, translucent, convex or slightly umbonate, with finely granular surface and lobate margins after incubation for 24 hours.

Biochemical Reactions

The gonococcus is oxidase positive and resembles meningococci except in the fermentation of maltose. Gonococci ferment only glucose and not maltose. This can be remembered by G for gonococcus and **M+G for meningococcus.**

Antigenic Structure

The structure of *N. gonorrheae* is typical of gram-negative bacteria. The surface structures include the following:
A. **Pili:** Pili are hair-like appendages that extend up to several micrometers from the gonococcal surface. They act as virulence factors by promoting attachment to host cells and inhibiting phagocytosis. The pili are composed of repeating protein subunits (pilins).
B. **Por proteins (protein I):** Form pores or channels in the outer membrane.
C. **Opa protein (protein II):** These proteins facilitate bacterial adherence.
D. **Rmp (protein III):** These proteins stimulate antibodies.
E. **Lipooligosaccharide (LOS):** This antigen possesses endotoxic activity.

Resistance

The gonococcus is a very delicate organism, readily killed by drying, soap and water, and many other cleansing or antiseptic agents at their correct use-dilution. Organisms may remain viable for a day or so in pus contaminating linen or other fabrics. In cultures, the coccus dies in 3–4 days at room temperature. Freeze-drying is the most reliable method for long-term storage of gonococci but storage at −70°C or in liquid nitrogen may be more convenient for intermediate storage.

Pathogenesis

Gonorrhea

Gonorrhea is a venereal disease and is acquired by sexual contact. The incubation period is 2–8 days.
A. **Disease in men:** The most common clinical presentation is **acute urethritis** in the male. The infection extends along the urethra to the prostate, seminal vesicles, and epididymis. Proctitis occurs in both the sexes.
B. **Disseminated gonococcal disease** may lead to metastatic lesions, such as arthritis, ulcerative endocarditis, and very rarely meningitis.
C. **Disease in children**
   i. **Ophthalmic neonatorum:** A nonvenereal infection is **ophthalmia neonatorum** in the newborn, in which the eyes are coated with gonococci as the baby passes down the birth canal.
   ii. **Vulvovaginitis**

Laboratory Diagnosis

Diagnosis can be established readily in the acute stage but chronic cases sometimes present great difficulties.

1. Specimens

A. Specimens in men
1. **Urethra:** In men, urethral samples usually suffice. In **acute gonorrhea** the urethral discharge contains gonococci in large numbers. In **chronic infections**, there may not be any urethral discharge. The morning drop of secretion may be examined or some exudate may be obtained after prostatic massage. It may also be possible to demonstrate gonococci in the centrifuged deposits of urine in cases where no urethral discharge is available.
2. **Anal canal** in homosexual males.

B. **Specimens in women:** In women urethral, cervical, and rectal specimens should always be examined.

C. **Blood, swabs of skin lesions, or pus aspirated from a joint**

D. **Conjunctival swab:** Particularly in neonatal ophthalmia.

E. **Urine specimen**

2. Transport

For culture, specimens should be inoculated on prewarmed plates, immediately on collection. If this is not possible, specimens should be collected with charcoal impregnated swabs and sent to the laboratory in Stuart's transport medium.

3. Direct Microscopy

Gram staining shows characteristic kidney-shaped gram-negative diplococci. Approximately, 95% of infected men will yield a positive smear. It has to be emphasized that diagnosis of gonorrhea by smear examination is unreliable in women as some of the normal genital flora have an essentially similar morphology.

Immunologic methods include coagglutination and fluorescent antibody testing.

4. Culture

In acute gonorrhea, cultures can be obtained readily on chocolate agar or Mueller–Hinton agar incubated at 35–36°C under 5–10% CO_2. In chronic cases, where mixed infection is usual, it is better to use a selective medium such as the Thayer–Martin medium. Examine plates after 24 hours incubation and the growth is identified by morphology and biochemical reactions.

Colonies are small, round, translucent, convex or slightly umbonate, with finely granular surface and lobate margins.

Smear is made from the colony and Gram staining is done. Gonococci are gram-negative cocci arranged in pairs (diplococci) with adjacent sides concave (pear or bean-shaped).

5. Identification

Neisseria species: *N gonorrheae* is oxidase positive. It ferments glucose with acid only. It does not ferment maltose unlike meningococci.

6. Genetic Probes

Treatment

Penicillin is no longer the antibiotic of choice for treatment of gonorrhea.

Penicillinase producing gonococci (PPNG) have appeared, rendering penicillin treatment ineffective.

Currently **ceftriaxone, cefixime, ciprofloxacin, or ofloxacin are** used as the initial therapy for cases of **uncomplicated gonorrhea.**

KEY POINTS

Neisseria meningitidis
- Gram-negative diplococci with fastidious growth requirements.
- **Diseases:** Meningitis, meningoencephalitis, bacteremia, pneumonia, arthritis, and urethritis

N. gonorrhoeae
- Gram-negative diplococci.
- **Diseases:** Urethritis, cervicitis, salpingitis, pelvic inflammatory disease, proctitis, bacteremia, arthritis, conjunctivitis, pharyngitis

IMPORTANT QUESTIONS

1. Describe laboratory diagnosis of meningococcal meningitis.
2. Discuss laboratory diagnosis of gonorrhea.

MULTIPLE CHOICE QUESTIONS

1. All of the following bacteria are oxidase positive, *except*:
   a. *Neisseria gonorrhoeae*
   b. *Neisseria meningitidis*
   c. *Vibrio cholerae*
   d. *Enterobacter*
2. The most common infective cause of vaginal discharge in a sexually promiscuous female is:
   a. *Trichomonas vaginalis*
   b. *Gardnerella vaginalis*
   c. *Neisseria gonorrhoeae*
   d. *Candida albicans*
3. The specimen of choice for isolation of gonococci from women with gonorrhea is:
   a. Vaginal swab
   b. Cervical swab
   c. Urethral swab
   d. Urine
4. *Neisseria meningitidis* shows all the following characteristics, *except*:
   a. Oxidase test positive
   b. Catalase test positive
   c. Ferments maltose with production of acid
   d. Ferments sucrose with production of acid
5. Waterhouse–Friderichsen syndrome is caused by:
   a. *Neisseria meningitidis*
   b. *Leptospira*
   c. *Streptococcus pyogenes*
   d. *Neisseria gonorrheae*
6. Causative agent of nongonococcal urethritis is caused by:
   a. *Chlamydia trachomatis*
   b. *Ureaplasma urealytium*
   c. *Mycoplasma hominis*
   d. All of the above
7. Following statements are true for quadrivalent meningococcal polysaccharide vaccine (MPSV4), *except*:
   a. The vaccine is given intramuscularly
   b. Prevents disease caused by A, C, Y, and W135 serogroups of meningococci
   c. Indicated for at risk population during outbreak of meningococcal infection
   d. Produce good antibody response in children below 2 years of age

ANSWERS

1. d   2. c   3. a   4. d
5. a   6. d   7. d

CHAPTER 20

Corynebacterium

LEARNING OBJECTIVES

After reading and studying this chapter, you should be able to:
- Describe morphology, cultural characteristics, biochemical characters, toxin production, and pathogenesis of diphtheria.
- Differentiate among three different biotypes: gravis, intermedius, and mitis of *Corynebacterium diphtheriae*.
- Discuss diphtheria toxin.
- Discuss laboratory diagnosis of diphtheria.
- Toxigenicity tests/virulence tests of *C. diphtheriae*.
- Describe the following: Schick test; DPT vaccine or triple vaccine.
- Diphtheroids.
- Differentiate between of *C. diphtheriae* and diphtheroids. Describe species of *Staphylococcus*.

INTRODUCTION

Corynebacteria are gram-positive, nonacid fast, nonmotile rods with irregularly stained segments, and sometimes granules. They frequently show club-shaped swellings and hence, the name corynebacteria (from *coryne*, meaning club).

CORYNEBACTERIUM DIPHTHERIAE

Morphology

They are thin, slender **gram-positive bacilli**, measuring approximately 3–6 µm × 0.6–0.8 µm and have a tendency to **clubbing** at one or both ends. They are highly **pleomorphic**, nonmotile, nonspore forming, and nonacid fast.

The bacilli are arranged in a characteristic fashion in smears. They are usually seen in pairs, palisades (resembling stakes of a fence) or small groups or as individual cells lying at sharp angles to another, resembling the letters V or L. This particular arrangement with *C. diphtheriae* has been called the ***Chinese letter*** or ***cuneiform arrangement***.

When stained with methylene blue or toluidine blue, the granules in the cell stain metachromatically reddish-purple. These granules are known as **metachromatic granules or volutin granules or Babes-Ernst granules**. They are often situated at the poles of the bacilli and are called **polar bodies**. With Albert's stain, the granules stain **bluish black** and the protoplasm green **(Fig. 20.1)**.

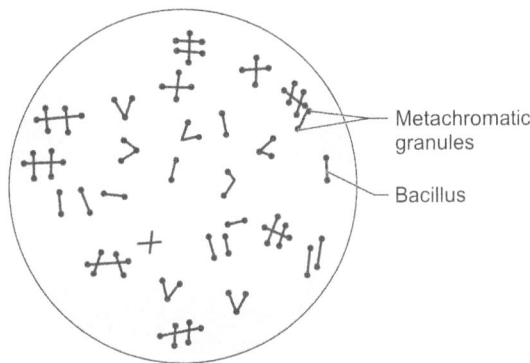

Fig. 20.1: *Corynebacterium diphtheriae* showing metachromatic granules and Chinese letter arrangement.

Cultural Characteristics

Corneybacterium diphtheriae is an aerobe and facultative anaerobe; the optimum temperature for growth is 37°C and optimum pH 7.2. Two media are useful for this purpose:
1. Loeffler's serum slope.
2. **Blood agar containing fresh, lysed, or heated blood.**

1. **Loeffler's serum slope:** Diphtheria bacilli grow on Loeffler's serum slope very rapidly and colonies can be seen in 6-8 hours. Colonies are at first small, circular white opaque disks but enlarge on continued incubation and may acquire a distinct yellow tint.
2. **Tellurite blood agar:** The addition of potassium tellurite (0.03-0.04%) makes the medium selective for corynebacteria. On this medium, *C. diphtheriae* give grey/black, shiny, or dull black colonies because the tellurite ion is reduced to the metal tellurium. Based on colonial morphology on the tellurite medium and other properties three different biotypes— ***gravis, intermedius,*** and ***mitis*** (Table 20.1).

Biochemical Reactions

Corneybacterium diphtheriae ferments glucose and maltose with the production of acid (but no gas) not lactose, mannitol, trehalose, or sucrose. Starch and glycogen are used for biochemical differentiation of three biotypes of *C. diphtheriae* (Table 20.1). *Gravis* strains utilize glycogen and starch, while *mitis* and *intermedius* do not.

Table 20.1: Type differentiation of *Corynebacterium diphtheriae.*

		Gravis	Intermedius	Mitis
1.	Morphology	i. Usually short rods, with uniform staining ii. Few or no granules iii. Pleomorphism (some degree)	i. Long barred forms with clubbed ends ii. Poor granulation iii. Very pleomorphic	i. Long, curved, rods ii. Prominent granules iii. Pleomorphic
2.	Colony on tellurite blood agar	i. In 18 hours: Colony is 1–2 mm in size, greyish black center, paler, semitranslucent periphery and commencing crenation of edge ii. In 2-3 days: 3–5 mm in size, flat colony with raised dark center and crenated edge with radial striation—'daisy head' colony	i. 18 hour—small, 1 mm in size, misty ii. In 48 hours does not enlarge, dull granular center with smoother, more glistening periphery and a lighter ring near the edge—'frog's egg' colony	i. Size variable, shiny black ii. In 2–3 days—colonies become flat, with a central elevation 'poached egg' colony
3.	Consistency of colonies	i. Brittle, moves as a whole on the plate like 'cold margarine' ii. Not easily picked out or emulsifiable	Intermediate between gravis and mitis	i. Soft, buttery ii. Easily emulsifiable
4.	Hemolysis	Variable	Nonhemolytic	Usually hemolytic
5.	Growth in broth	Surface pellicle. Deposit granular. Turbidity little or no	Turbidity in 24 hours, clearing in 48 hours, with fine granular sediment	Turbidity diffuse with soft pellicle later
6.	Glycogen and starch fermentation	Positive	Negative	Negative
7.	Toxigenic strains	Almost 100%	95–99%	80–85%
8.	Predominant strains in	Epidemic areas	Epidemic areas	Endemic areas

C. diphtheriae is H$_2$S positive and reduces nitrate to nitrite. It does not liquefy gelatin or hydrolyze urea or form of phosphatase.

Toxin

Toxigenic strains of *C. diphtheriae* produce a very powerful exotoxin. The toxicity observed in diphtheria is directly attributed to the toxin secreted by the bacteria at the site of infection.

Properties of Toxin

Diphtheria toxin is an iron-free, crystalline, heat-labile protein.

The toxin consists of two fragments **A (active)** and **B (binding)** of MW 24,000 and 38,000, respectively. Inhibition of protein synthesis is probably responsible for both the necrotic and neurotoxic effects of the toxin.

Clinical Diseases

The organism is carried in the upper respiratory tract and spread by droplet infection or hand-to-mouth contact. The incubation period of diphtheria is 2–5 days. Diphtheria, which occurs in two forms **(respiratory and cutaneous).**
Respiratory diphtheria: The most common site of infection is the **tonsils or pharynx.** The combination of cell necrosis and exudate forms a tough gray to white **pseudomembrane.**

The exotoxin is produced locally and is spread by the bloodstream to distant organs, with a special affinity for heart muscle, the peripheral nervous system, and the adrenal glands.

Laboratory Diagnosis

Diagnostic laboratory tests serve to confirm the clinical impression and are of epidemiologic significance but not for the treatment of individual cases. Specific treatment should be instituted *immediately* on suspicion of diphtheria without waiting for laboratory tests. Any delay may be fatal. Laboratory diagnosis consists of isolation of the diphtheria bacillus and demonstration of its toxicity.

1. Specimens

Swabs from the nose, throat, or other suspected lesions must be obtained before antimicrobial drugs are administered. In suspected cases, swabs should be taken both from the throat and from the nose. Swabs should also be taken from skin lesions and wounds where diphtheritic infection is suspected, and both throat and nose swabs should be taken from suspected carriers.

2. Microscopy

Direct microscopy of a smear is unreliable since C. *diphtheriae* is morphologically similar to other coryneforms. Hence, smear examination alone is not sufficient for diagnosing diphtheria but is important in identifying **Vincent's angina**. For this, a Gram or Leishman stained smear is examined for Vincent's spirochetes and fusiform bacilli. Toxigenic diphtheria bacilli may be identified in smears by immunofluorescence.

3. Culture

The swab should be inoculated on Loeffler's serum slope, tellurite blood agar, and blood agar. The cultures should be incubated aerobically at 37°C.
  i. **Loeffler's serum slope:** After incubation for 6 hours or overnight, make a smear of growth, stain by the Albert-Laybourn method and look for the presence of slender green-stained bacilli containing the purple-black granules characteristic of *C. diphtheriae.*
  ii. **Tellurite blood agar:** Blood tellurite agar is examined after 24 hours and after 48 hours, as growth may sometimes be delayed.
  iii. **Blood agar:** It is used for differentiating streptococcal or staphylococcal pharyngitis, which may simulate diphtheria.

4. Identification Tests

Corneybacterium diphtheriae ferments glucose and maltose, producing acid but not gas, and is catalase positive.

5. Virulence Tests

Any diphtheria-like organism cultured must be submitted to a "virulence" test. Diagnosis of diphtheria depends on showing that the isolate produces diphtheria toxin. Virulence testing may be by **in vivo** or **in vitro methods.**

A. In Vivo Tests

i. **Subcutaneous test:** The growth from an overnight culture on Loeffler's slope is emulsified in 2–4 mL broth and 1 mL of the emulsion injected **subcutaneously** into two guinea pigs or rabbits, one of which has been protected with the diphtheria antitoxin (500–1000 units) 18–24 hours previously and was used as control. If the strain is virulent, the unprotected animal will die within four days. Postmortem examination would show hemorrhage at the site of injection and injected blood vessels, with typically hemorrhagic adrenal necrosis.
   The method is not usually employed as it is wasteful of animals.

ii. **Intracutaneous (intradermal) test:** The broth emulsion of the culture is inoculated **intracutaneously** into two guinea pigs (or rabbits) so that each receives 0.1 mL in two different sites. One animal acts as the **control** and should receive antitoxin (500 units) the previous day. After four hours of the skin test, the other is given 50 units of antitoxin intraperitoneally in order to prevent death. In the test animal, toxigenicity is indicated by inflammatory reaction at the site of injection, progressing to necrosis in 48–72 hours and in **the control animal** no change.

Advantage in the intracutaneous test
   a. The animals do not die.
   b. As many as ten strains can be tested at a time on a rabbit.

B. In Vitro Test

i. **Elek's gel precipitation test:** The in vitro diphtheria toxin detection procedure is an **immunodiffusion test**.
   A rectangular strip of filter paper impregnated with diphtheria antitoxin **(1,000 units/mL)** is placed on the surface of a 20% normal horse serum agar in a Petri dish while the medium is still fluid. When the agar has set, the surface is dried. The plate should be streaked with the **test strain** as well as the **control positive** and **negative strains** at right angles to the strip in a single straight line parallel to each other. The plate is incubated at 37°C and examined after 24 and 48 hours.
   Toxins produced by the bacterial growth will diffuse in the agar and where it meets the antitoxin at optimum concentration will produce a line of precipitation (**Fig. 20.2**). No precipitate will form in the case of nontoxigenic strains.

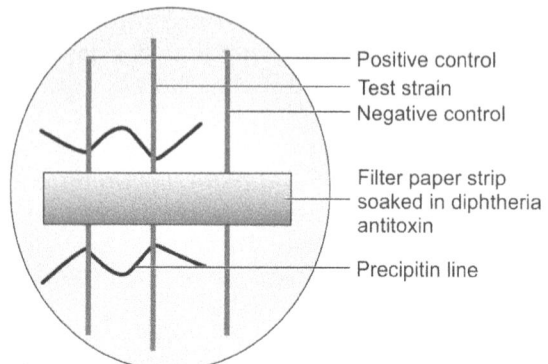

Fig. 20.2: Elek's test.

ii. **Tissue culture test**
iii. **Enzyme-linked immunosorbent assays (ELISA)**
iv. **Polymerase chain reaction (PCR)**

SCHICK TEST

Schick (1913) introduced an **intradermal test** (Schick test) for distinguishing between susceptible and immune persons.

Principle

This test depends upon the principle of toxin-antitoxin neutralization, in vivo, and the test is carried out by injecting one Schick test dose of diphtheria toxin (0.2 mL) intradermally on the anterior surface of the left forearm and a control injection in the right forearm contains a heat-inactivated dose of purified diphtheria toxoid. Readings are taken after 1, 4, and 7 days. Four types of reactions may occur:

1. **Negative reaction:** There is no reaction of any kind in either arm. This indicates that the toxin has been neutralized by the circulating

antitoxin and the person is immune to diphtheria.
2. **Positive reaction:** In the test arm there appears erythema and swelling at the site of inoculation in 24-36 hours. On the control arm there is no reaction.
   A positive Schick test indicates that the individual is susceptible to diphtheria and little or no antitoxin is present. The subject is not immune and should be immunized.
3. **Pseudo-reaction:** There is erythema occurring within 6-24 hours and disappearing within four days. The reaction is the same on both arms. This indicates that the individual is immune to diphtheria and also that he is hypersensitive to one or more antigens in the toxin preparation.
4. **Combined reaction:** Here the initial picture is that of pseudo-reaction, but while the erythema in the control arm fades, within four days, it progresses in the test arm to a typical positive reaction. This indicates that the individual is susceptible to diphtheria and is sensitive to one or more antigens in the toxin preparation.

Prophylaxis

The methods of immunization available are **active, passive, or combined**.

A. **Active immunization—DPT (diphtheria-pertussis-tetanus) vaccine:** Diphtheria toxoid is usually given in children as a trivalent preparation containing tetanus toxoid and **pertussis vaccine** also as the **DPT or triple vaccine**. The schedule of primary immunization of infants and children consists of **DPT given** at the age of 6 weeks, 10 weeks, 14 weeks, and 16-24 months followed by booster dose **DT** at the age of **5-6 years (school entry)**.

B. **Passive immunization:** This is an emergency measure to be employed where susceptibles (nonimmunized) are exposed to infection, as when a case of diphtheria is admitted to general pediatric wards. It consists of the subcutaneous administration of 500-1000 units of antitoxin (antidiphtheritic serum, ADS).

C. **Combined immunization:** This consists of administration of the first dose of adsorbed toxoid, while ADS is given on the other arm, to be continued by the full course of active immunization.

Treatment

Antitoxin should be given immediately as soon as clinical diagnosis is made to neutralize the toxin being produced.

C. diphtheriae is sensitive to most antibiotics, including **penicillin** and **erythromycin**. The antibiotics do not neutralize circulating toxin. They prevent further toxin production by killing diphtheria bacilli. Penicillin-sensitive individuals can be given erythromycin.

DIPHTHEROIDS

Corynebacteria resembling C. diphtheriae, occur as normal commensals in the throat, skin, and other areas. These may be mistaken for diphtheria bacilli and are known as **diphtheroids.** They stain more uniformly than diphtheria bacilli, are arranged in V forms or palisades rather than Chinese letter arrangement and possess few or no metachromatic granules. They can be differentiated from C. diphtheriae on the basis of biochemical characters and toxigenicity tests **(Table 20.2)**. The common diphtheroids are C. pseudodiphtheriticum and C. xerosis.

KEY POINTS

Corynebacterium diphtheriae
- Gram-positive bacilli with Chinese letter or cuneiform arrangement, granules in the cell are known as metachromatic granules volutin granules or Babes-Ernst granules.
- **Toxin:** Toxigenic strains of C. diphtheriae produce a very powerful exotoxin.
- **Clinical diseases:** Diphtheria, which occurs in two forms **(respiratory and cutaneous)**

- **Prophylaxis:** Administration of diphtheria vaccine and booster shots are given.

IMPORTANT QUESTIONS

1. Describe laboratory diagnosis and prophylaxis of diphtheria.
2. Write short notes on:
   a. Diphtheria toxin.
   b. Toxigenicity tests/Virulence tests of *C. diphtheriae*.

MULTIPLE CHOICE QUESTIONS

1. *Corynebacterium diphtheriae* is classified into three distinct biotypes (mitis, intermedius, and gravis) based on the morphologies of the colonies on:
   a. Tellurite blood agar
   b. Loeffler's serum slope
   c. Blood agar
   d. All of the above media
2. Diphtheria toxin shows following features, *except*:
   a. It is a protein with a molecular weight of 58,300 Da
   b. It consists of two functionally distinct polypeptide chain fragments, A and B protein
   c. It inhibits synthesis of fatty acids
   d. It is a very potent toxin
3. Which of the following sites is most commonly affected by diphtheria bacilli?
   a. Upper respiratory tract
   b. Skin
   c. Cornea
   d. Conjunctiva
4. Diphtheroids show following features, *except*:
   a. They possess few or no metachromatic granules
   b. They are usually arranged in parallel rows
   c. Most of them do not produce toxins
   d. They do not ferment sucrose
5. A positive Schick test implies that the person is:
   a. Immune and nonhypersensitive
   b. Susceptible and non-hypersensitive
   c. Immune and hypersensitive
   d. Nonimmune and hypersensitive

ANSWERS

1. a   2. c   3. a   4. d
5. b

CHAPTER 21

Bacillus

LEARNING OBJECTIVES

After reading and studying this chapter, you should be able to:
- Describe the morphology, cultural characters, and pathogenicity of *Bacillus anthracis*
- Discuss laboratory diagnosis of anthrax.
- Describe the following: Anthracoid bacilli; *Bacillus cereus* food poisoning.

INTRODUCTION

The genus *Bacillus* consists of aerobic gram-positive bacilli forming heat-resistant spores. Their spores are ubiquitous, being found in soil, dust, water, and air and constitute the most common contaminants in bacteriological culture media.

Species: The species that are of medical interest are:
1. ***Bacillus anthracis:*** The organism is responsible for anthrax and is the most important member of this genus.
2. ***Bacillus cereus:*** It is commonly implicated in episode of food poisoning.

BACILLUS ANTHRACIS

The disease caused by *B. anthracis* is anthrax.

Morphology

Bacillus anthracis is one of the largest of pathogenic bacteria, gram-positive 3-8 by 1-1.3 mm and is gram positive nonacid fast, nonmotile straight, sporing bacillus. A chain of bacilli presents a **"bamboo-stick" appearance**. The entire chain is being surrounded by a **capsule**. **The spore** is oval (ellipsoidal), refractile, central in position and of the same diameter as the bacillus and not swelling the mother cell **(Fig. 21.1)**.

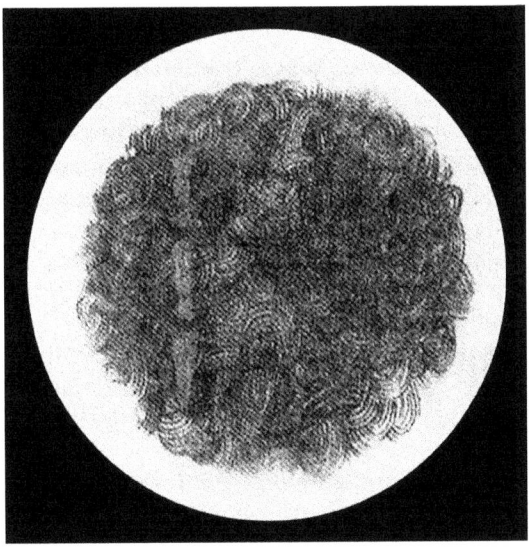

Fig. 21.1: Medusa head appearance of anthrax bacilli.

Cultural Characteristics

It is aerobe and facultative anaerobe. Temperature range for growth is 12-45°C (optimum 37°C). Good growth occurs on ordinary media.

1. **Nutrient agar:** Colonies are irregularly round, 2-3 mm in diameter, raised, dull, opaque, grayish white, with a frosted glass appearance. It grows on all ordinary media as typical colonies with a wavy margin and small projections, resembling locks of matted hair, the socalled *medusa head* appearance.

2. **Blood agar:** Colonies on horse or sheep **blood agar** are virtually nonhemolytic, though occasional strains produce a narrow zone of hemolysis.
3. **In broth:** Growth develops as silky strands, a surface pellicle and a floccular deposit.
4. **Gelatin stab culture:** There is growth giving an **'inverted fir tree' appearance**.
5. **Selective medium: A selective medium (PLET medium)**, consisting of polymyxin, lysozyme, ethylenediamine tetra acetic acid (EDTA), and thallous acetate added to heart infusion agar.

Pathogenicity

Anthrax is primarily a disease of herbivores. Cattle and sheep, goats, pigs, and other herbivores are naturally affected.

Animal anthrax: Anthrax is a zoonosis. Animals are infected by the ingestion of the spores present in the soil. Infected animals shed in the discharges from the mouth, nose, and rectum, large numbers of bacilli, which sporulate in soil and remain as the source of infection.

Human anthrax: Humans are infected through exposure to contaminated animals or animal products.

Based on the mode of infection, human anthrax presents in one of three ways: (1) cutaneous (2) pulmonary, or (3) intestinal. All types are leading to fatal septicemia or meningitis.

1. **Cutaneous anthrax:** Cutaneous anthrax used to be caused by shaving brushes made with animal hair. Rupture of the vesicle reveals a **black eschar** at the base. This is sometimes referred to as a **malignant pustule**.
   Was known as the **"hide porter's disease"**.
2. **Pulmonary anthrax:** Pulmonary anthrax, known as **"wool-sorter's" disease**, because it used to be common in workers in wool factories, due to inhalation of dust from infected wool.
3. **Intestinal anthrax:** Intestinal anthrax is rare and occurs mainly in **primitive communities** who eat the carcasses of animals dying of anthrax.

Laboratory Diagnosis

1. **Specimens:** Material from a malignant pustule, sputum from pulmonary anthrax, gastric aspirates feces or food in intestinal anthrax and in the blood in the septicemic stage of all forms of the infection.
2. **Microscopy:** Prepare smears of each specimen and stain with **Gram's method** and **McFadyean's method** or with **Giemsa stain.** Gram's stain may show typical large gram-positive bacilli. Capsule appears as a clear halo around the bacterium by India-ink staining.
   Direct fluorescent antibody test (DFA) for capsule-specific staining and for polysaccharide (cell wall) antigen confirms the identification.
3. **Culture**: Culture the exudate on **nutrient agar, blood agar, PLET medium**, and **nutrient broth**. Examine plates for the medusa-head colonies characteristic of *B. anthracis,* nonhemolytic on the blood agar plate. Prepare a smear, stain it by Gram's method, and look for tangled chains of large gram-positive bacilli.
4. **Confirmatory tests:**
   i. **Biochemical and physiological reactions**
   ii. **Animal inoculation:** Inoculate intraperitoneally in mice a 24-hours broth culture. The animal dies in 48–72 hours. Make smears from heart blood and spleen, stain by Gram's and McFadyean's methods, and look for typical anthrax bacilli.
5. **Serological diagnosis** is seldom used diagnostically.
   Treatment: Ciprofloxacin is the drug of choice.

ANTHRACOID BACILLI

Aerobic spore bearing bacilli morphologically having a general resemblance to anthrax bacilli have been collectively called **pseudo anthrax or anthracoid bacilli. These** large number and variety of nonpathogenic bacilli appear as common contaminants in cultures. The important species include *B. cereus, B. subtilis,*

Table 21.1: Differentiating features between *B. anthracis* and *Anthracoid bacilli*.

Features	*B. anthracis*	*Anthracoid bacilli*
1. Motiliy	Nonmotile	Generally motile
2. Capsule	Capsulated	Noncapsulated
3. Chain formation	Grow in long chains	Grow in short chains
4. Colony on nutrient agar	Medusa head colony	Not present
5. Growth in penicillin agar (10 units/mL)	No growth	Grow usually
6. Hemolysis on blood agar	Hemolysis absent or weak	Usually well marked
7. Gelatin stab culture	Inverted fir tree growth and slow gelatin liquefaction	Rapid liquefaction
8. Turbidity in broth	No turbidity	Turbidity usual
9. Salicin fermentation	Negative	Usually positive
10. Growth at 45°C	No growth	Grows usually
11. Growth inhibition by chloral hydrate	Growth inhibited	Not inhibited
12. Susceptible to gamma phage	Susceptible	Not susceptible
13. Pathogenic to laboratory animals	Pathogenic	Not pathogenic
14. Mc Fadyean's reaction	Positive	Negative
15. Ascoli's precipitin test	Positive	Negative
16. Fluorescent antibody test with antrax antiserum	Positive	Negative

B. licheniformis, B. pumilus. **Table 21.1** lists the main differentiating features between them.

BACILLUS CEREUS

Bacillus cereus has recently assumed importance as a cause of food poisoning. It is widely distributed in nature may be readily isolated from soil, vegetables, and a wide variety of foods including milk, cereals, spices, meat, and poultry.

Pathogenesis

Infections include emetic (vomiting) and diarrheal forms of gastroenteritis.
1. **Emetic form (the short incubation type):** The emetic form results from the consumption of contaminated rice. After 1–5 hours after meal symptoms consist of vomiting, nausea, and abdominal cramps. Fever and diarrhea are generally absent.
2. **Diarrheal form:** The diarrheal form of *B. cereus* food poisoning results from the consumption of contaminated meat, vegetables, or sauces. There is a longer incubation period occurring 8–24 hours after ingestion. Diarrhea, nausea, and abdominal cramps develop.

Diagnosis

Isolation of the organism in implicated food product or nonfecal specimens.

TREATMENT

Both the emetic and diarrheal syndromes are shortlived and no specific treatment is needed.

KEY POINTS

- *Bacillus anthracis*
- Spore-forming gram-positive bacilli.
- **Diseases:** Cutaneous anthrax, inhalation anthrax, and gastrointestinal anthrax.

IMPORTANT QUESTION

1. Write short notes on:
   a. Anthracoid bacilli
   b. *Bacillus cereus* food poisoning

MULTIPLE CHOICE QUESTIONS

1. Mc Fadyean's reaction is employed for the presumptive diagnosis of:
   a. Anthrax
   b. Tetanus
   c. Diphtheria
   d. Typhoid
2. 'Medusa head' appearance of the colonies is characteristic of:
   a. *Proteus mirabilis*
   b. *Clostridium tetani*
   c. *Bacillus anthracis*
   d. *Pseudomonas aeruginosa*
3. Malignant pustule is characteristic of:
   a. Cutaneous anthrax
   b. Pulmonary anthrax
   c. Intestinal anthrax
   d. All of the above

ANSWERS

1. a   2. c   3. a

CHAPTER 22

Clostridium

LEARNING OBJECTIVES

After reading and studying this chapter, you should be able to:
- Discuss morphology, cultural characteristics of *C. welchii*.
- Discuss Nagler's reaction.
- Discuss laboratory diagnosis and prophylaxis of gas gangrene.
- Describe toxins produced by *C. tetani*.
- Describe the following: Pathogenesis of tetanus; prophylaxis of tetanus.
- Discuss morphology and cultural characteristics of *C. botulinum*.
- Discuss laboratory diagnosis of botulinum.
- Describe the following: Gas gangrene; botulinum toxin; *Clostridium difficile*.

INTRODUCTION

The genus *Clostridium* includes all anaerobic, gram-positive bacilli capable of forming endospores. The name *Clostridium* is derived from the word "**Kloster**" (meaning a spindle).

Diseases produced: Clostridia are more commonly associated with skin and soft tissue infections, food poisoning, and antibiotic-associated diarrhea and colitis **(Table 22.1)**.

Table 22.1: Clostridia as human pathogens.

A. The gas gangrene group
1. Established pathogens — *C. perfringens*
    C. septicum
    C. novyi
2. Less pathogenic — *C. histolyticum*
    C. fallax
3. Doubtful pathogens — *C. bifermentans*
    C. sporogenes
B. Tetanus: — *C. tetani*
C. Food poisoning:
  1. Gastroenteritis — *C. perfringens (Type A)*
  2. Necrotising enteritis — *C. perfringens (Type C)*
  3. Botulism — *C. botulinum*
D. Acute colitis — *C. diflicile*

CLOSTRIDIUM PERFRINGENS (CLOSTRIDIUM WELCHII)

Clostridium perfringens is a normal inhabitant of the large intestines of human beings and animals. The spores are commonly found in soil, dust, and air.

Morphology

It is a relatively large gram-positive bacillus (about 4–6 × 1 μm). It is capsulated and nonmotile. Spores are typically oval, central, or subterminal and not bulging.

Cultural Characteristics

It is an anaerobe but can also grow under microaerophilic conditions. It grows over a pH range of 5.5–8.0 and temperature range of 20–50°C (optimum temperature range 37–45°C). It grows on blood agar, Robertson's cooked meat broth (CMB) and thioglycolate broth. Good growth occurs in **Robertson's cooked meat medium**. The meat is turned pink but is not digested.

On blood agar, colonies of most strains demonstrate a "**target hemolysis**" after overnight

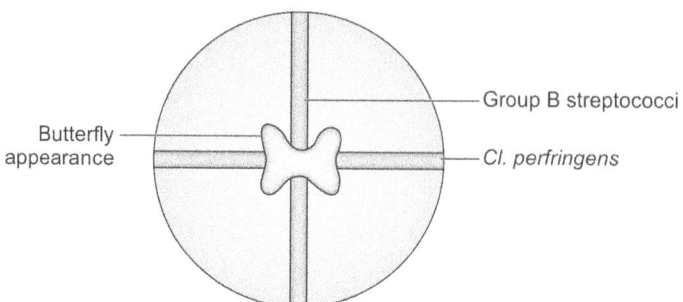

Fig. 22.1: Reverse CAMP test.

incubation on blood agar. It results from a narrow zone of complete hemolysis due to theta toxin and a much wider darker zone of incomplete hemolysis due to the α-toxin.

Biochemical Reactions

It is actively saccharolytic. Glucose, maltose, lactose, and sucrose are' fermented with the production of acid and gas. It is indole negative, MR positive, and VP negative (**Fig. 22.1**). Hydrogen sulfide is produced abundantly; sulfite is actively reduced; most strains reduce nitrates to nitrites.

In litmus milk medium, fermentation of lactose leads to formation of acid, which is indicated by the change in the color of litmus from blue to red. The acid clots the milk – casein- (acid clot) and the clotted milk is disrupted due to the vigorous gas production. This is known as "**stormy fermentation** or **stormy clot**" reaction.

Resistance

Spores are usually destroyed within five minutes by boiling but those of the 'food poisoning' strains of type A and certain Type C strains resist boiling for 1–3 hours. Autoclaving at 121°C for 15 minutes is lethal. Spores generally resist routinely used antiseptics and disinfectants.

Toxins

Clostridium perfringens is forming at least 12 distinct soluble substances or toxins. The four "major toxins", alpha, beta, epsilon, and iota, are predominantly responsible for pathogenicity.

C. perfringens can be divided into five types, A to E on the basis of four major toxins.

Alpha Toxin

The alpha (α) toxin is produced by all types of *C. perfringens* and most abundantly by Type A strains. It is a lecithinase (phospholipase C) that lyses erythrocytes, platelets, leukocytes, and endothelial cells.

Nagler's Reaction

Basis: The alpha (α) toxin is lecithinase C (or phospholipase C) splits lecithin into phosphorylcholine and diglyceride, in the presence of Ca^{++} and Mg^{++} ions. This reaction is seen as opalescence in serum or egg yolk media and is specifically neutralized by the antitoxin. This is the basis of Nagler's reaction.

Procedure: For rapid detection of *C. perfringens*, a culture plate containing 6% agar, 5% peptic digest of sheep blood, and 20% human serum or 5% egg-yolk is prepared. On one half of the plate, 2–3 drops of *C. perfringens* antitoxin are spread and allowed to dry. The plate is then inoculated with the test organisms or the exudate under investigation and incubated anaerobically at 37°C for 18 hours.

Interpretation: On the section containing no antitoxin, *C. perfringens* colonies show surrounding **zone of opalescence, i.e., Nagler's reaction.** There will be **no opacity** around the colonies on the half of the plate with the antitoxin, due to the specific neutralization of the alpha toxin (**Fig. 22.2**).

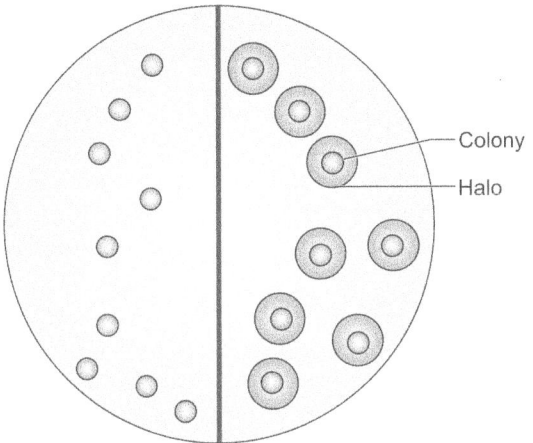

Fig. 22.2: Negler reaction. *C. perfringens* colonies on the right half of the plate are surrounded by haloes, while colonies on the left half (containing antiserum to alpha toxin) have no haloes around them.

Other Major Toxins

Beta (β), Epsilon (ε), and iota (ι) toxins have lethal and necrotizing properties.

Enterotoxin

Clostridium perfringens type A strains produce a potent enterotoxin, which causes diarrhea and other symptoms of food poisoning.

Pathogenesis

1. **Soft tissue infections:** Soft tissue infections caused by *C. perfringens* are subdivided into (1) cellulitis, (2) fasciitis or suppurative myositis, and (3) myonecrosis or gas gangrene.
2. **Food poisoning**
3. **Enteritis necroticans (*necrotizing jejunitis, necrotic enteritis*)**
4. ***Clostridium perfringens* colitis**
5. **Clostridial endometritis**

Laboratory Diagnosis

Gas gangrene is a medical emergency. The diagnosis of gas gangrene must be made primarily on clinical grounds, and the function of the laboratory is only to provide confirmation of the clinical diagnosis as well as identification and enumeration of the infecting organisms.

A. **Specimens:** (1) Edge of the affected muscles; (2) Exudates from the wound; and (3) Necrotic tissue and muscle fragments.
B. **Microscopy:** Gram-stained films give presumptive information. Thick, stubby, gram-positive rods suggest *C. perfringens*.
C. **Culture: Fresh** and **heated-blood agar** are used for aerobic and anaerobic cultures. Four tubes of **CMB** are inoculated, incubated, and subcultured on **blood agar plates** after 24–48 hours. A plate of **serum or egg yolk agar (EYA)** with *C. perfringens* antitoxin spread on one half is used for the "Nagler reaction". **Blood cultures** are often positive.
D. **Identification:** Examine plates for typical colonies. The isolates are identified based on their morphological, cultural, biochemical and toxigenic characters. Toxigenicity of the strain can be done by animal pathogenicity.

Prophylaxis and Therapy

1. Surgery
2. Antibiotics
3. Passive immunization
4. Hyperbaric oxygen
5. Active immunization.

CLOSTRIDIUM TETANI

Clostridium tetani is the causative agent of tetanus.

Morphology

It is a gram positive, slender bacillus, 2–5 × 0.4–1 mm. The spores are spherical, terminal and twice the diameter of vegetative cells giving them typical **drumstick appearance (Fig. 22.3)**. It is noncapsulated and motile by peritrichate flagella (except *C. tetani* type VI) with peritrichate flagella.

Cultural Characteristics

Clostridium tetani is an obligate anaerobe. The optimal temperature for growth is 37°C, and the optimal pH is 7.4. It can grow well in CMB, thioglycolate broth, nutrient agar, and blood agar.

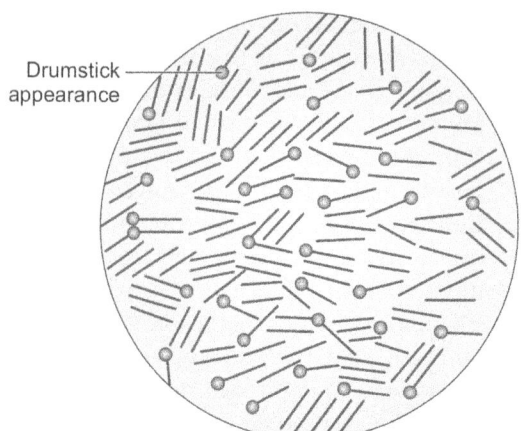

Fig. 22.3: *C. tetani*, some with spores and some without spores.

In **CMB**, growth occurs as turbidity and there is also some gas formation. The meat is not digested but becomes black on prolonged incubation.

On **blood agar** the bacilli produce a swarming (thin-spreading film) growth.

Biochemical Reactions

Clostridium tetani has feeble proteolytic but no saccharolytic property. It does not attack any sugar. Gelatin liquefaction occurs very slowly.

Resistance

Most of the strains are killed by boiling for 10–15 minutes but some resist boiling for up to 3 hours. They can, however, be killed by autoclaving at 121°C for 15 minutes. Spores are able to survive in soil for years.

Tetanus Toxin

Clostridium tetani produces at least two distinct toxins—an oxygen-labile **hemolysin (tetanolysin)** and a powerful plasmid-encoded, heat-labile **neurotoxin (tetanospasmin).**

Pathogenicity

Tetanus develops following the contamination of wound with *C. tetani* spores. The most typical focus of infection in tetanus is a puncture wound. Germination of spores is dependent upon the reduced oxygen tension occurring in devitalized tissue. Infection strictly remains localized in the wound and the disease is due to the effect of a potent diffusible exotoxin (tetanospasmin). **Generalized tetanus** is the most common form.

In cephalic tetanus, the primary site of infection is the head and has high mortality. The most feared form of tetanus is **tetanus neonatorum.**

Laboratory Diagnosis

The diagnosis of tetanus is made on clinical grounds. Laboratory tests only help in confirmation.

A. **Specimen:** Wound exudate or tissue removed from the wound.
B. **Microscopy:** Microscopy is unreliable and the demonstration of the typical 'drumstick' bacilli in wounds in itself is not diagnostic of tetanus.
C. **Culture:** The material is inoculated on one half of a blood agar plate. *C. tetani* produces a swarming growth.
   The material is also inoculated into three tubes of CMB.
D. **Toxigenicity test:** Toxigenicity is best tested in animals.

Prophylaxis

The available methods of prophylaxis are:
1. Surgical attention
2. Antibiotics
3. Immunization—passive, active, or combined.

1. Surgical Prophylaxis

This includes prompt and adequate wound toilet and proper surgical debridement of wound, removal of foreign material, necrotic tissue and blood clots. This ensures an anaerobic environment for the growth of *C. tetani* is not provided.

2. Antibiotic Prophylaxis

Long-acting penicillin injection is the drug of choice. An alternative is erythromycin. Antibiotic prophylaxis does not replace immunoprophylaxis but serves as a useful adjunct.

3. Immunoprophylaxis

It includes three types of immunization:

A. Active Immunization

Tetanus is best prevented by active immunization with tetanus toxoid. Two preparations are available for active immunization are:

Tetanus toxoid **(formol toxoid)**, which is available either as 'plain toxoid', or adsorbed on aluminum hydroxide or phosphate (APT), is commonly used for active immunization. Three doses of 0.5 mL tetanus toxoid each are given intramuscularly, with an interval of 4–6 weeks between first two doses and 6–12 months between the second and third dose. A full course of three doses confers immunity for a period of at least 10 years. A 'booster dose' of toxoid is recommended after 10 years.

Tetanus toxoid is given along with diphtheria toxoid and pertusis vaccine called **DPT** in children as **triple vaccine**. Pertusis vaccine acts as adjuvant. Three doses are given intramuscularly at interval of 4-6 weeks, starting at age as early as 6 weeks. Booster doses are given at age of 18 months and then at 5 years. Thereafter, booster doses of tetanus toxoid (TT) are given at the age of 10 and 16 years. Subsequently, immunity to tetanus can be maintained by booster doses of toxoid every 10 years.

B. Passive Immunization

- **Antitetanus serum (ATS):** ATS from hyperimmune horses was the preparation originally used.
- **Disadvantages of ATS:** Equine ATS carried two disadvantages implicit in the use of any heterologous serum—'**immune elimination** and **hypersensitivity reactions.**
- **Human antitetanus immunoglobulin (HTIG):** Passive immunity without risk of hypersensitivity can be obtained by the use of **HTIG**. This is effective in smaller doses.

C. Combined Immunization

It consists of administering to a nonimmune person ATS or HTIG at one site, along with the first dose of a course of active immunization with adsorbed toxoid at the same time at another site, followed by second and third doses of TT at appropriate intervals.

CLOSTRIDIUM BOTULINUM

Clostridium botulinum causes **botulism,** which is a severe form of food poisoning. Botulism is caused by the action of a neurotoxin that is one of the most potent poisons known.

Morphology

Clostridium botulinum is a strictly anaerobic gram-positive bacillus (about 5 × 1 mm). It is noncapsulated, motile with peritrichous flagella and produces spores which are oval, subterminal, and bulging.

Cultural Characteristics

It is a strict anaerobe. Optimum temperature is 35°C. Surface colonies are large, irregular, semitransparent, with fimbriae border. On **horse blood agar**, all strains except those of type G are β-hemolytic. On **EYA** all types except G produce opalescence and a pearly effect.

Resistance

Spores are heat and radiation resistant, surviving several hours at 100°C and for up to 10 minutes at 120°C.

Classification

The species *C. botulinum* has been divided into eight serologically distinct types—A, B, C1, and C2, D, E, F, and G—on the basis of the type of toxin produced.

Botulinum Toxin

A powerful exotoxin produced by *C. botulinum* is responsible for its pathogenicity. It differs, however, from a classic exotoxin in that it is not released during the life of the organism but appears in the medium only after death and autolysis of the organism. It is a neurotoxin and acts slowly, taking several hours to kill.

Pathogenicity

It is noninvasive and its pathogenicity is entirely due to the toxin produced by it. The disease caused by this organism is known as **botulism.**

It is of three types—food-borne botulism, wound botulism, and infant botulism.

1. **Food-borne botulism:** It is due to the ingestion of preformed toxin. The causative organism, *C. botulinum,* multiplies in the food before it is consumed, and produces a powerful soluble toxin. The source of botulism is usually preserved food such as meat and meat products, fish, and vegetables. Symptoms usually begin 18–36 hours after ingestion of food and may include nausea, vomiting, thirst, constipation, double vision, difficulty in swallowing, speaking, and breathing. This may be followed by muscular weakness, blurred vision, and death as a result of respiratory failure.
2. **Wound botulism:** *Wound botulism* is a very rare condition resulting from wound infection with *C. botulinum.*
3. **Infant botulism:** The disease typically affects infants below 6 months. The most common food source in infant botulism is **honey** contaminated with botulinum spores.

Laboratory Diagnosis

Botulism confirmed by isolating the organism or detecting the toxin in food products or the patient's feces or serum.

1. **Specimens:** Feces, food, vomitus, gastric fluid, serum, environmental samples, and occasionally wound exudate.
2. **Culture:** For the isolation of *C. botulinum,* the specimen is inoculated on **EYA, blood agar, and CMB.**
3. **Demonstration of toxin:** Demonstration of toxin production must be done with a **mouse bioassay.**

Prophylaxis

Control can be achieved by proper canning and preservation. Children younger than 1 year should not eat honey. A prophylactic dose of polyvalent antitoxin should be given intramuscularly to all persons who have eaten food suspected of causing botulism.

Active immunization should be considered for laboratory staff. Two injections of aluminum sulfate adsorbed toxoid may be given at an interval of ten weeks, followed by a booster a year later.

CLOSTRIDIUM DIFFICILE

Clostridium difficile was so named because of the unusual difficulty in isolating

Morphology

Clostridium difficile is a motile gram-positive rod. Spores are large, oval, and terminal.

Toxins

The organism produces an **enterotoxin (toxin A)** and a **cytotoxin (toxin B). Toxin A** is an enterotoxin that is primarily responsible for diarrhea.

Pathogenesis

It is a proven cause of **antibiotic associated diarrhea (AAD)**, and **pseudomembranous colitis (PMC)**—a life-threatening condition. The three drugs most commonly implicated are **clindamycin, ampicillin, and the cephalosporins.**

Laboratory Diagnosis

1. **Isolation of bacilli:** *C. difficile* can be isolated from the feces by enrichment and selective culture procedures.
2. **Demonstration of toxin:** Toxin B can be demonstrated in the feces of patients by its characteristic effect on **Hep-2 and human diploid cell cultures** or both toxins may be demonstrated by immunological methods, e.g., enzyme-linked immunosorbent assay (ELISA).

Treatment and Prophylaxis

The disease is treated by discontinuing the antibiotic that is presumed to have precipitated the disease of *C. difficile* by giving oral metronidazole or vancomycin. The spores of *C. difficile* are difficult to destroy.

KEY POINTS

The genus *Clostridium* includes all anaerobic, gram-positive bacilli capable of forming endospores.

Clostridium perfringens

Diseases:
1. Soft tissue infections (cellulitis, suppurative, myositis, myonecrosis).
2. Food poisoning.
3. Septicemia.

Clostridium tetani

Pathogenicity: Tetanus develops following the contamination of wound with C. *tetani* spores.

Clostridium botulinum

Diseases: The disease caused by this organism is known as **botulism**.

Clostridium difficile

Diseases:
1. Asymptomatic colonization
2. Antibiotic-associated diarrhea (AAD)
3. Pseudomembranous colitis.

IMPORTANT QUESTIONS

1. Describe the laboratory diagnosis and prophylaxis of gas gangrene.
2. Describe laboratory diagnosis and prophylaxis of tetanus.
3. Write short notes on:
   a. Nagler's reaction
   b. Botulism
   c. *Clostridium difficile*

MULTIPLE CHOICE QUESTIONS

1. Which of the following types of *Clostridium perfringens* produces alpha toxin most abundantly?
   a. Type A
   b. Type B
   c. Type C
   d. Type D

2. Nagler's reaction is useful for the identification of:
   a. *Clostridium tetani*
   b. *Clostridium perfringens*
   c. *Clostridium botulinum*
   d. *Clostridium difficile*

3. All the following species cause gas gangrene, *except*:
   a. *Clostridium perfringens*
   b. *Clostridium novyi*
   c. *Clostridium sordelli*
   d. *Clostridium histolyticum*

4. Food poisoning is caused by *Clostridium perfringens*:
   a. Type A
   b. Type B
   c. Type C
   d. Type D

5. Typical drumstick appearance of bacilli is observed in:
   a. *Clostridium perfringens*
   b. *Clostridium tetani*
   c. *Clostridium botulinum*
   d. *Clostridium histolytieum*

6. Antibiotics-associated diarrhea is caused by:
   a. *Clostridium perfringens*
   b. *Clostridium tetani*
   c. *Clostridium botulinum*
   d. *Clostridium difficile*

7. Which of the following bacteria is responsible for pseudomembranous enterocolitis?
   a. *Clostridium perfringens*
   b. *Clostridium tetani*
   c. *Clostridium botulinum*
   d. *Clostridium difficile*

ANSWERS

1. a   2. b   3. d   4. a
5. b   6. d   7. d

CHAPTER 23

Nonsporing Anaerobes

 LEARNING OBJECTIVES

After reading and studying this chapter, you should be able to:
- Describe classification of nonsporing anaerobes.
- List infections caused by nonsporing anaerobes.
- Discuss laboratory diagnosis of infections caused by nonsporing anaerobes.

INTRODUCTION

The anaerobic bacteria are widespread in nature. A bewildering range of anaerobes is found in the mouth and oropharynx, gastrointestinal tract, and female genital tract of healthy individuals as part of the commensal flora. Many of these anaerobic organisms are now recognized as opportunistic pathogens.

CLASSIFICATION

Medically important anaerobes may be broadly classified as shown in **Box 23.1**.

LABORATORY DIAGNOSIS

As anaerobes form part of the normal flora of the skin and mucous surfaces, their isolation from specimens has to be interpreted cautiously. The mere presence of an anaerobe does not prove its causal role.
  A. **Specimen collection and transport:** Specimens should be collected in such a manner as to avoid resident flora. For example, from a suspected case of lung abscess the sputum is unsatisfactory for culture and only material collected by aspiration would be acceptable. In general, material for anaerobic culture is best obtained by tissue biopsy or by aspiration using a needle and syringe.

Box 23.1 Classification of nonsporing anaerobes.

I. **Cocci**
  1. Gram positive
     a. *Peptostreptococcus*
     b. *Peptococcus*
  2. Gram negative
     a. *Veillonella*
II. **Bacilli**
  1. Endospore forming
     a. Clostridia
  2. Nonsporing
     A. Gram positive
        a. *Eubacterium*
        b. *Propionibacterium*
        c. *Lactobacillus*
        d. *Mobiluncus*
        e. *Bifidobacterium*
        f. *Actinomyces*
     B. Gram negative
        a. *Bacteroides*
        b. *Prevotella*
        c. *Porphyromonas*
        d. *Fusobacterium*
        e. *Leptotrichia*
III. **Spirochetes**
  1. *Treponema*
  2. *Borrelias*

Ideally, specimens should be placed in an anaerobic transport device. Specimens should be delivered immediately (within 20 minutes) for culture.

B. **Direct microscopy:** Examination of a Gram stained smear is very useful. Pus in anaerobic infection usually shows a large variety of different organisms and numerous pus cells. Examination of specimen under ultraviolet light may show bright red fluorescence of *Prevotella melaninogenica*.
C. **Culture:** Freshly prepared blood agar with neomycin, yeast extract, hemin, and vitamin K is adequate. Plates are incubated at 37°C in an anaerobic jar, with 10% CO_2. **The Gas-Pak system** provides a convenient method of routine anaerobic cultures.
Other anaerobic media, such as **cooked meat broth (CMB)** and **thioglycollate broth**, may also be used for inoculating the specimens. Parallel aerobic cultures, such as *Pseudomonas aeruginosa* should always be set up.
D. **Identification:** Colony morphology, pigmentation, and fluorescence are helpful in identifying anaerobes. Biochemical activities and chromatography for fatty acids are used for laboratory confirmation.
E. **Antibiotic sensitivity tests:** Antibiotic sensitivity tests can be done by disk diffusion or dilution methods.

KEY POINTS

- Many anaerobic bacteria are pathogenic for human beings.

- **Laboratory diagnosis:** Specimens should be placed in an anaerobic transport device. Examination of a Gram stained smear is very useful. Other anaerobic media, such as **CMB** and **thioglycollate broth**, may also be used.

IMPORTANT QUESTION

1. Classify nonsporing anaerobes. Discuss the laboratory diagnosis of infections caused by nonsporing anaerobes.

MULTIPLE CHOICE QUESTIONS

1. The following is an example of gram-negative anaerobic cocci:
    a. Veillonella
    b. Peptococcus
    c. Peptostreptococcus
    d. Bacteroides
2. Which of the following bacterial colonies fluorescence. bright-red in UV light?
    a. Bacteroides fragilis
    b. Prevotella melaninogenica
    c. Bacteroides gingivalis
    d. Bacteroides levii

ANSWERS

1. a   2. b

Mycobacterium I: Mycobacterium tuberculosis

CHAPTER 24

LEARNING OBJECTIVES

After reading and studying this chapter, you should be able to:
- Classify mycobacteria.
- Discuss morphology and culture characteristics and biochemical characteristics of *Mycobacterium tuberculosis*.
- Describe pathogenesis of *Mycobacterium tuberculosis*.
- Discuss the laboratory diagnosis of pulmonary tuberculosis.
- Describe the following: Koch's phenomenon; Tuberculin test; BCG vaccine.

INTRODUCTION

The genus *Mycobacterium* belongs to the family Mycobacteriaceae. The most familiar of the species are **Mycobacterium tuberculosis (MTB)** and **Mycobacterium leprae,** the causative agents of tuberculosis (TB) and Hansen's disease (leprosy), respectively.

They are aerobic, nonmotile, noncapsulated, and nonsporing. Growth is generally slow. They do not stain readily, but once stained with hot carbol fuchsin or other aryl methane dyes, they resist decolorization with dilute mineral acids (or alcohol). Mycobacteria are, therefore, known as acid-fast bacilli (AFB).

MYCOBACTERIUM TUBERCULOSIS

Morphology

Mycobacterium tuberculosis is a slender, straight, or slightly curved rod with rounded ends, about 3 μm × 0.3 μm, in pairs or as small clumps. The bacilli are nonmotile, nonsporing, noncapsulated, and acid-fast.

When stained with carbol fuchsin by the Ziehl–Neelsen method or by fluorescent dyes (auramine O, rhodamine), they resist decolorization by 20% sulfuric acid and absolute alcohol for 10 minutes **(acid and alcohol fast)**. The Ziehl–Neelsen acid-fast stain is useful in staining organisms either from cultures or from clinical material. With this stain, the tubercle bacilli stain **bright red,** while the tissue cells and other organisms are stained blue.

Acid fastness has been ascribed variously to the presence in the bacillus of an **unsaponifiable wax (mycoloic acid)** or to **a semipermeable membrane around the cell.** It is related to the **integrity of the cell** and appears to be a property of the lipid-rich waxy cell wall. Staining may be uniform or granular. In *M. tuberculosis* beaded or barred forms are frequently seen.

Cultural Characteristics

Mycobacterium tuberculosis is an obligate aerobe. The optimal growth temperature of tubercle bacilli is 35–37°C. Optimum pH is 6.4–7.0. The bacilli grow slowly.

Solid Medium

Tubercle bacilli are able to grow on a wide range of enriched culture media. The solid medium most widely employed for routine culture is **Lowenstein–Jensen (LJ) medium.** This consists of coagulated hens' egg, mineral salt solution, and asparagine and malachite green, the last acting as a selective agent inhibiting other bacteria and to provide a contrasting color against which colonies of mycobacteria are easily seen. In this medium egg acts as a solidifying agent. The addition of 0.5% glycerol improves the growth of *M. tuberculosis*.

Human tubercle bacilli produce visible growth on LJ medium in about 2 weeks, although on primary isolation from clinical material colonies may take up to 8 weeks to appear. On solid media, *M. tuberculosis* forms dry, rough, raised, irregular colonies with a wrinkled surface. They are tenacious and not easily emulsified. *M. tuberculosis* has a luxuriant growth (**eugenic growth**) as compared to *M. bovis*, which grows poorly on LJ glycerol medium (**dysgonic growth**).

Liquid Media

In liquid media the growth forms a prominent surface pellicle. Virulent strains tend to form long serpentine cords in liquid media, while avirulent strains grow in a more dispersed manner.

Biochemical Reactions

Several biochemical tests are used in identifying and differentiation of mycobacterial species.
1. **Niacin test:** The test is positive with human type and negative with bovine type of bacilli.
2. **Nitrate reduction test:** *M. tuberculosis*, give positive reaction.

Constituents of Tubercle Bacilli

The cell wall consists of lipids, proteins, and polysaccharides.

Pathogenesis

The mode of infection is by direct inhalation of aerosolized bacilli contained in droplet nuclei of expectorated sputum Tubercle bacilli are acquired from persons with active disease who are excreting viable bacilli by means of coughing, sneezing, or talking. Infection also occurs infrequently by ingestion, e.g., through infected milk, and rarely by inoculation.

The initial infection with *M. tuberculosis* is referred to as a **primary infection**. Subsequent disease in a previously sensitized person, either from an exogenous source or by reactivation of a primary infection, is known as **postprimary (secondary or reinfection) tuberculosis** with quite different pathological features.

After infection, *M. tuberculosis* cells are phagocytized by alveolar macrophages and are capable of intracellular multiplication. In a person with adequate cellular immunity, T cells arrive within 4–6 weeks with macrophage-activating polypeptides called *lymphokines*. This enables the macrophage in the area of infection to destroy the intracellular mycobacteria.

Laboratory Diagnosis

The definitive diagnosis of tuberculosis is based on:
- Microscopy
- Culture
- By transmitting the infection to experimental animals.
- Demonstration of hypersensitivity to tuberculoprotein
- Molecular diagnostic methods

Pulmonary Tuberculosis

A. Specimens

- **Sputum:** The most usual specimen for diagnosis of pulmonary tuberculosis is sputum. Patient is instructed to cough up the sputum into a clean wide-mouthed container. If sputum is scanty, a 24-hour sample may be tested. Three or more consecutive samples should be examined collected first in the morning, if possible.
- **Laryngeal swabs or bronchial washings:** These may be collected where sputum is not available.
- **Gastric lavage:** It can be examined in small children who tend to swallow the sputum.

B. Microscopy

Direct or concentration smears of sputum are examined. Smears are dried, heat fixed, and stained by the **Ziehl–Neelsen technique (hot-stain procedure)**.

Under the oil immersion objective, acid-fast bacilli are seen as bright red rods while the background is blue.

It is more convenient to use fluorescent microscopy when several smears are to be examined daily. Smears are stained **with auramine phenol or auramine rhodamine fluorescent dyes**. The fluorescent bacilli stand out brightly against the background.

C. Concentration Methods

Several methods have been described for the homogenization and concentration of sputum and other specimens. Concentration methods that do not kill the bacilli and so can be used for culture and animal inoculation. Several methods are in use:

i. **Petroff's method:** This simple method is widely used. Equal volumes of sputum and 4% sodium hydroxide are mixed and incubated at 37°C with frequent shaking till it gets liquefied and becomes clear. On the average, it takes 20–30 minutes. It is then centrifuged at 3,000 rpm for 30 minutes. The supernatant fluid is pipetted off and the deposit is neutralized by adding 8% hydrochloric acid in the presence of a drop of phenol red indicator and used for smear, culture, and animal inoculation.

ii. **Other methods:** Instead of alkali, homogenization can be achieved by treatment with dilute acids (6% sulfuric acid, 3% hydrochloric acid, or 5% oxalic acid), N acetyl cysteine with NaOH, pancreatin, desogen, zephiran and cetrimide. Flocculation methods have also been described.

D. Culture

It is a very sensitive diagnostic technique for tubercle bacilli, detecting as few as 10–100 bacilli per mL. The concentrated material is inoculated onto at least two bottles of LJ medium. Inoculated media are incubated at 35–37°C. Growth of most strains of *M. tuberculosis* may appear in 2–8 weeks.

Any bacterial growth is stained by the Ziehl–Neelsen method and, if acid-fast, it is subcultured for further identification. For routine purposes, a slow growing, nonpigmented, niacin positive acid-fast bacillus is taken as *M. tuberculosis*. Confirmation is by detailed biochemical studies.

In recent years, isolation of mycobacteria from clinical samples has been improved by newer techniques, notably radiometric respirometry. This is usually by means of the BACTEC radiometric technique, using the BACTEC 460 TB instrument. The procedure utilizes vials containing a 14C-labeled palmitic acid substrate, which during microbial growth releases $^{14}CO_2$ into the atmosphere above the medium. The $^{14}CO_2$ is detected by the instrument.

E. Sensitivity Testing

Several methods have been described.

F. Animal Inoculation

Two healthy, tuberculin-negative guinea-pigs are used.

G. Hybridization and Nucleic Acid Technology

1. Nucleic acid probes
2. Polymerase chain reaction (PCR) and ligase chain reaction
3. Transcription-mediated amplification targeting ribosomal RNA
4. DNA fingerprinting

H. Immunodiagnosis

1. **Serology:** Various serological tests, such as enzyme-linked immunosorbent assay (ELISA), radioimmunoassay (RIA) and latex agglutination have been tried for the serodiagnosis of tuberculosis.
2. **Tuberculin testing**

I. Chromatography

Extrapulmonary Tuberculosis
For diagnosis of extrapulmonary tuberculosis, microscopy, culture, and occasionally animal inoculation are also used.

Koch Phenomenon

Robert Koch (1890-1891) originally described the response of a tuberculous animal to reinfection. In a normal guinea pig subcutaneous injection of virulent tubercle bacillus produces no immediate response, but after 10-14 days a nodule develops at the site, which breaks down to form an ulcer that persists till the animal dies of progressive tuberculosis. The draining lymph nodes are enlarged and caseous. If on the contrary, virulent tubercle bacillus is injected in a guinea pig, which had received a prior injection of the tubercle bacillus 4-6 weeks earlier, an indurated lesion appears at the site in a day or two. This undergoes necrosis in another day or so to form a shallow ulcer, followed by rapid healing and no lymph node involvement or other tissues. This is known as the *Koch phenomenon* and is a combination of hypersensitivity and immunity.

Tuberculin Test

Principle: The principle of this test is delayed (Type IV) hypersensitivity reaction.

Reagents

1. **'Original' or 'old tuberculin' (OT):** Koch prepared a protein extract of tubercle bacillus. It was soon given up as it was not only of no benefit but also caused serious reactions in some.
2. **Purified protein derivative (PPD):** A partially purified protein antigen was introduced by Seibert. This is known as the PPD.

Method

1. **Mantoux test:** In the Mantoux test, 0.1 mL of PPD containing 5 TU is injected intradermally on the flexor aspect of the forearm, when properly performed, will produce a discrete pale elevation of the skin (a wheal). Tuberculin tests should be read 48-72 hours after injection. Induration of diameter 10 mm or more is considered positive, 5 mm or less negative, and 6-9 mm is of doubtful significance because it may be due to other mycobacterial infections. A positive tuberculin test indicates hypersensitivity to tuberculoprotein denoting infection with tubercle bacillus or BCG immunization, recent or past, with or without clinical disease.
2. **Heaf test**

Prophylaxis

In the prevention of tuberculosis general measures, such as adequate nutrition, good housing, and health education are as important as specific antibacterial measures. The latter consists of early detection and treatment of cases, BCG vaccination, and by chemoprophylaxis.

BCG Vaccination

Immunoprophylaxis is by intradermal injection of the live-attenuated vaccine developed by Calmette and Guerin (1921), the Bacille Calmette-Guerin (BCG). This is a strain of *M. bovis* attenuated by 239 serial subcultures in a glycerine-bile-potato medium over a period of 13 years between the years 1908 and 1920, which was avirulent for man while retaining its capacity to induce an immune response.

Dose and administration: BCG vaccine is given in a dose of 0.1 mL intradermally. BCG vaccine should be administered soon after birth failing which it may be given at any time during the first year of life.

Protective Value

Studies have shown that the range of protection offered by BCG varied from **0 to 80%** in different parts of the world.

The consensus opinion is that BCG may not protect from the risk of tuberculosis infection, but gives protection to infants and young children against the more serious types of the disease, such as meningitis and disseminated tuberculosis.

Treatment

The **bactericidal drugs,** rifampicin (R), isoniazid (H), pyrazinamide (Z), and streptomycin along with the **bacteristatic drug** ethambutol (E) thiacetazone, ethionamide, para-aminosalicyclic acid (PAS), and cycloserine constitute the **first-line drugs** in antituberculous therapy. The old practice of daily administration of drugs for two years or so has been replaced by short course regimens of 6–7 months, which are effective and convenient.

Multidrug-resistant *Mycobacterium tuberculosis* (MDR-TB)

A very serious consequence of unchecked drug resistance has been the emergence and spread of "**MDR-TB**". WHO defines a MDR strain as one that is at least resistant to rifampicin(R) and isoniazid (H).

Another serious condition *extensively drug resistant-tuberculosis* (XDR-TB) has emerged recently.

If compliance is an issue, a single daily dose of all first-line antitubercular drugs is preferred, and "**directly observed treatment strategy (DOTS)**" has been recommended.

KEY POINTS

Mycobacterium tuberculosis
- *Mycobacterium tuberculosis* is weakly gram-positive, strongly acid-fast, aerobic bacilli.
- The solid medium most widely employed for routine culture is **LJ medium**.
- Diseases: *M. tuberculosis* causes primarily **pulmonary tuberculosis**.

IMPORTANT QUESTIONS

1. Describe the laboratory diagnosis of pulmonary tuberculosis.

2. Write short notes on:
   a. Koch's phenomenon
   b. Tuberculin test
   c. Mantoux test
   d. BCG vaccine

MULTIPLE CHOICE QUESTIONS

1. Eugonic growth on Lowenstein-Jensen medium is produced by:
   a. *Mycobacterium tuberculosis*
   b. *M. bovis*
   c. Both of the above
   d. None of the above

2. LJ medium consists of the following ingredients, except:
   a. Egg yolk
   b. Agar
   c. Mineral salts
   d. Malachite green

3. Culture of tubercle bacilli maybe positive if number of bacteria in the specimen is:
   a. As few as 1–4 per mL
   b. As few as 5–9 per mL
   c. As few as 10–100 per mL
   d. As few as 150–200 per mL

4. Multidrug resistance tuberculosis (MDR-TB) is due to *M. tuberculosis* strain as one that is:
   a. Resistant to rifampicin only
   b. Resistant to isoniazid only
   c. Resistant to at least rifampicin and isoniazid
   d. None of the above

ANSWERS

1. a   2. b   3. c   4. c

Mycobacterium III: Mycobacterium leprae

LEARNING OBJECTIVES

After reading and studying this chapter, you should be able to:
- Describe morphology of *M. leprae*.
- Discuss cultivation of lepra bacilli.
- Explain animal models in leprosy.
- Describe pathogenesis of leprosy.
- Describe the following: Lepromatous leprosy; tuberculoid leprosy; lepromin test.
- Discuss laboratory diagnosis of leprosy.

INTRODUCTION

Leprosy is probably the oldest disease known to mankind. Leprosy was described as "kushta" in Sushruta Samhita written in India in 600 BC. It is caused by *Mycobacterium leprae,* which was discovered by Hansen in 1874 in Norway.

MYCOBACTERIUM LEPRAE

Morphology

Mycobacterium leprae is a straight or slightly curved rod, 1–8 × 0.2–0.5 mm in size, showing considerable morphological variations.

They are gram-positive and stain more readily than *M. tuberculosis*. With **Ziehl-Neelsen stain**, they are less acid-fast than tubercle bacilli, so 5% sulfuric acid is employed for decolorization after staining with carbol fuchsin. The bacilli are seen singly and in groups, intracellularly or lying free outside the cells. Inside the cells, they are present as bundles of organisms bound together by a lipid-like substance, the glia. These masses are known as *globi*. The parallel rows of bacilli in the globi give appearance of a *cigar bundle*. In tissue sections, the globi are present in Virchow's *lepra cells* or *foamy cells,* which are large undifferentiated histiocytes.

Cultivation

There have been several reports of successful cultivation but none has been confirmed.

There have been many attempts to transmit leprosy to experimental animals. However, the real break through was in 1960, when Shepard discovered that *M. leprae* could multiply in the footpads of mice kept at a low temperature (20°C). **Nine-banded armadillo:** The **nine-banded armadillo** *(Dasypus novemcinctus)* is highly susceptible to infection with lepra bacilli.

Classification

Classification system of Ridley and Jopling: The spectrum of disease activity in leprosy is very broad, characterized by pronounced variations in clinical, histopathologic, and immunologic findings. On the basis of these properties, Ridley and Jopling (1966) have established a classification scheme consisting of five forms of leprosy:
- Tuberculoid (TT)
- Borderline tuberculoid (BT)
- Borderline (BB)
- Borderline lepromatous (BL)
- Lepromatous (LL)

Pathogenesis

Leprosy (Hansen's disease) is a chronic granulomatous disease of humans primarily involving the skin, peripheral nerves, and nasal mucosa but capable of affecting any tissue or organ.

The two extreme or polar forms of the disease are the lepromatous and tuberculoid types.
1. **Lepromatous leprosy:** Lepromatous form is the generalized form of the disease and is found in individuals where the host resistance is low. This is known as "**multibacillary disease**".
2. **TT leprosy:** At the other end of the spectrum is hyper-reactive TT leprosy, which is seen in patients with high degree of resistance where cell-mediated immunity is intact. There are very few acid-fast bacilli (AFB), so that they are generally not seen microscopically (**paucibacillary disease**) and infectivity is minimal.

Lepromin Test

The lepromin test was first described by Mitsuda in 1919.

Lepromins: The lepromins used as antigen in lepromin test may be of human origin (lepromin-H) or of armadillo origin (lepromin-A):

Procedure

The test is performed by injecting intradermally 0.1 mL of lepromin into the inner aspect of the forearm of the individual. The response to the intradermal injection of lepromin is typically biphasic:
1. **Early or Fernandez reaction:** It consists of erythema and induration at the site of inoculation developing in 24-48 hours and usually remaining for 3-5 days.
2. **Late or Mitsuda reaction:** The reaction develops late, becomes apparent in 7-10 days following the injection and reaching its maximum in 3 or 4 weeks. At the end of 21 days, if there is a *nodule* at the site of inoculation, the reaction is said to be positive.

Uses of Lepromin Reaction

1. **To classify the lesions of leprosy patients:** The reaction is positive in tuberculoid and negative in lepromatous leprosy patients.
2. **To assess the prognosis and response to treatment:** A positive reaction indicates good prognosis and a negative one indicates bad prognosis.
3. **To assess the resistance of individuals to leprosy:** It is desirable to recruit only lepromin positive persons for work in leprosaria.
4. **To verify the identity of candidate lepra bacilli.**

Laboratory Diagnosis

The diagnosis consists of demonstration of AFB in the lesions.

1. Specimens

For routine examination, specimens are collected from the nasal mucosa, skin lesions, and ear lobules. Biopsy of the nodular lesions and thickened nerves, and lymph node puncture may be necessary in some cases.

Skin Smears
Slit and scrape method: About 5-6 different areas of the skin should be sampled, including the skin over the buttocks, forehead, chin, cheek, and ears.

Nasal Scrapings
The nose and the internal septum scraped sufficiently to remove a piece of mucus membrane.

2. Microscopy

Smears are stained by Ziehl-Neelsen method using 5% sulfuric acid for decolorization. AFB arranged in parallel bundles within macrophages *(Lepra-cell)* confirms the diagnosis of lepromatous leprosy. The viable bacilli stain uniformly and the dead bacilli are fragmented, irregular, or granular.

The smears are graded, based on the number of bacilli as follows:

- 1–10 bacilli in 100 fields = 1+
- 1–10 bacilli in 10 fields = 2+
- 1–10 bacilli per field = 3+
- 10–100 bacilli per field = 4+
- 100–1,000 bacilli per field = 5+
- More than 1,000 bacilli,
- Clumps and globi in every field = 6+

i. **Bacteriological index (BI):** The bacteriological index is the number of bacilli in a tissue.

ii. **Morphological index (MI):** It is defined as the percentage of uniformly stained bacilli out of the total number of bacilli counted.

3. Animal Inoculation

Foot pad of mouse or **nine-banded armadillo** are the animals used for inoculation of material.

4. Lepromin Test

The test can be used to assess the prognosis and response to treatment.

5. Serological Test

Various serological tests like latex agglutination, *Mycobacterium leprae* particle agglutination (MLPA) and enzyme-linked immunosorbent assay (ELISA) have been described.

6. Molecular Diagnostic Methods

Polymerase chain reaction (PCR).

Treatment

Due to emergence of dapsone resistance, WHO recommended multiple drug therapy (MDT) for all leprosy cases based on dapsone, rifampicin and clofazimine. Patients with paucibacillary (I, TT, BT) leprosy are given rifampicin 600 mg once a month (supervised) and dapsone 100 mg daily (unsupervised) for 6 months. For multibacillary (BB, BL, LL leprosy, rifampicin 600 mg once a month (supervised, dapsone 100 mg daily (unsupervised), clofazimine 300 mg once monthly supervised and 50 mg daily, unsupervised are given for 2 years or until skin smears are negative.

KEY POINTS

- *Mycobacterium leprae* are weakly gram-positive, strongly AFB.
- **Diseases:** Leprosy is classifies into five types.

IMPORTANT QUESTION

1. Write short notes on:
   a. Lepromin test
   b. Laboratory diagnosis of leprosy

MULTIPLE CHOICE QUESTIONS

1. All the following are used as animal models for leprosy, *except*:
   a. Rhesus monkey
   b. Nine-banded armadillo
   c. Slender loris
   d. Indian pangolin

2. The most infectious form of leprosy is:
   a. Tuberculoid leprosy
   b. Borderline tuberculoid leprosy
   c. Mid-borderline leprosy
   d. Lepromatous leprosy

3. Tuberculoid form of leprosy is seen in patients with:
   a. Good cell-mediated immunity
   b. Good humoral immunity
   c. Deficient cell-mediated immunity
   d. Poor humoral immunity

4. Lepromin test is used for all of the following, *except*:
   a. Determine the type of leprosy
   b. Confirm diagnosis of leprosy
   c. Monitor leprosy patients to treatment with chemotherapy
   d. Evaluate host resistance to leprosy

5. All the following statements are true for Mitsuda reaction, *except*:
   a. A nodule develops after 3–4 weeks of injection of lepromin antigen
   b. Manifestation of cell-mediated immunity
   c. Negative in tuberculoid leprosy
   d. Negative in lepromatous leprosy

ANSWERS

1. a 2. d 3. a 4. b
5. c

CHAPTER 26

Nontuberculous Mycobacteria

LEARNING OBJECTIVES

After reading and studying this chapter, you should be able to:
- Classify nontuberculous mycobacteria (NTM) and examples of different groups of nontuberculous mycobacteria.
- Name the diseases caused by nontuberculous mycobacteria.
- Discuss the clinical significance of nontuberculous mycobacteria.

INTRODUCTION

Mycobacteria other than human or bovine tubercle bacilli may occasionally cause human disease resembling tuberculosis. This large group of mycobacteria has been known by several names; **atypical, anonymous, unclassified, paratubercle, tuberculoid, environmental or nontuberculous mycobacteria (NTM), opportunistic mycobacteria other than tubercle bacilli (MOTT)**. The names "**environmental**" or "**opportunistic mycobacteria**" are better suited.

CLASSIFICATION

Runyon (1959) classified NTM into four groups (**Table 26.1**) based on phenotypic characteristics of the various species, most notably pigment (yellow or orange) production and rate of growth.

Group 1: Photochromogens

Photochromogens, which are colorless when incubated in the dark, but develop a bright yellow or orange coloration, if young cultures are exposed to a light source.

Group II: Scotochromogens

The scotochromogens are slow-growing NTM whose colonies are pigmented (yellow-orange-red) when grown in the dark or the light.

Table 26.1: Runyon classification scheme of nontuberculous mycobacteria.

Runyon group	Name	Species
I	Photochromogens	• M. kansasii • M. marinum • M. simiae
II	Scotochromogens	• M. scrofulaceum • M. gordonae • M. szulgai
III	Nonphotochromogens	• M. avium • M. intracellulare • M. xenopi • M. ulcerans • M. ulcerans • M. malmoense
IV	Rapid growers	• M. chelonei • M. chelonei

Group III: Nonphotochromogens

The nonphotochromogens are slow-growing NTM whose colonies produce no pigment whether they are grown in the dark or the light.

Group IV: Rapid Growers

This is a heterogeneous group of mycobacteria capable of rapid growth, colonies appearing within seven days of incubation at 37°C or 25°C.

Chapter 26: Nontuberculous Mycobacteria

Table 26.2: Principal types of opportunist mycobacterial disease in man and the usual causative agents.

Disease	Usual causative agent
A. Lymphadenopathy	M. avium complex M. scrofulaceum
B. Skin lesions	
1. Post-trauma abscesses	M. chelanae M. fortuitum M. terrae
2. Swimming pool granuloma	M. marinum
3. Buruli ulcer	M. ulcerons
C. Pulmonary disease	M. avium complex M. kansasii M. xenopi M. malmoense
D. Disseminated disease	
1. AIDS-related	M. avium complex M. genevense
2. Non-AIDS-related	M. avium complex M. chelonae

(AIDS: acquired immunodeficiency syndrome)

PATHOGENESIS

Four main types of opportunist mycobacterial disease have been described in man **(Table 26.2)**.

LABORATORY DIAGNOSIS

Ziehl–Neelsen staining of smear shows acid fast bacilli. They grow well on LJ medium. There is no universally recognized identification scheme.

KEY POINTS

- Mycobacteria other than the *tubercle and leprae bacilli* are known as NTM.
- Classification—Runyon (1959) classified NTM into four groups.

IMPORTANT QUESTION

1. Write short notes on atypical mycobacteria.

MULTIPLE CHOICE QUESTIONS

1. All the following are scotochromogens, *except*:
   a. Mycobacterium kansasii
   b. Mycobacterium scrofulaceum
   c. Mycobacterium gordonae
   d. Mycobacterium szulgai
2. All the following species are rapid growers, *except*:
   a. Mycobacterium fortuitum
   b. Mycobacterium chelonae
   c. Mycobacterium abscessus
   d. Mycobacterium ulcerans
3. Which of the following bacteria *cause/s* pulmonary disease?
   a. Mycobacterium avium-intracellulare
   b. M. kansasii
   c. M. xenopi
   d. All of the above
4. Swimming pool granuloma is caused by:
   a. Mycobacterium ulcerans
   b. Mycobacterium marinum
   c. Mycobacterium chelonei
   d. Mycobacterium fortuitum
5. Buruli ulcer is caused by:
   a. Mycobacterium marinum
   b. Mycobacterium fortuitum
   c. Mycobacterium ulcerans
   d. Mycobacterium xenopi

ANSWERS

1. a   2. d   3. d   4. b
5. c

CHAPTER 27

Actinomycetes: Actinomyces, Nocardia

LEARNING OBJECTIVES

After reading and studying this chapter, you should be able to:
- Describe morphology of actinomyces.
- Explain clinical forms of actinomyces.
- Discuss laboratory diagnosis of actinomycosis.
- Describe the following: Nocardiosis

INTRODUCTION

The family *Actinomycetes* contains three major medically important genera, *Actinomyces*, *Nocardia*, and *Actinomadura*. *Actinomyces* is anaerobic or microaerophilic and non-acid-fast, while *Nocardia* is acid-fast and aerobic. *Actinomadura* is non-acid-fast and aerobic.

ACTINOMYCES

Morphology

Actinomyces are gram-positive, nonmotile, nonsporing, non-acid-fast. They often grow in mycelial forms and break up into coccoid and bacillary forms. Most show true branching.

Cultural Characteristics

They grow best under anaerobic or microaerophilic conditions with the addition of 5–10% CO_2. The optimum temperature for growth is 35–37°C. They can be grown on brain heart infusion (BHI) agar, heart infusion agar supplemented with 5% defibrinated horse, rabbit, or sheep blood, BHI broth and thioglycolate broth.

Pathogenesis

Actinomyces colonize the upper respiratory tract, gastrointestinal tract, and female genital tract. These bacteria are not normally present on the skin surface. The organisms have a low virulence potential and cause disease only when the normal mucosal barriers are disrupted by trauma, surgery, or infection.

Actinomycosis

The *Actinomyces* causes the disease known as actinomycosis. Actinomycosis is a chronic disease characterized by multiple abscesses and granulomata, tissue destruction, extensive fibrosis, and the formation of sinuses. Within diseased tissues the actinomycetes form large masses of mycelia embedded in an amorphous protein-polysaccharide matrix and surrounded by a zone of gram-negative, weakly acid-fast, club-like structures. The mycelial masses may be visible to the naked eye and are called *sulfur granules*, as they are often light yellow in color (Fig. 27.1). Human actinomycosis may take several forms such as—(1) cervicofacial; (2) thoracic; (3) abdominal; (4) pelvic.

Laboratory Diagnosis

1. **Specimens:** Pus, sinus discharge, bronchial secretions, sputum, or infected tissues are collected aseptically.
2. **Microscopy:** "Sulfur granules" may be demonstrated in pus by shaking it up in a

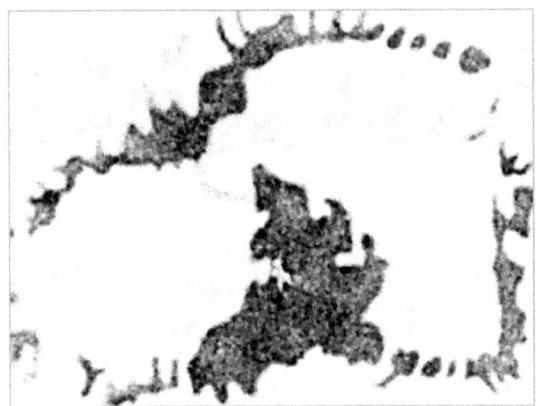

Fig. 27.1: Sulfur granules. Section of tissue showing an actinomycotic clolony, the clubs at the periphery giving a "sun ray" appearance.

test tube with some saline. On standing, the granules sediment may be withdrawn with a capillary pipette. Granules may also be obtained by applying gauze pads over the discharging sinuses.

Granules are crushed between two slides and stained with Gram and Ziehl-Neelsen (ZN) staining using 1% sulfuric acid for decolorization. Gram staining shows a dense network of thin gram-positive filaments, surrounded by a peripheral zone of swollen radiating club-shaped structures, presenting a *sun-ray appearance* (**Fig. 27.1**). The "clubs" are believed to be antigen-antibody complexes.

3. **Culture:** Sulfur granules or pus containing actinomycetes are washed and inoculated into thioglycolate liquid medium or streaked on BHI agar, blood agar, and incubated anaerobically at 37°C. On solid media, *A. israelii* may form so-called *spider colonies* that resemble molar teeth in 48-72 hours.
4. **Identification:** The identity may be confirmed by direct fluorescence microscopy and biochemical tests or by gas chromatography of metabolic products of carbohydrate fermentation.
5. **Biopsy:** In hematoxylin and eosin-stained sections, the sulfur granules are deeply stained with hematoxylin except in the periphery which is stained by eosin, which shows short, radiate, club-like structures.

Treatment

Treatment for actinomycosis involves the combination of surgical debribement of the involved tissues and the prolonged administration of antibiotics with penicillin or tetracycline.

NOCARDIA

Nocardia resemble *Actinomycetes* morphologically but are aerobic.

Species: The species most commonly associated with human disease are *N. asteroides, N. brasiliensis, N. farcinica. N. otitidiscaviarum, N. nova,* and *N. transvalensis.*

Morphology

Nocardiae are gram-positive bacteria and form a mycelium that fragments into rod-shaped and coccoid elements. *Nocardia* resembles *Actinomyces,* but some species are acid-fast, and a few are non-acid-fast.

Cultural Characteristics

Nocardiae readily grow in ordinary media. Nocardiae readily grow on nutrient agar, Sabouraud dextrose agar, BHI agar and yeast extract-malt extract agar. In addition, the technique of *paraffin baiting* may be used.

Colonies of nocardiae are cream, orange or pink-colored.

Pathogenesis

Nocardiae produce opportunistic pulmonary disease known as *nocardiosis* in immunocompromised individuals including those with acquired immunodeficiency syndrome (AIDS). Soil is known to be natural habitat of *Nocardia.* Man acquires infection by inhalation of the bacteria from environmental sources.

Bronchopulmonary disease: Systemic nocardiosis manifests primarily as pulmonary disease, pneumonia, lung abscess, or other lesions resembling tuberculosis.

Cutaneous infection: Primary or secondary cutaneous infection may lead to mycetoma, lymphocutaneous infections, cellulites, subcutaneous abscesses.

Laboratory Diagnosis
1. **Specimens:** Pus or purulent sputum
2. **Microscopy:** The smears are stained with Gram staining and ZN technique using decolorization with 1% sulfuric acid. Gram positive filamentous bacteria can be seen on Gram staining. Acid-fast bacilli are detected on ZN technique.
3. **Culture:** The specimens are inoculated on nutrient agar, Sabouraud's dextrose agar (SDA) and BHI agar and incubated at 36°C for 3 weeks. Colony morphology is seen and bacteria are identified by staining.
   Nocardia can be isolated from sputum by *paraffin bait* technique.

Treatment
Sulfonamide are the antibiotics of choice. They are also susceptible to amikacin, imipenem, minocycline, tobramycin and vancomycin.

KEY POINTS

- The *Actinomyces* causes the disease known as actinomycosis.
- *Nocardia* species cause primary cutaneous nocardiosis, bronchopulmonary infection, and secondary CNS infection.

IMPORTANT QUESTION
1. Write short notes on:
   a. Actinomycosis
   b. Nocardiosis

MULTIPLE CHOICE QUESTIONS
1. Which of the following bacteria is/are acid fast?
   a. *Actinomyces*
   b. *Nocardia*
   c. *Streptomyces*
   d. All of the above
2. Molar-teeth-like colonies are produced by:
   a. *Nocardia asteroides*
   b. *Actinomyces israelii*
   c. *Actinomadura madurae*
   d. *Tropheryma whipplei*
3. Paraffin bait technique is used for the isolation of Nocardia from:
   a. Soil
   b. Sputum
   c. Both of the above
   d. None of the above

ANSWERS
---
1. b   2. b   3. c

Enterobacteriaceae: Escherichia, Klebsiella, Proteus, and other Genera

LEARNING OBJECTIVES

After reading and studying this chapter, you should be able to:
- Describe general characters of the family *Enterobacteriaceae*.
- Classify the family *Enterobacteriaceae*.
- Describe morphology, cultural characteristics, and biochemical reactions of *Escherichia coli*.
- Discuss pathogenicity of *Escherichia coli*.
- Discuss various groups of *Escherichia coli* producing diarrhea.
- Discuss laboratory diagnosis of urinary tract infections caused by *Escherichia coli*.
- Discuss morphology, cultural characteristics and biochemical reactions of *Klebsiella* sp.
- Differentiate between *E. coli* and *Klebsiella sp.*
- Describe morphology, cultural characteristics and biochemical reactions of *Proteus* sp.

The family *Enterobacteriaceae* is the largest, most heterogeneous collection of medically important gram-negative bacilli.

CHARACTERISTICS OF THE FAMILY ENTEROBACTERIACEAE

1. They are gram-negative bacilli.
2. They are aerobes or/and facultative anaerobes and grow readily on ordinary laboratory media.
3. All species ferment glucose with the production of acid or acid and gas.
4. Either nonmotile or motile with peritrichous flagella.
5. They are catalase positive (except for *Shigella dysenteriae* type 1 which is catalase-negative)
6. They are oxidase-negative.
7. They reduce nitrate to nitrites.
8. They are typically intestinal parasites of humans and animals.

CLASSIFICATION OF ENTEROBACTERIACEAE

The classification of *Enterobacteriaceae* has been controversial and there have been successive changes in their grouping and nomenclature (**Table 28.1**).

ESCHERICHIA COLI

Morphology

Escherichia coli is a gram negative, straight, rod measuring 1–3 × 0.4–0.7 µm. It is motile by peritrichous flagella, though some strains may be nonmotile. It is nonsporing and noncapsulated.

Table 28.1: Classification of the family *Enterobacteriaceae*.

Tribe	Genus
1. Escherichiae	• Escherichia • Shigella
2. Edwardsielleae	Edwardsiella
3. Salmonelleae	Salmonella
4. Citrobactereacae	Citrobacter
5. Klebsielleae	• Klebsiella • Enterobacter • Serratia • Hafnia
6. Proteeae	• Proteus • Morganella • Providencia
7. Yersinieae	Yersinia

Cultural Characteristics

It is an aerobe and a facultative anaerobe. The temperature range is 10–40°C (optimum 37°C). It can grow on the ordinary media like **nutrient agar**. Colonies are large, thick, grayish white, moist, smooth opaque or partially translucent disks. Some strains may occur in the 'mucoid' form. On **blood agar,** many strains are hemolytic. On **MacConkey's medium**, colonies are red or pink due to lactose fermentation. In broth, growth occurs as general turbidity and a heavy deposit.

Biochemical Reactions

1. *E. coli* ferments glucose, lactose, mannitol, maltose, and many other sugars with the production of acid and gas. Typical strains do not ferment sucrose.
2. Indole and MR positive, and VP and citrate negative (IMViC + + – –)
3. It is negative for phenylalanine deaminase test, urease test, H_2S production.

Antigenic Structure

Serotyping of *E. coli* is based on three antigens—the flagellar antigen H, somatic antigen O and the capsular antigen K as detected in agglutination assays with specific rabbit antibodies.
1. **H antigens:** 75 antigens.
2. **Somatic antigen (O antigen):** Over 170 O antigens
3. **Capsular antigen (K antigen):** 103 K antigens.
4. **Fimbrial antigen (F antigen):** It has no role in antigenic classification.

Toxins

Exotoxins: *E. coli* produces two kinds of exotoxins *hemolysins* and *enterotoxins*.
   a. **Hemolysins:** Hemolysins do not appear to be relevant in pathogenesis.
   b. **Enterotoxins:** Three distinct types of *E. coli* enterotoxins have been identified:
      i. Heat-labile toxin (LT)
      ii. Heat-stable toxin (ST)
      iii. Verocytotoxin or verotoxin (VT)

Clinical Infections

Four main types of clinical syndromes are caused by *E. coli*:
1. Diarrhea
2. Urinary tract infection
3. Pyogenic infections
4. Septicemia

1. Diarrhea

At least five different types of diarrheagenic *E. coli* are now recognized, each associated with specific serotypes and with different pathogenic mechanisms.

A. **Enteropathogenic *E. coli* (EPEC):** These have been associated mainly with diarrhea in infants and children. In infantile enteritis, the bacilli are seen to be adherent to the mucosa of the upper small intestine, causing disruption of the brush border microvilli.

B. **Enterotoxigenic *E. coli* (ETEC):** In developing countries 'ETEC are a major cause of mortality in children under the age of 5 years. Persons from developed countries visiting endemic areas often suffer from ETEC diarrhea—a condition known as "**traveler's diarrhea**".

C. **Enteroinvasive *E. coli* (EIEC):** EIEC, like those of *Shigella* species, can penetrate the epithelial cells of the large intestine and multiply intracellularly, giving rise to blood and mucus in the stool. Clinically, EIEC infection resembles shigellosis, ranging from mild diarrhea to frank dysentery, and occurs, in children as well as adults.

D. ***E. coli* verocytotoxin or verotoxin (VT):** *E. coli* verocytotoxin or verotoxin (VT) was so named because it was first detected (1977) by its cytotoxic effect on Vero cells and cause **hemorrhagic colitis** and **hemolytic uremic syndrome**.

E. **Enteroaggregative *E. coli* (EAEC):** They have been associated with persistent diarrhea, especially in developing countries.

Laboratory Diagnosis of Diarrhea

1. **Laboratory diagnosis of EPEC:** Fresh diarrheal feces are plated on blood agar

and MacConkey media. *E. coli* colonies are examined by slide agglutination with polyvalent rabbit antisera.
2. **Laboratory diagnosis of ETEC:** Demonstration of enterotoxin in *E. coli* isolates either LT or ST or both.
3. **Laboratory diagnosis of EIEC:**
   a. Sereny test
   b. Tissue culture and DNA hybridization methods
   c. Enzyme-linked immunosorbent assay (ELISA)
4. **Laboratory diagnosis of VTEC:** By demonstration of the bacilli or VT in feces directly or in culture.

2. Urinary Tract Infection

E. coli and coliforms account for the large majority of naturally acquired urinary tract infections (UTIs). UTI occurs more often in females than in males.

Laboratory Diagnosis of UTI
A. **Collection of specimen:**
   i. **Catheter specimen:** It is no longer considered justifiable.
   ii. **Midstream urine specimen:** In, male patients, retract the prepuce and clean the glans penis with wet cotton. In case of female, anogenital toilet is more important and should consist of careful cleaning with soap and water. Separate labia majora with fingers of one hand and collect midstream urine in a sterile wide-mouthed container. The first portion of urine that flushes out commensal bacteria from the anterior urethra is discarded. The next portion of the urine (midstream sample) is collected directly into a sterile wide-mouthed container.
   iii. **Suprapubic stab:** In children and young infants.
B. **Transport:** Urine is a good medium for the growth of coliforms and other urinary pathogens. If delay of more than 1–2 hours is unavoidable, the specimen should be refrigerated at 4°C.
C. **Microscopy of urine:** In the past, the microscopical examination was commonly done on a wet film or Gram-stained film of deposit centrifuged from the urine to find out the presence of pus cells, red blood cells, and bacteria in it.
D. **Culture:** Semiquantitative culture—semiquantitative techniques (standard loop method) are used for urine specimens.
   Standard loop method: Measured quantity of urine with the help of standardized loop is inoculated on blood agar and another loopful on MacConkey agar and incubated overnight at 37°C. Blood agar medium gives a quantitative measurement of bacteriuria, while MacConkey agar enables a presumptive diagnosis of the bacterium.
   Interpretation of results: Kass (1956) gave a criterion for active bacterial infection of urinary tract as follows:
   - **Significant bacteriuria:** When bacterial count is >10^5/mL of a single species.
   - **Doubtful significance:** Between 10^4 and 10^5 bacteria per mL. Specimen should be repeated for culture.
   - **No significant growth:** When the bacterial count is <10^3 bacteria per mL and are regarded as contaminant.
E. **Identification:** The organisms are identified by colony characters, Gram's staining, motility, biochemical reactions, and slide agglutination test.
F. **Antibiotic sensitivity test:** *E. coli* and other common urinary pathogens develop drug resistance so frequently that no antibacterial therapy can be instituted meaningfully without testing individual strains.

3. Pyogenic Infections

Escherichia coli form of intra-abdominal infections, such as peritonitis and abscesses pyogenic infections in the perianal area neonatal meningitis. The specimens are usually pus and wound swab. Cultures are made on MacConkey's agar.

The isolate is identified by colony morphology, staining, motility and biochemical reactions.

4. Septicemia

Blood stream invasion by *E. coli* may lead to fatal conditions like septic shock and "systemic inflammatory response syndrome" (SIDS). Diagnosis depends on the isolation of the organism by blood culture and its identification by colony morphology, staining, motility, and biochemical reactions.

EDWARDSVILLE

The genus contains the species *Edwardsiella tarda*. It mainly causes wound infection, but meningitis and septicemia have also been reported.

CITROBACTER

Clinical Infection

Citrobacter spp. may cause infections of the urinary tract, gallbladder, middle ear, and meninges. *C. koseri* occasionally causes neonatal meningitis.

KLEBSIELLA

Introduction

Members of the genus *Klebsiella* are gram-negative, nonsporing, nonmotile bacilli that grow well on ordinary media, produce pink mucoid colonies on MacConkey's agar. They are usually found in the intestinal tract of humans and animals or free-living in soil, water, and on plants.

Classification

The name *K. pneumoniae* is used for the species as a whole. It is further divided into four sub-species. *K. pneumoniae* subsp. *ozaenae*, *K. pneumoniae* subsp. *Pneumoniae*, *K. pneumoniae* subsp. *Rhinoscleromatis*.

Morphology

They are short, plump, gram-negative, nonsporing, capsulated, nonmotile bacilli, 1–2 μm long and 0.5–0.8 μm.

Cultural Characteristics

Klebsiellae grow well on ordinary media at optimum temperature 37°C in 18–24 hours. On MacConkey agar, the colonies typically appear large, mucoid, and red in color. Mucoid nature of colonies is due to capsular material produced by the organism.

Biochemical Reactions

They ferment sugars (glucose, lactose, sucrose, and mannitol) with production of acid and gas. They are urease positive, indole negative, MR negative, VP positive, and citrate positive (IMViC – – + +). These reactions are typical of *K. pneumoniae* subsp. *aerogenes*.

Antigenic Structure

Klebsiella possess capsular (K) and somatic (O) antigens.
1. **Capsular (K) antigen:** On the basis of capsular (K) antigens, the *Klebsiellae* have been differentiated, into, 80 serotypes.
2. **Somatic (O) antigen:** Five different somatic or O antigens (01–05) occur.

KLEBSIELLA PNEUMONIAE

It is the second most populous member of the aerobic bacterial flora of the human intestine. It has become a very important cause of nosocomial infections, even replacing *E. coli* in some centers.

Pathogenicity: *Klebsiella pneumoniae* can cause a primary community-acquired pneumonia, nosocomial infections, UTIs, wound infections, bacteremia and meningitis, and rarely diarrhea.

Pneumonia: *Klebsiella pneumoniae* is a serious disease with high-case fatality.

Diarrhea: Some strains of *K. pneumoniae* isolated from cases of diarrhea.

Laboratory Diagnosis

Diagnosis is made by culturing appropriate specimens on blood agar and MacConkey agar and identifying the isolate by biochemical reactions. Antibiotic sensitivity should invariably be done.

K. ozaenae: It is associated with ozena, an uncommon, chronic disease in which there is atrophy of the nasal mucosa.

Chapter 28: Enterobacteriaceae: Escherichia, Klebsiella, Proteus, and other Genera

K. rhinoscleromatis: It causes rhinoscleroma, a chronic granulomatous hypertrophy of the nose.

Treatment
They are normally susceptible to cephalosporins, and to fluoroquinolones. They are often sensitive to gentamicin and other aminoglycosides.

ENTEROBACTER
They may cause UTIs and hospital infections.

HAFNIA
They are occasionally encountered as an opportunistic pathogen that has been recovered from infected wounds, abscesses, sputum urine, blood, and other sites.

SERRATIA
Nosocomial infections due to *S. marcescens* are being reported with increasing frequency.

TRIBE PROTEAE: *PROTEUS, MORGANELLA,* AND *PROVIDENCIA*

Classification
The tribe Proteae is classified into three genera *Proteus, Morganella,* and *Providencia.* A characteristic feature, which distinguishes tribe proteae from other enterobacteria is the presence, in all members of the tribe, of the enzyme phenylalanine deaminase, which converts phenyl alanine to phenyl pyruvic acid (PPA reaction).

Proteus

Introduction
Proteus bacilli are normal intestinal commensals and opportunistic pathogens like coliforms.

Classification
Genus *Proteus* has four species: *P. mirabilis, P. vulgaris, P. myxofaciens,* and *P. penneri.*

Morphology
They are gram-negative coccobacilli. Pleomorphism is frequent. They are actively motile with peritrichous flagella and are noncapsulated.

Cultural Characteristics
They are aerobe and facultative anaerobes. All grow well on laboratory **nutrient media.** *Proteus* organisms are usually first recognized by their characteristic putrefactive odor described as **'fishy' or 'seminal'** and **swarming appearance** on noninhibitory solid media such as **nutrient agar and blood agar.** Swarming is a striking feature of *P. mirabilis* and *P. vulgaris.* Swarming of *Proteus* appears to be due to vigorous motility of the organism although the exact cause is not yet established.

Swarming does not occur on MacConkey's medium, on which smooth colorless (NLF) formed.

Dienes phenomenon: It has been used to determine the identity or nonidentity of various strains of *Proteus.*

Biochemical Reactions
1. **PPA test:** Deamination of phenyl alanine to phenyl pyruvic acid (PPA test) is always positive.
2. **Urea hydrolysis:** Urea hydrolysis by enzyme urease is another characteristic of *Proteus*, but is negative in some Providencia strains.
3. All species of *Proteus* produce acid from glucose.
4. Lactose is not fermented.
5. They are malonate utilization negative.
6. Indole is formed by *P. vulgaris* but is negative in *P. mirabilis.*
7. They are MR positive and VP negative.
8. H_2S is produced by *P. vulgaris* and *P. mirabilis.*
9. Nitrate reduction positive.

Antigenic Structure
Proteus bacilli possess **somatic O** and **flagellar H** antigens, which are of considerable historical interest.

Pathogenesis

Proteus bacilli are widely distributed in nature as saprophytes. They are frequently present on the moist areas of the skin. They are opportunistic pathogens, commonly responsible for urinary and septic infections, often nosocomial. All members of the tribe can cause **UTI, wound infections, pneumonia, infection of the ear, respiratory tract infection, septicemia,** and **nosocomial infections**.

Laboratory Diagnosis

A. **Specimen:** Pus in pyogenic lesions midstream urine in UTI
B. **Culture:** Laboratory diagnosis of the infections caused by species *Proteus* can be carried out by culture of the specimen on MacConkey agar or blood agar culture media are incubated at 37°C for 18–24 hours. Swarming does not occur on MacConkey's medium, on which smooth colorless (NLF) formed. *Proteus* produces uniform turbidity with a slight powdery deposit and an ammoniacal odor in liquid medium (peptone water).
C. **Identification:** The isolate is identified by its morphological, biochemical, and agglutination reactions.
D. **Antibiotic susceptibility test**

Treatment

Proteus bacilli are resistant to many of the common antibiotics. An exception is *P. mirabilis*, which is sensitive to ampicillin and cephalosporins.

MORGANELLA

M. morganii causes urinary infection and nosocomial wound infections.

PROVIDENCIA

Providencia species may be recovered from feces may be associated with diarrhea, hospital-acquired urinary tract, wound, and other infections, infection of burns and pneumonia and septicemia.

ERWINIA

E. herbicola has occasionally been isolated from respiratory and urinary infections.

KEY POINTS

Escherichia coli
- **Toxins (Exotoxins):** *Hemolysins* and *enterotoxins*.

Klebsiella
- *Klebsiella pneumoniae* can cause a primary community-acquired pneumonia, nosocomial infections, UTI, wound infections, bacteremia and meningitis, and rarely diarrhea.
- Genus *Proteus* has four species: *P. mirabilis, P. vulgaris, P. myxofaciens,* and *P. penneri.*
  All members of the tribe proteae can cause UTI, wound infections, and pneumonia.

IMPORTANT QUESTIONS

1. Describe the laboratory diagnosis of bacterial diarrheas caused by *Escherichia coli*.
2. Discuss the pathogenesis and laboratory diagnosis of urinary tract infections caused by *Escherichia coli*.
3. Write briefly about:
   a. *Klebsiella pneumoniae*
   b. *Proteus* species.

MULTIPLE CHOICE QUESTIONS

1. Which of the following properties is/are shown by the organisms belonging to the family Enterobacteriaceae?
   a. They are catalase positive
   b. They are oxidase negative
   c. They ferment glucose
   d. All of the above
2. Which of the following bacteria is/are known as coliform bacilli?
   a. *Escherichia*
   b. *Klebsiella*
   c. *Enterobacter*
   d. All of the above
3. Traveler's diarrhea is caused by:
   a. Enteropathogenic *Escherichia coli*
   b. Enterotoxigenic *Escherichia coli*

Chapter 28: Enterobacteriaceae: Escherichia, Klebsiella, Proteus, and other Genera

    c. Enteroinvasive *Escherichia coli*
    d. Verotoxigenic *Escherichia coli*
4. Hemolytic uremic syndrome is caused by:
    a. Enteropathogenic *E. coli*
    b. Enterotoxigenic *E. coli*
    c. Enteroinvasive *E. coli*
    d. Verocytotoxin producing *E. coli*
5. The bacterium that shows swarming on blood agar is:
    a. *Proteus stuartii*
    b. *Proteus mirabilis*
    c. *Providencia rettgeri*
    d. *Morganella morganii*

6. Diene's phenomenon is used to detect identity of strains of:
    a. Klebsiella
    b. Salmonella
    c. Shigella
    d. Proteus

ANSWERS

1. d   2. b   3. b   4. d
5. b   6. d

CHAPTER 29

Shigella

LEARNING OBJECTIVES

After reading and studying this chapter, you should be able to:
♦ Describe morphology and various culture media for the isolation of Shigella.
♦ Discuss the antigenic structure and toxins of Shigella.
♦ Discuss laboratory diagnosis of bacillary dysentery.

INTRODUCTION

The genus *Shigella* is named after the Japanese microbiologist Kiyoshi Shiga, who first isolated the organism in 1896. All *Shigella* species can cause **bacillary dysentery**.

MORPHOLOGY

Shigellae are nonsporing, noncapsulated, gram-negative rods, 2–4 × 0.6 μm, nonmotile, and nonflagellate.

CULTURAL CHARACTERISTICS

They are aerobes and facultative anaerobes, with a growth temperature range of 10–40°C and optima of 37°C and pH 7.4. They grow well on conventional media.

After overnight incubation, colonies are smooth, greyish or colorless, translucent, often 2–3 mm in diameter, circular, convex, resembling those of salmonellae **on nutrient agar and blood agar**. Colonies on **MacConkey agar** and **deoxycholate citrate agar (DCA)** are colorless [nonlactose fermenting (NLF)] except in case of *S. sonnei*, which becomes pink due to late fermenter of lactose. DCA is an excellent selective plating medium. However, xylose lysine deoxycholate (XLD is probably the best selective medium for shigellae).

Enrichment broths are selenite F broth and gram-negative (GN) broth.

ANTIGENIC STRUCTURE

The shigellae are divided into four "major" **O antigenic groups**, designated A, B, C, and D.

CLASSIFICATION

Shigellae are classified into four species or subgroups (A, B, C, D) based on a combination of biochemical and serological characteristics.

Fermentation of mannitol is of importance in classification and shigellae have traditionally been divided into mannitol fermenting species (*S. flexneri, S. boydii,* and *S. sonnei*) ferment mannitol, and mannitol nonfermenting species (*S. dysenteriae*) *which* does not ferment mannitol.

Group A (S. dysenteriae)

This species of mannitol nonfermenting bacilli consists of 12 serotypes. **Serotypes 1 and 2** are the organisms formerly called **S. shigae** and *S. schmitzii*. *S. shigae* is indole negative and is the only member of the family that is always catalase negative.

Exotoxin: *S. dysenteriae* type 1 produces a powerful exotoxin (**Shiga toxin**).

Group B (S. flexneri)

This group is biochemically heterogeneous and antigenically the most complex among shigellae. Based on type-specific and group-specific antigens, they have been classified into six serotypes (1-6) and several subtypes (1a; 1b; 2a, 2b; 3a, 3b, 3c; 4a, 4b; 5a, 5b). In addition, two antigenic "variants" called X and Y are recognized, which have lost their type antigens.

Serotype 6 is always indole negative and occurs in three biotypes: Boyd 88, Manchester and Newcastle, some of which form gas from sugars.

Group C (S. boydii)

This group consists of dysentery bacilli that resemble S. flexneri biochemically but not antigenically. Eighteen different serotypes of S. boydii are recognized.

Group D (S. sonnei)

It is indole negative. It may, however undergo an antigenic variation and may occur in two forms, **phase I and phase II**.

PATHOGENIC MECHANISMS

1. **Surface properties:** Lipopolysaccharide (LPS) enable these bacteria to enter intestinal cells.
2. **Invasiveness:** S. dysenteriae type 1 forms an exotoxin, which appears to be much less important in pathogenesis than the ability of the bacillus to penetrate and multiply in colonic mucosa.
3. **Toxins:** S. dysenteriae type 1 produces a powerful exotoxin (**Shiga toxin**).

Pathogenicity

Shigellae cause bacillary dysentery. Humans are the only known reservoir of *Shigella* organisms. Infection occurs by ingestion. The infection is highly communicable because of the low infective dose required to produce the disease (10-100 bacilli).

Bacillary dysentery has a short-incubation period (1-7 days, usually 48 hours). The clinical manifestations of shigellosis vary from asymptomatic to severe forms of the disease.

Complications are most often seen in patients with S. dysenteriae serotype 1 infection.

LABORATORY DIAGNOSIS

Diagnosis depends on isolating the bacillus from feces.

A. Specimens

1. **Feces:** A specimen of feces is always preferable to a rectal swab.
2. **Rectal swabs:** A direct swab may be taken from the ulcer by sigmoidoscopic examination.

B. Transport

Fresh feces should be inoculated without delay or transported in a suitable medium such as Sachs' buffered glycerol saline.

C. Microscopy

Make a wet film of a suspension of the feces in saline. This will show numerous erythrocytes and polymorphs and some macrophages.

D. Culture

The feces are inoculated on **MacConkey agar** and **DCA**. **SS agar** and **XLD medium** can also be used. After overnight incubation at 37°C, the plates are inspected for pale (nonlactosefermenting) colonies on MacConkey agar and DCA, and red and colorless colonies with no blackening on XLD and SS agar, respectively.

Identification

1. **Biochemical reactions:** Any nonmotile bacillus that is urease, citrate, H_2S, and KCN negative should be further investigated by biochemical tests.
2. **Slide agglutination:** Identification is confirmed by slide agglutination with polyvalent and monovalent sera and then with type-specific sera.

E. Colicine Typing

Plasmid pattern analysis and colicine typing may help elucidate patterns of spread of S. sonnei.

F. Serology
Serology has no place in diagnosis of disease.

TREATMENT
Most of the cases of bacillary dysentery especially those due to *S. sonnei,* are mild and self-limiting and do not require antibiotic therapy. Replacement of fluids and electrolytes by oral rehydration salt solution is all that is required.

Treatment with a suitable antibiotic is necessary in the very young, the aged, or the debilitated, and in severe infections. Ampicillin, cotrimoxazole, tetracycline, the quinolone antibiotics, such as nalidixic acid and ciprofloxacin are appropriate choices.

KEY POINTS
- The genus *Shigella* is gram-negative bacilli, non-motile.
- **Classification:** The shigellae are divided into four **groups** or **species**. It causes dysentery.

IMPORTANT QUESTION
1. Discuss laboratory diagnosis of bacillary dysentery.

MULTIPLE CHOICE QUESTIONS
1. All *Shigella* species ferment mannitol, *except:*
   a. *Shigella dysenteriae*
   b. *Shigella boydii*
   c. *Shigella flexneri*
   d. *Shigella sonnei*
2. **Shiga toxin is produced by:**
   a. *Shigella dysenteriae* serotype 1
   b. *Shigella dysenteriae* serotype 2
   c. *Shigella dysenteriae* serotype 8
   d. *Shigella dysenteriae* serotype 10

ANSWERS
1. a   2. a

Enterobacteriaceae III: Salmonella

LEARNING OBJECTIVES

After reading and studying this chapter, you should be able to:
- Describe morphology, culture characteristics and biochemical reactions of *Salmonella* sp.
- Discuss laboratory diagnosis of enteric fever.
- Describe vaccination against enteric fever.

INTRODUCTION

Genus *Salmonella* consists of bacilli that parasitize the intestines of a large number of vertebrate species and infect human beings, leading to enteric fever, gastroenteritis, septicemia with or without focal suppuration, and the carrier state. Typhi is the causative agent of typhoid.

SALMONELLA

Morphology

Salmonellae are gram-negative bacilli, 2–4 × 0.6 µm in size. They are motile with peritrichous flagella except *S. Gallinarum—Pullorum*, which is nonmotile. They are non-acid-fast, noncapsulate, and nonsporing.

Cultural Characteristics

Salmonellae are aerobes and facultative anaerobes, growing readily over a range of pH 6–8 and temperature 15–45°C (optimum 37°C). They can grow on simple laboratory media. Colonies of most strains are 2–3 mm in diameter, gray-white, moist, circular disks with a smooth convex surface, and entire edge after 24 hours at 37°C **on nutrient agar and blood agar**. On MacConkey agar and **deoxycholate-citrate agar (DCA), colonies are** colorless due to nonlactose fermentation (NLF). **On Wilson and Blair's brilliant-green bismuth sulfite agar (which is selective media for salmonellae),** jet black colonies with a metallic sheen are formed due to production of H_2S. **On Xylose lysine deoxycholate (XLD) agar,** most salmonellae produce hydrogen sulfide to produce black centers in their red colonies. The H_2S-negative salmonellae form red colonies without black centers.

Enrichment media: Tetrathionate broth and Selenite F broth are commonly used enrichment media for inoculation of specimens especially feces.

Biochemical Reactions

1. Salmonellae ferment glucose, mannitol, arabinose, maltose, dulcitol and sorbitol, forming acid and gas except *S. typhi, Gallinarum.*
2. Lactose, sucrose, salicin, or adonitol are not fermented.
3. Indole is not produced. They are MR positive, VP negative and citrate positive (IMViC - + - +) except by *S. typhi* and *S. paratyphi A* which are citrate negative.
4. Hydrogen sulfide is produced except by *S. paratyphi A, S. choleraesuis, S. typhisuis,* and *S. sendai.*
5. Urease is not hydrolyzed.
6. Salmonellae decarboxylate the amino acids lysine, ornithine, and arginine.

Resistance

Salmonellae are readily killed by moist heat, at 55°C in 1 hour or at 60°C in 15 minutes and most strong disinfectants. Boiling or chlorination of water and pasteurization of milk destroy the bacilli. In polluted water and soil, they survive for weeks and in ice for months.

Antigenic Structure

Salmonellae possess the following antigens based on which they are classified and identified:
1. Flagellar antigen H
2. Somatic antigen O
3. Surface antigen Vi, found in some species.

Pathogenesis

Salmonellae are strict parasites of animals or humans.

Host-adapted Serotypes

S. typhi, S. paratyphi A and usually, but not invariably *S. paratyphi B* are confined to human beings. Other salmonellae are parasitic in various animals—domestic animals, rodents, reptiles, and birds.

Clinical Syndromes

Salmonellae cause the following four major syndromes:
1. Enteric fever
2. Septicemia with or without metastatic infection
3. Gastroenteritis or food poisoning
4. Asymptomatic carrier state

1. Enteric Fever

The term enteric fever includes typhoid fever caused by *S. typhi* and *paratyphoid* fever caused by paratyphi A, B, or C.

Typhoid Fever
Clinical course: The infection is acquired by ingestion. The incubation period is usually 7–14 days. The clinical course may vary from mild undifferentiated pyrexia to a rapidly fatal fulminating disease.

In the untreated case, the temperature shows a step ladder rise. Physical signs include a relative bradycardia at the height of the fever, hepatomegaly, splenomegaly, and often a rash of *rose spots,* found on the front of the chest during the second or third week and fade on pressure.

Paratyphoid Fever
S. paratyphi A and *B* cause paratyphoid fever, which resembles typhoid fever but is generally milder.

2. Bacteremia with Focal Lesion

This is associated with *S. choleraesuis* but may be caused by any salmonella serotype.

3. Gastroenteritis or Food Poisoning

This is the most common manifestation of salmonella infection (For detail see under the heading, **"Salmonella gastroenteritis"**).

4. Asymptomatic Carrier State

A few patient continue to excrete the Salmonella for long period after complete clinical recovery.

Laboratory Diagnosis

Bacteriological diagnosis of enteric fever consists of:
A. Isolation and identification of the bacilli
B. Demonstration of circulating antigen
C. Demonstration of antibodies in patient's serum
D. Other laboratory tests

A. Isolation and Identification of the Bacilli

It may be done by culture of specimens such as patient's blood, feces, urine, bone marrow, duodenal drainage rose spots, etc. For the laboratory diagnosis of enteric fever, selection of relevant specimens depends upon duration of illness, e.g., blood for culture must be taken repeatedly. Urine culture may be positive after second week and stool second or third week (**Fig. 30.1 and Table 30.1**).

Blood Culture
Blood cultures are positive in approximately 90% cases in the first week of fever, in approximately

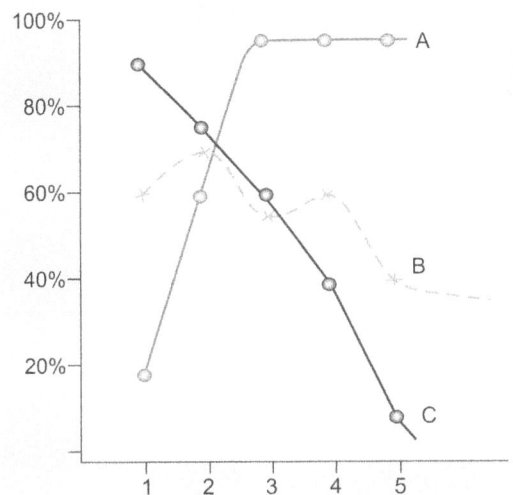

Fig. 30.1: Laboratory diagnosis of typhoid fever. The approximate percentages of test found positive during different stages of the disease (from 1st to 5th week). A. Widal agglutination; B. Feces culture; C. Blood culture.

Table 30.1: Positivity of various specimens at different phases of enteric fever.		
Duration	Specimen	% positivity
1st week	Blood culture	90
	Feces culture	–
	Widal test	–
2nd week	Blood culture	75
	Faeces culture	50
	Widal test	Low titer
3rd week	Blood culture	60
	Feces culture	80
	Widal test	80–100

75% of cases in the second week, 60% in the third week and 25% thereafter till the subsidence of pyrexia **(Fig. 30.1 and Table 30.1)**.

With all aseptic precautions, about 5–10 mL of blood is collected by venipuncture and inoculated into a culture bottle containing 50–100 mL of 0.5% bile broth. Blood contains substances that inhibit the growth of the bacilli and hence it is essential that this effect may be annulled by diluting of blood between 1 in 5 and 1 in 10 in culture medium. The addition of liquid (sodium polyanethol sulfonate) counteracts the bactericidal action of blood.

After overnight incubation at 37°C, the bile broth is subcultured on MacConkey agar and blood agar media. These plates are incubated at 37°C for 24 hours. Pale NLF colonies that may appear on MacConkey agar medium are picked out for biochemical tests and motility. If no growth is obtained after 5–7 days, then the culture is declared negative.

Castaneda's method of culture: Castaneda's method of culture may be adopted to eliminate the risk of introducing contamination during repeated subculture, and also for economy and safety.

Subcultures repetition: If salmonellae are not obtained from the first subculture from bile broth.

Clot Culture
An alternative to blood culture is the clot culture. Here, with strict aseptic precautions, 5 mL of blood is withdrawn from the patient into a sterile test tube and allowed to clot. The serum is pipetted off and used for Widal test. The clot is broken up with a sterile glass rod and added to a bottle of bile broth incorporating streptokinase (100 units/mL). Streptokinase in the broth facilitates lysis of the clot with release of bacteria trapped in the clot.

Advantage of clot culture
  a. Clot cultures with streptokinase yields a higher rate of isolation than blood cultures.
  b. A sample of serum also becomes available for Widal test. Widal test provides a baseline titer against which the results of tests performed later may be evaluated.

Feces Culture
Salmonellae are shed in the feces throughout the course of the disease and even in convalescence, with varying frequency. Hence, fecal cultures are almost as valuable as blood cultures in diagnosis. A positive fecal culture may occur in carriers as well as in patients.

Fecal samples are plated directly on MacConkey agar, DCA, and Wilson and Blair's brilliant-green bismuth sulfite agar media. On MacConkey and DCA media, salmonellae appear as pale colonies. On Wilson and Blair's brilliant-green bismuth sulfite agar media, *S. typhi* forms large black colonies with a metallic sheen. *S. paratyphi A* produces green colonies due the absence of H_2S production.

For enrichment, one tube each of selenite F and tetrathionate broth are also inoculated. These are also incubated at 37°C **for 8–12** hours with subsequent subculture on MacConkey agar and DCA media.

Urine Culture
Urine culture is less useful than the culture of blood and feces because salmonellae are shed in the urine irregularly and infrequently. Generally, cultures are positive only in the second and third weeks and then only in about 25% of cases. The rate of isolation is improved by repeated sampling.

Other Materials for Culture
Bone marrow culture is valuable and it is positive in most cases even when blood culture is negative. **Culture of bile** may be employed for the detection of carries.

Colony morphology: Pale NLF colonies that may appear on MacConkey agar or DCA medium after incubating at 37°C for 24 hours are picked out for biochemical tests and motility. Salmonellae will be gram negative and motile bacilli.

Biochemical reactions: Salmonellae will be indole and urease negative, catalase positive, oxidase negative, **nitrate reduction positive** and ferment glucose, mannitol and maltose but not lactose or sucrose. *S. typhi* will be anaerogenic and ferments glucose and mannitol with production of acid only, while paratyphoid bacilli (*S. paratyphi A, B, and C*) will form acid and gas from sugars.

Identification: Identification of the isolate is by slide agglutination.

Slide agglutination test: A loopful of the growth from an agar slope is emulsified in two drops of saline on a slide. One emulsion acts as a control to show that the strain is not autoagglutinable. If *S. typhi* is suspected, a loopful of typhoid O antiserum is added to one drop of bacterial emulsion. Prompt agglutination indicates that the isolate belongs to *Salmonella* group D. Its identity as *S. typhi* is established by agglutination with the flagellar antiserum (anti-d serum).

Where the isolate is nontyphoid *Salmonella*, it is tested for agglutination with O and H antisera for groups A, B and C.

B. Demonstration of Circulating Antigen
In the early phase of the disease, typhoid bacillus antigens are consistently present in the blood and also in the urine of patients.

C. Demonstration of Antibodies in Patient's Serum
1. Widal test
2. Other serological tests

1. Widal Test
The patient's serum is tested by tube agglutination for its titers of antibodies against H, O, and Vi suspensions of the enteric fever bacteria likely to be encountered, e.g., *S. typhi and S. paratyphi A* in India

Usually, agglutinins appear by the end of first week (seventh to tenth day) of the illness. Demonstration of a rise in titer of antibodies by testing two or more samples is more meaningful than a single test.

2. Other Serological Tests
Enzyme-linked immunosorbent assay (ELISA), indirect hemagglutination test and counter immunoelectrophoresis (CIEP) are other serological methods of diagnosis.

Prophylaxis
Control depends essentially on safe water supply, proper sewage disposal, handling of food hygienically, and periodic examination of food handlers to ascertain that they are not carriers.

VACCINES AGAINST TYPHOID FEVER

1. Killed Whole Cell Vaccine: TAB Vaccine
Heat-killed, phenol-preserved whole-cell vaccines containing a mixture of cultures of

S. typhi 1,000 million and S. Paratyphi A and B, 750 million each per mL killed by heating at 50–60°C and preserved in 0.5% phenol.

Dose schedule: The vaccine is given in 2 doses of 0.5 mL subcutaneously at an interval of 4–6 weeks followed by a booster dose every 3 years.

2. Oral Vaccine—Live Oral (Ty21) Typhoid Vaccine

The live oral vaccine (**typhoral**) is a stable mutant of *S. typhi* strain (Ty21a). On ingestion, it initiates infection but 'self destructs' after four or five cell divisions, and therefore, it cannot induce any illness.

Dose schedule: Three doses of the vaccine are given on alternate days to children.

Protection: It is safe and confers 65–96% protection for 3–5 years.

3. Vaccine of Purified Vi Antigen (Typhim-Vi)

Treatment

Specific antibacterial therapy for enteric fever is chloramphenicol, but resistance became common. Ampicillin, amoxicillin, and trimethoprim-sulfamethoxazole have been used successfully.

Ciprofloxacin has emerged as the drug of choice for the treatment of adult typhoid. At present, the drugs useful in treatment of such multiresistant typhoid cases are the later fluoroquinolones (such as ciprofloxacin, pefloxacin, ofloxacin) and the third generation cephalosporin (such as ceftazidime, ceftriaxone, cefotaxime).

SALMONELLA GASTROENTERITIS

Salmonella gastroenteritis (more appropriately **enterocolitis**) or *food* **poisoning** is generally a zoonotic disease. The source of infection being animal products. It may be caused by any *Salmonella* except *S. typhi*. In most parts of the world, *S. typhimurium* is the most common (30–40%) species. Some other common species have been *S. enteritidis, S. Haldar, S. Heidelberg, S. Agona, S. Virchow, S. Seftenberg, S. Indiana, S. Newport,* and *S. Anatum. S. Dublin*

KEY POINTS

- *Salmonella*: Gram-negative bacilli, motile bacilli
- **Diseases:** Asymptomatic colonization. Enteric fever; enteritis; bacteremia.

IMPORTANT QUESTIONS

1. Name the *Salmonellae* causing enteric fever. Describe in detail the laboratory diagnosis of enteric fever.
2. Write short notes on:
   a. Widal test
   b. Vaccination against enteric fever.

MULTIPLE CHOICE QUESTIONS

1. All the following enrichment media are used for isolation of *Salmonella*, *except*:
   a. Alkaline peptone water
   b. Selenite F broth
   c. Brilliant green tetrathionate broth
   d. Tetrathionate broth
2. The selective medium used for isolation of *Salmonella* is:
   a. Wilson and Blair's brilliant-green bismuth sulfite agar
   b. Cary-Blair medium
   c. Thiosulfate citrate bile salt agar
   d. Xylose, lysine deoxycholate agar
3. All the following *Salmonella* serotypes are motile, *except*:
   a. *Salmonella typhi*
   b. *Salmonella typhimurium*
   c. *Salmonella choleraesuis*
   d. *Salmonella gallinarum*
4. Which of the following Salmonella is/are primarily human pathogens?
   a. *S. typhi.*
   b. *S. paratyphi A.*
   c. *S. paratyphi B.*
   d. All of the above.

Section 3: Systemic Bacteriology

5. The most important specimen for isolation of *Salmonella typhi* culture in first week of enteric fever?
   a. Blood
   b. Urine
   c. Feces
   d. CSF.

6. All the following are the examples of killed vaccines used against typhoid fever, *except*:
   a. TAB vaccine
   b. Vi capsular polysaccharide antigen vaccine
   c. Acetone-inactivated parenteral vaccine
   d. Ty21a vaccine

ANSWERS

1. a 2. a 3. d 4. d
5. a 6. d

CHAPTER 31

Vibrio

LEARNING OBJECTIVES

After reading and studying this chapter, you should be able to:
- Describe morphology, cultural characteristics, and biochemical reactions of *Vibrio cholerae*.
- Discuss antigenic structure of *Vibrio cholerae*.
- Describe the following: Pathogenesis of cholera; mechanism of action of cholera toxin.
- Differentiate between classical and El Tor vibrios.
- Discuss laboratory diagnosis of cholera.
- Describe the following: Cholera vaccine; halophilic vibrios.

INTRODUCTION

Vibrio: Of the 35 *Vibrio* species recognized, 12 have been implicated in gastrointestinal and extraintestinal infections in man. The most important member of the genus is *Vibrio cholerae*, the causative agent of cholera.

VIBRIO CHOLERAE

Morphology

These are gram-negative, short, curved, cylindrical rods, about 1.5 µm × 0.2–0.4 µm in size. The cell is typically comma shaped (hence the old name *V. comma*). It is actively motile, by means of a single, polar sheathed flagellum. The motility is of the **darting type**. They are nonsporing, noncapsulated, and nonacid-fast **(Fig. 31.1)**.

Cultural Characteristics

The cholera vibrio is strongly aerobic, growth being scanty and slow anaerobically. It grows within a temperature range of 16–40°C (optimum 37°C). Growth is better in an alkaline medium and it occurs freely between pH 7.4 and 9.6 (optimum pH 8.2).

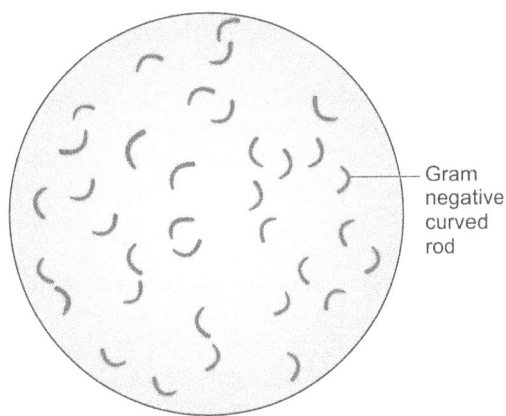

Fig. 31.1: Cholera vibrios.

A. Ordinary Media

1. **Nutrient agar:** After overnight growth, colonies are moist, translucent, round disks, about 1–2 mm in diameter, with a bluish tinge in transmitted light.
2. **MacConkey agar:** The colonies are smaller than those on nutrient agar and are colorless, but become reddish on prolonged incubation due to the late fermentation of lactose.
3. **Blood agar:** Colonies are initially surrounded by a zone of greening, which later becomes clear due to hemodigestion.

4. **Gelatin stab culture:** At first a white line of growth appears along the track of the inoculating wire.
5. **Peptone water:** It forms a fine surface pellicle because of its affinity for oxygen.

B. Special Media
They may be classified as follows:
  a. **Holding or transport media**
     1. **Venkatraman–Ramakrishnan (VR) medium:** A simple modified form of this medium is prepared by dissolving 20 g crude sea salt and 5 g peptone in one liter of distilled water and adjusting the pH to 8.6–8.8. Vibrios do not multiply in this medium but remain viable for several weeks.
     2. **Cary-Blair medium:** This is a buffered solution of disodium hydrogen phosphate, sodium thioglycolate, sodium chloride, and agar to 1 liter of distilled water and pH 8.4.
  b. **Enrichment media:** These are good transport as well as enrichment media.
     1. **Alkaline peptone water-**Alkaline peptone water at pH 8.6 is useful for preliminary enrichment of vibrios from feces or other contaminated materials.
     2. **Monsur's taurocholate tellurite peptone water at pH 9.2**.
  c. **Plating media**
     1. **Alkaline bile salt agar (BSA); pH 8.2:** This simple medium has stood the test of time and is still widely used. This is modified nutrient agar medium containing 0.5% sodium taurocholate. The colonies on BSA are similar to those on nutrient agar medium.
     2. **Monsur's gelatin taurocholate trypticase tellurite agar (GTTA) medium; pH 8.5:** After 24 hours incubation, vibrios produce small (1–2 mm) translucent colonies with grayish black center and a turbid halo, due to hydrolysis and denaturation of gelatin. After 48 hours incubation, colonies increase in size to 3–4 mm.
     3. **Thiosulfate-citrate-bile-sucrose (TCBS) agar; pH 8.6:** This is most used selective plating medium for vibrios. Constituents of this medium are sodium thiosulfate, sodium citrate, ox bile, sucrose, yeast extract, peptone, sodium chloride, ferric citrate, thymol blue, bromothymol blue (indicator) and water. This medium resembles DCA except that it has high pH value of 8.6 and contains sucrose instead of lactose. On this differential medium, the colonies of sucrose-fermenting vibrios, e.g., *V. cholerae*, are yellow, those of sucrose-nonfermenting vibrios, e.g., *V. parahaemolyticus*, are green.

Biochemical Reactions
1. **Sugar fermentation:** It ferments glucose, mannitol, maltose, mannose and sucrose and ferments lactose only after several days (late lactose-fermenter). Arabinose and dulcitol are not fermented.
2. **Cholera red reaction:** *V. cholerae* is strongly indole positive and reduces nitrates to nitrites. These two properties contribute to the "**cholera red reaction**".
3. It is **catalase and oxidase-positive**, **methyl red, and urease negative**.
4. It decarboxylates lysine and ornithine but does not utilize arginine.
5. Gelatin is liquefied.
6. Voges–Proskauer reaction and hemolysis of sheep RBCs are positive in El Tor biotype and both these reactions are negative in classical biotype.

String test: Vibrio colonies may be identified by the 'string test'.

Antigenic Structure
1. **Flageller antigen (H antigen):** Many vibrios share a single heat-labile flagellar antigen.
2. **O antigen (LPS, endotoxin):** *V. cholerae* has O lipopolysaccharides (LPS, endotoxin) that confer serologic specificity.

Classification
Serological Classification
Cholera vibrios and biochemically similar vibrios, possessing a **common flagellar (H)**

Table 31.1: Differences between classical cholera and El Tor vibrios.		
Test	Classical cholera	El Tor
Hemolysis	−	+*
Voges–Proskauer	−	+*
Chick erythrocyte agglutination	−	+
Polymyxin B sensitivity[†]	+	−
Group IV phage susceptibility	+	−
El Tor phage 5 susceptibility	−	+

* Strains isolated after 1961 give variable results;
† 50 IU disk

antigen were classified as **Group A vibrios**, and the rest as **Group B vibrios** comprising a heterogeneous collection.

Based on the major somatic (O) antigen, Group A vibrios were classified into '**subgroups**' (now called **O serogroups or serovars**), more than 200 of which are currently known. All isolates from epidemic cholera (till 1992) belonged to serogroup 0-1 which are referred to as "**agglutinable vibrios**". Other vibrio isolates, which were not agglutinated by the 0-1 antiserum came to be called **nonagglutinable (NAG) vibrios**. They were considered nonpathogenic and hence also called **noncholera vibrios (NCV)**.

Biotypes of V. cholerae 01

There are two biotypes of *V. cholerae* 01: *classical* and *El Tor* biotypes. The differences between classical and El Tor biotypes *V. cholerae* are shown in **Table 31.1**.

Subtypes of V. cholerae 01

Strains of *V. cholerae* 01 may be further subdivided Ogawa, Inaba, and Hikojima on the basis of differences in minor 0 antigens (A, B and C). Antigen A is present in all the three subtypes. O antigens present in Ogawa (AB), Inaba (AC) and Hikojima (A BC) **(Table 31.2)**.

Table 31.2: Serotypes of *Cholera vibrios*.	
Serotype	O antigens
Ogawa	AB
Inaba	AC
Hikojima	ABC

V. cholerae 0139

It closely resembles *V. cholerae* 01 El Tor biochemically and physiologically.

Pathogenesis

In human infection, the vibrios enter orally through contaminated water or food.

After passing the acid barrier of the stomach the organisms begin to multiply in the alkaline environment of the small intestine. The incubation period varies from less than 24 hours to about five days. The clinical illness may begin slowly with mild diarrhea and vomiting in 1-3 days or abruptly with sudden massive diarrhea. The cholera stool is typically a colorless watery fluid with flecks of mucus called, "rice water stool".

Cholera Toxin (CT)

Vibrios multiplying on the intestinal epithelium produce a toxin (choleragen, cholera enterotoxin, cholera toxin, CT, or CTX).

Mechanism of Action

The toxin molecule, of approximately 84,000 MW consists of one A and 5 B subunits. The B (binding) subunit of cholera toxin binds to the ganglioside GM_1 receptors on the intestinal epithelial cells, which promotes entry of subunit A into the cell. The A (active) subunit, on being transported into the enterocyte dissociates into two fragments A_1 and A_2. The active portion (A_1) of the A subunit enters the cell and activates adenyl cyclase. This in turn converts ATP into cyclic adenosine monophosphate (cAMP). The result is irreversible activation of adenylate cyclase and overproduction of cAMP. This in turn causes inhibition of uptake of Na+ and Cl⁻ ions by cells lining the villi, together with hypersecretion of Cl⁻ and HCO_3 ions leading to serious loss of water and electrolytes.

All the clinical features of severe cholera result from this massive loss of fluid and electrolytes. There is rapid loss of fluid and electrolytes, which leads to profound dehydration, circulatory collapse, and anuria.

Laboratory Diagnosis

A. Specimen
a. Watery stool
b. Rectal swabs

B. Collection of Specimen
Stool: A fresh specimen of stool should be collected for laboratory examination. Sample should be collected before the person is treated with antibiotics. Collection may be made generally in one of the following ways:
  i. Rubber catheter
  ii. Rectal swab

C. Transportation
Stool samples may be preserved in VR fluid or Cary–Blair medium for long periods.

If the specimen can reach the laboratory in a few hours, it may be transported in enrichment media, such as alkaline peptone water or Monsur's medium. The specimen should be transported in alkaline peptone water or Cary–Blair medium, if it is collected by a rectal swab. Strips of blotting paper may be soaked in the watery stool and sent to the laboratory packed in plastic envelopes, if transport media are not available.

D. Microscopy
Direct microscopic examination of feces is not recommended as the results are not reliable. For rapid diagnosis, the characteristic motility of the vibrio and its inhibition by antiserum can be demonstrated under the dark field or phase contrast microscope.

E. Culture
In the laboratory, the sample should be plated both directly and after enrichment culture, on to the suitable solid media.

Selective Media
The plating media used are bile salt agar (BSA), MacConkey agar for nonselective and GTTA and TCBS agar for selective plates. Generally, the plates are examined after overnight incubation at 37°C.

Colony morphology: On **MacConkey medium**, they form translucent colonies, on GTTA medium they form translucent colonies with grayish-black center and a turbid halo and on TCBS, they form yellow colonies.

Identification: Do the Gram staining from the suspected colonies and look for gram-negative curved or comma-shaped rods. Perform motility and oxidase tests. Cholera vibrios show characteristic motility and are oxidase positive.

Slide agglutination: Pick up colonies with a straight wire and test by slide agglutination with *V. cholerae* 01 antiserum. If positive, agglutination may be repeated using specific Ogawa and Inaba antisera. Hikojima strains will agglutinate well with both Ogawa and Inaba antisera.

Biochemical Reactions
The identity of the organism should be confirmed biochemically in a set of conventional tests.

For further characterization of the biotype of the *V. cholerae* 01 isolate, do VP test, agglutination of fowl RBCs, hemolysis of sheep RBCs, and sensitivity to polymyxin B, Mukerjee phages IV and V **(Table 31.1)**.

F. Serological Diagnosis
A retrospective diagnosis of infection can be made.

Treatment
1. **Oral rehydration therapy (ORT):** In cholera absolute priority must be given to the life-saving replacement of fluid and electrolytes. ORT is often sufficient, but severe cases may require intravenous rehydration.
2. **Antibacterial therapy:** Antibacterial therapy is of secondary importance. Oral tetracycline was recommended for reducing the period of vibrio excretion and the need for parenteral fluids.

Prophylaxis
1. **General measures:** Most important are the provision of safe drinking water supplies and the proper disposal of human feces. Control rests on education and on improvement of sanitation, particularly of food and water.

2. **Specific measures—vaccines**: Following vaccines are available:
   a. **Killed whole organism vaccine:** It is killed suspension containing 8,000 million *V. cholerae* per mL, composed of equal numbers of Ogawa and Inaba serotypes. Primary immunization consists of two equal doses, injected subcutaneously, at an interval of 4-6 weeks.
   b. **Oral vaccine:** Two types of oral cholera vaccines are available in some countries.
      i. **Nonliving oral B subunit-whole cell (BS-WC) vaccine:** This vaccine contains CT subunit B heat-killed vibrios each of Ogawa and Inaba serotypes of classical biotype and equal number of formalin killed vibrios each of Ogawa and Inaba serotypes of El Tor biotype.
      ii. **Live oral vaccine:** Recombinant DNA vaccine with expression of *V. cholerae* 01 in attenuated strain of *S. typhi* Ty21 as a carrier bacterium has been developed.

HALOPHILIC VIBRIOS

Vibrios that have a high requirement of sodium chloride are known as *halophilic vibrios*. Their natural habitat is sea water and marine life. Some halophilic vibrios have been shown to cause human disease—*V. parahaemolyticus, V. alginolyticus* and *V. vulnificus*.

KEY POINTS

- *Vibrio cholerae is* the causative agent of cholera.
- **Disease:** Cholera toxin is primarily responsible for the watery diarrhea characteristic of this species.

IMPORTANT QUESTIONS

1. Discuss laboratory diagnosis of cholera.
2. Write short notes on:
   a. Noncholera vibrios
   b. Differences between classical and El Tor vibrios
   c. *Halophilic vibrios*

MULTIPLE CHOICE QUESTIONS

1. **All the following *Vibrio* species require sodium chloride as a growth factor, *except*:**
   a. *Vibrio cholerae*
   b. *Vibrio parahaemolyticus*
   c. *Vibrio vulnificus*
   d. *Vibrio alginolyticus*
2. **Which of the following media can serve a transport medium for *Vibrio cholerae*?**
   a. Selenite-F broth
   b. Tetrathionate broth
   c. Venkatraman-Ramakrishnan medium
   d. Nutrient broth
3. **Classical and *El Tor* biotypes of *Vibrio cholerae* can be differentiated by which of the following tests?**
   a. Sensitivity to polymyxin B
   b. Agglutination of fowl RBCs
   c. Sensitivity to Mukerjee group IV phage
   d. All of the above
4. **Stools from suspected cholera cases can be transported to the laboratory in:**
   a. Venkatraman–Ramakrishnan medium
   b. Cary–Blair medium
   c. Thick blotting paper
   d. All of the above
5. **Which of the following vaccines is/are available for prophylaxis against cholera?**
   a. Killed parenteral vaccine
   b. Live oral vaccine
   c. All of the above
   d. None of the above

ANSWERS

1. a   2. c   3. d   4. d
5. c

Campylobacter and Helicobacter

LEARNING OBJECTIVES

After reading and studying this chapter, you should be able to:
- Describe morphology, culture characteristics and biochemical reactions of *Campylobacter*.
- Discuss morphology, culture characteristics and biochemical reactions of *Helicobacter*.
- Discuss laboratory diagnosis of *Helicobacter pylori* infections.

INTRODUCTION

Campylobacter and *Arcobacter* are grouped into the family **Campylobacteriaceae**; *Helicobacter, Wolinella,* and *Flexispira* are grouped into **an unnamed family**.

Species: A total of 18 species and subspecies are now recognized; *C. jejuni* is a very common cause of diarrhea in humans.

CAMPYLOBACTER JEJUNI AND CAMPYLOBACTER COLI

Campylobacter jejuni and *Campylobacter coli* have emerged as common human pathogens, causing mainly enteritis and occasionally systemic infection.

Morphology

The genus *Campylobacter* consists of small, comma-shaped, gram-negative bacilli that microscopically resemble vibrios. They are motile by means of a single polar flagellum. They are nonsporing.

Cultural Characteristics

Most species are microaerobic, requiring an atmosphere with decreased oxygen (5% oxygen) and increased hydrogen and carbon dioxide (CO_2) level for aerobic growth. Many pathogenic species are thermophilic, growing well at 42°C.

Selective media for isolation of *C. jejuni* are Butzler's selective medium, Skirrow's *Campylobacter* selective medium, Preston *Campylobacter* selective medium, and Blaser's medium (Campy-BAP). Plates are incubated for 48 hours. Colonies are circular and convex but those of thermophilic group, particularly *C. jejuni,* are flat and tend to swarm on moist agar.

Biochemical Reactions

Campylobacters do not ferment carbohydrates and utilize a respiratory (oxidative) pathway. They are strongly oxidase positive. They are catalase positive and reduce nitrates to nitrites. *C. jejuni* has the ability to hydrolyze sodium hippurate.

Pathogenesis

Campylobacters are important veterinary pathogens. Humans acquire the infections after consumption of contaminated food, milk, or water. **Heat-labile enterotoxin** along with the **invasive property** of this organism may contribute to the production of the damage.

Clinical manifestations: Clinical manifestations are acute onset of crampy abdominal pain, profuse diarrhea that may be grossly bloody, headache, malaise, and fever. Usually, the illness is self-limited to a period of 5–8 days.

Laboratory Diagnosis

A. **Specimens:** Diarrheal stool is the usual specimen.
B. **Microscopy: Gram-stained smears** of stool may show the typical "gull wing" -shaped rods. **Dark-field or phase contrast microscopy** may show the typical darting or tumbling motility of the spiral rods.
C. **Culture:** Feces or rectal swabs are plated on selective media. Selective media for isolation of *C. jejuni* are Butzler's selective medium, Skirrow's *Campylobacter* selective medium, Preston *Campylobacter* selective medium, and Blaser's medium (Campy-BAP). Skirrow's medium contains vancomycin, polymyxin B, and trimethoprim to inhibit growth of other bacteria.
Inoculated plates are incubated at 42°C to favor growth of the thermophilic campylobacters over that of other fecal bacteria. Incubation must be done in an atmosphere of 5% O_2, 10% CO_2, and 85% N_2. Plates are incubated for 48 hours.
Colonies are typically flat and effuse, with a tendency to spread on moist agar. They are nonhemolytic, gray or colorless, moist, and flat or convex.
D. **Identification:** Suggestive colonies are screened by Gram staining, motility, and oxidase tests. Confirmation is by further biochemical tests, including positive catalase and nitrate reduction tests.
E. **Serology:** Complement fixation test and **enzyme-linked immunosorbent assay (ELISA)** can detect recent infection.

HELICOBACTER

These are strict microaerophiles with a spiral or helical morphology. They possess sheathed flagella. **Species: Three** medically important species of this genus are: *H. pylori, H. cinaedi,* and *H. fennelliae.*

Helicobacter pylori

Warren and Marshall in Australia in 1983 observed spiral, *Campylobacter*-like bacteria in close apposition to the gastric mucosa in several cases of gastritis and peptic ulcer. They and now redesignated as ***Helicobacter pylori.***

Morphology

Helicobacter pylori is a gram-negative spirally-shaped bacterium, 0.5–0.9 mm wide by 2–4 mm long. It is motile by means of a tuft of sheathed unipolar flagella. It is nonsporing.

Cultural Characteristics

Like campylobacters, *H. pylori* is microaerophilic. The optimum temperature for its growth is 35–37°C. It can grow in an atmosphere of 5% O_2, 10% CO_2, and 85% N_2. It does not grow anaerobically or in air. It can be grown on moist freshly prepared **chocolate agar** and **Skirrow's *Campylobacter* selective medium**. *H. pylori* produces circular, convex, and translucent colonies after incubation at 35-37°C in a microaerophilic atmosphere for 3-5 days.

Biochemical Reactions

i. **Abundant urease production:** A distinctive feature is the production of **abundant urease**. The urease enzyme produced by *H. pylori* is almost 100 times more active than that of *Proteus vulgaris*.
ii. It produces oxidase, catalase, phosphatase, and H_2S.

Pathogenesis

Helicobacter pylori is associated with **antral gastritis, duodenal (peptic) ulcer disease, gastric ulcers.** It is also recognized as a risk factor for **gastric malignancies**, namely, "adenocarcinoma" and "**mucosa associated lymphoid tissue" (MALT) lymphomas.**

Laboratory Diagnosis

Diagnostic tests are of two kinds:
A. Noninvasive tests
 1. Serology
 2. Urea breath test
 3. Fecal antigen test
 4. Polymerase chain reaction (PCR)
B. Invasive tests
 1. Specimens
 2. Microscopy

3. Culture
4. Biopsy urease test

A. Noninvasive Tests
1. **Serology:** ELISA test.
2. **Urea breath test:** This test detects bacterial urease activity in the stomach by measuring the output of CO_2 resulting from the splitting of urea into CO_2 and ammonia. Urea tagged with an isotope of carbon (carbon-14 or -13) is fed to the patient. If the patient's stomach is colonized with *H. pylori*, urea is converted into ammonia and tagged CO_2. The latter appears in the breath where it can be measured. Patients infected with *H. pylori* give high readings of the isotope.
3. **Fecal antigen test**
4. **Polymerase chain reaction (PCR)**

B. Invasive Tests
1. **Specimens:** Endoscopic biopsy of gastric mucosa for examination by microscopy, culture, and urease tests.
2. **Microscopy:** The biopsy specimen can be examined by microscopic examination of Gram's staining, silver staining, hematoxylin and eosin (H and E) staining, Giemsa staining or immunofluorescence for the presence of bacteria. Warthin-Starry silver stain is the most sensitive.
3. **Culture:** Culture is done on nonselective medium such as **chocolate agar** and a selective medium. Plates are incubated for 2-7 days in a moist, microaerophilic atmosphere at 35-37°C in the presence of 5-10% CO_2. The organism is identified on the basis of its colonial morphology, Gram staining, biochemical properties, and positive urease tests.
4. **Biopsy urease test:** The biopsy urease test can be performed by crushing biopsy tissue in 0.5 mL urea solution with an indicator and incubated at 37°C. If *H. pylori* is present, the pH changes within a few minutes to 2 hours due to the production of ammonia.

Treatment

The standard treatment is a combination of bismuth subsalicylate, tetracycline (or amoxicillin) and metronidazole for two weeks. An alternative schedule employs a proton pump inhibitor like omeprazole and clarithromycin.

KEY POINTS

- Campylobacters are thin, curved gram-negative bacilli.
- Diseases: *C. jejuni* is associated with gastroenteritis, septicemia, meningitis, spontaneous abortion, proctitis, Guillain-Barre syndrome.
- *Helicobacter pylori* causes gastritis, peptic ulcers, gastric adenocarcinoma.

IMPORTANT QUESTION

1. Write short notes on:
   a. *Campylobacter* infections
   b. *Helicobacter pylori*
   c. Urea breath test.

MULTIPLE CHOICE QUESTIONS

1. Most common *Campylobacter* species known to cause diarrhea in humans is:
   a. *Campylobacter lari*
   b. *Campylobacter fetus*
   c. *Campylobacter jejuni*
   d. *Campylobacter coli*
2. All the following media are commonly used for cultivation of *Campylobacter*, except:
   a. Butzler medium
   b. Skirrow's medium
   c. Preston's campylobacter selective medium
   d. TCBS medium
3. *Campylobacter* and *Helicobacter* can be differentiated on the basis of:
   a. Multiple sheathed flagella
   b. Strong hydrolysis of urea
   c. Both of the above
   d. None of the above
4. *Helicobacter pylori* have been implicated in all of the following clinical conditions, *except*:
   a. Chronic gastritis
   b. Peptic ulcer disease
   c. Septicemia
   d. Idiopathic thrombocytopenic purpura

ANSWERS

1. c   2. d   3. c   4. c

Pseudomonas, Stenotrophomonas, and Burkholderia

LEARNING OBJECTIVES

After reading and studying this chapter, you should be able to:
- Describe morphology, cultural characteristics, biochemical reactions and laboratory diagnosis of *Pseudomonas aeruginosa*.
- Describe the following: Pigments of *Pseudomonas*; pathogenicity of *Pseudomonas aeruginosa*; *Burkholderia mallei*.

INTRODUCTION

The term pseudomonads describe a large group of aerobic, nonfermentative, nonsporing gram-negative bacilli, motile by polar flagella. They belong to over 100 species.

Pseudomonas aeruginosa is the most common pseudomonad. *Burkholderia* (previously *Pseudomonas*) *cepacia*, an important pathogen in immunocompromised patients, particularly in individuals with cystic fibrosis or chronic granulomatous disease. *Stenotrophomonas maltophilia* also infects immunocompromised patients.

PSEUDOMONAS AERUGINOSA

Morphology

It is a slender gram-negative bacillus, 1.5–3 µm × 0.5 µm, actively motile usually with a single polar flagellum. It is nonsporing, noncapsulated but many strains have a mucoid slime layer.

Cultural Characteristics

It is a strict aerobe. Growth occurs at a wide range of temperatures, 6–42°C, the optimum being 37°C. Optimum pH 7.4–7.6. It grows well on ordinary media.

1. **Nutrient agar:** The colonies are large, 2–3 mm in diameter, smooth, translucent, irregularly round, and emit a characteristic fruity odor.
2. **MacConkey and DCA media:** It grows on **MacConkey and DCA media,** forming nonlactose-fermenting colonies.
3. **Blood agar:** Colonies may be surrounded by a zone of hemolysis.
4. **In broth:** It forms a dense turbidity with a surface pellicle.
5. **Cetrimide agar** is selective medium for *P. aeruginosa*.

Pigment Production

Pseudomonas aeruginosa produces at least four distinct pigments:

i. **Pyocyanin:** It is a bluish-green phenazine pigment soluble in chloroform and water. This pigment is not produced by other species of this genus and the presence of it is the major diagnostic test.
ii. **Pyoverdine (fluorescein):** The yellow/green pigment pyoverdin (fluorescein) is also produced by most strains.
iii. **Pyorubrin:** It is a bright red water soluble pigment.
iv. **Pyomelanin:** It is a brown to black pigment.

Biochemical Reactions

Pseudomonas aeruginosa derives energy from carbohydrates by an oxidative rather than a fermentative metabolism. It utilizes glucose oxidatively with the production of acid only. MR, VP, and H_2S tests are negative. However, all strains give a rapid positive oxidase reaction and utilize citrate as sole source of carbon. It reduces nitrates to nitrites and further to gaseous nitrogen. It is catalase, arginine dihydrolase and gelatinase positive.

Resistance

The bacillus is being killed at 55°C in one hour but exhibits a high degree of resistance to chemical agents. It is resistant to the common antiseptics and disinfectants, such as quaternary ammonium compounds, chloroxylenol and hexachlorophene. It is sensitive to a 2% aqueous alkaline solution of glutaraldehyde (Cidex), acids, silver salts, and strong phenolic disinfectants.

Pathogenesis

Pseudomonas aeruginosa can infect almost any external site or organ. Individuals most at risk include those with impaired immune defenses.

A. Community Infections

1. Otitis externa and varicose ulcers
2. Corneal infections
3. Jacuzzi rash or whirlpool rash (an acute self-limiting folliculitis)
4. Panophthalmitis

B. Hospital Infections

1. **Localized lesions: Infections of wounds and bedsores, eye infections, and urinary infections following** catheterization, infection in burns, iatrogenic meningitis, post-tracheostomy pulmonary infection.
2. Septicemia and endocarditis
3. Ecthyma gangrenosum and many other types of skin lesions
4. Infection of the nail bed
5. Infantile diarrhea and sepsis
6. Shanghai fever
7. **Other infections:** Localized in the gastro-intestinal tract, central nervous system, and musculoskeletal system.

Laboratory Diagnosis

1. **Specimens:** Pus, wound swab, urine, sputum, CSF or blood.
2. **Microscopy:** Gram-negative rods are often seen in smears.
3. **Culture:** They grow easily on common isolation media, such as **blood agar** and **MacConkey agar**. It may be necessary to use selective media, such as **cetrimide agar** for isolation of *P. aeruginosa* from feces or other samples with mixed flora such as wound swab.
4. **Identification:** The colonial morphology combined with the results of selected rapid biochemical tests (e.g., positive oxidase reaction) is sufficient for the preliminary identification of these isolates.
5. **Typing method**
6. **Antibiotic sensitivity tests:** It is useful to select out proper antibiotic as multiple resistance to antibiotics is quite common in *P. aeruginosa*.

Treatment

Pseudomonas aeruginosa is intrinsically resistant to most commonly employed antimicrobial agents. Many strains are, however, susceptible to carbenicillin, azlocillin, ticarcillin, cefotaxime, ceftazidime, gentamicin, and tobramycin. Ciprofloxacin exhibits good activity against *P. aeruginosa*.

STENOTROPHOMONAS MALTOPHILIA

The spectrum of nosocomial infections with *S. maltophilia* includes **bacteremia, pneumonia, meningitis, wound infections**, and **urinary tract infections**.

BURKHOLDERIA CEPACIA

Infections caused by this organism include:
1. Respiratory tract infections
2. Urinary tract infections in catheterized patients
3. Septicemia
4. Endocarditis

BURKHOLDERIA MALLEI

It is the causative agent of glanders *(malleus, in Latin)*, a disease primarily of equine animals—horses, mules, and asses—but capable of being transmitted to other animals and to human beings.

BURKHOLDERIA PSEUDOMALLEI

Burkholderia pseudomallei is the causative agent of melioidosis, a glanders-like disease.

KEY POINTS

Pseudomonas aeruginosa
- Small gram-negative bacilli. Strict aerobe.
- **Diseases:** Burn wound infections and other skin and soft tissue infections, urinary tract infections, pulmonary infections (common in patients with cystic fibrosis), external otitis, eye infections.

IMPORTANT QUESTION

1. Write short notes on:
   a. *Pseudomonas aeruginosa*

MULTIPLE CHOICE QUESTIONS

1. All the following statements are true for *Pseudomonas aeruginosa* except that they:
   a. Are catalase positive
   b. Are oxidase positive
   c. Are fermenters
   d. Reduce nitrates to nitrogen gas

2. Which of the following pigments is diagnostic of *Pseudomonas aeruginosa*?
   a. Pyocyanin
   b. Pyoverdin
   c. Pyomelanin
   d. Pyorubin

3. Which of the following infections can be caused by *Pseudomonas aeruginosa*?
   a. Urinary tract infection
   b. Wound and bum infection
   c. Respiratory tract infection
   d. All of the above

ANSWERS
1. c   2. a   3. d

Chapter 34: Legionella

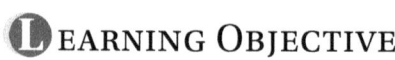 EARNING OBJECTIVES

After reading and studying this chapter, you should be able to:
- Describe morphology, culture characteristics, and biochemical reactions of *Legionella pneumophila*.
- Describe the following: *Legionella pneumophila*; diseases caused by *Legionella*.

INTRODUCTION

The family *Legionellaceae* consists of one genus, *Legionella* with 40 species and more than 60 serogroups. The original isolate in this genus is designated as *L. pneumophila* serogroup 1 (SG1), which accounts for nearly all severe infections.

LEGIONELLA PNEUMOPHILA

Morphology

Legionellae are thin, noncapsulated bacilli. Most are motile with polar or subpolar flagella. They are gram negative but stain poorly.

Culture

Legionellae have fastidious requirements and grow on complex media such as buffered charcoal yeast extract (BCYE) agar, with L-cysteine and antibiotic supplements, with 5% CO_2, at pH 6.9, 35°C, and 90% humidity. Growth is slow and colonies take 3–6 days to appear.

Biochemical Reactions

Most species are motile and catalase-positive, liquefy gelatin, and do not reduce nitrate or hydrolyze urea.

Pathogenesis

Respiratory tract disease caused by *Legionella* species develops in susceptible people who inhale infectious aerosols. Dissemination occurs by endobronchial, hematogenous, lymphatic, and contiguous spread.

Clinical Diseases

Symptomatic infections primarily affect the lungs and present in one of two forms:
1. **Pontiac fever:** An influenza-like illness
2. **Legionnaires' disease:** A severe form of pneumonia

Laboratory Diagnosis

1. **Microscopy:** *Legionellae* in clinical specimens stain poorly with Gram stain. The most sensitive way of detecting legionellae microscopically in clinical specimens is to use the direct fluorescent antibody (DFA) test.
2. **Culture:** The medium most commonly used for the isolation of legionellae is BCYE agar. Legionellae grow in air or 3–5% CO_2 at 35°C after 3–5 days.
3. **Antigen detection:** By enzyme-linked immunosorbent assays (ELISA), radio-immunoassays, the agglutination of antibody-coated latex particles, and nucleic acid analysis.
4. **Serology:** ELISA or indirect immunofluorescence assay.

KEY POINT

L. pneumophila causes Legionnaire's disease and Pontiac fever.

IMPORTANT QUESTIONS

1. Discuss pathogenicity and laboratory diagnosis of Legionnaire's disease.
2. Write short notes on:
   a. *Legionella pneumophila*
   b. Legionnaire's disease
   c. Pontiac fever

MULTIPLE CHOICE QUESTIONS

1. The causative agent of Pontiac fever is:
   a. *Legionella pneumophila*
   b. *Pseudomonas putida*
   c. *Yersinia pseudotuberculosis*
   d. *Francisella tularensis*
2. **Respiratory tract disease caused by *Legionella* species develops by:**
   a. Inhaling infectious aerosols
   b. Ingestion
   c. Injection
   d. Insects

ANSWERS

1. a   2. a

Chapter 35: Yersinia, Pasteurella and Francisella

LEARNING OBJECTIVES

After reading and studying this chapter, you should be able to:
- Describe morphology, culture characteristics and biochemical reactions of *Yersinia pestis*.
- Describe laboratory diagnosis of plague.
- Describe the following: *Yersinia enterocolitica*; *Yersinia pseudotuberculosis*.

INTRODUCTION

Genus *Yersinia*: The genus *Yersinia* currently has medically important species: *Y. pestis*; *Y. pseudotuberculosis*; *Y. enterocolitica*.

YERSINIA PESTIS

Morphology

Yersinia pestis is a gram-negative, short, oval coccobacilli with rounded ends and convex sides, about 1.5 × 0.7 µm, occurring singly, in short chains or in small groups. In smears stained with Giemsa or methylene blue, it shows **bipolar staining (safety-pin appearance)** with the two ends densely stained and the central area is clear **(Fig. 35.1). Pleomorphism** is marked in culture. The bacillus is surrounded by a **slime layer (envelope or capsule)**. It is nonmotile, nonsporing, and nonacid fast.

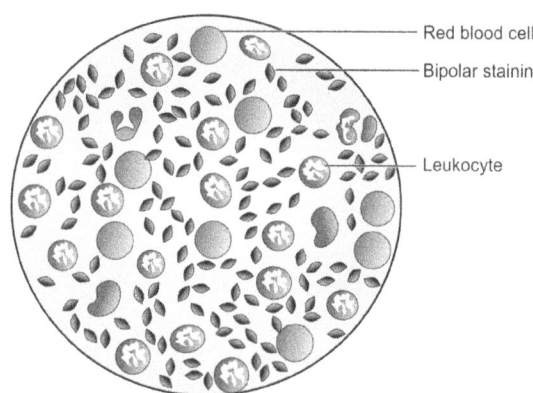

Fig. 35.1: Smear from gland puncture in a case of plague showing *Y. pestis* with bipolar staining (safety-pin appearance), a few red blood cell and leukocytes.

Cultural Characteristics

The plague bacillus is aerobe and facultative anaerobe. Growth occurs over a wide range of pH 5–9.6 (optimum pH 7.2). Optimum temperature for primary culture is 27°C (range 14–37°C).

It can grow on ordinary laboratory media.
1. **Nutrient agar:** Colonies are small, delicate, and transparent disks.
2. **Blood agar:** Colonies are dark brown due to absorption of the hemin pigment.
3. **DCA** and **MacConkey agar:** On **DCA** and **MacConkey agar** produce pin-point, reddish colonies.
4. In **broth,** a flocculent growth occurs at the bottom and along the sides of the tube, with little or no turbidity. A delicate pellicle may form later.
5. **Ghee broth:** If grown in a flask of **broth with sterile oil or ghee** (clarified butter) floated on top (ghee broth) a characteristic growth occurs, resembling stalactites **(stalactite growth)**.

Biochemical Reactions

It ferments glucose, mannitol, and maltose with the production of acid but no gas. Lactose and sucrose or rhamnose are not fermented. It is catalase positive, indole negative, MR positive, VP and citrate negative (IMViC - + - -), nitrate reduction positive, aesculin positive, and oxidase and urease negative.

Pathogenesis

Plague is a **zoonotic** disease. The plague bacillus is naturally parasitic in rodents. Infection is transmitted among them by **rat fleas.** When a rat flea, commonly *Xenopsylla cheopis*, bites a diseased rat, it sucks blood.

Forms of human plague: Traditionally, three severe forms of human plague are described.

1. **Bubonic plague:** As the plague bacillus usually enters through the bite of infected flea on the legs, the inguinal lymph nodes are involved, hence the name bubonic plague (**bubo** means enlarged gland in groin). The glands become enlarged and suppurate.
2. **Pneumonic plague:** It may also be acquired as a primary infection by inhalation of droplets infected with *Y. pestis*. This type of plague is highly contagious and is almost invariably fatal.
3. **Septicemia plague:** This may occur as a primary infection or as a complication of bubonic or pneumonic plague. Purpura may develop in the skin, giving the skin a blackish coloration which, in the past, led to the name "black death". **Disseminated intravascular coagulation** is usually present. **Meningitic involvement** may occur rarely.

Laboratory Diagnosis

1. **Specimens**
   i. Bubonic plague—pus or fluid aspirated.
   ii. Pneumonic plague—sputum and blood.
   iii. Septicemic plague—blood.
   iv. Meningeal plague—cerebrospinal fluid (CSF).
   v. On postmortem—splenic tissue.
2. **Microscopy:** Smears of exudate or sputum are stained with methylene blue or Giemsa stain. Characteristic gram-negative coccobacilli and bacilli show bipolar staining with methylene blue. The fluorescent antibody technique may be of use in identifying plague bacilli.
3. **Culture:** Culture the samples on **blood agar plates**, **MacConkey agar, nutrient agar** and **ghee broth** and incubated at 27°C. The growth is identified by biochemical tests and slide agglutination tests.
4. **Animal inoculation**
5. **Antigen detection:** By immunospecific staining and ELISA test.
6. **Serology**
7. **Polymerase chain reaction (PCR)**

Yersiniosis

The term *yersiniosis* denotes infection with *Yersinia* species other than *Y. pestis*, namely, *Y. pseudotuberculosis* and *Y. enterocolitica*. These are nonlactose fermenting (NLF) gram-negative rods that are urease-positive and oxidase-negative. They resemble *Y. pestis* because they are small, gram-negative rods with bipolar staining and rodents, wild and domestic animals are reservoirs of infection. They differ from *Y. pestis* by motility when grown at 22°C (nonmotile at 37°C), noncapsulated, urease positive, oxidase negative and insusceptible to *Y. pestis* bacteriophage.

YERSINIA PSEUDOTUBERCULOSIS

Yersinia pseudotuberculosis is a small, oval, gram-negative, bipolar-stained bacillus. It is motile when grown at 22°C and urease positive.

Pathogenesis

Animal infection: It causes pseudotuberculosis, which is a **zoonotic diseases**.

Human infection: Human infection probably results from ingestion of materials contaminated with animal feces. Infection results in a **severe**

typhoid-like illness, mesenteric lymphadenitis, and **terminal ileitis**.

Laboratory Diagnosis

Laboratory diagnosis may be made by isolation of the organism in culture from blood, local lesions, or mesenteric nodes, or demonstration of antibodies in patient serum during the acute phase of the illness.

YERSINIA ENTEROCOLITICA

It is a gram-negative coccobacillus showing pleomorphism in older cultures.

Cultural Characteristics

It is aerobe and facultative anaerobe. Optimum temperature for growth is 22–29°C. On **blood agar**, it forms nonhemolytic, smooth, translucent colonies, 2–3 mm in diameter in 48 hours. On **MacConkey medium**, it forms pinpoint NLF colonies.

Pathogenesis

Human disease usually results from ingestion of contaminated food or from contact with the environment. Blood transfusion is a significant hazard. Diseases in humans are:
1. Gastroenteritis or enterocolitis
2. Mesenteric lymphadenitis and terminal ileitis in older children
3. Septicemia
4. Pneumonia and meningitis
5. Postinfectious complications

Laboratory Diagnosis

Laboratory diagnosis may be made by isolation of the organism in culture from feces, blood, or from mesenteric nodes, or demonstration of antibodies in patient serum during the acute phase of the illness.

KEY POINTS

- *Yersinia pestis* is a gram-negative, shows **bipolar staining (safety pin appearance)**, **pleomorphic** and is capsulated. It causes *plague*.
- *Yersinia pseudotuberculosis* causes pseudotuberculosis.
- *Yersinia enterocolitica* produces in humans—gastroenteritis or enterocolitis, mesenteric lymphadenitis, and terminal ileitis, septicemia, pneumonia, and meningitis.

IMPORTANT QUESTION

1. Write short notes on:
   a. *Yersinia pestis*
   b. *Yersinia pseudotuberculosis*
   c. *Yersinia enterocolitica*

MULTIPLE CHOICE QUESTIONS

1. Bipolar staining is characteristic of:
   a. *Yersinia pestis*
   b. *Yersinia enterocolitica*
   c. *Yersinia pseudotuberculosis*
   d. *Proteus mirabilis*
2. Bubonic plague is transmitted by:
   a. Inoculation
   b. Inhalation
   c. Ingestion
   d. All of the above routes
3. Pneumonic plague is transmitted to humans by:
   a. Rat flea
   b. Droplet infection
   c. Ingestion
   d. Inoculation
4. The name *Black Death* is given to which of the following diseases?
   a. Tuberculosis
   b. Diphtheria
   c. Plague
   d. AIDS
5. Which of the following diseases is/are caused by *Yersinia enterocolitica* in man?
   a. Gastroenteritis
   b. Mesenteric lymphadenitis
   c. Septicemia
   d. All of the above

ANSWERS

1. a   2. a   3. b   4. c
5. d

CHAPTER 36

Haemophilus

LEARNING OBJECTIVES

After reading and studying this chapter, you should be able to:
- Describe morphology and culture characteristics of *Haemophilus influenzae*.
- Describe the following: X and V factors; Satellitism; Antigenic structure of *Haemophilus influenzae*.
- Describe pathogenicity of *H. influenzae*.
- Discuss laboratory diagnosis of infections caused by *Haemophilus influenzae*.
- Describe morphology and culture characteristics of *Haemophilus ducreyi*.
- Discuss *Haemophilus ducreyi* or Chancroid or soft sore and its laboratory diagnosis.

INTRODUCTION

The genus *Haemophilus* comprises a group of small, nonmotile, nonsporing, nonacid-fast, gram-negative coccobacilli or rods, often markedly pleomorphic are characterized by their requirement of one or both of two accessory growth factors (X and V) present in blood.

Species: ***Haemophilus influenzae*; *Haemophilus ducreyi*; *Haemophilus aphrophilus*.**

HAEMOPHILUS INFLUENZAE

Morphology

Haemophilus influenzae is a small, gram-negative rods or coccobacilli (0.3-0.5 × 1-2 mm size), exhibiting considerable pleomorphism. It is nonmotile, nonsporing, and nonacid-fast.

Cultural Characteristics

Haemophilus influenzae is an aerobe and facultative anaerobe. Growth is enhanced by a moist atmosphere supplemented with 5-10% CO_2. The optimum temperature is 37°C. The accessory growth factors: named X and V, present in blood are essential for growth.

X factor: X factor (hemin) is required for the synthesis of the iron-containing respiratory enzymes cytochrome *c*, cytochrome oxidase, peroxidase, and catalase.

V Factor

V factor is present in red blood cells and in many other animal and plant cells. The V factor is present inside the RBC. **Chocolate agar (heated blood agar)** is superior to plain blood agar for the growth of *H. influenzae*, because V factor is released from within the erythrocytes during heating (80-90°C) of blood agar. The colonies are small, translucent and nonhemolytic on blood agar. Capsulated strains produce larger, distinctive iridescent colonies.

Satellitism

The V factor is present inside the RBC. It is synthesized by some fungi and bacteria such as *S. aureus* in excess of their requirements and released into the surrounding medium. When *S. aureus* is streaked across a plate of blood agar on which a specimen containing *H. influenzae* has been inoculated, after overnight incubation, the colonies of *H. influenzae* will be large and well-developed alongside the streak of staphylococcus, and smaller farther away. This phenomenon is called **satellitism** and demonstrates the dependence of *H. influenzae*

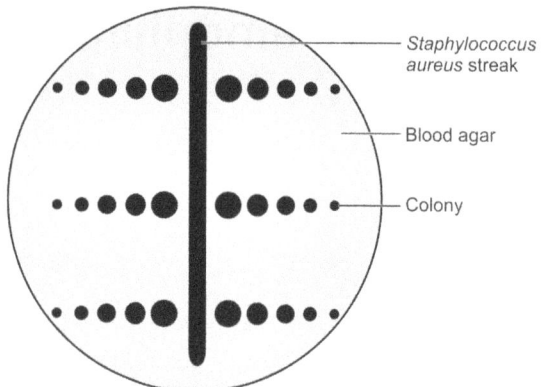

Fig. 36.1: Satellitism. *H. influenzae* colonies are large near growth of staphylococcus, and smaller away from it.

on the V factor, which is available in high concentrations near the staphylococcal growth and only in smaller quantities away from it (**Fig. 36.1**).

Biochemical Reactions

Haemophilus influenzae ferments glucose and galactose but does not ferment sucrose, lactose and mannitol. Catalase and oxidase reactions are positive. It reduces nitrates to nitrites.

Resistance

Haemophilus influenzae is a delicate organism. It is readily killed by moist heat (at 55°C in 30 minutes), refrigeration (4°C), drying and disinfectants.

Antigenic Structure

1. **Capsular antigens:** The major antigenic determinant of capsulated strains is the capsular polysaccharide based on which *H. influenzae* strains have been classified by Pittman into six capsular types—types a to f. *H. influenzae* strains lacking a capsule cannot be typed and are called "nontypable strains".
2. **Somatic antigens** consist of outer membrane proteins.

Pathogenesis

Haemophilus influenzae is exclusively a human parasite, which resides principally in the upper respiratory tract. Noncapsulate organisms are present in the nasopharynx or throat of healthy people. Capsulate strains (about half of which are capsular type b) are present in 5–10%.

H. influenzae causes **invasive** and **noninvasive infections.**

A. Invasive Infections

1. **Meningitis:** The most serious of the diseases produced by *H. influenzae* is acute bacterial meningitis. The disease is more common in children between 2′months and 3 years of age.
2. **Epiglottitis:** This is an acute inflammation of the epiglottis, with obstructive laryngitis, seen in children above 2 years.
3. **Pneumonia:** It typically occurs in infants.
4. **Suppurative lesions:** Suppurative lesions, such as arthritis, endocarditis, and pericarditis may result from hematogenous dissemination.
5. **Cellulitis:** It is seen in young children.

B. Noninvasive Disease

1. **Acute sinusitis and otitis media**.
2. **Acute exacerbations of chronic obstructive airway disease**
3. **Conjunctivitis**

Laboratory Diagnosis

1. Specimens

The specimens may be collected depending upon the type of lesion, such as:
i. Blood culture
ii. Cerebrospinal fluid
iii. Throat swabs
iv. Sputum
v. Pus
vi. Aspirates from joints, middle ears, or sinuses, etc.

2. Collection and Transport

Specimens should be transported to the laboratory and seeded on to appropriate culture media without delay. As haemophili are poorly viable in clinical specimens particularly at

4°C, therefore, the specimens should never be refrigerated.

3. Direct Microscopy
i. **Gram-stained smear:** Gram-stained smear of clinical material show poorly stained gram-negative coccobacilli and occasionally slender filamentous forms.
ii. **Immunofluorescence and Quellung reaction:** These can be employed for direct demonstration of *H. influenzae* after mixing with specific rabbit antiserum type b.
iii. **Antigen detection:** Type b capsular antigen can be detected in patient serum, urine, CSF or pus by latex agglutination, coagglutination **(COA)**, countercurrent immunoelectrophoresis **(CIE)**, radioimmunoassay (RIA), and ELISA.

4. Culture
i. **CSF culture:** CSF should be plated promptly on blood agar or chocolate agar. A strain of *S. aureus* should be streaked across the blood agar plate on which the specimen has already been inoculated. Plate is then incubated at 37°C with 5–10% CO_2 and high humidity overnight. The growth is identified by colony morphology, Gram staining, satellite phenomenon, biochemical reactions, and serotyping.
ii. **Blood culture:** Blood cultures are often positive in cases of epiglottitis and pneumonia.
iii. **Sputum culture:** The rate of isolation is increased by culturing several samples of sputum from the patient.

5. Identification
H. influenzae colonies have a characteristic seminal odor. Confirmation of the identity depends on demonstrating a requirement for one or both of the growth factors, X and V *H. influenzae* requires both.

6. Molecular Techniques
Polymerase chain reaction (PCR)

7. Antibiotic Sensitivity Tests
Treatment
Haemophilus influenzae is susceptible to sulfonamides, trimethoprim, ampicillin, chloramphenicol, tetracycline, coamoxiclav, ciprofloxacin, cefuroxime, cefotaxime, and ceftazidime.

Prophylaxis
Active Immunization
i. A purified type b capsular polysaccharide vaccine
ii. **Conjugate vaccines**
iii. Household contacts of patients Rifampicin given for four days
Haemophilus influenzae **biogroup aegyptius Diseases:** It causes **purulent conjunctivitis** and *Brazilian purpuric feve* **(BPF)**.

HAEMOPHILUS DUCREYI

Morphology
Haemophilus ducreyi is a gram-negative short, ovoid bacillus (1–1.5 μm × 0.6 mm) with a tendency to occur in end-to-end pairs or short chains and frequently shows bipolar staining. The bacilli may be arranged in small groups or whorls or in parallel chains giving a "**school-of fish**"; or "**rail road track**" appearance.

Cultural Characteristics
Primary isolation is difficult. It requires X factor but not V factor for its growth. It can be grown on **rabbit-blood agar, fresh clotted rabbit blood** or **chocolate agar enriched with 1% Iso Vitalex, and** containing **vancomycin** as a selective agent. It requires 10% CO_2 and high humidity for primary isolation. Cultures should be incubated for up to 5 days at 35–37°C.

The colonies of *H. ducreyi* are small, pinpoint to 0.5 mm in diameter, nonmucoid, grey, yellow, or tan, translucent or semiopaque after 24 hours incubation.

Pathogenicity

Haemophilus ducreyi is the etiologic agent of a highly communicable sexually transmitted disease (STD) **chancroid or soft sore** characterized by tender nonindurated irregular ulcers on the genitalia. Genital lesions caused by *H. ducreyi* are also known as **soft chancres or soft sores**. The lesions are generally on the penis in male and they may be present on the labia and within the vagina in females. The infection remains localized, spreading only to the inguinal lymph nodes which are enlarged and painful.

KEY POINTS

- The genus *Haemophilus* comprises a group of small, pleomorphic, gram-negative bacilli or coccobacilli. Most species require X and/or V factor for growth.
- *Haemophilus ducreyi* is the etiologic agent of a highly communicable STD *chancroid or soft sore*.

IMPORTANT QUESTIONS

1. Discuss pathogenesis and laboratory diagnosis of infections caused by *Haemophilus influenzae*.
2. Write short notes on:
   a. X and V factors
   b. Satellitism
   c. *Haemophilus ducreyi* or Chancroid or soft sore.

MULTIPLE CHOICE QUESTIONS

1. Following statements are true for morphology of *Haemophilus influenzae*, *except*:
   a. It is a gram-negative coccobacillus
   b. It rarely shows pleomorphism
   c. It is nonmotile
   d. The capsule may be present
2. All the following *Haemophilus* species require both X and V factors for their growth, *except*:
   a. *Haemophilus influenzae*
   b. *Haemophilus aegyptius*
   c. *Haemophilus haemolyticus*
   d. *Haemophilus ducreyi*
3. *Haemophilus influenzae* shows the phenomenon of satellitism on:
   a. Blood agar
   b. Chocolate agar
   c. Nutrient agar
   d. All of the above
4. Chancroid is caused by:
   a. *Haemophilus influenzae*
   b. *Haemophilus aegyptius*
   c. *Haemophilus ducreyi*
   d. *Haemophilus parainfluenzae*

ANSWERS

1. b   2. d   3. a   4. c

Chapter 37: Bordetella

LEARNING OBJECTIVES

After reading and studying this chapter, you should be able to:
- Describe culture media for *Bordetella pertussis*.
- Discuss pathogenesis of pertussis.
- Discuss laboratory diagnosis of pertussis.
- Describe the following: Cough plate method; vaccination against pertussis.

INTRODUCTION

The genus *Bordetella* constitutes a group of minute, gram-negative, non-acidfast, nonsporing, coccobacilli.

Species: The genus contains four species.
1. *Bordetella pertussis*
2. *Bordetella para pertussis*
3. *Bordetella bronchiseptica*
4. *Bordetella avium*

BORDETELLA PERTUSSIS

Morphology

The bacteria are small, gram-negative coccobacilli measuring 0.2–0.3 μm × 0.5–1.0 mm. It is nonmotile, nonsporing, and capsulated. **Bipolar metachromatic staining** may be demonstrated with toluidine blue. In culture films, the bacilli give a **"thumb print" appearance**.

Cultural Characteristics

It is an obligate aerobe. The optimum temperature for growth is 35–36°C. Complex media are necessary for primary isolation. The medium in common use is the **Bordet-Gengou medium (potato-blood-glycerol agar)**. The plates are incubated at 35–36°C in a moist environment. After incubation for 48–72 hours, colonies are small, dome-shaped, smooth, opaque, viscid, grayish white, refractile and glistening, resembling **"bisected pearls" or "mercury drops"**. Colonies are surrounded by a hazy zone of hemolysis. Confluent growth presents an **"aluminum paint"** appearance.

Biochemical Reactions

It is biochemically inactive. It produces oxidase and usually catalase also.

Pathogenesis

Whooping cough is predominantly a pediatric disease.

Stages of disease: In **human beings**, after an incubation period of about 1–2 weeks, the disease takes a protracted course comprising three stages— the catarrhal, paroxysmal and convalescent—each lasting approximately 2 weeks.

The disease usually lasts 6–8 weeks though in some it may be very protracted.

Laboratory Diagnosis

1. **Microscopy:** Microscopic diagnosis depends on demonstration of the bacilli in respiratory secretions by the fluorescent antibody technique.

2. **Culture:** For culture, following methods have been used for collection of specimens.
   a. **The cough plate method:** Here a culture plate is held about 10–15 cm in front of the patient's mouth during a bout of coughing so that droplets of respiratory exudates impinge directly on the medium.
   b. **The postnasal (peroral) swab:** Secretions from the posterior pharyngeal wall are collected with a cotton swab on a bent wire passed through the mouth. A West's postnasal swab may be conveniently employed.
   c. **The pernasal swab:** A sterile swab on a flexible wire is passed gently along the floor of the nose.

   The swab is inoculated immediately on charcoal-horse blood agar and Bordet-Gengou medium both. Plates are incubated in high humidity at 35–36°C and colonies appear in 48–72 hours. Typical 'bisected pearl' colonies appearing after 3–5 days must be investigated further.
3. **Identification:** Identification is confirmed by microscopy and slide agglutination with specific antisera.
4. **Detection of bacterial antigens.**
5. **Polymerase chain reaction (PCR).**
6. **Serology:** By ELISA, agglutination, complement fixation, immunoblotting, indirect hemagglutination, and toxin neutralization.

Treatment

The drug of choice is erythromycin.

Prophylaxis Vaccination

Specific immunization with killed *B. pertussis* vaccine has been found very effective. Immunization against diphtheria, whooping cough, and tetanus (DPT) is done simultaneously, by administering three doses of DPT vaccine intramuscularly, at 1–2 months interval, when the infant is about 6 weeks old. A booster dose of DPT is indicated at the age of 18–24 months.

KEY POINTS

- *Bordetella pertussis* is extremely small, ovoid, gram-negative coccobacilli.
- Diseases: Pertussis.

IMPORTANT QUESTION

1. Write short notes on:
   a. *Bordetella pertussis*
   b. *Laboratory diagnosis of pertussis*
   c. *Vaccination against pertussis*

MULTIPLE CHOICE QUESTIONS

1. Which of the following species of *Bordetella* is the most important human pathogen?
   a. *Bordetella pertussis*
   b. *Bordetella parapertussis*
   c. *Bordetella bronehiseptiea*
   d. *Bordetella avium*
2. Which of the following methods is suitable for culture of *Bordetella pertussis*?
   a. Pernasal swab culture
   b. Postnasal swab culture
   c. Cough plate method
   d. All of the above

ANSWERS

1. a   2. d

CHAPTER 38

Brucella

LEARNING OBJECTIVES

After reading and studying this chapter, you should be able to:
- Describe culture characteristics and biochemical reactions of *Brucella* spp.
- Discuss pathogenesis of brucellosis.
- Discuss laboratory diagnosis of brucellosis.
- Describe Castaneda method of blood culture.

INTRODUCTION

The genus *Brucella* consists of very small, nonmotile, aerobic, gram-negative coccobacilli that grow poorly on ordinary media.

Species: Six species are currently recognized: *B. melitensis, B. abortus, B. suis, B. ovis, B. neotomae* (isolated from desert wood rats), and *B. canis*.

Morphology

Brucellae are coccobacilli or short rods 0.5–0.7 mm × 0.6–1.5 mm. They are arranged singly and, less frequently, in pairs, short chains, or small groups. They are gram-negative non-acid-fast, nonmotile, noncapsulated, and nonsporing.

Cultural Characteristics

Brucellae are strict aerobes and do not grow anaerobically. Many strains of *B. abortus* and nearly all of *B. ovis* are capnophilic, requiring 5–10% CO_2 for growth. The optimum temperature is 37°C (range 20–40°C) and pH 6.6–7.4. They may grow on simple media, though growth tends to be slow and scanty. The media employed currently are **serum dextrose agar, serum potato infusion agar, trypticase soy agar, or tryptose agar.** The addition of bacitracin, polymyxin, and cycloheximide to the above media makes them selective. On solid culture media, colonies are small, smooth, transparent, low convex with an entire margin. In **liquid media**, growth is uniform.

Biochemical Reactions

The metabolism is oxidative and not fermentative. They are catalase-positive, urease positive and usually oxidase-positive.

Pathogenesis

All three major species of brucellae are pathogenic to human beings. *B. melitensis* is the most pathogenic, *B. abortus* and *B. suis* of intermediate pathogenicity.

Mode of infection:
i. **Ingestion:** The most important vehicle of infection is raw milk.
ii. **Contact:** Contact infection is especially important as an occupational hazard in agricultural workers, veterinarians, butchers, animal handlers, and others in occupations
iii. **Inhalation or accidental inoculation:** Infection is transmitted by inhalation of dried material of animal origin, such as dust from wool. Infection by inhalation is a serious risk in laboratory workers handling brucellae.

Types of Human Infection

Human infection may be of three types:
1. **Latent or subclinical infection**

2. **Acute brucellosis:** It is associated with prolonged bacteremia and irregular fever. It is also known as **undulant fever or Malta fever.**
3. **Chronic brucellosis**

Laboratory Diagnosis

A. **Specimens:** Blood culture is most important. Material from bone marrow or liver biopsy, lymph nodes, cerebrospinal fluid, urine, and abscesses can be collected.
B. **Culture:**
   a. Because the organisms may be scanty, at least 10 mL of blood should be withdrawn, 5 mL being added to each of two blood culture bottles containing **serum dextrose (SD) broth.** One of these bottles should be incubated in an atmosphere containing 10% carbon dioxide at 37°C. Subcultures are made on solid media (serum dextrose agar) every 3–5 days, beginning on the fourth day.
   b. **Castaneda's method of blood culture:**
      i. Here, both liquid and solid media are available in the same bottle. The blood is inoculated into the broth and the bottle incubated in the upright position. For subculture, it is sufficient if a bottle is tilted so that the broth flows over the surface of the agar slant. It is again incubated in an upright position. Colonies appear on the slant (Fig. 38.1).
      ii. This method **minimizes materials and manipulation.**
      iii. Reduces chances of contamination and risk of infection to laboratory workers.
   c. **Bone marrow or liver biopsy**
   d. **Other material:** Cultures may also be obtained from lymph nodes, cerebrospinal fluid, urine, and abscesses, if present.
C. **Serological tests:** In the absence of positive cultures, the diagnosis of brucellosis usually depends on serological tests, the results of which tend to vary with the stage of the infection.
   i. **Standard agglutination test (SAT):** This is a tube agglutination test in which equal

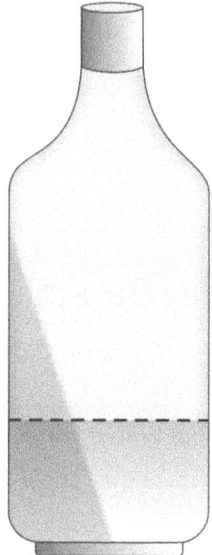

Fig. 38.1: Castaneda's method of blood.

volumes of serial dilutions of the patient's serum and the standardized antigen (a killed suspension of a standard strain of *B. abortus*) are mixed and incubated at 37°C for 24 hours or 50°C for 18 hours. A titer of 160 or more is considered significant.
   ii. **Two-mercaptoethanol (2ME) agglutination test.**
   iii. **Complement fixation test**
   iv. **Enzyme-linked immunosorbent assay (ELISA)** and radioimmunoassay (RIA).
   v. **Rose Bengal plate test**
   vi. **Rapid dipstick assay**
D. **Polymerase chain reaction (PCR)**
E. **Hypersensitivity test (Brucellin skin test)** This test, similar to the tuberculin test, is no longer recommended.

Prophylaxis

1. Prevention consists of checking brucellosis in dairy animals.
2. Control of this disease in cattle has been achieved by serologic surveillance, vaccination, and elimination of reactor cattle.
3. Pasteurization of infected milk or milk products.
4. The live-attenuated *B. abortus* vaccine.
5. Human vaccination is not recommended.

Treatment

Brucella infections respond to a combination of streptomycin or gentamicin and tetracycline or to rifampicin and doxycycline.

KEY POINTS

- The genus *Brucella* consists of very small, non-motile, aerobic, and gram-negative coccobacilli.
- **Disease:** Human brucellosis is primarily a zoonotic bacterial infection.

IMPORTANT QUESTIONS

1. Discuss laboratory diagnosis of brucellosis.
2. Write short notes on:
   a. Castaneda method of blood culture.
   b. Serodiagnosis of brucellosis.

MULTIPLE CHOICE QUESTIONS

1. All the following statements are true regarding cultural characteristics of *Brucella*, except:
   a. They are strict aerobes
   b. They require 5–10% of CO_2 for better growth
   c. Castaneda's method of blood culture cannot be used for them
   d. They may grow on simple media
2. Brucellae are transmitted to humans by:
   a. Direct contact with animal tissues
   b. Ingestion of contaminated meats
   c. Ingestion of raw infected milk
   d. All of the above
3. The most common *Brucella* species causing human infection in India is:
   a. *Brucella melitensis*
   b. *Brucella abortus*
   c. *Brucella suis*
   d. *Brucella canis*
4. The specimen of choice for isolation of *Brucella* is:
   a. Blood
   b. Bone marrow
   c. Urine
   d. Stool

ANSWERS

1. c   2. d   3. a   4. a

Spirochetes

CHAPTER 39

LEARNING OBJECTIVES

After reading and studying this chapter, you should be able to:
- Describe diseases caused by different spirochetes.
- Name various pathogenic treponemes.
- Describe morphology of *Treponema pallidum*.
- Discuss pathogenesis of syphilis.
- Describe diseases caused by *Treponema pallidum* their laboratory diagnosis.
- Explain serological tests for syphilis.
- Discuss standard tests for syphilis (STS)
- Describe the following: Fluorescent treponemal antibody-absorption (FTA-ABS) test; TPHA (or) *T. pallidum* hemagglutination test.
- Discuss biological false positive (BFP) reactions.
- Describe the following: (i) Endemic syphilis or Bejel; (ii) Yaws; (iii) *Treponema pertenue*; (iv) Pinta; (v) *Borrelia recurrentis*; (vi) *Borrelia vincentii*; (vii) *Borrelia burgdorferi* or Lyme disease; (viii) Leptospirosis; (ix) Weil's disease.

INTRODUCTION

The spirochetes are elongated, motile, slender, helically coiled, flexible organisms with one or more complete turns in the helix.

Diseases caused by spirochetes are shown in **Table 39.1**.

Species designation of spirochetes based on morphology is shown in **Figure 39.1**.

TREPONEMA

Treponema pallidum

Treponema pallidum is the causative agent of syphilis.

Morphology

It is a very delicate, spiral filament 6–14 μm (average 10 μm) by 0.2 μm, with 6–12 coils, which are comparatively small, sharp, and regular. The length of the coils is about 1 μm and the depth 1–1.5 μm. The ends are pointed and tapering.

Spirochetes show rotary corkscrew-like motility and also movements of flexion **(Fig. 39.1)**.

Treponema pallidum cannot be seen under the light microscope in wet films but can be made out by negative staining with **Indian ink**. Its morphology and motility can be seen under the dark ground or phase contrast microscope **(Fig. 39.2)**. It can be stained by **silver impregnation methods. Fontana's method** is useful for staining films and **Levaditi's method** for tissue sections. **Immunofluorescence methods** can now be used to detect treponemes in tissues and body fluids.

Cultivation

There have been many claims of cultivation of *T. pallidum* in cultures but none has been substantiated. Virulent *T. pallidum* strains have been maintained by serial testicular passage in rabbits for many decades. One such strain is **Nichol's strain.**

Chapter 39: Spirochetes

Table 39.1: Diseases caused by spirochetes.

Genus	Species	Diseases	Transmission
Treponema	T. pallidum	Syphilis	Sexual contact or congenital
	T. pertenue	Yaws	Traumatized skin comes in contact with an infected lesion
	T. caratem	Pinta	Traumatized skin comes in contact with an infected lesion
	T. endemicum	Endemic syphilis	Mouth to mouth by utensils
Borrelia	B. recurrentis	• Epidemic releasing fever • Endemic releasing fever	• Body louse • Soft-shelled tick
	B. vincentii	Vincent's angina	
	B. burgdorferi	Lyme disease	Tick bites
Leptospira	L. interrogans	• Leptospirosis	
	L. biflexa	• Saprophytes	

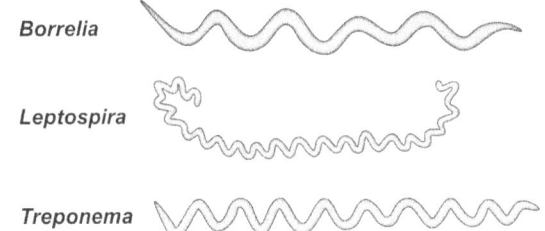

Fig. 39.1: Species designation of spirochetes based on morphology.

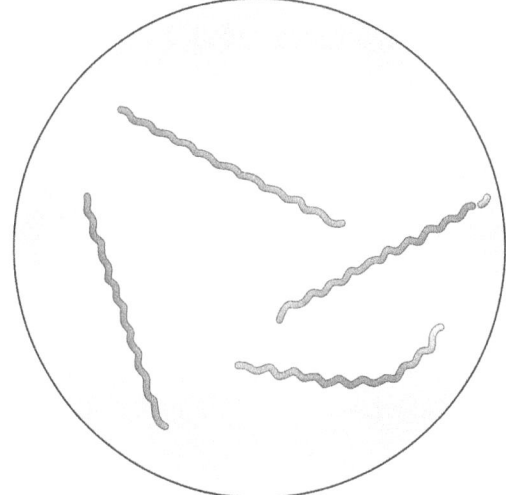

Fig. 39.2: *Treponema pallidum*—dark ground illumination.

Antigenic Structure
A. Nonspecific Antigen
The first is the *reagin* antibody in which a hapten extracted from the beef heart is used as the antigen. This lipid hapten is known as *cardioliom*.

B. Specific Antigens
- **Group-specific antigen:** It is a protein antigen present in *T. pallidum* as well as in nonpathogenic treponemes, such as Reiter treponeme.
- **Species-specific treponemal antigen**.

Pathogenesis
Treponema pallidum subsp. *pallidum* causes syphilis. Venereal syphilis is acquired by sexual contact. *T. pallidum* enters tissues by penetration of intact mucosae or through abraded skin. Clinical disease sets in after an incubation period of about a month (range 10–90 days). The natural course of syphilis can be divided into **primary, secondary, and tertiary stages** based on the clinical manifestations.
- **Primary disease:** The bacteria multiply at the initial entry site and the primary lesion in syphilis is the **chancre.** The chancre is a painless, relatively avascular, circumscribed, indurated, superficially ulcerated lesion. It is known as **'hard chancre'** and is most frequently on the external genitalia. **The regional lymph nodes** are swollen, discrete, rubbery, and nontender. The chancre invariably heals in **about 10–40 days,** even without treatment, leaving a thin scar.
- **Secondary syphilis:** Secondary syphilis sets in 1–3 months after healing of primary lesion. The secondary lesions are due to

widespread multiplication of the spirochetes and their dissemination through the blood.
- **Latent syphilis:** After the secondary lesions disappear there is a period of quiescence known as 'latent syphilis'.
- **Tertiary syphilis or late syphilis:** The three most common forms of late syphilis are cardiovascular syphilis, gummatous syphilis and neurosyphilis.

Congenital syphilis: In congenital syphilis infection is transmitted from mother to fetus transplacentally. The lesions of congenital syphilis usually develop only after the fourth month of gestation, the time when fetal immune competence starts appearing.

Laboratory Diagnosis

Laboratory diagnosis consists of **demonstration of the spirochetes** under the microscope and of **antibodies in serum or CSF.**

A. Specimen Collection and Handling
Specimens should be collected with care as the lesions are highly infectious.

- **Direct microscopy: Dark field microscopy**—This bacterium is too thin to be visualized with a standard Gram stain so two techniques to visualize it with a light microscope are **dark field microscopy** and **immunofluorescence**.
- Direct fluorescent-antibody staining for *Treponema pallidum* (DFA-Tp).

B. Demonstration of Treponemes in Tissues

C. Demonstration of Treponemal Antigen in the Lesion
By enzyme immunoassay and polymerase chain (PCR) reaction.

D. Serological Tests
These tests form the mainstay of laboratory diagnosis **(Table 39.2)**. Two major types of serologic tests exist: **nontreponemal tests or standard tests for syphilis (STS)** where cardiolipin or lipoidal antigen is used and **treponemal tests** (treponemes are used as the antigen).

Table 39.2: Diagnostic tests for syphilis.

A. Demonstration of treponemes in the exudate	1. Dark-ground microscopy 2. Direct fluorescent-antibody staining for *Treponema pallidum* (DFA-Tp)
B. Demonstration of treponemes in tissues	By immunofluorescence staining Silver impregnation method (Levaditi's stain)
C. Demonstration of treponemal antigen in the lesions	Enzyme immunoassay Polymerase chain reaction (PCR)

D. Serological diagnosis of syphilis	1. Nontreponemal tests
	   a. Venereal disease research laboratory (VDRL) test
	   b. Rapid plasma reagin (RPR) test
	2. Treponemal tests
	   a. Group specific test
	      I. Reiter protein CF (RPCF) test
	   b. Specific tests
	      I. Test using live *T. pallidum*
	         Treponema pallidum immobilization (TPI) test
	      II. Tests using killed *T. pallidum*
	         a. *Treponema pallidum* agglutination (TPA) test
	         b. *Treponema pallidum* immune adherence (TPIA) test
	         c. Fluorescent treponemal antibody absorption (FTA-ABS) test
	      III. Tests using *T. pallidum* extract
	         a. *Treponema pallidum* hemagglutination assay (TPHA)
	         b. *Treponema pallidum* enzyme immunoassays (TP-EIA)

1. Nontreponemal Tests or STS

Reagin antibodies are detected by cardiolipin antigen in STS. The antigen used in these tests is an alcoholic extract of beef heart tissue (cardiolipin) to which lecithin and cholesterol are added. The STS includes Wassermann, Kahn, Venereal Diseases Research Laboratory (VDRL) and the rapid plasma reagin (RPR) tests. All these tests are *flocculation tests* except Wassermann reaction. The Wassermann reaction is no longer in use. Similarly, Kahn test is rarely done these days.

The two nontreponemal tests widely used today are the **VDRL** and **RPR tests.**

- *Venereal disease research laboratory (VDRL) test:* It is the most widely used, simple, cheaper, and rapid test, which requires only a small quantity of serum. The VDRL test uses a cardiolipin antigen that is mixed with the patient's serum or CSF. Flocculation occurs in a positive reaction and is observed microscopically.
- *Rapid plasma reagin (RPR) test:* Rapid plasma reagin test is the most popular modifications of the VDRL test. RPR test employs stabilized VDRL carbon antigen, which make the result more clear cut and is read macroscopically.

Toluidine red unheated serum test (TRUST): A modification of the RPR test has been used.

Automated RPR test (ART) is available for large scale tests.

VDRL-ELISA test, which can measure IgG and IgM antibodies separately and is suitable for large-scale testing of sera.

Disadvantages of STS

Since cardiolipin antigen tests detect antibodies against a nonspecific antigen, a positive result is sometimes obtained with sera from healthy individuals or patients without clinical evidence of syphilis. These reactions are termed Biological False Positives (BFP) reactions. These are not caused by technical faults. BFP reactions may be classified as acute or chronic.

a. **Acute BFP reactions:** Acute BFP reactions are usually associated with acute infections, injuries or inflammatory conditions and occur in patients with other acute illnesses, especially pneumonia, hepatitis, vaccinations, and viral exanthematous disease.

b. **Chronic BFP reactions:** These are typically seen in—(1) SLE and other collagen diseases; (2) Leprosy; (3) Malaria; (4) Relapsing fever; (5) Infectious mononucleosis; (6) Hepatitis; (7) Tropical eosinophilia.

2. Treponemal Tests

Treponemal tests in which treponemes are used as the antigen. These are of two types.

a. Group-specific tests using Reiter treponeme:

Reiter Protein Complement Fixation (RPCF) Test—The principle of this test is the same as that of Wassermann test.

b. Species tests using pathogenic *T. pallidum* (Nichol's strain): These tests use the virmulent Nichol's strain of *T. pallidum.*

i. **Using Live *T. pallidum***

Treponema pallidum immobilization (TPI) test: The first in this group is the *Treponema pallidum immobilization* (TPI) test. The test serum is incubated with complement and *T. pallidum* anaerobically. If antibodies are present, the treponemes are immobilized, that is, rendered nonmotile, when examined under dark ground illumination.

ii. **Using killed *T. pallidum*:** The *Treponema pallidum* immune adherence (TPIA) test and *Treponema pallidum* agglutination (TPA) test were used for some time but have now been given up.

Treponema pallidum immune adherence (TPIA) test: A suspension of *T. pallidum,* inactivated by formalin, is mixed with the test serum and examined under dark ground microscopy. The treponemes are found agglutinated in the presence of antibodies.

Treponema pallidum agglutination (TPA) test: A suspension of inactivated *T. pallidum* is mixed with the test serum, complement, and fresh heparinized whole blood from a normal individual and incubated. The treponemes will be found to adhere to the erythrocytes in the presence of antibodies.

Fluorescent treponemal antibody (FTA) test: It is an indirect immunofluorescence test using as antigen, smears prepared on slides with Nichol's strain of *T. pallidum*. The slides can be stored for several months in deep freeze. The currently used modification of the test is the fluorescent treponemal antibody-absorption (FT A-ABS).

Fluorescent treponemal antibody-absorption (FTA-ABS) test: It is an indirect immunofluorescence test. Smears are prepared on slides with Nichol's strain of *T. pallidum* as antigen. The currently used modification of the test is the FTA-Absorption (FT A-ABS) test in which the test serum is preabsorbed with a sonicate of the Reiter treponemes (sorbent) to eliminate group specific reactions. After specific antibody from the patient is allowed to react with the organisms, unbound antibodies in the serum are removed by washing. The presence of anti-*T. pallidum* antibody is then detected by application of fluorescein-labeled, anti-human globulin and examination of the slide with an ultraviolet (UV) microscope. Positive results are indicated by fluorescence of the *T. pallidum* organisms. An FTA-ABS 19S-lgM test has also been developed for evaluation of congenital syphilis.

iii. Using an extract of *T. pallidum*
- ***T. pallidum* hemagglutination assay (TPHA):** The (TPHA) uses tanned erythrocytes sensitized with a sonicated extract of *T. pallidum* as antigen. When these sensitized erythrocytes are mixed with patient's serum (test sera) containing antitreponemal antibodies it causes hemagglutination.
- **Enzyme immunoassays (EIA):** Table 39.3 shows the relative sensitivities of the serological tests in common use.

Interpretation of Various Serological Tests

1. **Serological screening:** VDRL and TPHA tests provide a highly efficient screen for the detection or exclusion of treponemal infection.
2. **Response to treatment:** VDRL testing provides the best means of measuring response to treatment in most stages of treponemal infection.
3. **Biological false positive (BFP) reactions:** TPHA and FTA-ABS are helpful in excluding or confirming the diagnosis of syphilis and for identifying BFP reactions.
4. **Diagnosis of congenital syphilis.**

Table 39.3: Frequency of reactive serological tests in untreated syphilis (percentage) in common use.

Stage	VDR/RPR	FTA-ABS	TPHA
Primary	70–80	85–100	65–85
Secondary	100	100	100
Latent/late	60–70	95–100	95–100

Treatment

Penicillin is the drug of choice for treating infections with *T. pallidum*. **In early cases**, a single injection of 2.4 million units of benzathine penicillin is adequate. **For late syphilis**, this may be repeated weekly for 3 weeks. In patients allergic to penicillin, **erythromycin or tetracycline** may be used.

Jarisch–Herxheimer reaction: Antibiotic therapy of syphilitics, particularly with penicillin, characteristically induces a systemic response called the **Jarisch-Herxheimer reaction.**

Nonvenereal Treponematoses

Nonvenereal treponemal diseases are found in developing countries where hygiene is poor, little clothing is worn, and direct skin contact is common because of overcrowding.

The three nonvenereal treponemal diseases are: **Endemic syphilis, Yaws, and Pinta.**

1. Endemic Syphilis (Bejel)

Endemic syphilis or *bejel* syphilis, transmitted nonvenereally, was endemic in several foci.

Etiologic agent is *T. pallidum* subspecies *endemicum*.

Transmission is by direct person-to-person contact and by sharing of contaminated eating or drinking utensils.

Clinical manifestations: The primary chancre is not usually seen, except sometimes on the nipples of mothers infected by their children. The disease is usually seen with manifestations of secondary syphilis, such as mucous patches in the mouth and skin eruptions. The disease progresses to tertiary lesions.

The laboratory diagnosis and treatment are as for venereal syphilis.

2. Yaws (Frambesia)

Yaws is a disease that is endemic also known as **frambesia, Rian, parangi** and by many other synonyms.

Causative agent—is *T. pallidum* subspecies *pertenue* (still known as *T. pertenue*) which is morphologically and antigenically indistinguishable from *T. pallidum*.

Clinical manifestations: The primary lesion (mother yaw) is an extragenital papule. It enlarges and breaks down to form an ulcerating granuloma. As in syphilis, secondary and tertiary manifestations follow.

Transmission: Infection is acquired by direct contact with open ulcers. Flies may act as mechanical vectors.

Laboratory diagnosis and treatment are similar to those of venereal syphilis.

3. Pinta

Pinta is caused by *T. carateum*. Spread of infection is by direct contact with infectious lesions. Transmission appears to require direct person to person contact. The skin bears the brunt of the disease. Incubation ranges from 7 to 21 days. **The primary lesion** is an extragenital papule, which does not ulcerate but develops into a lichenoid or psoriasiform. **Secondary skin lesions** are characterized by hyperpigmentation or hypopigmentation. Tissues other than skin are seldom affected.

The laboratory diagnosis and treatment are similar to those of venereal syphilis.

Nonpathogenic Treponemes

Several commensal treponemes occur on the buccal and genital mucosa and may cause confusion in the diagnosis of syphilis by dark field examination. Best known among them is the oral spirochete, *T. dentium,* which can be readily cultivated. *T. refringens* and *T. gracilis* may be found as normal commensal in genitalia.

BORRELIA

Borreliae are large, motile, refractile spirochetes with irregular, wide, open coils. They are readily stained by ordinary methods and are gram negative. Members of the genus *Borrelia* can be easily distinguished from spirochetes of the genera *Leptospira* and *Treponema* by their much larger size (10–30 in length by 0.3–0.7 in width), by their irregular, wide-open, loosely wound primary coils and by the ease with which they can be stained with the usual laboratory aniline dyes **(Table 39.2)**.

Species of *Borrelia*: Borreliae of medical importance are:
1. *B. recurrentis* causing relapsing fever.
2. *B. vincentii* causes fusospirochetosis.
3. *B. burgdoiferi* causes Lyme disease.

Morphology

Borreliae are helical organisms 0.2–0.5 µm wide and 8–20 µm in length. They are gram negative, actively motile and possess 5–8 irregular spirals with pointed ends **(Fig. 39.1)**. They can be seen with light microscopy in preparations stained with Wright's or Giemsa stains.

Cultural Characteristics

Borreliae are microaerophilic. Optimum temperature for growth is 28–30°C. The organism can be grown on Noguchi's medium (ascitic fluid containing rabbit kidney), chorioallantoic membrane (CAM) of chick embryos and in mice or rats intraperitoneally.

Pathogenicity

Relapsing Fever

Relapsing fever (RF) is an **arthropod-borne infection**, and two types of which occur—**louse-borne** and **tick-borne**.

1. Epidemic or Louse-borne Relapsing Fever

The causative agent of louse-borne or epidemic RF is *B. recurrentis*. It is an exclusive human pathogen, being transmitted from person to person through body lice *(Pediculus humanus corporis)* and disease is found worldwide.

2. Endemic or Tick-borne Relapsing Fever

The second form of RF is endemic and **tick-borne**. It is spread by infected soft ticks of the genus *Ornithodoros*.

After an incubation period of 2-10 days RF sets in as fever of sudden onset. The fever subsides in 3-5 days. The disease ultimately subsides after 3-10 relapses.

Laboratory Diagnosis

Routine laboratory diagnosis of relapsing fever depends on demonstrating the spirochetes in peripheral blood samples.
  i. **Dark ground microscopy:** A drop of blood may be examined as a wet film under the dark ground or phase contrast microscope and borreliae detected by their lashing movements.
  ii. **Giemsa or Leishman stain:** Blood smears are stained with Giemsa or Leishman stain and examined for borreliae.
  iii. **Animal inoculation:** Inoculate intraperitoneally blood into six young white mice. Examine by darkfield microscopy for living spirochetes or after staining by Giemsa.
  iv. **Culture and serology:** Cultivation of the borreliae and demonstration of antibodies are too difficult and unreliable to be used in diagnosis.

Treatment: Tetracycline, chloramphenicol, penicillin, and erythromycin are effective.

BORRELIA VINCENTII (TREPONEMA VINCENTII)

Treponema vincentii (old name *Borrelia vincentii*) is a motile spirochete, about 5-20 µm long and 0.2-0.6 µm wide, with 3-8 coils of variable size. It is easily stained with dilute carbol fuchsin and is gram negative.

Treponema vincentii is a normal commensal of mouth. It may give rise to **ulcerative gingivostomatitis or oropharyngitis (Vincent's angina)** under predisposing conditions, such as malnutrition or viral infections. In Vincent's angina, *T. vincentii* is often associated with anaerobic gram negative fusiform bacillus known as *Fusobacterium fusiforme* (now known as *Leptotrichia buccalis)*. This symbiotic infection is known as **fusospirochetosis.**

Diagnosis

1. **Microscopic examination:** Diagnosis may be made by demonstrating spirochetes and fusiform bacilli in stained smears of exudates from the lesions.
2. **Culture:** *B. vincentii* may be cultivated with difficulty in enriched media anaerobically.

Treatment: Penicillin and metronidazole are effective in treatment.

Lyme Disease: Borrelia burgdorferi

It is caused *by Borrelia burgdorferi* transmitted by the bite of ixodid ticks.

Morphology: It measures 4-30 mm × 0.2-0.25 µm. It is flexible, helical, and gram negative.

Culture: It is a microaerophilic spirochete. It is fastidious bacterium and can be grown in a modified Kelley's (BSK) medium, after incubation for 2 weeks or more. Optimum temperature for growth is 33°C.

Pathogenesis

The natural hosts for *B. burgdorferi* are wild and domesticated animals, including mice and other rodents, deer, sheep, cattle, horses and dogs.

B. burgdorferi is transmitted to man by ixodid ticks that become infected while feeding on infected animals. The bacterium grows primarily in the midgut of the tick, and transmission to man occurs during regurgitation of the gut contents during the blood meal. Lyme disease may be a progressive illness, and is divided into three stages.

Laboratory Diagnosis
A. **Isolation of the borrelia**
B. **Serology:** ELISA and immunofluorescence (IF) have been described and immunoblotting recommended for confirmation.

Treatment
Penicillins, the newer macrolides, cephalosporins and tetracyclines have all been used successfully in Lyme disease.

LEPTOSPIRA

Classification
The genus *Leptospira* is now classified into two species *L. interrogans*, and *L. biflexa*.
1. ***Leptospira interrogans***: It comprises the parasitic and pathogenic leptospires. *L. interrogans* is classified into 23 serogroups (**Icterohemorrhagiae, Canicola, Pyogenes, Autumnalis, Australis, Pomona, Hebdomadal, Grippotyphosa, etc.**). Within each serogroup over 200 serovars are recognized.
2. ***L. biflexa:*** It contains saprophytic leptospires.

Morphology
Leptospires are delicate spirochetes about 6–20 µm long and 0.1 µm thick. They have numerous closely wound primary coils. Their ends are hooked and resemble umbrella handles (**Fig. 39.3**). They are actively motile, gram-negative, but take up conventional stains poorly. They can be visualized by Giemsa or silver deposition methods or by use of fluorescent antibody.

Cultural Characteristics
They are aerobic and microaerophilic. Optimum temperature is 25–30°C and optimum pH 7.2–7.5. Leprospires can be grown in media enriched with rabbit serum.

Liquid medium is Stuart's or Korthofs medium. **Semisynthetic media,** such as EMJH (Ellinghausen, McCullough, Johnson, Harris) medium are now commonly used. A simple **semisolid medium** is Fletcher's medium. Leptospires may be grown on the **CAM** of chick embryos.

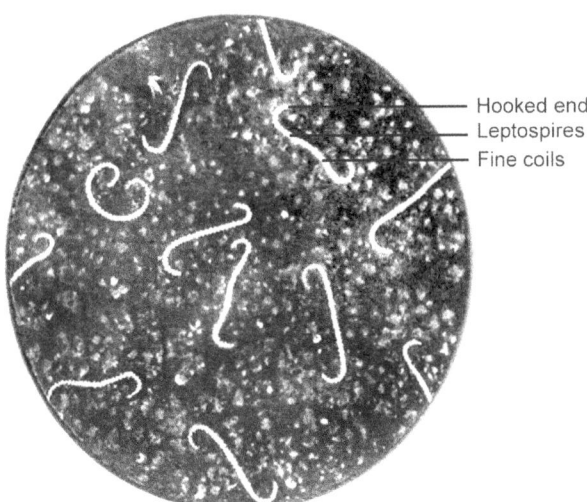

Fig. 39.3: Dark ground microscopy shows the appearance of living leptospira.

Pathogenesis

Leptospirosis is most common **zoonotic bacterial disease** throughout the world. Rodents are most important reservoirs. Several animals act as carriers. **Rats** are particularly important.

In natural reservoir hosts, leptospiral infection is asymptomatic. It is transmitted to humans when the leptospires in water contaminated by the urine of carrier animals enters the body through cuts or abrasions on the skin or through intact mucosa of mouth, nose, or conjuctiva. During the acute phase of the disease, leptospires are seen in the blood but can seldom be demonstrated after 8–10 days. They persist in the internal organs, and most abundantly in the kidneys, so that they may be demonstrated in the urine in the later stages of the disease.

Diseases: Mild virus-like syndrome. The incubation period is usually about 10 days (range 2–26 days). The onset of clinical illness is usually abrupt, with nonspecific, influenza-like constitutional symptoms.

The patient may develop more advanced disease-including **aseptic meningitis**.

Severe systemic disease (Weil's disease) includes renal failure, hepatic failure, and intravascular disease, and may result in death.

Duration of the illness varies from less than 1–3 weeks.

Serious cases of leptospirosis are caused most often by serotype **icterohemorrhagiae**.

Laboratory Diagnosis

Diagnosis may be made by—(1) demonstration of the leptospires microscopically in blood or urine; (2) isolation in culture; (3) animal inoculation; (4) serological tests.
1. **Demonstration of leptospiras in blood or urine**
   i. **Microscopy:** As leptospires disappear from the blood after the first week, blood examination is helpful only in the early stages of the disease. Leptospires may be demonstrated by examination of the blood under the dark field microscope or by immunofluorescence. Leptospires may be found in the urine during the second week and intermittently for 4–6 weeks or even longer. Centrifuged deposit of the urine may be examined under dark ground illumination.
2. **Culture:** Three or four drops of blood are inoculated into each of several bijou bottles containing medium. The bottles are incubated at 37°C. Samples from the cultures are examined every third day for the presence of leptospires under dark ground illumination for 2 weeks.
3. **Animal inoculation:** The blood or urine from the patient is inoculated intraperitoneally into young guinea pigs. The animals develop fever and die within 8–12 days with jaundice and hemorrhage into the lungs and serous cavities with virulent serotypes, such as icterohemorrhagiae.
4. **Serological diagnosis:** Tests for detection of leptospiral antibodies in sera are of two kinds:
   i. **Genus-specific tests:** The tests employed include **sensitized erythrocyte lysis (SEL), complement fixation, agglutination,** and **indirect immunofluorescence**. **ELISA** has been used to detect IgM and IgG antibodies separately. A simple and rapid **dip-stick assay** has been developed for the assay of leptospira-specific IgM antibody in human sera.
   ii. **Serogroup-specific tests:** Serogroup-specific tests are reactive mainly with strains of the same serogroup as the infecting strain. They comprise agglutination tests that are either **macroscopic,** or **microscopic. The microscopic agglutination test (MAT)** is more specific and is generally accepted as **"gold standard".**

KEY POINTS

- *Treponema pallidum:* It is the causative agent of syphilis. It is a sexually transmitted disease (STD).
- *Borrelia: Borrelia recurrentis* is the causative agent of *relapsing fever, B. vincentii* causes *vincent's angina* and *B. burgdorferi* causes Lyme disease.

- **Leptospira:** Leptospirosis is most common zoonotic bacterial disease. Rodents are most important reservoirs.

IMPORTANT QUESTIONS

1. Classify spirochetes. Name different spirochetes and diseases caused by them. Discuss the laboratory diagnosis of syphilis.
2. Write short notes on:
   a. VDRL test
   b. Fluorescent treponemal antibody-absorption (FTA-ABS) test.
   c. TPHA (or) *T. pallidum* hemagglutination test.
   d. *Borrelia vincentii*
   e. Lyme disease

MULTIPLE CHOICE QUESTIONS

1. *Treponema pallidum* can be cultivated in:
   a. Thayer–Martin medium
   b. Blood agar medium
   c. Chocolate agar medium
   d. Rabbit testes
2. Hard chancre is characteristic of:
   a. Primary syphilis
   b. Secondary syphilis
   c. Latent syphilis
   d. Tertiary syphilis
3. Which of the following serological tests is employed for diagnosis of congenital syphilis?
   a. FTA-ABS test
   b. IgM FTA-ABS test
   c. TPHA test
   d. Reiter protein complement fixation test
4. Jarisch–Herxheimer reaction is a complication observed following therapy with antibiotics in:
   a. Syphilis
   b. Relapsing fever
   c. Lyme disease
   d. Leptospirosis
5. The causative agent of louse-borne relapsing fever is:
   a. *Borrelia recurrentis*
   b. *B. duttoni*
   c. *B. vincentii*
   d. *B. burgdroferi*
6. All the following diseases are transmitted non-venereally, *except*:
   a. Syphilis
   b. Pinta
   c. Yaws
   d. Congenital syphilis
7. Which serogroup of *Leptospira interrogans* is responsible for causing Weil's disease?
   a. *Icterohemorrhagiae*
   b. *Hebdomadis*
   c. *Australis*
   d. *Canicola*
8. Which of the following tests can be performed for the serodiagnosis of leptospirosis?
   a. Macroscopic agglutination test
   b. Microscopic agglutination test
   c. Complement fixation test
   d. All of the above

ANSWERS

1. d 2. a 3. b 4. a
5. a 6. a 7. a 8. d

Mycoplasma and Ureaplasma

LEARNING OBJECTIVES

After reading and studying this chapter, you should be able to:
- Describe morphology and cultural characteristics of *Mycoplasma* spp.
- Describe pathogenicity of *Mycoplasma pneumoniae*.
- Describe laboratory diagnosis of mycoplasmal and ureaplasmal infections.
- Discuss the use of serologic tests for diagnosing *M. pneumoniae* infections.
- Describe *Ureaplasma urealyticum* and *Mycoplasma hominis*.

INTRODUCTION

Mycoplasmas are the smallest prokaryotes capable of self-replication.

"Mycoplasma" (Greek: *mykes* = fungus; *plasma* = something molded) refers to the filamentous (fungal-like) nature of the organisms of some species and the plasticity of the outer membrane resulting in pleomorphism.

CLASSIFICATION

Mycoplasmas are members of the class Mollicutes (*mollis,* soft; *kutis,* skin), and the order Mycoplasmatales. The class Mollicutes contains five families.

Family *Mycoplasmataceae*: It is subdivided into two genera:
1. **Genus *Mycoplasma*** utilizes glucose or arginine but do not split urea. It has more than 110 named species.
2. **Genus *Ureaplasma*** hydrolyzes urea. It has six species. Found in insects and plants.

MORPHOLOGY

Mycoplasmas are the smallest free-living microorganisms. They can pass through bacterial filters. They lack cell wall but are bounded by a trilaminar membrane, which is rich in cholesterol and other lipids. They are very small pleomorphic cells, which may range from spherical through to short- and long-branching filaments. Mycoplasmas are gram negative but are better stained by Giemsa stain.

Replication is basically by binary fission. Mycoplasmas do not possess spores, flagella, or fimbria. Some mycoplasmas, including *M. pneumoniae,* exhibit a gliding motility.

CULTURAL CHARACTERISTICS

Most mycoplasmas are facultative anaerobic. They grow within a temperature range of 22–41°C, the parasitic species growing optimally at 35–37°C.

Media for cultivating mycoplasma are enriched with 20% horse or human serum and yeast extract. Mycoplasmas may be cultivated in liquid or solid media. A medium widely used for the isolation of mycoplasmas consists of bovine heart infusion broth [pleuropneumonia-like organism (PPLO) broth) to which are added 20% horse serum and 10% fresh yeast extract along with glucose and phenol red as a pH indicator. This medium can be solidified by the addition of agar. Penicillin, ampicillin, and polymyxin

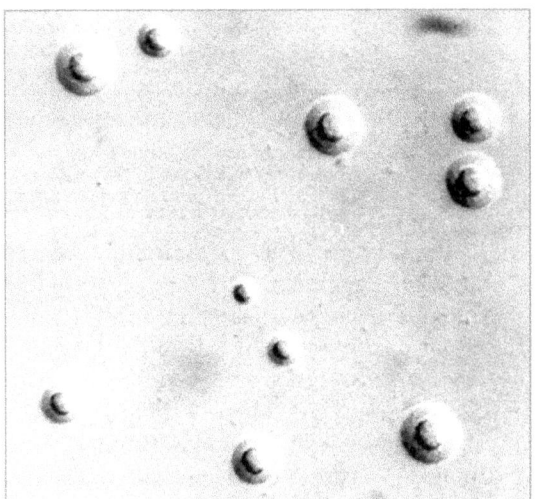

Fig. 40.1: Colonies of *M. hominis* with typical "fried egg" appearance.

B may be added in the medium to inhibit contaminating bacteria and amphotericin B to inhibit fungi. Colonies appear after incubation for 2-6 days and are about 10-600 μm in size. On agar, colonies are typically biphasic that have a **"fried egg" appearance**, with an opaque central zone of growth within the agar and a translucent peripheral zone on the surface **(Fig. 40.1)**.

Colonies may be seen with a hand lens but are best studied after staining by Dienes method. Colonies cannot be picked with platinum loops. Subculture is done by cutting out an agar block with colonies and rubbing it on fresh plates. Most *Mycoplasma* colonies are hemolytic.

PATHOGENICITY

Mycoplasma causes two types of diseases in humans—pneumonia and genital infections.

Mycoplasma pneumoniae

Infection with *M. pneumoniae* typically produces mild **upper respiratory tract disease.** More severe diseases with **lower respiratory tract infections** include **tracheobronchitis, pneumonia (referred to as primary atypical pneumonia or walking pneumonia)**. Transmission is probably through aerosol droplet spray produced while coughing.

Ureaplasma urealyticum

Some strains of *Mycoplasma* frequently isolated from the urogenital tract of human beings and animals form very tiny colonies, generally 15-50 μm in size. They were called **T strain or T form mycoplasmas (T for tiny)**. They are peculiar in their ability to **hydrolyze urea,** which is an essential growth factor in addition to cholesterol. Human T strain mycoplasmas have been reclassified as *Ureaplasma urealyticum.*

Clinical Manifetations

1. *U. urealyticum* may cause nonchlamydial, nongonococcal urethritis (NGU), epididymitis, vaginitis, and cervicitis.
2. They may cause chorioamnionitis, prematurity, postpartum endometritis, chronic lung disease of the premature infant and infection of wounds and soft tissues.
3. Male and female infertility and low-birth weight.

Mycoplasma hominis

Mycoplasma hominis is found in the lower genitourinary tracts of approximately 50% of healthy adults and has not been reported as a cause of **NGU**. The organism may cause salpingitis, pyelonephritis, pelvic inflammatory disease (PID), or postpartum fevers.

LABORATORY DIAGNOSIS

Laboratory diagnosis of may be established either by isolation of the mycoplasma or by serological methods.

1. **Specimens:** *M. pneumoniae* may be recovered from throat swabs, nasopharyngeal swabs, sputum, throat washings, bronchoalveolar lavage, tracheal aspirate, and lung tissue specimens. **Genital mycoplasmas** may be isolated from urethral, vaginal and cervical swabs, and other specimens.
2. **Culture:** In the laboratory, if inoculation is not possible immediately, then the specimen may be held up to 24 hours at 4°C. If delay more than 24 hours is expected, then the specimen should be frozen at −70°C. A widely

used isolation medium contains bovine heart infusion (PPLO broth) with fresh yeast extract and horse serum supplemented with penicillin, thallium acetate, glucose and with phenol red as a pH indicator. For genital mycoplasma, polymyxin B and amphotericin B and lincomycin are also added to mycoplasmal broth.

3. **Isolation and identification:** Broth cultures are incubated at 35°C with the caps tightened. A slight, gradual shift in the pH indicator (from salmon to yellow) over an 8–15 day period without gross turbidity suggests a true-positive culture. The broth must be subcultured to appropriate agar medium as soon as color changes in the medium are apparent.
    i. **Colonies:** Colonies of *M. pneumoniae* are small, beta-hemolytic and have a homogeneous granular appearance (**"mulberryshaped"**), unlike the fried-egg morphology of other mycoplasmas. *M. hominis* colonies have a typical large **"fried egg" appearance (Fig. 40.1)**. *Ureaplasma* spp. form extremely small colonies (15–60 μm in diameter) that are difficult to see with the naked eye.
    ii. **Species identification:**
        a. Hemadsorption test
        b. Tetrazolium reduction test
        c. Growth inhibition test
        d. **Polymerase chain reaction (PCR) amplification.**
4. **Antigen detection techniques:** By direct immunofluorescence and counter immuno-electrophoresis techniques, immunoblotting with monoclonal antibodies and antigen capture enzyme immunoassay (EIA).
5. **DNA probes**
6. **Serological tests**
    A. Specific tests using mycoplasmal antigens
    B. Nonspecific methods.

A. Specific Tests Using Mycoplasmal Antigens

The development of antibody to *M. pneumoniae* by infected subjects may be measured by a range of techniques, viz. complement fixation, metabolic inhibition, inhibition of tetrazolium reduction, immunofluorescence, direct or antibody capture enzyme-immunosorbent assays (EIA), or agglutination of antigen-coated erythrocytes, latex or gelatin particles.

B. Nonspecific Serological Tests

The nonspecific serological tests are *Streptococcus* MG and cold agglutination tests.
- **Sterptococcus MG test:** It is done by mixing serial dilutions of the patient's unheated serum and a heat killed suspension of *Streptococcus MG,* and observing agglutination after overnight incubation at 37°C. A titer of 1:20 or over is considered suggestive.
- **Cold agglutination test:** The cold agglutination test is based on the appearance in a high proportion of cases with primary atypical pneumonia, of macroglobulin antibodies that agglutinate human group O cells at low temperature. This test is easily performed by mixing serial dilutions of the patient's serum with an equal volume of a 0.2% washed human O group erythrocytes and clumping observed after incubating the mixture overnight. The test is based on the development of hemagglutination, which can be reversed by placing the tubes at 37°C. A titer of 1:32 or over is suggestive but demonstration of rise in titer in paired serum samples is more reliable.

TREATMENT

Mycoplasmas and ureaplasmas are sensitive to tetracycline and erythromycin, which inhibit protein synthesis.

KEY POINTS

- Mycoplasmas are the smallest free-living bacterium.
- *Mycoplasma pneumoniae:*
    - **Diseases:** Upper respiratory infections.
    - Lower respiratory infections, including tracheobronchitis and **pneumonia.**
- *Ureaplasma urealyticum* was called **T strain or T form mycoplasmas**, peculiar in their ability to hydrolyze urea.

IMPORTANT QUESTION

1. Write short notes on:
   a. *Mycoplasma pneumoniae*
   b. *Streptococcus MG* agglutination test
   c. *Ureaplasma urealyticum*

MULTIPLE CHOICE QUESTIONS

1. Which of the following media is/are used for isolation of *Mycoplasma*?
   a. PPLO broth
   b. PPLO agar
   c. Both of the above
   d. None of the above
2. Which of the following statements are true for *Ureaplasma urealyticum*, *except*:
   a. They do not hydrolyze urea
   b. They require supplementation with urea for their growth
   c. They may cause nongonococcal urethritis (NGU)
   d. They are called T strain or T form mycoplasmas
3. Which of the following pathogens cause nongonococcal urethritis, *except*:
   a. *Mycoplasma hominis*
   b. *Chlamydia trachomatis*
   c. *Ureaplasma urealyticum*
   d. *Mycoplasma genitalium*
4. Which of the following tests can help in the laboratory diagnosis of primary atypical pneumonia?
   a. Cold agglutination test
   b. *Streptococcus MG* agglutination test
   c. Culture on *Mycoplasma* broth medium
   d. All of the above

ANSWERS

1. c   2. a   3. b   4. d

Miscellaneous Bacteria

LEARNING OBJECTIVES

After reading and studying this chapter, you should be able to:
- Describe morphology and culture characteristics of *Listeria*.
- Describe infections caused by *Listeria monocytogenes* and their laboratory diagnosis.
- Discuss rat bite fever.
- Describe *Klebsiella granulomatis* and disease caused by it.
- Describe the following: *Acinetobacter* spp.; **rat-bite fever**; *Gardnerella vaginalis*.

LISTERIA MONOCYTOGENES

Morphology

Listeria monocytogenes is a small, coccoid, gram-positive bacillus measuring approximately 0.5 × 2–3 μm. They occur singly or in pairs which are often angled at the point of contact and may resemble diphtheroids or diplococci. It exhibits a characteristic, slow, tumbling motility when grown at 25°C but at 37°C is nonmotile. They are non-capsulate, nonsporing, and nonacid-fast.

Cultural Characteristics

Listeriae are aerobes and facultative anaerobes. They can grow over a temperature range of 2–43°C, the optimum temperature for the growth is 35–37°C. They can grow on ordinary media containing fermentable carbohydrate, but growth is better on blood agar or tryptose phosphate agar. After 24 hours incubation at 37°C, colonies are 0.5–1.5 mm in diameter, smooth, translucent, and emulsifiable and non-pigmented.

On blood agar, *L. monocytogenes* develops zones of slightly hazy β-hemolysis.

Biochemical Reactions

Listeria monocytogenes ferments glucose, maltose, L-rhamnose, and alpha methyl D-mannoside, producing acid without gas. It is catalase positive. It grows in the presence of 0.1% potassium tellurite, 10% salt, and at pH 9.6.

Pathogenicity

The genus contains eight species, but almost all cases of human listeriosis are caused by *L. monocytogenes*. *Listeria monocytogenes* is commonly ingested in food, and is usually a harmless transient in the intestinal tract and *L. seeligeri* have been associated with a very small number of human infections.

Clinical Features

1. **Intrauterine and neonatal infection:** Intrauterine infection of the fetus may result in abortion, stillbirth, premature delivery, or acute-onset disseminated infection in the newborn infant. Meningitis or septicemia may occur in neonates.
2. **Adult and juvenile infection:** It may cause meningitis or meningoencephalitis.
3. **Disease in healthy adults:** Several food-borne outbreaks of acute gastroenteritis with fever have been described.
4. **Other infections:** Listeriosis may also present as abscesses, conjunctivitis, pharyngitis, urethritis, pneumonia, infectious mono-

nucleosis like syndrome, endocarditis or septicemia.

Laboratory Diagnosis

1. **Specimens:** Blood, CSF, amniotic fluid, placenta, pus, and biopsy material from the organs involved may be collected. Specimens may also be collected from neonate, stillbirth, or products of conception.
2. **Microcopy:** If the Gram stain shows organisms, they are intracellular and extracellular gram-positive coccobacilli.
3. **Culture:** Specimens should be inoculated on blood agar, chocolate agar and tryptose phosphate agar, and incubated at 35–37°C for 1–3 days. Uncentrifuged CSF and blood may be added to nutrient broth and incubated at 35–37°C for 5 days followed by subculture on solid media.

Blood agar shows small colonies surrounded by a narrow zone of β-hemolysis. The bacteria are actively motile when grown at 25°C. The isolate is identified by its morphology and biochemical tests.

Treatment

Currently, penicillin or ampicillin, either alone or with gentamicin, is the treatment of choice for infections with *L. monocytogenes*. Erythromycin can be used in patients allergic to penicillin.

ERYSIPELOTHRIX RHUSIOPATHIAE

The genus *Erysipelothrix* contains two species, of which *Erysipelothrix rhusiopathiae* is responsible for human disease.

Morphology

Erysipelothrix rhusiopathiae is a slender, nonmotile, nonsporing, non-capsulated, straight or slightly curved, gram-positive rod, with tendency toward formation of long filaments.

Pathogenicity

Human infection: Disease is common in swine but rare in humans. Three forms of human infection:

1. Localized skin infection (erysipeloid)
2. Generalized cutaneous form
3. Septicemia

ALCALIGENES FAECALIS

Alcaligenes faecalis refers to gram-negative, short, nonsporing bacilli, which are strict aerobes and do not ferment sugars. They are motile by means of peritrichous flagella. They are usually oxidase positive.

They have been considered responsible for a typhoid-like fever, urinary infections, infantile gastroenteritis, and suppuration in various parts of the body.

CHROMOBACTERIUM VIOLACEUM

Chromobacrium violaceum is a gram-negative, nonsporing bacillus, motile by means of single polar and scanty lateral flagella. It causes rare but dangerous infection and consists of skin lesions with pyemia and multiple abscesses.

FLAVOBACTERIUM MENINGOSEPTICUM

Flavobacterium meningosepticum is a gram-negative nonmotile rod. It has been responsible for outbreaks of meningitis in newborn infants. Infection in adults leads to a mild febrile illness.

DONOVANIA GRANULOMATIS (CALYMMATOBACTERIUM GRANULOMATIS) OR KLEBSIELLA GRANULOMATIS

The etiologic agent of granuloma inguinale, a granulomatous disease affecting the genitalia and inguinal area, has been called historically *Calymmatobacterium (Donovania) granulomatis*. Recently, this organism was transferred into the genus *Klebsiella*.

Morphology

Klebsiella granulomatis is a small, capsulate, gram-negative, coccobacillus. They show bipolar condensation of chromatin, giving a closed **safety-pin appearance** in stained smears. They are, nonmotile, nonsporing, and non-acid-fast.

Culture
It can be cultured readily in the egg yolk medium and on a modified Levinthal agar.

Pathogenicity
Donovanosis is a venereal disease. It can be transmitted after repeated exposure through sexual intercourse or nonsexual trauma to the genitalia. A chronic granulomatous disease known as *granuloma inguinale, granulomatous venereum*, or *donovanosis*.

Laboratory Diagnosis
Laboratory confirmation of granuloma inguinale is made by scraping the border of the lesion, by spreading the collected tissue on a slide, and by staining it with Giemsa or Wright's stain. Pathognomonic **Donovan bodies** are observed within mononuclear phagocytes.

Treatment
Cases of donovanosis respond well to tetracycline, chloramphenicol, erythromycin, clindamycin, cotrimoxazole, streptomycin, and other aminoglycosides.

ACINETOBACTER (MIMA POLYMORPHA; BACTERIUM ANITRATUM)

The genus *Acinetobacter* contains strictly aerobic short, stout, often capsulate, nonmotile gram-negative bacilli or coccobacilli. They are oxidase negative,

The most important species currently are *Acinetobacter baumannii* and *Acinetobacter lwoffii*.

Pathogenesis
Serious infections, including meningitis, pneumonia and septicemia, are most commonly associated with *Acinetobacter baumannii*. Patients in intensive care units are at particular risk.

RAT BITE FEVER (STREPTOBACILLUS MONILIFORMIS AND SPIRILLUM MINUS)

Streptobacillus moniliformis is a long, thin, gram-negative bacillus. *Spirillum minus* is a short, spiral, gram-negative organism. *Streptobacillus moniliformis* and *Spirillum minus* are the causative agents of two distinct diseases referred to collectively as **rat-bite fever**.

GARDNERELLA VAGINALIS

Gardnerella vaginalis is a small, gram-negative, nonmotile, pleomorphic rod, which shows metachromatic granules.

G. vaginalis is considered responsible for bacterial vaginosis, a mild but common condition characterized by raised vaginal pH >4.5, foul smelling discharge and the presence of 'clue cells', which are vaginal epithelial cells with their surface studded with numerous small bacteria. Bacterial vaginosis is also associated with anaerobic bacteria, particularly *Mobiluncus*. Metronidazole is effective in treatment.

KEY POINTS

- ***Listeria*:** The disease chiefly affects pregnant women, unborn or newly delivered infants, the immunosuppressed and elderly.
- ***Erysipelothrix rhusiopathiae*:** Disease is common in swine but rare in humans.
- ***Alcaligenes faecalis*:** It causes urinary tract infection, infantile gastroenteritis, and typhoid-like fever in humans.
- ***Calymmatobacterium (Donovania) granulomatis*** is the causative agent of granuloma inguinale, a sexually transmitted disease.
- ***Gardnerella vaginalis*** is considered responsible for bacterial vaginosis.

IMPORTANT QUESTION

1. Write short notes on:
   a. *Listeria monocytogenes*
   b. Donovan bodies
   c. Rat-bite fever

MULTIPLE CHOICE QUESTIONS

1. Tumbling motility is seen in:
   a. Listeria monocytogenes
   b. Enterobacter cloacae
   c. Proteus vulgaris
   d. Salmonella typhi
2. In adults, listeriosis may lead to:
   a. Meningitis
   b. Meningoencephalitis
   c. None of the above
   d. All of the above
3. Which of the following bacteria can cause rat bite fever?
   a. Streptobacillus moniliformis
   b. Listeria monocytogenes
   c. Chromobacterium violaceum
   d. Flavobacterium meningosepticum
4. Causative agent of donovanosis is:
   a. Klebsiella pneumoniae
   b. Klebsiella oxytoca
   c. Klebsiella granulomatis
   d. None of the above

ANSWERS

1. a   2. d   3. a   4. c

CHAPTER 42

Rickettsiaceae, Bartonellaceae, and Coxiella

LEARNING OBJECTIVES

After reading and studying this chapter, you should be able to:
- Describe diseases caused by different rickettsiae.
- Discuss the laboratory diagnosis of rickettsial infections.
- Describe Weil-Felix reaction.
- Discuss Q fever, Trench fever, and Oroya fever.

INTRODUCTION

Rickettsiae are small, gram-negative bacilli adapted to obligate intracellular parasitism, and transmitted by arthropod vectors.

CLASSIFICATION

The family Rickettsiacae currently comprises three genera—***Rickettsia*, *Orientia*,** and ***Ehrlichia*** (Table 42.1).

GENUS *RICKETTSIA*

Morphology

In smears from infected tissues, rickettsiae appear as pleomorphic coccobacilli, 0.3–0.6 mm × 0.8–2 mm in size. They are nonmotile and noncapsulated. They are gram negative, though they do not take the stain well. They stain bluish purple with Giemsa and Castaneda stains and deep red with Machiavello and Gimenez stains.

Cultivation

Rickettsiae are unable to grow in cellfree media. The optimum temperature for growth is 32–35°C.
1. **Yolk sac:** They are readily cultivated in the **yolk sac** of developing chick embryos.
2. **Cell culture:** Many strains of rickettsiae also grow in **cell culture** such as mouse fibroblast, HeLa, HEp-2, Detroit 6, and other continuous cell lines.
3. **Laboratory animals** such as guinea pigs and mice are useful for the isolation of rickettsiae from patients. They may also be propagated in arthropods.

Pathogenesis

Rickettsiae normally enter the body through the bite or feces of an infected arthropod vector.

Human disease caused by rickettsia species is shown in **Table 42.2**.

Table 42.1: The family Rickettsiaceae causing human diseases.

Genus	Species
A. Rickettsia	R. prowazekii
	R. typhi
	R. rickettsii
	R. conorii
	R. australis
	R. sibirica
	R. akari
B. Orientia	O. tsutrugamushi
C. Ehrlichia	E. sennestu
	E. chaffeensis
	E. phagocytophila

Table 42.2: Human disease caused by *Rickettsia* and *Orientia* species.

Group	Species	Diseases	Vector	Vertebrate reservoir	Geographical distribution
Typhus group	R. prowazekii	Epidemic typhus	Louse	Human beings	Worldwide group
		Brill-Zinsser disease	"	Human beings	America, Europe
	R. typhi	Endemic typhus	Rat flea	Rat	Worldwide
	R. felis	Endemic typhus	Cat flea	Opossum	USA
Spotted fever group	R. rickettsii	Rocky Mountain spotted fever	Tick	Rabbit, dog	N. America
	R. siberica	Siberian tick typhus	"	Wild animals cattle	Russia, Mongolia
	R. conori	Boutonneuse fever	"	Dog, rodents	Mediterranean
		S. African tick typhus	"	"	S. Africa
		Kenyan tick typhus	"	Rodents	Kenya
		Indian tick typhus	"	? Rodents	India
	R. australis	Qeensland tick typhus	"	Bush rodents	N. Australia
	R. japonica	Oriental spotted fever	"	?	Japan
	R. akari	Rickettsial pox	Gamasid mite	Mouse	USA, Russia
Scrub typhus group:	O. tsutsugamushi	Scrub typhus	Trombiculid mite	Small rodents	East Asia, Pacific

A. Typhus Fever Group (Table 42.2)

Differences between R. typhi (R. mooseri) and R. prowazekii

Neill-Mooser or the tunica reaction: When male guinea pigs are inoculated intraperitoneally with blood from a case of endemic typhus or with a culture of *R. typhi*, they develop fever and a characteristic scrotal inflammation. The scrotum becomes enlarged and the testes cannot be pushed back into the abdomen because of inflammatory adhesions between the layers of the tunica vaginalis. This is known as the Neill-Mooser or the tunica reaction. The Neill-Mooser reaction is negative with *R. prowazekii*.

B. Spotted Fever Group

They are all transmitted by ticks, **except R. akari**, which is miteborne. Many species have been recognized in this group **(Table 42.2)**.

GENUS *ORIENTIA*

[Scrub typhus (chigger-borne typhus), tsutsugamushi disease]

Scrub typhus is caused by ***Orientia tsutsugamushi***. It was first observed in Japan where it was found to be transmitted by **mites.** The disease was therefore called ***tsutsugamushi*** (from *tsutsuga*, meaning dangerous, and Mushi meaning insect or mite).

Laboratory Diagnosis

Rickettsial diseases may be diagnosed in the laboratory either:
1. Isolation of rickettsiae
2. Direct detection of the organisms and their antigens
3. Serology.
   1. **Isolation of rickettsiae:** Rickettsiae can be isolated in **laboratory animals** such as **mice or guinea-pigs, in embryonated chicken eggs** and in **cell culture.**
      i. **Laboratory animals:** Rickettsiae may be isolated in male guinea pigs or mice from patients in the early phase of the disease. Blood clot ground in skimmed milk or any suitable suspending medium is inoculated intraperitoneally. The animals have to be observed for 3–4 weeks. Their response to rickettsial infection varies. Smears from peritoneum, tunica and spleen of infected animals may be stained by Giemsa or Gimenez methods to demonstrate the rickettsiae.
      ii. **Embryonated chicken egg:** *Rickettsiae* can also be grown in the yolk sac of chick embryo.
      iii. **Cell culture**
   2. **Direct detection of the organisms and their antigens:**
      i. **Detection of rickettsiae in tissue:** By immunofluorescence or immuno-enzyme methods.
      ii. **Polymerase chain reaction (PCR).**
   3. **Serology:** Serological diagnosis may be by the heterophile Weil-Felix (WF) reaction or by specific tests using rickettsial antigens.
      i. **Weil-Felix reaction:** The WF reaction is an agglutination test in which sera are tested for agglutinins to the antigens of certain nonmotile Proteus strains OX 19, OX 2, and OX K.
      Basis of the test: The basis of the test is the sharing of an alkali-stable carbohydrate antigen by some rickettsiae and by certain strains of Proteus, *P. vulgaris* OX 19, OX 2 and *P. mirabilis* OX K.

Table 42.3: Weil–Felix reaction in rickettsial diseases.

Disease	Agglutination pattern with		
	OX19	OX2	OXK
1. Epidemic typhus	+++	+	–
2. Brill-Zinsser disease	Usually negative	or	Weak positive
3. Endemic typhus	+++	+/–	–
4. Tickborne spotted fever	++	++	–
5. Scrub typhus	–	–	+++

Interpretation: Sera from epidemic and endemic typhus agglutinate OX 19 and sometimes OX 2 also. The test is negative or only weakly positive in Brill-Zinsser disease. In tick-borne spotted fever both OX 19 and OX 2 are agglutinated. OX K agglutinins are found only in scrub typhus **(Table 42.3)**.

   ii. **Specific tests using rickettsial antigens:** Serological methods using rickettsial antigens are specific, which include complement fixation test, latex agglutination test, and enzyme immuno assay.

Treatment

Rickettsial infections may be treated with tetracyclines or chloramphenicol.

GENUS *EHRLICHIA*

Ehrlichiae are small gram-negative, obligate intracelluar bacteria, which have an affinity toward blood cells that parasitize mononuclear and granulocytic phagocytes, but not erythrocytes.

Species: *Ehrlichia* species causing human infections:
Ehrlichia sennetsu causes Sennetsu fever;
E. chaffeensis causes monocyclic ehrlichiosis;
E. ewingii and *E. phagocytophila* causes granulocytic ehrlichiosis.

GENUS *COXIELLA*: Q FEVER

Q fever (Q for "query") is caused by *Coxiella burnetii*. *Coxiella burnetii*, is an obligately intracellular prokaryote.

Morphology
Coxiella burnetii is pleomorphic, occurring as small rods 0.2–0.4 μm × 0.4–1.0 μm or as spheres 0.3–0.4 μm in diameter. Generally regarded as gram negative.

Resistance
Coxiella burnetii may be the most infectious of all bacteria. In milk it may survive pasteurization by the holding method. It can survive in dust and aerosols, therefore, can be transmitted as an airborne infection. It can be inactivated by 2% formaldehyde, 5% hydrogen peroxide, and 1% lysol.

Pathogenesis
Coxiella burnetii causes Q fever, as a **zoonosis** solidly established in **domestic livestock**.

Reservoirs of the disease: The primary reservoirs of the disease are wild and domestic ungulates, including cattle, sheep, goats, rabbits, cats, and dogs. It is transmitted among them and to cattle, sheep, and poultry by ixodid ticks. They are shed in the milk of infected animals.

Animal infection: Domestic animals have inapparent infections but may shed large quantities of infectious organisms in their urine, milk, feces, and, especially, their placental products.

Human infection: Human infection may occur occupationally through consumption of infected milk, handling of contaminated wool or hides, soil contaminated by infected animal feces, infected straw, and even to dusty clothing. Incubation period is 2–4 weeks.

Laboratory Diagnosis
1. **Isolation:** Isolation of *C. burnetii* is not generally recommended because of the extremely infectious nature of the organism.
2. **Serology:** Complement fixation test (CFT) or indirect immunofluorescence assay.

Treatment
Tetracyclines are the drugs of choice for acute infections. Rifampin combined with either doxycycline or trimethoprim sulfamethoxazole is used to treat chronic infections.

BARTONELLA

Members of genus *Bartonella* are very small gram-negative bacilli. They grow in close association with the surfaces of vertebrate erythrocytes, including those of humans. They are mainly arthropod-borne. They cause feverish illness in humans involving red blood cells. The genus *Bartonella* contains species such as *B. bacilliformis, B. quintana,* and *B. henselae* which cause Oroya fever, trench fever, and cat-scratch disease in man, respectively.

KEY POINTS

- Genus *Rickettsia*
- **Pathogenesis:** A. typhus fever group—(1) Epidemic typhus; (2) Brill-Zinsser disease; (3) Endemic (Murine) typhus.
- *O. tsutsugamushi* causes scrub typhus.
- **Ehrlichia:** These tick-borne bacteria cause three human infections.
- *Coxiella burnetii causes* Q fever, which is a worldwide **zoonosis**.
- *Bartonella*: The genus *Bartonella* contains *B. bacilliformis, B. quintana* and *B. henselae* which cause Oroya fever, trench fever and cat-scratch disease in man respectively.

IMPORTANT QUESTIONS

1. Write short notes on:
   a. Neil-Mooser reaction or Tunica reaction
   b. *Coxiella burnetii* or Q fever
   c. Weil-Felix reaction
2. Discuss laboratory diagnosis of rickettsial infections.

MULTIPLE CHOICE QUESTIONS

1. The causative agent of epidemic typhus is:
   a. *Rickettsia prowazekii*
   b. *Rickettsia rickettsii*
   c. *Coxiella burnetii*
   d. *Rickettsia akari*
2. Human body louse is responsible for transmission of which of the following diseases?
   a. Epidemic typhus
   b. Murine typhus
   c. Rickettsial pox
   d. Q fever
3. The rickettsial disease transmitted by ixodid ticks is:
   a. Rickettsial pox
   b. Rocky Mountain spotted fever
   c. Trench fever
   d. Scrub typhus
4. Weil-Felix reaction is positive in all the following diseases, *except*:
   a. Epidemic typhus
   b. Endemic typhus
   c. Brill-Zinsser's disease
   d. Q fever
5. Human infections due to *Coxiella* can be acquired by:
   a. Consumption of infected milk
   b. Handling of infected wool or hides
   c. Soil contaminated with feces of infected animals
   d. All of the above
6. Oroya fever is caused by:
   a. *Capnocytophaga ochracea*
   b. *Legionella pneumophilia*
   c. *Streptobacillus moniliformis*
   d. *Bartonella bacilliformis*

ANSWERS

1. a 2. a 3. b 4. d
5. d 6. d

CHAPTER 43: Chlamydia and Chlamydophila

LEARNING OBJECTIVES

After reading and studying this chapter, you should be able to:
- Describe serotypes of various chlamydiae and diseases produced by them.
- Associate each of the major diseases with the three most important human species of *Chlamydia* and *Chlamydophila*.
- Discuss morphology and the unique growth cycle of *Chlamydia*, describing elementary (EB) and reticulate (RB) bodies.
- Discuss laboratory diagnosis of chlamydial infections.
- Describe the following: TRIC agents, inclusion conjunctivitis, lymphogranuloma venereum (LGV), Frei's test.

INTRODUCTION

Chlamydiaceae are a family of obligate intracellular bacterial parasites, small, nonmotile, and gram negative.

Classification

Genus *Chlamydia* is in the order Chlamydiales and the family Chlamydiaceae. The proposed taxonomic classification for the family Chlamydiaceae consists of two genera: (1) *Chlamydia* to include *C. trachomatis* and (2) *Chlamydophila* to include *C. pneumoniae*, *C. psittaci*, and *C. pecorum* (**Table 43.1**).

CHLAMYDIA

Morphology

Chlamydiae are small, nonmotile bacteria. There are two morphologically distinct forms of chlamydiae: Elementary body (EB) and reticulate body (RB).

1. **Elementary body:** It is a spherical particle, 200-300 nm in diameter. The EB is the extracellular, infective form.
2. **Reticulate bod:** The RB is the intracellular growing and replicative form, 500-1,000 nm in size (larger than the EB).

Growth Cycle

The *Chlamydia* growth cycle is initiated by the attachment of an infectious EB to the surface of a susceptible epithelial cell (**Fig. 43.1**). The EB undergoes transformation to the large RB, which begins to divide by binary fission and are converted to EBs. The developing chlamydial microcolony within the host cell is called the *inclusion body.* The mature inclusion body contains 100-500 EBs, which are ultimately released from the host cell and may infect new cells and cycle is repeated (**Fig. 43.1**).

Laboratory Propagation

Chlamydiae can be propagated in the mouse, chick embryo, or in cell culture. The presence of chlamydial inclusions is determined by

Table 43.1: Revised classification of the family Chlamydiaceae.

Genus Chlamydia	Genus Chlamydophila
C. trachomatis	C. pneumoniae
	C. psittaci
	C. pecorum

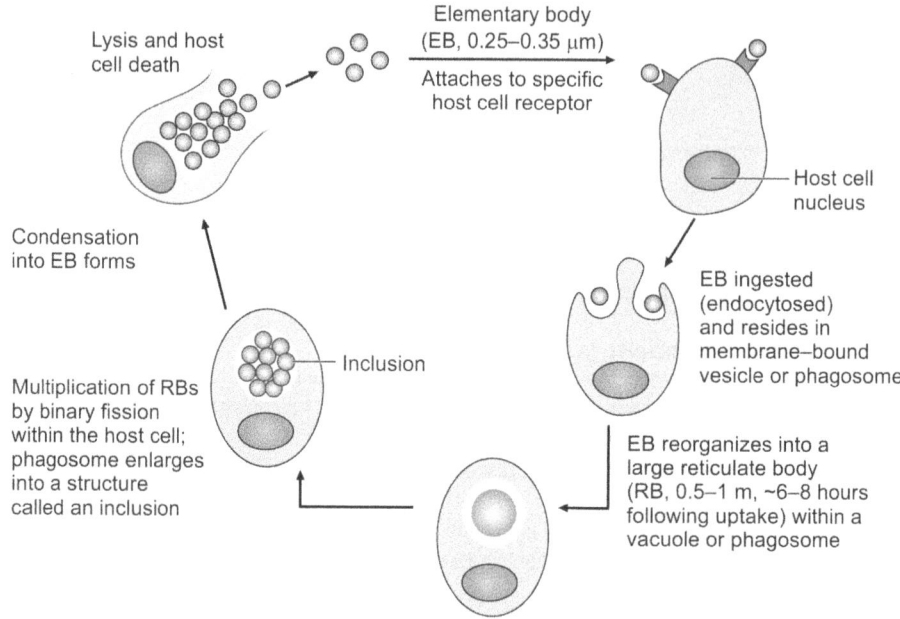

Fig. 43.1: The *Chlamydia* growth cycle.

microscopy in conjunction with a suitable staining method, preferably fluorescence microscopy with labeled monoclonal antibody.

Chlamydia trachomatis: *Chlamydia trachomatis* has been divided into three biovars, which cause trachoma, inclusion conjunctivitis (the so-called **TRIC agents**) and lymphogranuloma venereum (LGV). Both the trachoma and the LGV biovars can be divided into serotypes **(Table 43.2)**.

Chlamydia psittaci: The serological classification of *C. psittaci* is complex.

Chlamydia pneumonia: *C. pneumoniae* has not been subclassified yet **(Table 43.2)**.

CHLAMYDIA TRACHOMATIS

Chlamydia trachomatis has been divided into two biovars—those causing *trachoma, inclusion conjunctivitis* (the so-called **TRIC agents**) and oculogenital infection **(Table 43.2)**.
1. **Trachoma**
2. **Inclusion conjunctivitis:**
   - Inclusion blennorhea
   - Adult inclusion conjunctivitis

Table 43.2: Human diseases caused by Chlamydiae.

Species	Serotype*	Disease
C. trachomatis	A, B, Ba, C	Endemic blinding trachoma
C. trachomatis	D, E, F, G, H, I, J, K	Inclusion conjunctivities (neonatal and adult)
		Genital chlamydiasis
		Infant pneumonia
C. trachomatis	L1, L2, L3	Lymphogranuloma venereum
C. psittaci	Many serotypes	Psittacosis
C. pneumoniae	Only one serotype	Acute respiratory disease

*Predominant types associated with the disease

3. **Infant pneumonia**
4. **Genital infections:** *C. trachomatis* infections of the genital tract are of two types and are sexually transmitted:
   i. Those caused by the **oculogenital serotypes D through K** collectively referred to as 'genital chlamydiasis'
   ii. LGV caused by serotypes L1, L2, and L3.

Lymphogranuloma venereum: **Lymphogranuloma inguinale, climatic bubo, tropical bubo**, and **esthiomene** are synonyms of this sexually transmissible disease. It characterized by suppurative inguinal adenitis. Humans are the sole natural hosts of this infection caused by the LGV biovar of *C. trachomatis,* L1, L2, and L3 most commonly L2 **(Table 43.2)**.

CHLAMYDOPHILA PSITTACI

Chlamydophila psittaci is the cause of psittacosis *(psittacos* means parrot) among psittacine birds, also known as *ornithosis* (derived from the Greek word *ornithos* for "bird") or *parrot fever.*

Chlamydophila pneumoniae

Chlamydophila pneumoniae is recognized as a significant community acquired respiratory pathogen, has been implicated in other chronic afflictions such as asthma and cardiovascular diseases.

Laboratory Diagnosis of *Chlamydia* Infections

The laboratory diagnosis of *Chlamydia* infections can be accomplished by various approaches: (1) microscopic demonstration of inclusion or EBs, (2) isolation of the organisms, (3) demonstration of chlamydial antigen and (4) detection of specific antibodies (5) Skin test-hypersensitivity against these bacteria.

The specimens collected are conjunctival scrapings, sputum, throat swab, bubo pus, genital swabs and blood.

1. **Demonstration of inclusion or elementary bodies:** Smears may be prepared from conjunctival scrapings or bubo pus and stained by Giemsa, Castaneda, Machiavello or Gimenez stains to demonstrate characteristic inclusion bodies under light microscope. *Chlamydia* is gram negative.
   Glycogen-containing inclusions of *C. trachomatis* can be stained with Lugol's iodine. Immunofluresence (IF) can identify not only inclusions but also extracellular elementary bodies.
2. **Isolation of the organisms:** Traditionally the isolation of *Chlamydia* has been accomplished by the inoculation of infected material into either **embryonated eggs, experimental animals**, or selected **tissue culture cell lines**.
3. **Demonstration of chlamydial antigen**
   a. **Immunofluresence**
   b. **ELISA**
   c. **Molecular methods**
   Like **DNA probes** and amplification techniques (**polymerase chain reaction, ligase chain reaction**).
4. **Detection of specific antibodies or hypersensitivity response:** The diagnosis of chlamydial infections can be accomplished by either the group-specific **complement-fixation (CF) test** or type-specific **micro immunofluorescence (micro-IF) technique.**
5. **Skin test:** The **Frei test** is an intradermal skin test that detects a delayed hypersensitivity response to chlamydial antigen has been given up.

KEY POINTS

- The family Chlamydiaceae has been divided into two genera, ***Chlamydia*** and ***Chlamydophila***:
  1. *Chlamydia* to include *C. trachomatis*
  2. *Chlamydophila* to include *C. pneumoniae, C. psittaci,* and *C. pecorum.*
- **Chlamydia trachomatis infections:** Two human biovars—trachoma (with 15 serovars) and lymphogranuloma venereum (LGV; 4 serovars).
- *C. psittaci*—is the cause of psittacosis.
- *C. pneumoniae* is community acquired respiratory pathogen.

IMPORTANT QUESTIONS

1. Discuss laboratory diagnosis of chlamydial infections.
2. Write short notes on:
   a. TRIC agents
   b. Inclusion conjunctivitis

MULTIPLE CHOICE QUESTIONS

1. Trachoma is caused by *C. trachomatis* serotypes:
    a. A, B, Ba, C
    b. D-K
    c. Ll-L3
    d. All the serovars
2. Lymphogranuloma venereum (LGV) is caused by serotypes:
    a. A, B, Ba, C
    b. D-K
    c. L1, L2, and L3
    d. None of the above
3. Which of the following serotypes of *Chlamydia* are responsible for inclusion conjunctivitis?
    a. A, B, Ba, C
    b. D-K
    c. L1-L3
    d. None of the above

ANSWERS

1. a   2. c   3. b

Virology

SECTION OUTLINE
44. General Properties of Viruses
45. Laboratory Diagnosis, Prophylaxis and Chemotherapy of Viral Diseases
46. DNA Viruses
47. Hepatitis Viruses
48. RNA Viruses
49. Retroviruses: Human Immunodeficiency Virus

CHAPTER 44: General Properties of Viruses

LEARNING OBJECTIVES

After reading and studying this chapter, you should be able to:
- Describe size, shape, and symmetry of viruses.
- Describe cultivation of viruses.
- List various cell cultures.
- Discuss detection of virus growth in cell cultures.
- List DNA and RNA viruses.
- Describe prions and viroids.

INTRODUCTION

Viruses are the smallest known infective agents and are perhaps the simplest form of life known. Viruses do not possess a cellular organization and they do not fall strictly into the category of unicellular microorganisms.

MAIN PROPERTIES OF VIRUSES

1. Viruses do not have a cellular organization.
2. They contain only one type of nucleic acid, either DNA or RNA but never both.
3. They are obligate intracellular parasites.
4. They lack the enzymes necessary for protein and nucleic acid synthesis.
5. They multiply by a complex process and not by binary fission.
6. They are unaffected by antibacterial antibiotics.

The major differences between viruses and microorganisms are shown in **Table 44.1**.

MORPHOLOGY OF VIRUSES

Size

Viruses are much smaller than bacteria. The extracellular infectious virus particle is called the **virion.** Viruses vary widely in size from 20 to 300 nm. The largest among them is pox virus (300 nm). The smallest viruses are the parvovirus (about 20 nm).

Table 44.1: Properties of prokaryotes and viruses—Ananthnarayan.

	Cellular organization	Growth on inanimate media	Binary fission	Both DNA and RNA	Ribosomes	Sensitivity to antibacterial antibiotics	Sensitivity to interferon
Bacteria	+	+	+	+	+	+	–
Mycoplasmas	+	+	+	+	+	+	–
Rickettsiae	+	+	+	+	+	+	–
Chlamydiae	+	–	+	+	+	+	+
Viruses	–	–	–	–	–	–	+

Shape of the Virus

The overall shape of the virus particle varies in different groups of viruses. Poxviruses are brick-shaped, rabies virus is bullet-shaped.

STRUCTURE AND CHEMICAL COMPOSITION OF THE VIRUSES

Viral Capsid

Viruses consist of nucleic acid core surrounded by a protein coat called **capsid**. The capsid with the enclosed nucleic acid is known as **nucleocapsid**. The capsid is composed of a large number of **capsomers,** which form its morphological units. The chemical units of the capsid are polypeptide molecules, which are arranged symmetrically to form molecules to form an impenetrable shell around the nucleic acid core **(Figs. 44.1A and B)**.

Virus Symmetry (Fig. 44.2)

Viral architecture can be grouped into three types based on the arrangement of morphologic subunits: (1) Icosahedral symmetry, (2) helical symmetry, and (3) complex structures.

Viral Envelope

Virions may be **enveloped** or **nonenveloped (naked)**.

Viral Nucleic Acids

Viruses contain a single kind of nucleic acid—either DNA or RNA—that encodes the genetic information necessary for replication of the virus.

CULTIVATION OF VIRUSES

Because viruses are obligating intracellular parasites, their growth requires susceptible host cells capable of replicating them. They cannot be grown on any inanimate culture medium. Three methods are employed for the cultivation of viruses:

A. Animal inoculation
B. Embyronated eggs
C. Cell culture

A. Animal Inoculation

1. **Monkeys:** Monkeys were used for the isolation of the poliovirus.
2. **Mice: Infant (suckling) mice** are very susceptible to coxsackie and arboviruses, many of which do not grow in any other system. The growth of the virus in inoculated animals may be indicated by death, disease or visible lesions.

B. Embyronated Eggs

The embryonated eggs (8–11 days old) are inoculated by several routes for the cultivation of

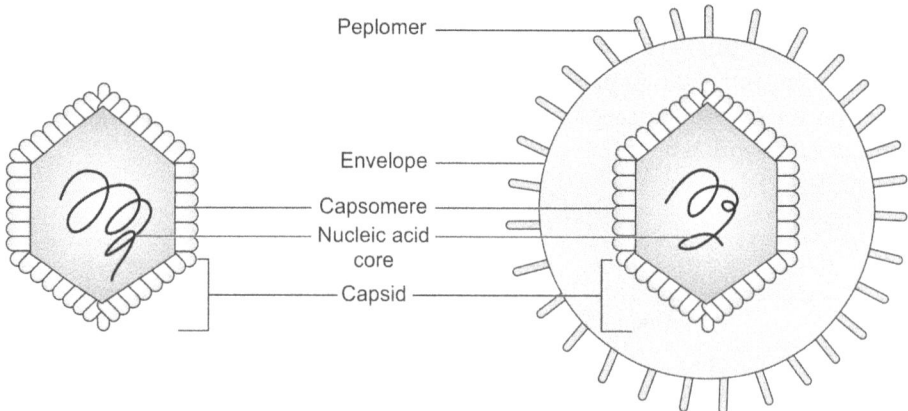

A. Naked icosahedron   B. Enveloped icosahedron

Figs. 44.1A and B: Schematic diagram illustrating the components of the complete virus particle (the virion). (A) Naked icosahedral virus, consisting of an inner core of nucleic acid enclosed by a capsid, which is made of capsomers; (B) Enveloped virus-differ from A in possessing envelope.

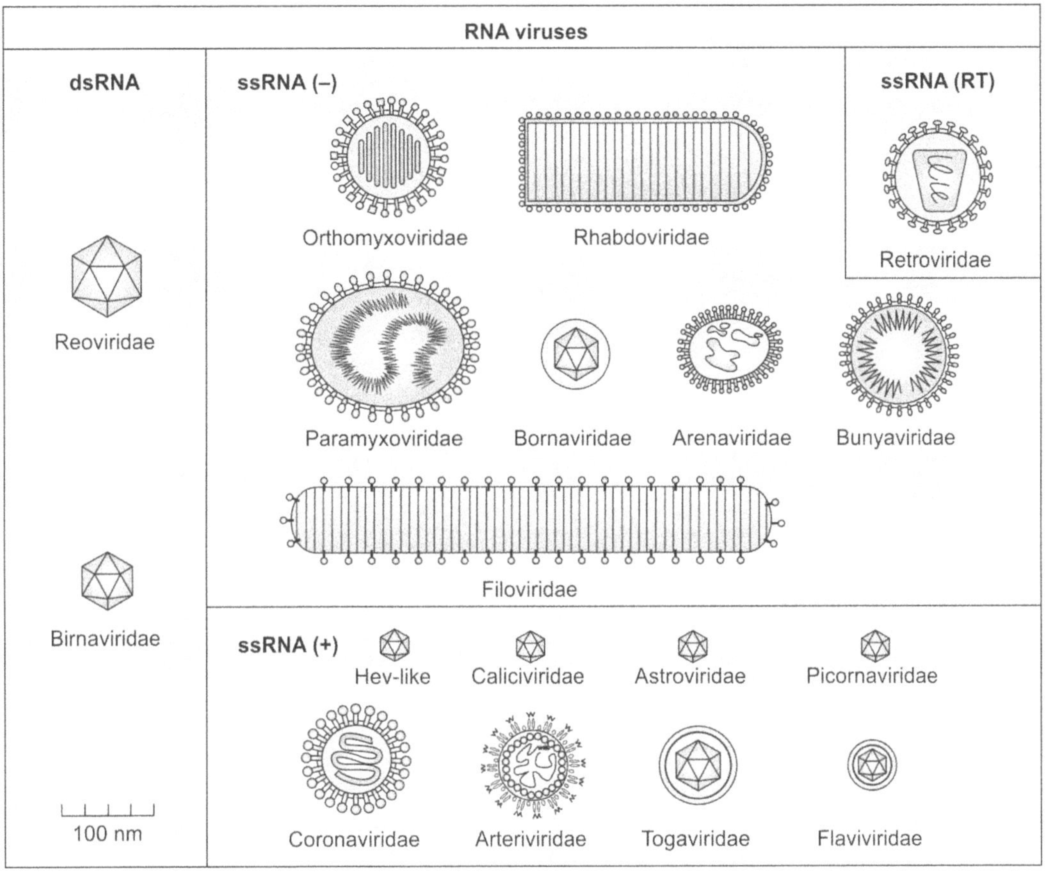

Chapter 44: General Properties of Viruses

Fig. 44.2: Shapes and relative sizes of viruses.

viruses, such as chorioallantoic membrane (CAM), allantoic cavity, amniotic cavity, and yolk sac (**Fig. 44.3**). After inoculated, eggs incubated for 2–9 days.

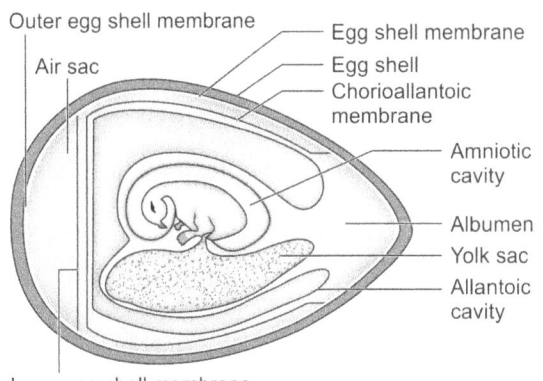

Fig. 44.3: Cross-section of an embryonated hen's egg.

1. **Chorioallantoic membrane:** Inoculation on the CAM produces visible lesions (**pocks**).
2. **Allantoic cavity:** Allantoic inoculation is employed for growing the influenza virus for vaccine production.
3. **Amniotic sac:** Inoculation into the amniotic sac is employed for the primary isolation of the influenza virus.
4. **Yolk sac:** Yolk sac inoculation is used for the cultivation of some viruses, **Chlamydiae, Coxiella burnetii,** and rickettsiae.

C. Cell cultures

Cell cultures are classified into three types (**Table 44.2**).

1. **Primary cell cultures:** These are normal cells freshly taken from the body and cultured. They are capable of only limited growth

Table 44.2: Some cell cultures in common use.

Type	Name of the cell culture
A. Primary cell cultures	1. Rhesus monkey kidney cell culture 2. Human amnion cell culture 3. Chick embryo fibroblast cell culture
B. Diploid cell strains	1. WI-38 (Human embryonic lung cell strain) 2. HL-8 (Rhesus embryo cell strain)
C. Continuous cell lines	1. HeLa (Human carcinoma of cervix cell line) 2. HEP-2 (Human epithelioma of larynx cell line) 3. KB (Human carcinoma of nasopharynx cell line) 4. McCoy (Human synovial carcinoma cell line) 5. Detroit-6 (Sternal marrow cell line) 6. Chang C/I/L/K (Human conjunctiva (C) Intestine (I), Liver (L) and Kidney (K) cell lines) 7. Vero (Vervet monkey kidney cell line) 8. BHK-21 (Baby hamster kidney cell line)

in culture (5–10 passages) and cannot be maintained in serial culture.

2. **Diploid (semicontinuous) cell strains:** These are cells of a single type that retain the original diploid chromosome number and karyotype during serial subcultivation for a limited number of times. They undergo 'senescence' after about fifty serial passages.
3. **Continuous cell lines:** These are cells of a single type, usually derived from cancer cells that are capable of continuous serial cultivation indefinitely. Standard cell lines derived from human cancers, such as HeLa, Hep-2, and KB cell lines have been used in laboratories throughout the world for many years.

DETECTION OF VIRUS GROWTH IN CELL CULTURE

Virus growth in cell cultures can be detected by the following methods:
1. **Cytopathic effect**
2. **Metabolic inhibition**
3. **Hemadsorption**
4. **Interference**
5. **Transformation**
6. **Immunofluorescence**
7. **Detection of virus-specific nucleic acid,** such as polymerase chain (PCR)
8. **Detection of enzymes**
9. **Electron microscopy**

CLASSIFICATION OF VIRUSES

Viruses are classified into two main divisions DNA and RNA viruses depending on the type of nucleic acid they possess: **deoxyriboviruses** are those containing DNA and **riboviruses** are those containing RNA and further classification is based on other properties, such as the strandedness of nucleic acid, symmetry of nucleocapsid, presence of envelope, size and shape of virion, and number of capsomers **(Fig. 44.2)**.

Viroids

The term "viroid" describes a new class of subviral agents characterized by the apparent absence of an extracellular dormant phase (virion) and by a genome much smaller than those of known viruses. They are small infectious agents that cause diseases of plants. None have been demonstrated to exist in animals or humans.

Prions

Prions (proteinaceous infectious particles) are infectious particles composed solely of protein with no detectable nucleic acid. Prion diseases, called "transmissible spongiform encephalopathies", include scrapie in sheep, mad cow disease in cattle, and kuru and Creutzfeldt–Jakob disease in humans. Unlike viruses, the agents are resistant to a wide range of chemical and physical treatments, such as formaldehyde, ultraviolet radiation, and heat to 80°C.

KEY POINTS

- The viruses are obligate intracellular parasites.
- Three methods are employed for cultivation of viruses namely *animal inoculation, embryonated egg inoculation,* and *tissue culture.*

IMPORTANT QUESTIONS

1. Give an account of cultivation of viruses.
2. Write short notes on:
   a. Cell cultures
   b. Detection of virus growth in cell cultures
   c. Prions

MULTIPLE CHOICE QUESTIONS

1. The viruses show all the following features, *except*:
   a. They are filterable agents
   b. They are obligate intracellular parasites
   c. They contain either DNA or RNA, but not both
   d. They multiply inside the living cells by using their synthesizing machinery
2. The symmetry of poxviruses is:
   a. Icosahedral
   b. Helical
   c. Complex
   d. None of the above
3. Which of the following is the largest virus?
   a. Smallpox virus
   b. Adenovirus
   c. Coronavirus
   d. Parvovirus
4. Which of the following viruses is/are relatively thermostable?
   a. Hepatitis A virus
   b. Human immunodeficiency virus
   c. Rubella virus
   d. All of the above
5. All the following are the examples of enveloped viruses, *except*:
   a. Polio virus
   b. Rubivirus
   c. Adenovirus
   d. Herpesvirus
6. Which of the following disinfectants is/are effective against viruses?
   a. Hypochlorite
   b. Formaldehyde
   c. Hydrogen peroxide
   d. All of the above
7. Suckling mice are used for the isolation of:
   a. Poxviruses
   b. Herpesviruses
   c. Arboviruses
   d. All of the above
8. All are continuous cell lines for growing viruses, *except*:
   a. HeLa
   b. HEp-2
   c. KB
   d. Rhesus monkey kidney cell culture
9. The following routes of inoculating embryonated hen's egg is/are used for cultivation of viruses:
   a. Chorioallantoic membrane
   b. Amniotic cavity
   c. Allantoic cavity
   d. All of the above
10. Which of the following agents is/are prions?
    a. Agent causing kuru
    b. Agent causing scrapie
    c. Agent causing Creutzfeldt–Jakob disease
    d. All of the above

ANSWERS

1. d   2. c   3. d   4. a
5. b   6. d   7. c   8. d
9. d   10. d

Laboratory Diagnosis, Prophylaxis, and Chemotherapy of Viral Diseases

LEARNING OBJECTIVES

After reading and studying this chapter, you should be able to:
- Describe laboratory diagnosis of viral infections.
- Describe immunoprophylaxis of viral diseases.

LABORATORY DIAGNOSIS OF VIRAL INFECTIONS

Specimens: The appropriate specimens should be collected from patients, preserved, and transported to the laboratory in the proper manner.

Laboratory diagnosis of viral infections can be carried out by the following methods:

A. **Cytological examination:** The cytologic examination of specimens provides a rapid initial diagnosis for viral infections.

B. **Direct detection of virus:**
 1. **Electron microscopy (EM):** Viruses that are difficult to culture can be recognized by EM. Clinical applications of EM include detection of rotavirus and hepatitis A virus in fecal specimens.
 2. **Immunoelectron microscopy:** This method is useful for the detection of enteric viruses, such as rotavirus.
 3. **Fluorescence microscopy**
 4. **Light microscopy:** Demonstration of the inclusion body is a routine diagnostic method. Rabies may be detected through the finding of Negri bodies (rabies virus inclusions) in brain cells of animals.

C. **Virus isolation:** The "gold standard" for proving a viral etiology of a syndrome is the recovery and growth of the infecting agent. In general the methods used for isolation consist of inoculation into **animals, eggs, or tissue culture,** after the specimen is processed to remove bacterial contaminants. The isolates are identified by neutralization or other suitable serological procedures.

D. **Detection of viral proteins**

E. **Detection of viral genetic material** by DNA probes and polymerase chain reaction (PCR).

F. **Serological diagnosis:** The demonstration of a rise in titer of antibodies to a virus during the course of a disease is strong evidence that it is the etiological agent. For this, it is essential to examine paired sera, the 'acute' sample collected early in the course of the disease and the "convalescent" sample collected 10–14 days later. Examination of a single sample of serum for antibodies may not be meaningful except when IgM specific tests are done generally indicates a recent primary infection. The serological techniques employed are neutralization, complement fixation, ELISA, hemagglutination inhibition tests, indirect fluorescent antibody test, and latex agglutination test.

IMMUNOPROPHYLAXIS OF VIRAL DISEASES

A. Active immunization
B. Passive immunization

Chapter 45: Laboratory Diagnosis, Prophylaxis, and Chemotherapy of Viral Diseases

Table 45.1: Viral vaccines.
1. **Live-virus vaccines**
    - Smallpox
    - Yellow fever
    - Poliomyelitis (Sabin type)
    - Measles
    - Mumps
    - Rubella
    - Varicella
2. **Inactivated virus vaccines**
    - Poliomyelitis (Salk type)
    - Rabies
    - Influenza
    - Hepatitis A
    - Hepatitis B
    - Japanese encephalitis
3. **Anti-idiotype and DNA vaccines**

A. Active Immunization

The World Health Organization (WHO) is now determined on global eradication of poliomyelitis. Viral vaccines are of three types **(Table 45.1)**.

B. Passive Immunization

Passive immunization with human gamma globulin, convalescent serum, or specific immune globulin gives temporary protection against many viral diseases.

CHEMOPROPHYLAXIS AND CHEMOTHERAPY OF VIRUS DISEASES

Because viruses are obligate intracellular parasites, antiviral agents must be capable of selectively inhibiting viral functions without damaging the host, making the development of such drugs very difficult.

The antiviral compounds include nucleoside analogues, synthetic oligonucleotides, oligosaccharides, and also natural products of plants and some inorganic and organic compounds.

Available antiviral agents can be considered under the various categories.

KEY POINTS

- Laboratory diagnosis of viral infections can be carried out by the methods, such as:
    - I. Direct detection of virus and its components;
    - II. Virus isolation;
    - III. Detection of specific antibodies; and
    - IV. Cytological examination.
- Immunoprophylaxis of viral diseases is by active and passive immunization.

IMPORTANT QUESTIONS

1. Discuss laboratory diagnosis of viral infections.
2. Discuss viral vaccines.

MULTIPLE CHOICE QUESTIONS

1. Electron microscopy can be used for the laboratory diagnosis of:
    a. Rotavirus infections
    b. Hepatitis A virus infections
    c. Adenovirus infections
    d. All of the above
2. Which of the following vaccines is/are live?
    a. Measles vaccine
    b. Mumps vaccine
    c. Rubella vaccine
    d. All of the above

ANSWERS

1. d   2. d

CHAPTER 46

DNA Viruses

LEARNING OBJECTIVES

After reading and studying this chapter, you should be able to:
- Describe morphology of Herpes virus.
- Classify of human herpes viruses.
- Describe infections caused by *Herpes simplex* virus type 1 and *Herpes simplex* virus type 2.
- Describe the following: Varicella-zoster virus; Cytomegalovirus.
- Discuss clinical manifestations of Epstein–Barr virus (EBV).
- Describe Paul-Bunnell test.
- Describe diseases associated with adenovirus.

INTRODUCTION

DNA Viruses

1. **Poxviridae family:** Smallpox virus, vaccinia virus.
2. **Herpesviridae family:** Herpes simplex types 1 and 2 (oral and genital lesions), varicella-zoster virus, cytomegalovirus (CMV), Epstein–Barr virus (EBV), human herpes viruses 6 and 7, and human herpes virus 8.
3. **Adenoviridae family:** Adenovirus
4. **Papovaviridae family:** JC virus, BK virus, SV40, papillomavirus
5. **Parvoviridae family:** Three genera have been described: *Parvovirus, Adenosatellovirus* and *Densovirus*.
6. **Hepadnaviridae family:** Hepatitis type B virus.

POXVIRUSES

Introduction

Poxviruses belong to family *Poxviridae* and cause a number of human diseases.

Morphology

The orthopoxviruses are brick-shaped. They measure about 230 × 270 nm and when suitably stained can just be seen with an ordinary light microscope.

Cultivation and Host Range

Virus isolation is carried out by inoculation of vesicular fluid onto the chorioallantoic membrane (CAM) of chick embryos, in tissue cultures of monkey kidney, HeLa, and chick embryo cells.

Comparison of Vaccinia and Variola Viruses

The variola *virus is the causative agent of smallpox*. Smallpox used to occur in two distinct clinical varieties:

1. **Variola major or classical smallpox:** The florid, highly fatal disease typically seen in Asia.
   The global eradication of smallpox, achieved after 10 years of concerted campaigns under the auspices of the WHO. Naturally occurring smallpox came to an end in 1977. On 8 May, 1980, the WHO formally announced the global eradication of smallpox.

2. **Variola minor or alastrim:** The mild, nonfatal disease (alastrim) typically seen in Latin America.

Vaccinia Virus

Vaccinia virus is the agent used for smallpox vaccination. Vaccinia virus is unique in that it is an 'artificial virus' and does not occur in nature as such.

Other Poxvirus Diseases

1. **Cowpox:** Cowpox lesions are seen on the udder and teats of cows and may be transmitted to humans during milking.
2. **Monkeypox:** Human-to-human transmission is more frequent than was at first thought, but control by vaccination is not difficult.
3. **Buffalopox:** Buffalopox was identified in cattle in India in 1934 and was considered an outbreak of vaccinia in them.
4. **Milker's node (paravaccinia):** Milker's node (paravaccinia) is a trivial occupational disease that humans get by milking infected cows.
5. **Orf (contagious pustular dermatitis or sore mouth):** It is an occupational disease of sheep handlers.
6. **Tanapox:** It appears to be spread by insect bites. Monkeys are the only animals susceptible. There is usually only one vesicular lesion.
7. **Molluscum contagiosum:** Molluscum contagiosum is a benign epidermal tumor that occurs only in humans. The disease is of two types: It is spread by direct and indirect contact (e.g., by barbers, common use of towels, swimming pools). The second type is common among young adults and is sexually transmitted.

HERPES VIRUSES

Introduction

The herpes virus family contains over a hundred species of enveloped DNA viruses that affect humans and animals.

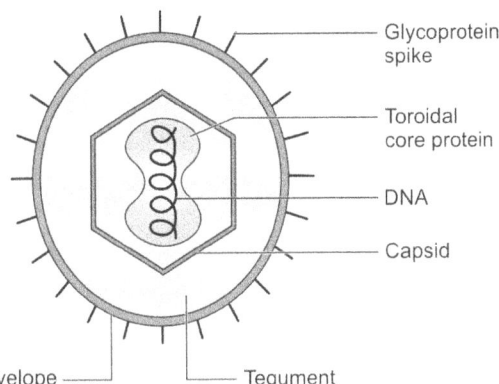

Fig. 46.1: Typical structure of the herpes viruses.

Structure

The herpesvirus capsid is icosahedral, composed of 162 capsomers, and enclosing the core containing the linear double-stranded DNA genome. The nucleocapsid is surrounded by the **lipid envelope**. Between the envelope and the capsid is an amorphous structure called the **tegument**, containing several proteins **(Fig. 46.1).**

Classification

The family Herpesviridae is divided into three subfamilies based on biological, physical, and genetic properties **(Table 46.1)**.

Herpes virus Infections in Humans

Herpes Simplex Virus

Herpes simplex virus (HSV) was the first human herpes virus to be recognized. The name herpes is derived from a Greek word meaning "to creep."

Pathogenesis

Herpes simplex virus generally causes disease at the site of infection. HSV-1 is usually associated with infections **above the waist,** and HSV-2 with infections **below the waist,** consistent with the means of spread for these viruses.

Clinical Features

1. **Cutaneous infections:**
   i. The most common site is the face.
   ii. Napkin rash

Table 46.1: Classification of human herpes viruses.

Subfamily	Virus	Primary target cell	Site of latency	Means of spread
A. Alpha herpes viriane				
Human herpesvirus 1	Herpes simplex type 1	Mucoepithelial cells	Neuron	Close contact
Human herpesvirus 2	Herpes simplex type 2	Mucoepithelial cells	Neuron	Close contact (sexually transmitted disease)
Human herpesvirus 3	Varicella-zoster virus	Mucoepithelial cells	Neuron	Respiratory and close contact
B. Beta herpesvirinae				
Human herpesvirus 5	Cytomegalovirus	Monocyte, lymphocyte, and epithelial cells	Monocyte, lymphocyte, and ?	Close contact, tansfusions, tissue transplant, and congenital
Human herpesvirus 6	Herpes lymphotropic virus	T cells and ?	T cells and ?	Respiratory and close contact?
Human herpesvirus 7	Human herpesvirus 7	T cells and ?	T cells and ?	?
C. Gamma herpes virinae				
Human herpesvirus 4	Epstein–Barr virus	B cells and epithelial cells	B cell	Saliva (kissing disease)
Human herpesvirus 8	Kaposi's sarcoma–related virus	Lymphocyte and other cells	?	Close contact (sexual), saliva

? indicates that other cells may also be primary target or the site of latency

   iii. 'Fever blister' or herpes febrilis
   iv. Herpetic whitlow—is an infection of the finger.
   v. Herpes gladiatorum
   vi. Eczema herpeticum
2. **Oral infection:** Acute gingivostomatitis, herpetic stomatitis, pharyngitis, tonsillitis, and localized lymphadenopathy.
3. **Ophthalmic:** Severe keratoconjunctivitis, follicular conjunctivitis with vesicle formation on the lids, dendritic keratitis or corneal ulcers or as vesicles on the eyelids, corneal scarring, and impairment of vision.
4. **Nervous system:**
   i. HSV encephalitis
   ii. Sporadic encephalitis
   iii. HSV meningitis
   iv. Sacral autonomic dysfunction
   v. Rarely transverse myelitis or the Guillain-Barre syndrome and Bell's palsy
5. **Visceral:**
   i. HSV esophagitis
   ii. Tracheobronchitis and pneumonitis
   iii. Hepatitis
   iv. Erythema multiforme
   v. Disseminated HSV infection
6. **Genital infections:** Genital disease is usually caused by HSV-2 genital herpetic ulcers.
   i. In male patients: The lesions typically develop on the glans or shaft of the penis and occasionally in the urethra.
   ii. In female patients: The lesions may be seen on the vulva, vagina, cervix, perianal area, or inner thigh.
   iii. Inguinal lymphadenopathy: In patients of both sexes.
   iv. Herpetic proctitis: Homosexuals
   v. Association between HSV-2 and carcinoma of the cervix uteri-has not been established.
7. **Neonatal herpes:** Congenital malformations
8. **Infections in immunocompromised hosts**

Laboratory Diagnosis

A. **Specimens:** Specimens include vesicle fluid, skin swab, saliva, corneal scrapings, brain biopsy, and CSF according to the site of involvement.

B. **Microscopy:**
   i. *Tzanck smear:* Characteristic cytopathologic effects (CPEs) can be identified in a **Tzanck smear** which is a scraping of the base of a lesion and stained with toluidine blue). Multinucleated giant cells with faceted nuclei and homogeneously stained 'ground glass' chromatin (Tzanck cells) constitute a positive smears. Cowdry type A intranuclear inclusion bodies may be seen in Giemsa stained smear.
   ii. *Electron microscopy*
   iii. *Fluorescent antibody technique:* The herpes virus antigen may be demonstrated in smears or sections from lesions by the fluorescent antibody technique.
C. **Virus isolation:** Human diploid fibroblasts are preferred.
D. **Serology:** Antibodies may be demonstrated by ELISA, neutralization, or complement fixation tests.
E. **Polymerase chain reaction (PCR)**

Treatment

Idoxuridine used topically in eye and skin infections. **Acyclovir** is currently the standard therapy. **Valaciclovir and famciclovir** are more effective oral agents.

VARICELLA-ZOSTER VIRUS

Varicella-zoster virus (VZV) causes chickenpox (varicella) and, with recurrence, causes **herpes zoster, or shingles**. Both diseases are caused by the same virus. Thus, chickenpox is 'caught' but not zoster.

Varicella (Chickenpox)

Varicella (chickenpox) is one of the mildest highly communicable and most common of childhood infections. The portal of entry of the virus is the respiratory tract or conjunctiva. After an incubation period of about two weeks, the skin lesions begin to appear macule, papule, vesicle, pustule and scab. The rash is characteristically centripetal in distribution.

Herpes Zoster (Shingles, Zona)

While varicella is typically a disease of childhood, herpes zoster is one of old age. Herpes-zoster usually occurs in persons who had chickenpox several years earlier. The virus remains latent in the sensory ganglia. When the immunity has fallen, the virus may be reactivated, and, travel along the sensory nerve to produce zoster lesions on the area of the skin or mucosa supplied by it. The attack is heralded by hyperesthesia and sometimes by pain in the affected area, followed within a day or so by a crop of typical herpetic vesicles, which eventually crust over and heal in the usual way.

Immunity

Varicella and zoster viruses are identical, the two diseases being the result of differing host responses. Previous infection with varicella is believed to confer lifelong immunity to varicella. Zoster occurs in the presence of neutralizing antibody to varicella. Increase in varicella antibody titer may occur in persons with HSV infections. **The development of varicella-zoster virus-specific cell-mediated immunity is important in recovery from both varicella and zoster.**

Laboratory Diagnosis

Diagnosis is usually clinical.

1. **Microscopy:** Multinucleated giant cells and **type A intranuclear inclusion bodies** may be seen in smears prepared by scraping the base of the early vesicles (Tzanck smear) and stained with toluidine blue, Giemsa, or Papanicolaou stain. Direct examination by electron microscopy will reveal herpes particles.
2. **Virus isolation:** Virus isolation can be attempted by inoculating human amnion, human fibroblast, HeLa, or Vero cells.
3. **Virus antigen:** Can be detected by **immunofluorescence, counterimmunoelectrophoresis, ELISA, and PCR**.
4. **Serological diagnosis:** By various tests, including **fluorescent antibody, latex agglutination, and enzyme immunoassay.**

Prophylaxis and Treatment
Active immunization by a live-attenuated varicella vaccine.
Passive immunization: *Varicella-zoster immunoglobulin* **(VZIG) is of no value for treating established infection.**
Treatment: Acyclovir and vidarabine are effective in the treatment of severe varicella and zoster infections.

CYTOMEGALOVIRUS
The name Cytomegaloviruses (CMV) means **"large cell virus"** and derives from the swollen cells containing large intranuclear inclusions that characterize these infections.

Pathogenesis
Transmission requires close person-to-person contact. The congenital, oral, and sexual routes, blood transfusion, and tissue transplantation are the major means by which CMV is transmitted.
- A. **Normal hosts:** Primary cytomegalovirus infection of older children and adults is usually asymptomatic.
- B. **Immunocompromised hosts:** CMV can cause severe and even fatal infections in the immunocompromised host.
- C. **Congenital and perinatal infections:** Intrauterine infection leads to fetal death or cytomegalic inclusion disease of the newborn which is often fatal.

Laboratory Diagnosis
- A. **Specimens:** CMV can be isolated from the urine, saliva, breast milk, semen, cervical secretions and blood leukocytes.
- B. **Histology:** The histologic hallmark of CMV infection is the cytomegalic cell, which is an enlarged cell that contains a dense, central, **"owl's-eye," basophilic intranuclear inclusion body.**
- C. **Isolation of virus:** by inoculating human fibroblast cultures.
- D. **DNA probes**
- E. **Polymerase chain reaction (PCR)**
- F. **Serology:** IgM antibodies suggest a current infection and can be detected in serum by ELISA.

Treatment and Prevention
Ganciclovir (dihydroxypropoxymethyl guanine) and **foscarnet** (phosphonoformic acid) have been approved for the treatment of CMV infections. No vaccine is available.

EPSTEIN–BARR VIRUS
Epstein–Barr virus is the most sinister herpesvirus, for its association with malignant disease. Only human and some subhuman primate B cells have receptors for the virus.

Epidemiology
The Epstein–Barr (EB) virus is ubiquitous in all human populations. Infection with EBV is transmitted by saliva, and requires intimate oral contact.

The source of infection is usually the saliva of infected persons who shed the virus in oropharyngeal secretions. Saliva sharing between adolescents and young adults often occurs during kissing; thus, the nickname **"kissing disease"** for infectious mononucleosis. Children can acquire the virus at an early age by sharing contaminated drinking glasses.

Clinical conditions
1. Infectious mononucleosis
2. EBV associated malignancies:
   a. Burkitt's lymphoma
   b. Lymphomas in immunodeficient persons, such as AIDS patients and transplant recipients.
   c. Nasopharyngeal carcinoma in persons of Chinese origin.

Infectious Mononucleosis (Glandular Fever)
This is an acute self-limited illness usually seen in nonimmune young adults following primary infection with the EB virus. The incubation period is 4–8 weeks. Infectious mononucleosis is characterized by high fever, malaise, pharyngitis,

lymphadenopathy (swollen glands), and often, hepatosplenomegaly. A mild transient rash may be present. In most patients the spleen is palpable and there is some liver dysfunction, occasionally with frank jaundice. The typical illness is self-limited and lasts 2–4 weeks.

Laboratory Diagnosis

1. **Differential white cell count:** Atypical lymphocytes are probably the earliest detectable indication of an EBV infection. Blood examination during the initial phase may show leucopenia due to a drop in the number of polymorphs. Later there is a prominent leukocytosis with the appearance of abnormal or atypical lymphocytes. These atypical cells are lymphoblast derived from T cells reactive to the virus infection.
2. **Paul–Bunnell test:** Infectious mononucleosis is accompanied by production of heterophile agglutinins. These antibodies are IgM heterophile antibodies elicited by EBV infection. These can be detected by the *Paul-Bunnell* test or a rapid slide agglutination test.
   Procedure: Inactivated serum (56°C for 30 minutes) in doubling dilutions is mixed with equal volumes of a 1% suspension of sheep erythrocytes. After incubation at 37°C for 4 hours the tubes are examined for agglutination. An agglutination titer of 100 or above is suggestive of infectious mononucleosis.
   Confirmation: For confirmation, differential absorption of agglutinins with guinea pig kidney and ox red cells is necessary. Forssman antibody induced by injection of horse. Serum is removed by treatment with guinea pig kidney and ox red cells. Infectious mononucleosis antibody is removed by ox red cells but not guinea pig kidney.
3. **EBV-specific antibodies:** The antibody to virus capsid antigen (VCA) can be demonstrated by immunofluorescence and ELISA.
4. **Antigen detection:** By immunofluorescence using monoclonal antibodies.
5. Nucleic acid hybridization
6. **Virus isolation:** By immortalization of normal human lymphocytes.
7. **Polymerase chain reaction (PCR)**

ADENOVIRUSES

Adenoviruses are a group of medium sized, nonenveloped, double-stranded DNA viruses. All human serotypes are included in a single genus within the **family Adenoviridae.**

Morphology

Adenoviruses are 70–90 nm in diameter and display icosahedral symmetry. The DNA is linear and doublestranded.

Pathogenesis

Adenoviruses infect and replicate in epithelial cells of the respiratory tract, eye, gastrointestinal tract, urinary bladder, and liver.

Several distinct clinical syndromes are associated with adenovirus infection:

A. Respiratory diseases:
   1. Pharyngitis
   2. Pneumonia
   3. Acute respiratory diseases (ARD)
B. Eye infections:
   1. Pharyngoconjunctival fever
   2. Epidemic keratoconjunctivitis (EKC)
   3. Acute follicular conjunctivitis
C. **Gastrointestinal disease: Diarrhea**
D. **Other diseases:** *Mesenteric adenitis* and intussusception in children.
E. **Systemic infection in immunocompromised patients**

Laboratory Diagnosis

A. **Specimens:** Stool urine throat, conjunctival, or rectal swab.
B. **Direct demonstration of virus**
   i. Electron microscopy
   ii. Virus antigen
   iii. Viral DNA
   iv. Latex agglutination method
C. **Virus isolation:** The clinical specimens are inoculated in tissue culture, such as HeLa, Hep, KB, and human embryo kidney cells.

D. **Polymerase chain reaction (PCR)**
E. **Serology:** Complement fixation and neutralization tests are may be used.

PAPOVAVIRUSES

The term "Papova" is a signal indicating the names of viruses included in this group: (*Pa, papilloma; po, polyoma; va, vacuolating* virus) belong to the family Papoviridae and has two genera—*Papillomavirus* containing human and animal papilloma viruses and *Polyomavirus*, which contains the simian vacuolating virus (SV 40) and polyomavirus.

They are small, nonenveloped (naked), have icosahedral nucleocapsids, and contain supercoiled, double-stranded, circular DNA.

PAPILLOMAVIRUSES

Papillomaviruses cause several different kinds of warts in humans, including cutaneous warts, genital warts, respiratory papillomatosis, oral papillomas, and cancer.

POLYOMAVIRUSES

The name is derived from "poly" (many) and "oma" (tumor). Tumor induction is well described in experimental animals.

PARVOVIRUS

The parvoviruses are the smallest of the DNA viruses (about 20 nm).

The family Parvoviridae is divided into two subfamilies: the Parvovirinae and the Densivirinae. The Parvovirinae contains three genera: *Parvovirus, Dependovirus,* and *Erythrovirus.*

Clinical diseases: Transmission of parvoviruses appears to be by the respiratory route. It may cause respiratory infection with an erythematous maculopapular rash, erythema infectiosum (slapped cheek disease), joint disease, aplastic crisis in children with chronic hemolytic anemia (sickle cell disease), nonimmune fetal hydrops following infection during pregnancy and persistent anemia in immunodeficient.

HEPATITIS B VIRUS

See Chapter 47

KEY POINTS

- **Herpes viruses:** Human herpes viruses include human herpes virus 1 (HVl) to human herpes virus 8 (HV-8).
- **Varicella-zoster virus (VZV):** Causes chickenpox (varicella) and herpes zoster or shingles, two distinct clinical entities in humans.
- **Cytomegalovirus:** CMV is the causative agent of mononucleosis syndrome in immunocompetent hosts.
- **Epstein-Barr virus:** Epstein–Barr virus causes infectious mononucleosis and has been causally associated with Burkitt's lymphoma, Hodgkin's disease, and nasopharyngeal carcinoma.

IMPORTANT QUESTION

1. Write short notes on:
    a. Herpes simplex virus
    b. Varicella-zoster virus
    c. Cytomegalovirus
    d. Epstein–Barr virus (EB virus)

MULTIPLE CHOICE QUESTIONS

1. Which of the following infection/s is/are caused by herpes simplex virus type I?
    a. Acute gingivostomatitis
    b. Keratoconjunctivitis
    c. Encephalitis
    d. All of the above
2. All the following infections are caused by HSV-2, *except*:
    a. Neonatal infection
    b. Aseptic meningitis
    c. Herpetic whitlow
    d. Genital herpes
3. All the following infections are caused by HSV-2, *except*:
    a. Neonatal infection
    b. Aseptic meningitis
    c. Herpetic whitlow
    d. Genital herpes

4. Ramsay–Hunt syndrome can be caused by:
    a. Herpes simplex virus
    b. Herpes-zoster virus
    c. Cytomegalovirus
    d. Epstein–Barr virus
5. Shingles is caused by:
    a. Varicella-zoster virus
    b. Cytomegalovirus
    c. Epstein–Barr virus
    d. Herpes simplex virus type 1
6. *Owl's eye* is the characteristic feature of the cell infected by:
    a. Herpes simplex virus
    b. Epstein–Barr virus
    c. Cytomegalovirus
    d. Human herpes virus 8
7. Which of the following malignancies is/are associated with Epstein–Barr virus?
    a. Burkitt's lymphoma
    b. Nasopharyngeal carcinoma
    c. B cell lymphoma
    d. All of the above
8. Paul–Bunnell test is used for serodiagnosis of:
    a. Infectious mononucleosis
    b. Genital herpes
    c. Neonatal infection
    d. Aseptic meningitis
9. Which of the following viruses is associated in causation of Kaposi's sarcoma?
    a. Herpes simplex virus
    b. Herpesvirus simiae
    c. Human herpesvirus 8
    d. Human herpesvirus 6

ANSWERS

1. d	2. c	3. c	4. b
5. a	6. c	7. d	8. a
9. c			

Hepatitis Viruses

LEARNING OBJECTIVES

After reading and studying this chapter, you should be able to:
- Classify various hepatitis viruses.
- Tabulate differences between various hepatitis viruses.
- Compare various features of hepatitis A virus (HAV) and hepatitis B virus (HBV).
- Describe the following: Morphology of hepatitis B virus; antigenic structure of hepatitis B virus; modes of transmission of hepatitis B virus; hepatitis B carriers.
- Describe laboratory diagnosis of hepatitis B virus.
- Discuss prophylaxis of hepatitis B infections or hepatitis B vaccine.
- Describe the following: Hepatitis C virus or type C hepatitis; hepatitis D virus or delta agent; hepatitis E virus; hepatitis G virus.

INTRODUCTION

Viral hepatitis is a systemic disease primarily involving the liver. At least six viruses, A through E (A, B, C, D, E, F) and a newly discovered G, are considered hepatitis viruses. **Hepatitis A virus (HAV)** and **hepatitis B virus (HBV)** are the best known, but three **non-A, non-B hepatitis (NANBH) viruses** (C, G, and E) have been described, as has **hepatitis D virus (HDV), the delta agent** (Table 47.1).

TYPE A HEPATITIS (INFECTIOUS HEPATITIS)

Hepatitis A virus causes infectious hepatitis and is spread by the fecal-oral route. It is a subacute disease of global distribution, affecting mainly children and young adults.

Morphology

Hepatitis A virus is a 27 nm nonenveloped RNA virus belonging to the picornavirus family. Only one serotype is known (**Fig. 47.1**).

Epidemiology

Hepatitis A virus transmission is by the fecal-oral route in contaminated water, in food, and by dirty hands. In India, type A hepatitis is the most common cause of acute hepatitis in children, but is much less frequent in adults.

Clinical Features

The incubation period is 2–6 weeks. The clinical disease consists of two stages: the **prodromal** or **preicteric** and the **icteric stages.** The onset may be acute or insidious, with fever, malaise, anorexia, nausea, vomiting, and liver tenderness. These usually subside with the onset of jaundice. Recovery is slow, over a period of 4–6 weeks.

Laboratory Diagnosis

Etiological diagnosis of type A hepatitis may be made by demonstration of the virus or its antibody.
  A. **Demonstration of the virus:** By immune electron microscopy (IEM) in fecal extracts.
  B. **Demonstration of antibody:** It is measured by an enzyme-linked immunosorbent assay (ELISA) or radioimmunoassay (RIA).

Chapter 47: Hepatitis Viruses

Table 47.1: Comparative features of hepatitis viruses.

	A	B	C	D	E
Virus structure	HAV, 27 nm RNA, picornavirus (hepatovirus)	HBV, 47 nm DNA (hepadnavirus)	HCV, 35–37 nm RNA, flavivirus (hepacivirus)	HDV, 35–37 nm Defective RNA Deltavirus	HEV, 32–34 nm RNA Herpesvirus
Modes of infection	Fecal-oral	Parenteral, vertical, sexual	Parenteral	Parenteral	Fecal-oral
Age affected	Children	Any age	Adults	Any age	Young adults
Incubation period (days)	15–45	30–180	15–160	30–180	15–160
Onset	Acute	Insidious	Insidious	Insidious	Acute
Illness	Mild	Occasionally severe	Moderate	Occasionally severe	Mild, except in pregnancy
Carrier state	Nil	Common	Present	Nil (only with HBV)	Nil
Oncogenicity	Nil	Present specially after neonatal infection	Present	Nil	Nil
Prevalence	Worldwide	Worldwide	Probably worldwide	Endemic areas (Mediterranean, N. Europe, Central and N. America)	Only developing countries (India, Asia, Africa, Central America)
Laboratory diagnosis Specific prophylaxis	Ig and vaccine	Ig and vaccine	Nil	HBV vaccine	Nil

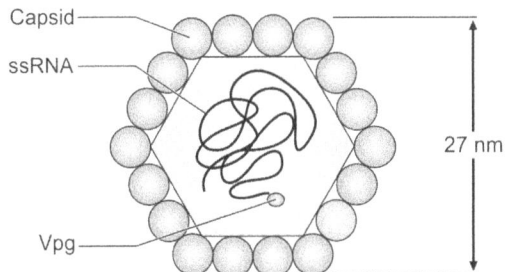

Fig. 47.1: The picornavirus structure of hepatitis A virus. The icosahedral capsid is made up of four viral polypeptides (VP1 to VP4). Inside the capsid is a single-stranded, positive-sense RNA (ssRNA) that has a genomic viral protein (VPg) on the 5′ end.

C. **Virus isolation** is not routinely performed.

Prophylaxis

A. **General measures:** Control of infection in the community depends on maintenance of hygiene.

B. **Immunization:** *Passive protection*—specific passive prophylaxis by pooled normal human immunoglobulin.

Hepatitis A Vaccine

1. **Formalin inactivated, alum conjugated vaccine**
2. **Live HAV vaccine:** A live HAV vaccine has been developed in China.

HEPATITIS B VIRUS (SERUM HEPATITIS)

Type B hepatitis is the most widespread and the most important type of viral hepatitis. It is a major factor in the eventual development of liver disease and hepatocellular carcinoma in those individuals.

Classification

Hepatitis B virus is assigned to a separate family *Hepadnaviridae* (*Hepatitis* DNA viruses).

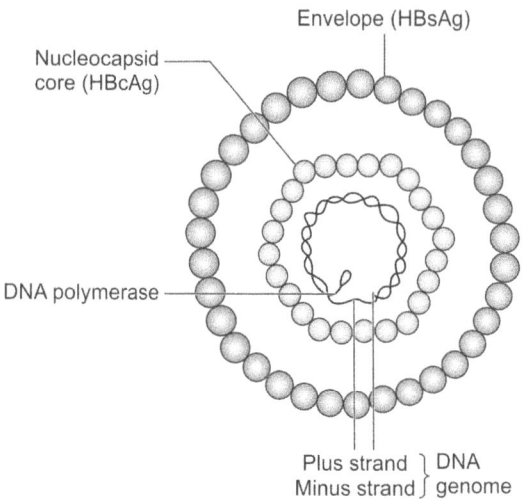

Fig. 47.2: Hepatitis B virus structure.

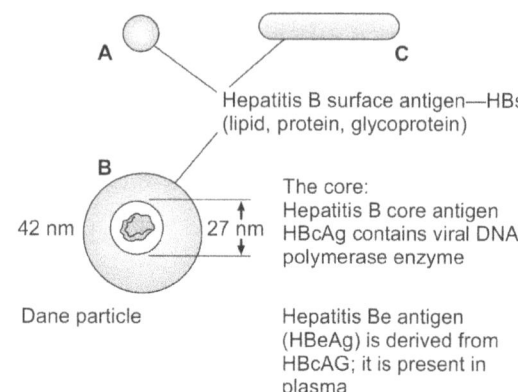

Fig. 47.3: Different types of particles of HBV: (A) Spherical 22 nm particle; (B) Double shelled 42 nm particle (Dane particle); (C) Tubular 22 nm particle.

Structure: HBV is a 42 nm DNA virus with an outer envelope and an inner core, 27 nm in diameter, enclosing the viral genome, and a circular double stranded DNA associated with a DNA polymerase **(Fig. 47.2)**.

Australia antigen: In 1965, Blumberg, studying human serum lipoprotein allotypes, observed in the serum of an Australian aborigine, a new antigen which gave a clearly defined line of precipitation with sera from two hemophiliacs who had received multiple blood transfusions. This was named the *Australia antigen*. By 1968 the 'Australia antigen' was found to be associated with serum hepatitis. It was subsequently shown to be the surface component of HBV. Therefore, the name Australia antigen was changed to *hepatitis B surface antigen* (HBsAg).

Types of particles: Under the electron microscope, sera from type B hepatitis patients show three types of particles **(Fig. 47.3)**.
1. **Spherical particle:** The predominant form is a small, spherical particle with a diameter of 22 nm.
2. **Tubular particle: The second type** of particle is filamentous or tubular with a diameter of 22 nm and of varying length.
3. **Dane particle: The third type of particle,** far fewer in number, is a double-walled spherical structure, 42 nm in diameter.

This particle is the complete hepatitis B virus. It was first described by Dane in 1970 and so is known as the **Dane particle**.

Antigenic Structure

1. **Hepatitis B surface antigen:** The envelope proteins expressed on the surface of the virion.
2. **Hepatitis B core antigen (HBcAg):** The antigen expressed on the core.
3. **Hepatitis B e antigen (HBeAg):** A third antigen called the *hepatitis B e antigen* is primarily secreted into serum, does not self-assemble like a capsid antigen.

Clinical Syndromes

Acute Infection

1. **Preicteric phase:** Symptoms during the prodromal period may include fever, malaise, and anorexia, followed by nausea, vomiting, abdominal discomfort, and chills.
2. **Icteric phase:** The classic icteric symptoms of liver damage (e.g., jaundice, dark urine, pale stools) follow soon thereafter.
3. **Convalescent phase:** About 90–95% of adults recover within 1–2 months of onset.

Chronic Infection

A proportion of cases (1–10%) remain chronically infected. Carriers or may progress to recurrent or chronic liver disease or cirrhosis. A few of them may develop hepatocellular carcinoma after many decades.

Mode of Transmission

Hepatitis B virus is a blood-borne virus and there are three important modes of transmission:
1. **Parenteral transmission:** HBV is transmitted only in blood and other body fluids. Professionals using sharp articles may unwittingly transmit the virus.
2. **Perinatal transmission:** Vertical transmission from mother to child is one of the most important routes. HBV can be transmitted to babies through contact with the mother's blood at birth and in mother's milk.
3. **Sexual transmission:** Since HBV is present in semen and vaginal secretions; therefore, it can be transmitted by sexual contact.

Laboratory Diagnosis

Specific Diagnosis

Specific diagnosis of hepatitis B rests on serological demonstration of the viral markers. These can be detected by sensitive and specific tests, such as ELISA and RIA.
1. **Detection of viral markers:**
   a. **HBsAg:** For the diagnosis of HBV infection, detection of HBsAg in blood is all that ordinarily necessary. The simultaneous presence of IgM anti-HBc indicates recent infection and the presence of IgG anti-HBc remote infection.
   b. **HBcAg:** Its appearance in the serum is indicative of viral replication. Initially, antiHBc is predominantly IgM, but after about 6 months, it is mainly IgG. Selective tests for IgM or IgG anti-HBc; therefore, enable distinction between recent or remote infection respectively.
   c. **HBeAg:** HBeAg presence denotes high infectivity and its absence, along with the presence of anti-HBe, indicates low infectivity. The disappearance of anti-HBe levels often is no longer detectable after 6 months.
2. **Viral DNA polymerase:** DNA polymerase activity, occur early in the incubation period.
3. **Polymerase chain reaction (PCR):** It is used for HBV DNA testing and is highly sensitive and quantitative.
4. **Biochemical tests:** Levels of serum transaminases (aminotransferases) are increased. Serum bilirubin levels may rise up to 25-fold.

Prophylaxis

Measures for the control of HBV infection are the same as those for HIV infection.

General Prophylaxis

General prophylaxis consists in avoiding risky practices like promiscuous sex, injectable drug abuse, and direct or indirect contact with blood, semen, or other body fluids of patients and carriers.

Immunization

Both passive and active methods of immunization are available.
1. **Passive immunization:** Hyperimmune hepatitis B immune globulin (HBIG) prepared from human volunteers with high titer anti-HBs, administered intramuscular (IM) in a dose of 300–500 iu.
2. **Active immunization:**
   a. **Plasma-derived hepatitis B vaccine:** The initial vaccine was prepared by purifying HBsAg associated with the 22-nm particles from healthy HBsAg-positive carriers and treating the particles with virus-inactivating agents (formalin, urea, heat). This was immunogenic, but became unacceptable.
   b. **Recombinant yeast hepatitis B vaccine:** The currently preferred vaccine is genetically engineered by cloning the S gene of HBV in baker's yeast. It consists of nonglycosylated HBsAg particles alone. This vaccine is safe, antigenic, free from side effects and as immunogenic as

plasma-derived vaccine. It is given with alum adjuvant, 1 M into the deltoid or, in infants into the anterolateral aspect of the thigh. Three doses given at 0, 1, and 6 months constitute the full course. Seroconversion occurs in about 90% of the vaccines.
3. **Recombinant Chinese hamster ovary (CHO) cell hepatitis vaccine.**
4. **Synthetic peptide vaccines:** These are still under experimental stage.
5. **Hybrid virus vaccine.**

HEPATITIS TYPE C

Hepatitis C Virus

Hepatitis C virus (HCV) has been classified as a new genus *Hepacivirus* in the family *Flaviviridae*. HCV is a 50–60 nm virus with a linear single-stranded RNA genome.

Mode of infection: Infection is mainly by blood transfusion and other modes of contact with infected blood or blood products. Injectable drug abusers, transplant recipients and immunocompromised persons are at high risk. The virus can be transmitted from mother to infant, though not as frequently as for HBV.

Clinical Features

Hepatitis C virus causes **three types of disease**:
1. **Acute hepatitis**
2. **Chronic persistent infection**
3. **Severe rapid progression to cirrhosis**

Laboratory Diagnosis

A. **Antibody detections** are based on ELISA recognition of antibody.
B. **HCV RNA identification:** Reverse transcriptase, PCR, branched-chain DNA, and other genetic techniques can detect HCV RNA.

Prophylaxis

Only general prophylaxis, such as screening of blood and blood products prior to transfusion, is possible.

TYPE D (DELTA) HEPATITIS

Delta or hepatitis D is a defective RNA virus dependent on the helper function of HBV for its replication and expression. It acquires an HBsAg coat for transmission.

Morphology

The HDV is a defective satellite virus requiring HBV as helper virus. HDV is a spherical, 36 nm particle with an outer coat composed of the hepatitis B surface antigen surrounding the circular single stranded RNA genome. The HDV RNA genome is very small, the single-stranded RNA and circular. Delta agent is thus an incomplete virus, reminiscent of the *Dependoviruses* (**Fig. 47.4**).

Pathogenesis

Its mode of transmission is the same as for HBV.

Types of infection: Two types of infection are recognized:
1. **Coinfection:** In coinfection, delta and HBV are transmitted together at the same time.
2. **Superinfection:** In superinfection, delta infection occurs in a person already harboring HBV.

Laboratory Diagnosis

The only way to determine the presence of the agent is by detecting the delta antigen or

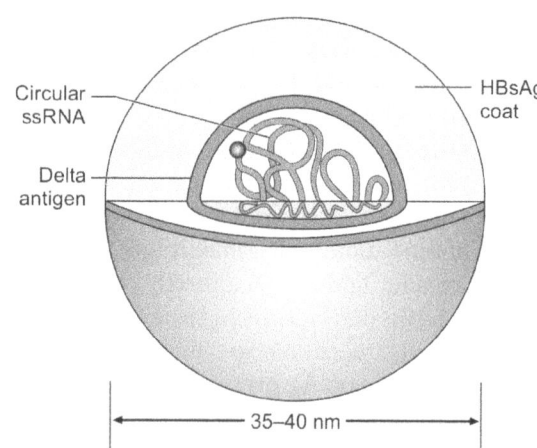

Fig. 47.4: The delta hepatitis virion.

antibodies by ELISA and RIA procedures. For the rapid identification of delta particles in circulation, RNA sequences have been cloned and DNA probes have been developed.

Prophylaxis

Because the delta agent depends on HBV for replication and is spread by the same routes, prevention of infection with HBV prevents HDV infection. Immunization with HBV vaccine protects against subsequent deltavirus infection.

HEPATITIS E VIRUS

Hepatitis E virus (HEV) has been provisionally classified in the genus *Hepevirus* under the **family Caliciviridae**. HEV is a spherical nonenveloped virus, 32–34 nm in diameter, with a single-stranded RNA genome.

Clinical Features

Hepatitis E virus is predominantly spread by the feco-oral route, especially in contaminated water. The symptoms and course of HEV disease are similar to those of HAV disease. HEV infection is especially serious in pregnant women.

Laboratory Diagnosis

1. **Exclusion of hepatitis A and hepatitis B:** Exclusion of hepatitis A by IgM serology and hepatitis B by absence of HBsAg and IgM anti-HBc.
2. **Immunoelectron microscopy:** Immunoelectron microscopic examination of patient feces for aggregated calicivirus-like particles using monoclonal antibodies.
3. **ELISA tests:** For IgM and IgG anti-HEV.
4. **Western blot assay:** A Western blot assay for IgM and/or IgG antiHEV.
5. **Polymerase chain reaction:** PCR assay for the detection of HEV RNA in patient feces or in acute-phase sera.

Prophylaxis

General measures: These depend on the maintenance of a clean water supply, and generally resemble those used to control HAV.

Immunization: Vaccines based on recombinant antigens are under development, and show some promise.

HEPATITIS G VIRUS

Hepatitis G virus (HGV) resembles HCV in many ways. HGV is a flavivirus, is transmitted in blood, and has a predilection for chronic hepatitis disease. It has not been grown, but its RNA genome has been cloned.

Laboratory Diagnosis

1. HGV is identified by detection of the genome by reverse transcriptase—PCR (RT-PCR) or other RNA detection methods.
2. Recently, an immunoassay has been developed to detect anti-HGV.

NON-A, NON-B (NANB) HEPATITIS

It refers to viral hepatitis resembling type A or type B clinically and epidemiologically but not caused by these viruses. **HAV** and **HBV** are the best known, but three **non-A, non-B hepatitis (NANBH) viruses** (C, G, and E) have been described. Diagnosis is possible with serological tests but a few are diagnosed by the process of exclusion.

KEY POINTS

- At least six viruses, A through G (A, B, C, D, E, and G) are hepatitis viruses.
- All the hepatitis viruses are RNA viruses, except the HBV, which is a DNA virus belonging to the family *Hepadnaviridae*.

IMPORTANT QUESTIONS

1. Classify hepatitis viruses. Discuss the laboratory diagnosis of infections caused by hepatitis B virus.
2. Write short notes on:
   a. Hepatitis A virus (HAV) or type A hepatitis or infectious hepatitis.
   b. Hepatitis B virus
   c. Hepatitis C virus (HCV).
   d. Hepatitis D virus or delta agent.

e. Non-A, non-B hepatitis.
f. Hepatitis E virus (HEV).
g. Prophylaxis of hepatitis B or hepatitis B vaccine.

MULTIPLE CHOICE QUESTIONS

1. Which of the following hepatitis viruses is DNA virus?
   a. Hepatitis A virus
   b. Hepatitis B virus
   c. Hepatitis C virus
   d. Hepatitis E virus

2. Which of the following hepatitis viruses can be transmitted by sexual route?
   a. Hepatitis A virus
   b. Hepatitis C virus
   c. Hepatitis E virus
   d. All of the above

3. Which of the following hepatitis viruses may cause hepatic carcinoma?
   a. Hepatitis A virus
   b. Hepatitis C virus
   c. Hepatitis E virus
   d. Hepatitis G virus

4. Which of the following antigens is present in the envelope of hepatitis B virus?
   a. HBsAg
   b. HBcAg
   c. HBeAg
   d. None of the above

5. Which statement is true for hepatitis D virus?
   a. An incomplete virus
   b. Related to hepatitis B
   c. A single-stranded DNA
   d. Transmitted by fecal-oral route

ANSWERS

1. b   2. b   3. b   4. a
5. a

RNA Viruses

LEARNING OBJECTIVES

After reading and studying this chapter, you should be able to:
- Describe enteroviruses
- Discuss prophylaxis against poliomyelitis.
- Differentiate live and killed polio vaccines.
- Describe the following: Hemagglutinin (H) and neuraminidase (NA); antigenic variation in influenza virus; antigenic shift and antigenic drift.
- Discuss laboratory diagnosis of influenza.
- Describe the following: Parainfluenza viruses; Measles virus; Respiratory syncytial virus (RSV).
- Describe neural and non-neural vaccines against rabies.
- Describe the following: Japanese B encephalitis; dengue fever or break bone fever; Kyasanur forest disease (KFD); Rubella virus.

PICORNAVIRUSES

Introduction

The family Picornaviridae comprises a large number of very small RNA (*pico,* meaning small, RNA: rna) viruses with a diameter of 27–30 nm and containing single-stranded RNA.

Classification

The Picornaviridae family has more than 230 members that are divided into six genera (**Box 48.1**).

> **Box 48.1:** Picornaviridae.
>
> - Enterovirus
>   - Poliovirus types 1, 2, and 3
>   - Coxsackie A virus types 1 to 22 and 24
>   - Coxsackie B virus types 1 to 6
>   - Echovirus (ECHO virus) types 1 to 9, 11 to 27, and 29 to 34
>   - Enterovirus 68 to 72
> - Rhinovirus types 1 to 100+
> - Cardiovirus
> - Aphthovirus
> - Heparnavirus: Hepatitis A virus
> - Parechovirus

POLIOVIRUS

Poliomyelitis is an acute infectious disease that in its serious form affects the central nervous system.

Morphology

Size: The virion is a spherical particle, about 27 nm in diameter.

Capsid: It is arranged in icosahedral symmetry.
Genome: The genome is a single strand of positive sense RNA.

Types

There are three types (1, 2, and 3) of poliovirus, identified by neutralization tests.

Pathogenesis

The virus is transmitted by the fecal-oral route through ingestion. Virus is ingested and multiplies initially in the lymphoid tissue of the tonsil or Peyer's patches in the small intestine. It then spreads to the regional lymph nodes and enters the blood stream (minor or primary viremia). *Primary viremia spreads the virus to target tissues, where a second phase of viral replication may occur, resulting in symptoms and a secondary viremia.*

Clinical Features

The incubation period is usually 7-14 days. Following exposure to poliovirus, 90-95% of susceptible individuals develop only **inapparent infection**. It is only in 5-10% that any sort of clinical illness results.
  A. **Asymptomatic illness:** At least 90% of poliovirus infections.
  B. **Abortive poliomyelitis, the minor illness**—in approximately 5%.
  C. **Nonparalytic poliomyelitis or aseptic meningitis**—in 1-2%.
  D. Paralytic poliomyelitis—in 0.1-2.0%.
  E. Progressive postpoliomyelitis muscle atrophy

Laboratory Diagnosis

  A. **Specimens:** Polioviruses may be isolated from the patient's pharynx during the first few days of illness, from the feces for as long as 30 days, but from the CSF only rarely.
  B. **Culture:** Primary monkey kidney cells are usually employed. The virus growth is indicated by typical cytopathic effects in 2-3 days.

Prophylaxis

Immunization

Two types of vaccines are used throughout the world; they are:
  1. **Inactivated polio vaccine (IPV)—Salk killed polio vaccine:** By 1953, Salk had developed a killed vaccine. Salk's killed polio vaccine is a formalin inactivated preparation of the three types of poliovirus grown in monkey kidney tissue culture.

Killed vaccine is given by injection and is therefore called inactivated or injectable poliovaccine (lPV). The primary or initial course of immunization consists of four inoculations. The first three doses are given at intervals of 1-2 months and 4th dose 6-12 months after the third dose. First dose is usually given when the infant is 6 weeks old. Additional doses are recommended prior to school entry and then every 5 years until the age of 18.

IPV induces humoral antibodies (lgM, IgG, and IgA serum antibodies) but does not induce intestinal or local immunity.

  2. **Oral polio vaccine (OPV)—Sabin live polio vaccine:** Oral polio vaccine was described by Sabin in 1957. It contains live attenuated virus (types 1, 2, and 3) grown in primary monkey kidney or human diploid cell cultures. The vaccine is issued either in the monovalent or trivalent form.

Immunization Schedule

The National Immunization Program in India recommends a primary course of three doses of OPV at one-month intervals, commencing the first dose when infant is 6 weeks old. One booster dose of OPV is recommended 12-18 months later.

ORTHOMYXOVIRUS

Orthomyxoviruses are spherical or filamentous, enveloped viruses with single stranded and segmented RNA genome. The family *Orthomyxoviridae* comprises influenza A, B, and C viruses.

Influenza Viruses

Morphology

Virus: The influenza virus is typically spherical, with a diameter of 80-120 nm but pleomorphism is common.
Genome: The virus core consists of ribonucleoprotein in helical symmetry. Single stranded RNA genome is segmented and exists as eight pieces.
Envelope: The nucleocapsid is surrounded by an M1 protein shell, immediately exterior to which is a lipid envelope.

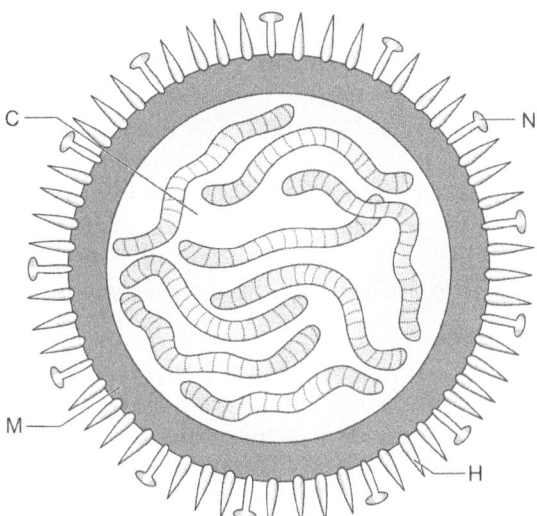

Fig. 48.1: Diagrammatic representation of influenza virus. (H—hemagglutinin; N—neuraminidase; C—core containing eight strands of RNA; M—membrane protein).

Peplomers: Projecting from the envelope are two types of spikes (peplomers): Hemagglutinin (HA) spikes which are triangular in cross-section and the mushroom-shaped *neuraminidase (NA)* peplomers, which are less numerous **(Fig. 48.1)**.

Antigenic Structure

The antigens of the influenza virus can be classified as the internal antigens and the surface antigens.
 A. **Internal antigens:**
  1. **Ribonucleoprotein (RNP) antigen-**based on its nature, influenza viruses are classified into types A, B, and C.
  2. **Matrix (M) protein**
 B. **Surface antigens:**
  1. **Hemagglutinin (HA)** is a glycoprotein composed of two polypeptides—HA1 and HA2. Fifteen distinct HA subtypes, named H1 to H15 have been identified in avian influenza viruses.
  2. **Neuraminidase (NA)** Nine different subtypes have been identified (N1-N9).

Antigenic Classification

Antigenic differences exhibited by two of the internal structural proteins, the nucleocapsid (NP) and matrix (M) proteins, are used to divide influenza viruses into types A, B, and C. These proteins possess no cross reactivity among the three types. Antigenic variations in the surface glycoproteins, HA, and NA, are used to subtype the viruses.

Antigenic Variation

Influenza viruses are remarkable because of the frequent 'antigenic changes that occur in HA and NA, which may be of two types *antigenic drift* (minor antigenic changes) *antigenic drift* (major antigenic changes).

Antigenic drift

Antigenic drift is the gradual sequential change in antigenic structure occurring regularly at frequent intervals.

Antigenic shift

Antigenic shift, on the other hand, is an abrupt, drastic, discontinuous variation in the antigenic structure, resulting in a novel virus strain unrelated antigenically to predecessor strains.

Pathogenesis

Influenza virus spreads from person-to-person by airborne droplets. Influenza initially establishes a local upper respiratory tract infection.

Clinical Features

 A. **Uncomplicated influenza:** The incubation period is 1–3 days. The disease varies in severity from a mild coryza to fulminating and rapidly fatal pneumonia.
 B. **Complications:** Complications of influenza include primary viral pneumonia, secondary bacterial pneumonia, myositis and cardiac complications, and, neurological involvement may occur.

Laboratory Diagnosis

Diagnosis of influenza relies on isolation of the virus, identification of viral antigens or viral nucleic acid, or demonstration of a specific immunologic response by the patient.
 1. **Demonstration of the virus antigen:** Rapid diagnosis of influenza may be made

by demonstration of the virus antigen on the surface of the nasopharyngeal cells by immunofluorescence.
Detection of influenza RNA by reverse transcriptase polymerase chain reaction (RTPCR) may be more sensitive than antigen detection.

2. **Isolation of the virus:** Nasal washings, gargles, and throat swabs are the best specimens for viral isolation and should be obtained within 3 days after the onset of symptoms but less often in later stages. Isolation may be made in eggs or in monkey kidney cell culture.
   a. The material is inoculated into the amniotic cavity of 11–13 day old eggs.
   b. For primary isolation the most suitable cells are primary monkey kidney or human embryo kidney cells. At 33°C in roller drum is recommended. The presence of virus may be detected by hemadsorption.
3. **Serology:** Complement fixation tests (CFTs) and hemagglutination inhibition (HI) tests are employed for the serological diagnosis of influenza. HI is a convenient and sensitive test for the serological diagnosis of influenza.

PARAMYXOVIRUSES

Paramyxoviruses belong to the family *Paramyxoviridae*. Paramyxoviruses resemble orthomyxoviruses in morphology but are larger and more pleomorphic.

Morphology and Structural Proteins

They are roughly spherical in shape and range in size from 100 to 300 nm. **The helical nucleocapsid** is much wider than in orthomyxoviruses, Genome of the *Paramyxoviruses* is an single-stranded (ssRNA) molecule. The nucleocapsid associates with the **matrix (M) protein** at the base of the lipid envelope. The virion envelope contains two glycoproteins, a **fusion (F) protein**, and a viral attachment protein [HN, hemagglutinin (H), or G protein].

Viruses of the Family Paramyxoviridae

1. Parainfluenza Viruses

Parainfluenza virus is transmitted by person-to-person contact and respiratory droplets. Parainfluenza viruses 1, 2, and 3 may cause respiratory tract syndromes ranging from a **mild cold-like upper respiratory tract infection** (coryza, pharyngitis, mild bronchitis, wheezing, and fever) to **bronchiolitis and pneumonia**.

2. Mumps Virus

Mumps is an acute contagious disease commonly affecting children characterized by nonsuppurative enlargement of one or both parotid glands. Infection is acquired by inhalation, and probably also through the conjunctiva. **Epididymo-orchitis** is a complication seen in postpubertal male patients.

3. Measles (Rubeoala)

Measles is one of the five classic childhood exanthems, along with rubella, roseola, fifth disease, and chickenpox.

Pathogenesis

The virus gains access to the human body via the respiratory tract, or the conjunctiva where it multiplies locally. After 2 days of illness, the typical mucous membrane lesions, known as **Koplik's spots,** appear most commonly on the buccal mucosa across from the molars. The prodromal illness subsides within a day or two of the appearance of the rash. The red maculopapular rash of measles typically appears on the forehead first and spreads downward, to disappear in the same sequence 3–6 days later, leaving behind a brownish discoloration and finely granular desquamation.

Prophylaxis

Measles vaccine is *a live attenuated vaccine*. Measles vaccine along with mumps and rubella *(MMR) vaccine* is currently used for universal immunization of the children.

4. Respiratory Syncytial Virus

Respiratory syncytial virus (RSV) is the most important cause of lower respiratory tract illness in infants and young children. It is the most important cause of viral pneumonia under age 5 years. The spectrum of respiratory illness ranges from the common cold in adults, through febrile bronchitis in infants and older children and pneumonia in infants, to bronchiolitis in very young babies. It may be the cause of some cases of sudden infant death syndrome.

The virus is transmitted by close contact and through contaminated fingers and fomites. RSV is highly contagious. It causes nosocomial infections in nurseries and on pediatric hospital wards.

RHABDOVIRUSES

Bullet-shaped, enveloped viruses with single-stranded RNA genome are classified as rhabdoviruses (from *rhabdos,* meaning rod) in the family Rhabdoviridae.

RABIES VIRUS

Morphology

1. **Virion:** The rabies **virion** consists of a helical nucleocapsid contained in a **bullet-shaped lipoprotein** envelope 180 × 75 nm, with one end rounded or conical and the other plane or concave.
2. **Proteins:** Protruding from the lipid envelope.
3. **Membrane or matrix (M) protein:** Beneath the envelope is the **membrane or matrix (M) protein** layer.
4. **Genome:** The core of the virion consists of helically arranged ribonucleoprotein. The genome is single-stranded RNA.

Pathogenesis

Rabies virus has a wide host range and is a natural infection of dogs, foxes, cats, and bats. Rabies infection usually results from the bite of rabid dogs or other animals. The virus present in the saliva of the animal is deposited in the wound. The virus appears to multiply in the muscles, connective tissue, or nerves at the site of deposition. Once the virus gains access to the spinal cord, the brain becomes rapidly infected. The clinical spectrum in humans can be divided into three phases: a short prodromal phase, an acute neurologic phase, and coma.

Laboratory Diagnosis
Human Rabies

A. **Rabies antigens by immunofluorescence:** The method most commonly used for diagnosis is the demonstration of rabies virus antigens by immunofluorescence. The specimens tested are corneal smears and skin biopsy or saliva antemortem, and brain postmortem by direct immunofluorescence.
B. **Virus isolation:**
   1. **Mouse inoculation:** Samples of brain tissue, saliva, CSF, or urine may be injected intracerebrally into newborn mice for isolation of the virus. The inoculated mice are examined for signs of illness and their brains are examined at death or at 28 days postinoculation for Negri bodies, or by immunofluorescence rabies antigen.
   2. **Isolation in cell culture**
C. **Serology:** Rabies antibodies can be detected in the serum and CSF by ELISA.
D. **Detection of nucleic acid: Reverse transcription-polymerase chain reaction (RTPCR)** testing.

Animal Rabies

1. **Demonstration of rabies virus antigen by immunofluorescence**
2. **Demonstration of inclusion bodies (Negri bodies):** A definitive pathologic diagnosis of rabies can be based on the finding of Negri bodies in the brain or the spinal cord. **Negri bodies** are seen as intracytoplasmic, round or oval, purplish pink structures with characteristic basophilic inner granules. Negri bodies vary in size from 3 to 27 μm.
3. **Isolation of the rabies virus (biological test)**
4. **Corneal test**

Prophylaxis

This may be considered under:
A. Post-exposure prophylaxis
B. Pre-exposure prophylaxis

A. Post-exposure Prophylaxis

a. Local Treatment of Wound
Immediate flushing and washing the wound(s), scratches, and the adjoining areas with plenty of soap and water is important in the prevention of human rabies. After cleansing, should be inactivated by irrigation either alcohol tincture or aqueous solution of iodine or povidone iodine. The local application of antirabies serum or its infiltration around the wound has been shown to be highly effective in preventing rabies.

b. Antirabic Vaccines
Antirabic vaccines fall into two main categories: neural and non-neural **(Box 48.2)**. Neural vaccines are associated with serious risk of neurological complications and have been replaced by the non-neural vaccines.

1. **Neural vaccines**
    a. *Semple vaccine:* It is a 5% suspension of sheep brain infected with fixed virus and inactivated with phenol at 37°C, leaving no residual live virus.
    b. *Beta propiolactone (BPL) vaccine:* This is a modification of the Semple vaccine, in which beta propiolactone is used as the inactivating agent instead of phenol.
    c. *Infant brain vaccines:* The encephalitogenic factor in brain tissue is a basic protein associated with myelin. To reduce the hazard from neuroparalytic factors, vaccines have been prepared from the brains of suckling mice. This vaccine is considered to be devoid of neuroparalytic effect because of the absence or low content of myelin in the neonatal animal.

2. **Non-neural vaccines**
    a. *Egg vaccines:*
        – Duck embryo vaccine (DEV): The rabies virus is grown in embryonated duck eggs and inactivated with beta propiolactone, but was discontinued because of its poor immunogenicity.
        – Live attenuated chick embryo vaccines: Two types of vaccines were developed with the Flury strain.
            i. **Low egg passage (LEP) vaccine** for immunization of dogs.
            ii. **High egg passage (HEP) vaccine** for cattle and cats. These are not in use now.
    b. *Cell culture vaccines:* The cell culture vaccines are of two types:
        i. Human diploid cell vaccine (HDCV)
            - First-generation cell culture vaccine
            - Human diploid cell vaccine (HDCV): The human diploid cell (HDC) vaccine is a purified and concentrated preparation of fixed rabies virus grown on human diploid and inactivated with beta propiolactone or tri-n-butyl phosphate. It is highly antigenic and free from serious side effects. Its only disadvantage is its high cost.
        ii. Second generation tissue culture vaccines **(Box 48.2):**
            - Purified chick embryo cell vaccine (PCEC)
            - Purified Vero cell rabies vaccine (PVRV). Second generation tissue culture vaccines are cheaper than HDC vaccines.

3. **Subunit vaccine**

Vaccination Schedules
a. **Neural vaccines:** The dosage of the vaccine depends on the degree of risk to which the

---

Box 48.2: Rabies vaccines.

- Neural vaccines:
    - Semple vaccine
    - Beta-propiolactone (8PL) vaccine
    - Suckling mouse brain vaccine
- Non-neural vaccines
    - Duck egg vaccine
    - Cell culture vaccines
        - First-generation cell culture vaccine
            – Human diploid cell vaccine (HDCV)
        - Second-generation cell culture vaccines
            – Purified chick embryo cell vaccine (PCEC)
            – Purified Vero cell rabies vaccine (PVRV)
- Third-generation rabies vaccine
Poxvirus-rabies glycoprotein recombinant vaccine (undergoing clinical trials in humans)

patient has been exposed. The ideal site for vaccination is the anterior abdominal wall. In India the following cell culture vaccines are available:
- Human diploid cell vaccine
- Purified chick embryo cell (PCEC) vaccine
- Purified vero cell (PVC) vaccine

b. **Cell culture vaccines:** All three cell culture vaccines available in India have the same dosage schedule, which is the same for both adults and children.

B. Pre-exposure Prophylaxis

Pre-exposure prophylaxis requires five or six doses, on days 0, 3, 7, 14, 30, and optionally 90. The vaccine is to be given IM or SC in the deltoid region, or in children on the anterolateral aspect of the thigh.

Passive Immunization

Two preparations of antirabies serum are available for passive immunization: (i) Horse anti-rabies serum (ii) Human rabies immune globulin (HRIG)

ARBOVIRUSES

Arboviruses (Arthropod-borne viruses) are defined as viruses that are transmitted by blood-sucking athropods from one vertebrate to another arthropods.

Laboratory Diagnosis

Diagnosis of arbovirus infections depends on: virus isolation, detection of arbovirus-specific RNA and serology.

A. **Specimen:** As all arbovirus infections are viremic, blood collected during the acute phase of the disease may yield the virus. Isolation may also be made from the CSF in some encephalitic cases but the best specimen for virus isolation is the brain.

B. **Virus isolation:**
  i. *Suckling mice:* Specimens are inoculated intracerebrally into suckling mice. The animals develop fatal encephalitis.
  ii. *Tissue cultures:* Some viruses may also be isolated in tissue cultures.
  iii. Virus isolation from insect vectors and reservoir animal

C. **Arbovirus-specific RNA detection:** By reverse transcriptase polymerase chain reaction (RTPCR).

D. **Serology:** Diagnosis may also be made serologically by demonstrating rise in antibody titer in paired serum samples by hemagglutination inhibition, complement fixation, or neutralization tests.

ALPHAVIRUS

Alphavirus (Mosquito-borne)

1. Encephalitis virus
2. Viruses causing febrile illness

Chikungunya Virus (CHIKV)

The vector is *Aedes aegypti*. In Swahili, "chikungunya" means "that which bends up", and refers to the posture assumed by patients suffering from severe joint pains.

FLAVIVIRUS

Mosquito-borne Group

a. **Japanese encephalitis:** Japanese encephalitis (JE) is mosquito-borne encephalitis caused by a group B arbovirus (Flavivirus) and transmitted by culicine mosquitoes.
b. **Yellow fever:** Yellow fever virus causes yellow fever, an acute, febrile, mosquito-borne illness that occurs only in Africa and Central and South America. **The disease yellow fever does not occur in India.**
c. **Dengue:** Dengue virus is widely distributed throughout the tropics and subtropics. Four types of dengue virus exist: DEN 1, DEN 2, DEN 3, and 4.

Clinical Findings

a. **Classic dengue fever:** Classic dengue usually affects older children and adults. After incubation period of 2–7 days, patient develops fever of sudden onset and often biphasic with severe headache, chills, retrobulbar pain, conjunctivitis, and severe pain in the back, muscles, and joints (**breakbone fever**). A maculopapular rash generally appears on the trunk in 3–5 days of illness and spreads later to the face and extremities. Lymph nodes are frequently enlarged. Leukopenia with a relative lymphocytosis is a regular occurrence.

Classic dengue fever is a self-limited disease.

b. **Other manifestations:** Dengue may also occur in more serious forms, with hemorrhagic manifestations (**dengue hemorrhagic fever**) or with shock (**dengue shock syndrome**).

Laboratory Diagnosis

A. **Virus detection** is difficult.
B. **Polymerase chain reaction (PCR)**
C. **Serology:** Demonstration of circulating IgM antibody provides early diagnosis, as it appears within two to five days of the onset of illness and persists for one to three months. IgM ELISA test offers reliable diagnosis. A strip immunochromatographic test for IgM is available for rapid diagnosis.

Control

Control depends upon antimosquito measures, e.g., elimination of breeding places and the use of insecticides as no vaccine is currently available.

Kyasanur Forest Disease

Kyasanur forest disease (KFD) is a febrile disease associated with hemorrhages caused by an arbovirus, flavivirus, and transmitted to man by bite of infective ticks.

RUBELLA (GERMAN MEASLES)

Rubella or German measles is a mild exanthematous fever characterized by transient macular rash and lymphadenopathy. *Rubella virus* has been classified in the family Togaviridae as the only member of the genus *Rubivirus*.

Morphology

Rubella virus is a pleomorphic, roughly spherical particle, 50–70 nm in diameter, with single-stranded RNA genome and surrounded by an envelope.

Clinical Features

Incubation period is 2–3 weeks. The characteristic clinical features are **rash**. A generalized rash develops first on the face and then spreads to the trunk and limbs sparing the palms and soles, **lymphadenopathy. Common complications** are arthralgia and arthritis.

CONGENITAL RUBELLA

Maternal viremia associated with rubella infection during pregnancy may result in infection of the placenta and fetus. Fetal damage caused by maternal rubella is related to the stage of pregnancy.

Laboratory Diagnosis

A. **Virus isolation:** The virus may be isolated from blood or more successfully from throat swabs in rabbit kidney or vero cells. Rubella virus isolation is not commonly employed for diagnosis because of the difficulties and delay involved.
B. **Serology:** Serological diagnosis is the method in routine use. ELISA for IgM and IgG antibodies gives valuable information. IgM antibody alone, without IgG means current acute infection.

Prophylaxis

Rubella vaccine: Several **live attenuated vaccines** have been developed. The vaccine in use is administered by subcutaneous injection in a single dose of 0.5 mL. The vaccine is available as a single antigen or combined with measles, mumps, rubella (MMR) vaccine.

ROTAVIRUSES

Morphology: Morphologically, rotaviruses are polyhedrons displaying characteristic sharp-edged double-shelled capsids, which look like spokes grouped around the hub of a wheel. The name is derived from *rota,* in Latin, meaning wheel. Both 'complete' and 'incomplete' particles are seen. The genome of rotaviruses and consists of double-stranded RNA.

Clinical Features

Rotavirus diarrhea is usually seen in children below the age of 5 years but symptomatic infections are most common in children between 6 months and 2 years.

Infection is by the fecal-oral route. The incubation period is 2–3 days. Vomiting and diarrhea occur with little or no fever. The disease is self-limited and recovery occurs within 5–10 days.

Laboratory Diagnosis

A. **Demonstration of virus:** At the peak of the disease as many as 10^{11} virus particles per milliliter of feces are present. Virus in stool is demonstrated by immune electron microscopy (IEM), latex agglutination tests, or ELISA.
B. **Genotyping:** By PCR
C. **Virus isolation:** Not used for routine diagnosis
D. **Serologic tests:** These can be used to detect after antibody titer rise, particularly ELISA.

KEY POINTS

- **Poliovirus** is the causative agent of *poliomyelitis.*
- Rubella or German measles is a mild exanthematous fever characterized by transient macular rash and lymphadenopathy.
- The family *Orthomyxoviridae* comprises four genera: influenza A, B, and C viruses.
- Mumps virus causes mumps.
- Measles virus causes measles.
- Respiratory syncytial virus (RSV) primarily causes infection of the respiratory tract, ranging from common cold to pneumonia.
- The rabies virus causes rabies in humans and a wide variety of animals.
- Japanese encephalitis (JE) is a mosquito-borne encephalitis.
- Dengue virus is causes classic dengue or breakdown fever, dengue hemorrhagic fever (DHF), and dengue shock syndrome (DSS).
- **Rotaviruses** are the most common cause of diarrhea in infants and children.

IMPORTANT QUESTIONS

1. Write short notes on:
   a. Prophylaxis against poliomyelitis
2. Discuss the morphology and pathogenesis of influenza virus infection.
3. Write short notes on:
   a. Parainfluenza viruses
   b. Mumps virus
   c. Measles virus
4. Write short notes on:
   a. Negri bodies
   b. Prophylaxis against rabies or rabies vaccines for human use.
5. Write short notes on:
   a. Arboviruses
   b. Dengue fever or break bone fever
6. Write short notes on:
   a. Rubella or German measles
   b. Rotaviruses

MULTIPLE CHOICE QUESTIONS

1. Which of the following vaccines induce/s production of local secretory IgA antibodies?
   a. Salk polio vaccine
   b. Sabin polio vaccine
   c. Both of the above
   d. None of the above
2. All the following statements are true for influenza viruses except that
   a. They are spherical or filamentous, enveloped particles, 80–120 nm in diameter.
   b. The virion contains an RNA-dependent RNA polymerase.
   c. Viral genome is a single-stranded unsegmented RNA.
   d. The virion has hemagglutinin and neuraminidase peplomers.
3. MMR vaccine is:
   a. A live attenuated vaccine.
   b. A killed vaccine.
   c. A subunit vaccine.
   d. A synthetic peptide vaccine.

Section 4: Virology

4. The inclusion bodies found in rabies are called:
   a. Bollinger bodies
   b. Councilman bodies
   c. Cowdry type a bodies
   d. Negri bodies
5. All of the following antirabies vaccine are inactivated vaccines, *except*:
   a. Human diploid cell strain vaccine
   b. Purified vero cell vaccine
   c. Purified chick embryo cell culture vaccine
   d. Chick embryo vaccine
6. The vaccine is not available for:
   a. Dengue fever
   b. Japanese encephalitis
   c. Yellow fever
   d. Russian spring-summer encephalitis
7. Which of the following can cause congenital infections?
   a. *Toxoplasma gondii*
   b. Rubella virus
   c. Cytomegalovirus
   d. All of the above

ANSWERS

| 1. b | 2. c | 3. a | 4. d |
| 5. d | 6. a | 7. d | |

CHAPTER 49

Retroviruses: Human Immunodeficiency Virus

Learning Objectives

After reading and studying this chapter, you should be able to:
- Describe morphology of human immunodeficiency virus.
- Describe modes of transmission of human immunodeficiency virus (HIV).
- Discuss opportunistic infections associated with human immunodeficiency virus infection.
- Discuss the laboratory tests for detection of specific antibodies in human immunodeficiency virus infection.

INTRODUCTION

Retroviruses are RNA viruses that belong to family *Retroviridae* (Re = Reverse, tr = transcriptase). Members of this family possess an RNA genome and the characteristic biochemical feature is the presence of RNA-dependent DNA polymerase (reverse transcriptase) within the virus.

HUMAN IMMUNODEFICIENCY VIRUS

Human immunodeficiency virus (HIV) types are the etiologic agents of *acquired immunodeficiency syndrome* (AIDS). The illness was first described in 1981, and HIV-1 was isolated by the end of 1983. HIV occurs in two main types: HIV-1 and HIV-2.

Structure

1. **Enveloped virus:** HIV is a spherical **enveloped virus,** about 90–120 nm in size **(Fig. 49.1).**
2. **Nucleocapsid:** The **nucleocapsid** has an outer icosahedral shell and an inner cone-shaped core, enclosing the ribonucleoproteins.
3. **Genome**: There are two identical copies of the positive sense, single-stranded RNA genome in the capsid (retroviruses are diploid). Also found within the capsid are the enzymes reverse transcriptase (which is a characteristic feature of retroviruses).
4. **Lipoprotein envelope:** Virus contains a **lipoprotein envelope**. The major virus coded envelope proteins are the projecting

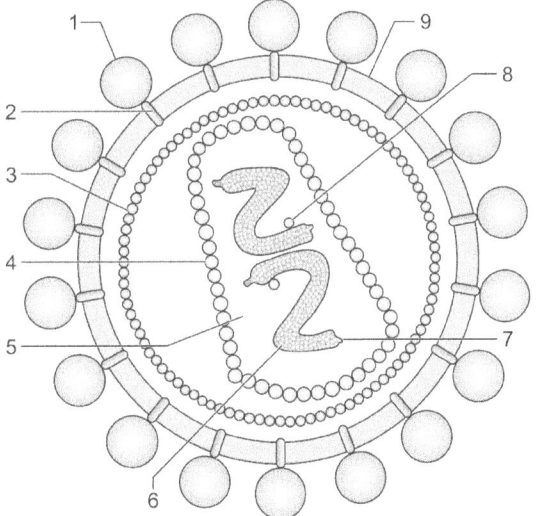

Fig. 49.1: Structure of HIV (diagrammatic representation). 1. Envelope glycoprotein spike (gp 120); 2. Transmembrance pedicle glycoprotein (gp 41); 3. Outer icosahedral shell of nucleocapsid (p18); 4. Cone-shaped core of nucleocapsid (p24); 5. Inner core; 6. Viral proteins associated with RNA; 7. Viral RNA; 8. Reverse transcriptase; 9. Envelope lipid bilayer.

knob-like spikes on the surface and the anchoring transmembrane pedicles. The env polypeptide is composed of two subunits—the outer glycoprotein knob (gpI20) and a transmembrane portion (gp41), which joins the knob to the virus lipid envelope.

Routes/Modes of Transmission

HIV is spread only by three modes:
1. **Sexual intercourse:** HIV is primarily a sexually transmitted infection. Both sexes are affected equally.
2. **Blood and blood products:** Transfusion of infectious blood or blood products is an effective route for viral transmission.
   a. *Contaminated needles:* Can transmit the infection. This is particularly relevant in drug addicts who share syringes and needles.
      The danger of needle-stick injury is present in medical and paramedical personnel.
3. **Mother to child transmission:** Transmission of infection from mother to baby can take place before, during or after birth. Transmission during breastfeeding usually occurs early (by 6 months).

Clinical Features of HIV Infection

The Centers for Disease Control (USA) have classified the clinical course of HIV infection under various groups. The natural evolution of HIV infection can be considered in the following stages:
- Group I: Acute HIV infection
- Group II: Asymptomatic or latent infection
- Group III: Persistent generalized lymphadenopathy (PGL)
- Group IV: AIDS-related complex (ARC)

This group includes patients with considerable immunodeficiency, suffering from various constitutional symptoms or minor opportunistic infections. The typical constitutional symptoms are fatigue, unexplained fever, persistent, diarrhea and marked weight loss of more than 10% of body weight.

Acquired Immune Deficiency Syndrome (AIDS)

This is the end-stage disease representing the irreversible breakdown of immune defense mechanisms, leaving the patient prey to progressive opportunistic infections and malignancies. Acquired Immune Deficiency Syndrome (AIDS) may be manifested in several different ways, including lymphadenopathy and fever, opportunistic infections, malignancies, and AIDS-related dementia **(Table 49.1)**.

Table 49.1: Opportunistic infections and malignancies commonly associated with HIV infection.

I. **Bacterial**
1. *M. avium* complex
2. *Mycobacterium tuberculosis*—disseminated or extrapulmonary
3. *Salmonella*—recurrent septicemia

II. **Viral**
1. Cytomegalovirus
2. Herpes simplex virus
3. Varicella-zoster virus
4. Epstein-Barr virus
5. Human herpesvirus 6
6. Human herpesvirus 8

III. **Fungal**
1. Candidiasis
2. Cryptococcosis
3. Aspergillosis
4. *Pneumocystis carinii pneumonia*
5. Histoplasmosis
6. Coccidioidomycosis

IV. **Parasitic**
1. Toxoplasmosis
2. Cryptosporidiosis
3. Isosporiasis
4. Microsporidiosis
5. Generalized strongyloidiasis

V. **Malignancies**
1. Kaposi's sarcoma
2. B cell lymphoma or non-Hodgkin's lymphoma

VI. **Slim disease**

Laboratory Diagnosis
A. Specific tests for HIV infection
B. Nonspecific tests
C. Tests for opportunistic infections and tumor

A. Specific Tests for HIV Infection
1. **Antigen detection:** The major core antigen p24 is the earliest virus marker to appear in blood. The p24 antigen capture assay (ELISA) can be used for this.
2. **Virus isolation:** It can be isolated from CD4 lymphocytes of peripheral blood, bone marrow and serum.
3. **Detection of viral nucleic acid:** As the most sensitive and specific test, PCR has become the gold standard for diagnosis in all stages of HIV infection. Two forms of PCR have been used, DNA PCR and RNA PCR.
4. **Antibody detection:** Demonstration of antibodies is the simplest and most widely employed technique for the diagnosis of HIV infection. Most individuals will have detectable antibodies within 6–12 weeks after infection, whereas virtually all will be positive within 6 months.

Serological tests for anti-HIV antibodies are of two type-screening and confirmatory tests.

A. Screening Tests
1. **Enzyme-linked immunosorbent assays (ELISA) tests:** HIV-I ELISA tests for HIV infection remain the most sensitive approved commercial assays for infection. ELISA specific for IgM antibody is also available.
2. **Rapid tests:** These tests take less than 30 minutes and do not require expensive equipment. A number of 'rapid tests' have been introduced for this purpose:
   - Dot blot assays
   - Particle agglutination (gelatin, RBC, latex, microbeads)
   - HIV spot and comb tests
   - Fluorometric microparticle technologies
   - Tests using finger-prick blood, saliva and urine have also been developed.
3. **Simple tests:** These tests are not as fast as rapid tests. They take 1–2 hours. They also do not require expensive equipment. These tests are also based on ELISA principle

B. Confirmatory Tests
1. **Western blot test:** In this test, HIV proteins separated according to their electrophoretic mobility by polyacrylamide gel electrophoresis are blotted onto strips of nitrocellulose paper. They retain their relative positions achieved on separation. Each strip is then incubated with a dilution of patient serum. Antibodies which attach to the separated viral antigens on the strip are detected by anti-human immunoglobulin antibody to which enzyme has been attached. Conjugate followed by application of a substrate. The substrate changes color in the presence of enzyme and permanently stains the strip. The location or position on the strip at which a patient's antibodies attach to viral antigens indicates whether antibody is specific for viral antigens (**Fig. 49.2**).

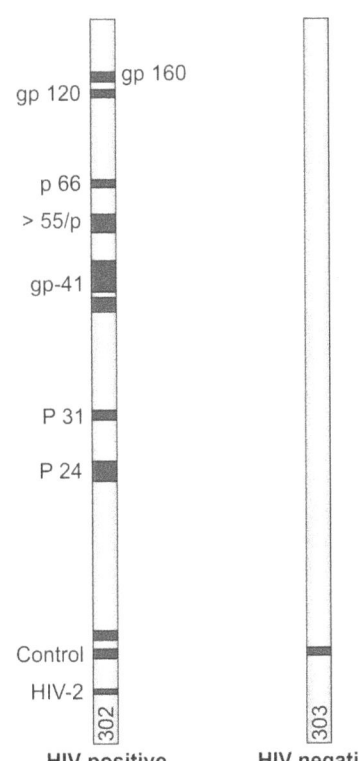

Fig. 49.2: HIV—Western blot test strips (positive and negative).

Interpretation of WB results: Western Blot results are scored as **negative, positive, or indeterminate**.
2. **Immunofluorescence test:** In this test, HIV infected cells are acetone fixed on to glass slides and then reacted with test serum followed by fluorescein conjugated anti-human gammaglobulin. A positive reaction appears as apple-green fluorescence of cell membrane under fluorescence microscope.
Strategies of HIV testing: As the Western blot technique is costly, the practice now is to perform either two different types of ELISA or an ELISA with any of the rapid tests. A serum positive in both tests is considered positive. When in doubt, retesting after 1 or 2 months may be useful.

There are three strategies of HIV testing:
Strategy I: The serum is tested with one E/R (ELISA/rapid) test and if reactive, sample is considered positive and if non-reactive it is considered negative. This strategy is used for transfusion safety.
Strategy IIA: The serum reactive with first E/R (ELISA/rapid) test is retested with a second E/R test based on a different antigen preparation and/or different test principle. If found reactive on second E/R test also, it is reported as positive, otherwise as negative.
Strategy IIB: The serum sample is processed as in strategy IIA, but a sample positive with first E/R test and negative with the second test is subjected to the third E/R test. If third test is positive, sample is considered equivocal.
Strategy III: It is similar to Strategy IIA, with the added confirmation by a third E/R test. The serum reactive with two E/R tests is retested with a third E/R test. The third test should again be based on different antigen preparation or test principle. A serum testing reactive with all three E/R tests is reported positive. A serum sample non-reactive in third E/R/S is considered equivocal/borderline.

B. Nonspecific Tests
Immunological Tests
- Total leukocyte and lymphocyte count to demonstrate leucopenia and a lymphocyte count usually below $2,000/mm^3$.
- T cell subset assays. Absolute CD4+ T cell count will be usually less than $200/mm^3$. T4:T8 cell ratio is reversed.
- Platelet count will show thrombocytopenia.
- Raised IgG and IgA levels.
- Diminished CMI as indicated by skin tests.
- Lymph node biopsy showing profound abnormalities.

C. Tests for Opportunistic Infections and Tumors
Apart from diagnosing HIV infection, the laboratory would be called upon to identify the opportunistic infections that are a feature of AIDS.

Applications of Serological Tests
Serological tests for HIV infection are employed in the following situations:
1. Screening
2. Seroepidemiology
3. Diagnosis
4. Prognosis

Control
1. **Sexual transmission:** The best method of checking sexual transmission of infection is health education regarding the danger of promiscuity and other high-risk activities. The use of condoms and vaginal antiseptics could have an impact.
2. **Exposure to blood:** All blood and blood products are to be screened for HIV. All organ donors must be screened. Occupational risk in the healthcare setting can be controlled by the implementation of safe working practices to prevent accidental injury and contamination with blood and body fluids.
3. **Mother to child transmission:** This can be reduced by identifying infected mothers and giving specific therapy in the later stages of pregnancy and to the baby after birth.

Prophylaxis
No specific vaccine is available.

Treatment

Antiretroviral treatment (ART) is the mainstay in HIV treatment. In the current guidelines, azidothymidine (AZT) is recommended for the treatment of asymptomatic or mildly symptomatic people with CD4 counts of less than 500/µL and for the treatment of infected pregnant women. A cocktail of several antiviral drugs (e.g., AZT, 3TC, protease inhibitor) termed **highly active antiretroviral treatment (HAART)**, has less potential to breed resistance and has become a recommended therapy. Although, HAART is a difficult drug regimen, many patients return to nearly normal on this therapy.

Postexposure Prophylaxis (PEP) Regimen for HIV

In contrast to the earlier recommendation of two antiretroviral drugs, recent guidelines prefer three antiretroviral drugs for PEP, irrespective of the degree of exposure (irrespective of percutaneous or mucous membrane exposure and irrespective of mild, moderate, or severe exposure). *See* Chapter 75 for details.

KEY POINTS

- Human immunodeficiency virus causes AIDS.
- There are three modes of transmission of HIV infection sexual contact, parenteral, and perinatal.

IMPORTANT QUESTIONS

1. Describe the structure and laboratory diagnosis of human immunodeficiency virus.
2. Discuss the modes of transmission and pathogenesis of human immunodeficiency virus (HIV).

MULTIPLE CHOICE QUESTIONS

1. HIV cannot be transmitted by:
   a. Sexual contact
   b. Kissing
   c. Intravenous drug abuse
   d. Blood transfusion
2. Which types of cells are most often infected by HIV?
   a. CD4+T lymphocytes
   b. CD8+T lymphocytes
   c. Null cells
   d. None of the above
3. Which of the following opportunistic parasitic infections is/are associated with HIV infection?
   a. Toxoplasmosis
   b. Cryptosporidiosis
   c. Isosporiasis
   d. All of the above
4. Which of the following tests is/are confirmatory testis for HIV infection?
   a. Virus isolation
   b. Detection of p24 antigen
   c. Detection of viral nucleic acid
   d. All of the above

ANSWERS

1. b   2. a   3. d   4. d

Medical Mycology

SECTION OUTLINE
50. General Properties, Classification and Laboratory Diagnosis of Fungi
51. Superficial, Cutaneous and Subcutaneous Mycoses
52. Systemic Mycoses
53. Opportunistic Mycoses

General Properties, Classification and Laboratory Diagnosis of Fungi

CHAPTER 50

LEARNING OBJECTIVES

After reading and studying this chapter, you should be able to:
- Differentiate between fungi and bacteria.
- Classify fungi.
- Describe laboratory diagnosis of fungal infections.
- Discuss diseases caused by fungi.

INTRODUCTION

Mycology is the study of fungi.

Beneficial effects of fungi: They reside in nature and are essential in breaking down and recycling organic matter, production of food and spirits, have served medicine, as model systems for the investigation. All fungi are eukaryotic protista. Most fungi are obligate or facultative aerobes.

Differences of Fungi from Bacteria

1. They possess rigid cell walls containing chitin, mannan, and other polysaccharides.
2. The cytoplasmic membrane contains sterols.
3. Cytoplasmic contents include mitochondria and endoplasmic reticulum.
4. They possess true nuclei with nuclear membrane and paired chromosomes.
5. They may be unicellular or multicellular.
6. They divide asexually, sexually, or by both processes.

GENERAL PROPERTIES OF FUNGI

Fungi grow in two basic forms, as yeasts and molds.
- **Yeast:** The simplest type of fungus is the unicellular budding yeast.
- **Hypha:** Elongation of the cell produces a tubular, thread-like structure called **hypha**.

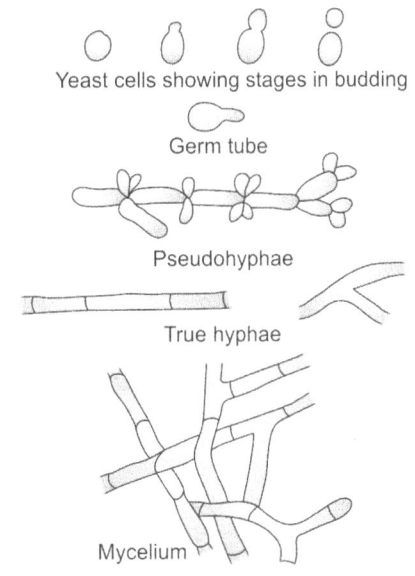

Fig. 50.1: Basic fungal morphology.

- Hyphae may be **septate or nonseptate**.
- **Mycelium:** A tangled mass of hyphae constitutes the **mycelium**. Fungi which form mycelia are called **molds or filamentous fungi (Fig. 50.1)**.

CLASSIFICATION OF FUNGI

Fungi are placed in the **phylum *Thallophyta***. It is divisible into two groups, **algae and fungi**.

A. Morphological Classification

On the basis of morphology, there are four groups of fungi:
1. Yeasts
2. Yeast-like fungi
3. Molds or filamentous fungi
4. Dimorphic fungi

B. Systematic Classification

On the basis of formation of sexual spores, fungi have been divided into four classes.

LABORATORY DIAGNOSIS

Collection and Processing of Specimens

A. Direct Microscopy

I. **Potassium hydroxide (KOH) preparation:** Most specimens can be examined satisfactorily in wet mounts after partial digestion of the tissue with 10–20% KOH.
II. **Potassium hydroxide with calcofluor white:** Addition of calcofluor white and subsequent examination by fluorescence microscopy enhances the detection of most fungi.
III. **Gram stain:** It id used for the diagnosis of yeast infections of mucous membranes.
IV. **India ink:** India ink preparations may be used for detecting encapsulated yeast *Cryptococcus neoformans* in cerebrospinal fluid (CSF).
V. **Histology**

B. Culture

1. **Culture media:** The most common culture media used in mycology Sabouraud's dextrose agar (SDA, pH 5.4). The antimicrobials usually included in SDA with antibiotics are chloramphenicol and gentamicin to inhibit bacterial growth and cycloheximide (actidione) to inhibit saprophytic fungi.
2. **Incubation:** Cultures are routinely incubated in parallel at room temperature 25°C (room temperature for weeks) and at 37°C for days.

C. Identification of Fungi

It is examined for characteristic **gross and microscopic structures**.

D. Serologic Tests

a. **For fungal antibodies** detection
   1. Immunodiffusion
   2. Countercurrent immunoelectrophoresis (CIE)
   3. Whole cell agglutination
   4. Complement fixation
   5. Enzyme-linked immunosorbent assay (ELISA).
b. **For antigen detection:**
   1. Latex particle agglutination
   2. ELISA.

E. Polymerase Chain Reaction (PCR)

Detection of fungal DNA by PCR in clinical material can be used for diagnosis

MYCOSES (FUNGUS INFECTIONS)

Infection caused by fungus is known as mycosis (*Pl. mycoses*).

Classification of Mycoses

Classification of fungal disease according to primary sites of infections are shown in **Table 50.1**.

KEY POINTS

- Mycology is the study of fungi.
- Fungi grow in two basic forms, as **yeasts and molds**.
- **Mycoses (fungus infections):** Infection caused by fungus is known as mycosis (plural—mycoses).

Chapter 50: General Properties, Classification and Laboratory Diagnosis of Fungi

Table 50.1: The major mycoses and causative fungi.

Type of mycosis	Causative fungal agents	Mycosis
A. Superficial	*Malassezia* species *Hortaea werneckii* *Trichosporon* species *Piedraia hortae*	Pityriasis versicolor Tinea nigra White piedra Black piedra
B. Cutaneous	*Microsporum* species, *Trichophyton* species, and *Epidermophyton floccosum* *Candida albicans* and other *Candida* species	Dermatophytosis Candidiasis of skin, mucosa, or nails
C. Subcutaneos	*Sporothrix schenckii* *Phialophora verrucosa, Fonecaea pedrosoi,* others *Pseudallescheria boydii, Madurella mycetomatis,* others *Exophiala, bipolaris, exserohilum,* and others	Sporotrichosis Chromoblastomycosis Mycetoma Phaeohyphomycosis
D. Systemic (primary, endemic)	*Coccidioides immitis, C. posadasii* *Histoplasma capulatum* *Blastomyces dermatitidis* *Paracoccidioides brasiliensis*	Coccidiodomycosis Histoplasmosis Blastomycosis Paracoccidioidomycosis
E. Opportunistic	*Candida albicans* and other *Candida* species *Cryptococcus neoformans* *Aspergillus fumigatus* and other *aspergillus* species Species of *Rhizopus, Absidia, Mucor,* and other *Zygomycets* *Penicillium marneffei*	Systemic candidiasis Cryptococcosis Aspergillosis Mucormycosis (zygomycosis) Penicilliosis

IMPORTANT QUESTIONS

1. Describe the laboratory diagnosis of fungal diseases.
2. Write short notes on classification of fungi.

MULTIPLE CHOICE QUESTIONS

1. All of the following fungi are mold, *except:*
    a. *Aspergillus fumigates*
    b. *Rhizopus*
    c. *Absidia*
    d. *Cryptococcus neoformans*
2. All the following are examples of dimorphic fungi, *except:*
    a. *Coccidioides immitis*
    b. *Cryptococcus neoformans*
    c. *Sporothrix schenkii*
    d. *Blastomyces dermatitidis*
3. Which of the following methods can be used for laboratory diagnosis of fungal infections?
    a. Direct microscopy of specimens
    b. Culture
    c. Histology
    d. All of the above
4. Which of the following culture media can be used for growing fungi?
    a. Sabouraud's dextrose agar
    b. Brain heart infusion agar
    c. Both of the above
    d. None of the above

ANSWERS

1. d   2. b   3. d   4. c

CHAPTER 51: Superficial, Cutaneous and Subcutaneous Mycoses

LEARNING OBJECTIVES

After reading and studying this chapter, you should be able to:
- List superficial, cutaneous, and subcutaneous mycoses.
- Describe causative agents of ectothrix and endothrix.
- Describe the following: Mycetoma; chromoblastomycosis; sporotrichosis; rhinosporidiosis.

A. SUPERFICIAL MYCOSES

These infections are limited to the outermost layers of the skin and hair. These include:
a. **Infection of skin:** It is caused by *Malassezia furfur* (pityriasis versicolor) and *Exophiala werneckii* (tinea nigra)
b. **Infection of hair:** It is caused by *Piedraia hortae* (black piedra) and *Trichosporon beigelii* (white piedra).

B. CUTANEOUS MYCOSES

Dermatophytes

The dermatophytes are a group of closely related filamentous fungi that infect only superficial keratinized tissues—the skin, hair, and nails. The term dermatomycosis is sometimes used as a synonym.

Classification

Dermatophytes have been classified into three genera:
A. **Trichophyton:** Trichophyton species infect hair, skin, or nails.
B. **Microsporum:** Microsporum species infect only hair and skin.
C. **Epidermophyton:** Epidermophyton attacks the skin and nails but not the hair.

Clinical Findings

Dermatophyte infections were mistakenly termed **ringworm or tinea** because of the raised circular lesions.

The clinical forms are based on the site of involvement.

Laboratory Diagnosis

A. **Specimens:** Specimens consist of scrapings from both skin and nails plus hairs.
B. **Microscopic examination:** Specimens are placed on a slide in a drop of 10–20% potassium hydroxide, with or without calcofluor white, viewed with a fluorescent microscope.
C. **Culture:** Specimens are inoculated onto inhibitory mold agar or Sabouraud's agar slant containing cycloheximide and chloramphenicol incubated for 1–3 weeks at room temperature. Species are identified on the basis of colonial morphology (growth rate, surface texture, and any pigmentation), microscopic morphology (macroconidia, microconidia), and, in some cases, nutritional requirements.

Treatment and Prevention

Topical therapy is satisfactory for most skin infections. Oral griseofulvin is useful for scalp, skin, and fingernail infections.

C. SUBCUTANEOUS MYCOSES

The principal subcutaneous mycoses are **mycetoma, chromomycosis, sporotrichosis, and rhinosporidiosis.**

1. Mycetoma

Mycetoma is a chronic, granulomatous infection of the skin, subcutaneous tissues, fascia, and bone, which most often affects the foot or the hand. The disease was originally reported by Gill (1842) from Madurai, south India, and Carter (1860) established its fungal etiology. It is therefore commonly known as Maduramycosis or Madura foot.

In India, it is quite common in Tamil Nadu but rare in Kerala.

Etiology

It can be divided into three types—eumycetomas, actinomycetomas and botryomycosis.

Pathogenesis

Triad of symptoms: Infection follows traumatic inoculation of the organism into the subcutaneous tissue from soil or vegetable sources, usually on thorns or splinters and results in tumefactions, deformities, and draining sinuses discharging fungal colonies called grains or granules (**triad of symptoms**). Subcutaneous tissues of the feet, lower extremities, hands, and exposed areas are most often involved. This process may spread to contiguous muscle and bone.

Grains: Within host tissues the organisms develop to form compacted colonies (grains), the color of which depends on the organism responsible.

Laboratory Diagnosis

The presence of grains in pus collected from draining sinuses or in biopsy material is diagnostic.

Treatment

The management of eumycetoma is difficult, involving surgical debridement or excision and chemotherapy. Actinomycetoma responds well to rifampicin in combination with sulfonamides or cotrimoxazole.

2. Chromoblastomycosis

This disease, also known as *chromomycosis,* is a chronic, localized disease of the skin and subcutaneous tissues, characterized by crusted, warty lesions usually involving the limbs. Like mycetoma, the disease is seen most often among males in rural areas.

3. Sporotrichosis

Sporotrichosis is a chronic, pyogenic granulomatous infection of the skin and subcutaneous tissues which may remain localized or show lymphatic spread.

Causative agent: It is caused by *Sporothrix schenckii,* a saprophyte in nature. Infection is acquired through thorn pricks or other minor injuries.

Laboratory Diagnosis

A. **Microscopic examination:** Direct microscopy is of little importance.
B. **Culture:** Sabouraud dextrose agar (SDA) or blood agar is the media used. *S. schenckii* is a dimorphic fungus occurring in the yeast phase in tissues and in cultures at 37°C, and in the mycelial phase in nature and in cultures at room temperature. The septate hyphae are very thin (1–2 mm diameter) and carry flower-like clusters of small conidia borne on delicate sterigmata (**Fig. 51.1**). Conidia are also produced along the sides of the hyphae.
C. **Serology:** A latex agglutination test.
D. **Skin test** is positive.
E. **Animal inoculation:** Rats are highly susceptible.

4. Rhinosporidiosis

Rhinosporidiosis is a chronic granulomatous disease characterized by the development of large polyps or wart-like lesions in the nose, conjunctiva and occasionally in ears, larynx,

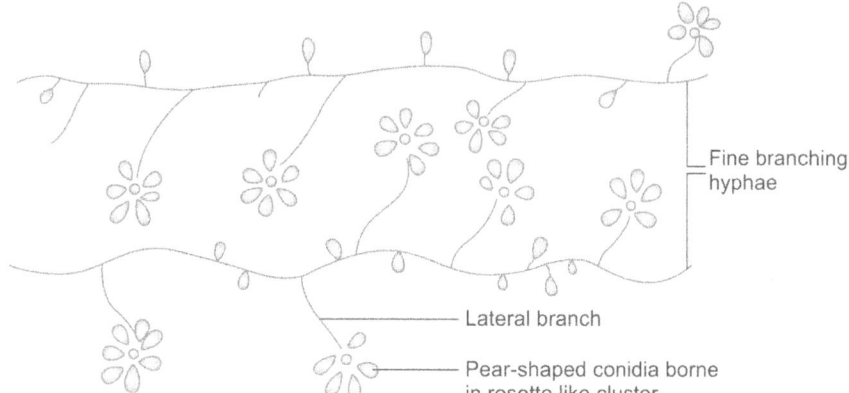

Fig. 51.1: *Sporothrix (Sporotrichum) schenkii*: Culture mounts showing fine branching hyphae and pear-shaped conidia borne in rossette like clusters at tips of lateral branches and singly along sides of hyphae.

bronchus, penile urethra, vagina, rectum, and skin. The large majority of cases come from India and Sri Lanka.

Etiology: The causative fungus *Rhinosporidium seeberi*.

Mode of infection: The mode of infection is not known though infection is believed to originate from stagnant water or aquatic life.

Laboratory Diagnosis

It has not been cultured and animal inoculation is also not successful.

5. Demonstration of Sporangia

Diagnosis depends on the demonstration of sporangia. Direct examination of the surface of the polypoid growth and histologic examination are the only ways to make a diagnosis. *R. seeberi* can be identified in hematoxylin and eosin stained sections, but sometimes one may need special stains. Histologically, the lesion is composed of large numbers of fungal spherules embedded in a stroma of connective tissue and capillaries. The spherules are 10–200 mm in diameter and contain thousands of endospores (6–7 mm in diameter) **(Fig. 51.2)**.

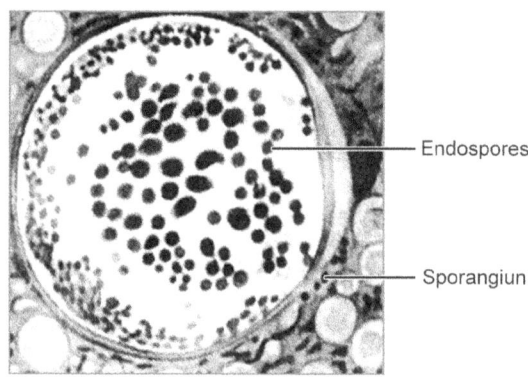

Fig. 51.2: Rhinosporidiosis: Sporangium with numerous endospores.

KEY POINTS

- Cutaneous mycoses
- The dermatophytes infect only superficial keratinized structure.
- **Subcutaneus mycosis**
- **Mycetoma** is a chronic, granulomatous infection of the skin, subcutaneous tissues, fascia and bone, which most often affects the foot or the hand.
- **Sporotrichosis** caused by *Sporothrix schenckii*.
- **Rhinosporidiosis:** The causative fungus is *Rhinosporidium seeberi*.

IMPORTANT QUESTION

1. Write short notes on:
   a. Dermatophytes
   b. Mycetoma or madura foot or maduramycosis
   c. Sporotrichosis
   d. Rhinosporidiosis

MULTIPLE CHOICE QUESTIONS

1. Black piedra is a superficial infection of the hair caused by:
   a. Malassezia furfur
   b. Cladosporium werneckii
   c. Trichosporon beigelli
   d. Piedraia hortae

2. Which of the following fungi has not been cultured?
   a. Sporothrix
   b. Rhinosporidium
   c. Blastomyces
   d. Acremonium

ANSWERS

1. d   2. b

Systemic Mycoses

LEARNING OBJECTIVES

After reading and studying this chapter, you should be able to:
- List of fungi causing systemic infections.
- Describe histoplasmosis.

SYSTEMIC MYCOSES

Systemic mycoses include blastomycosis, coccidioidomycosis, paracoccidioidomycosis, and histoplasmosis.

1. Blastomycosis

Blastomycosis is a chronic infection of the lungs which may spread to other tissues, particularly skin, bone and genitourinary tract.

It is caused by *Blastomyces dermatitidis,* a dimorphic fungus. The disease has been called **North American blastomycosis.**

Morphology

Blastomyces dermatitidis is a dimorphic fungus. In tissue and in cultures at 37°C, the fungus appears as budding yeast cells, which are large and spherical, with thick, double contoured walls. Each cell carries only a single broad-based bud **(Fig. 52.1).** At room temperature, the culture is filamentous with septate hyphae and many round or oval conidia, and in older cultures chlamydospores also.

Pathogenesis

1. Asymptomatic

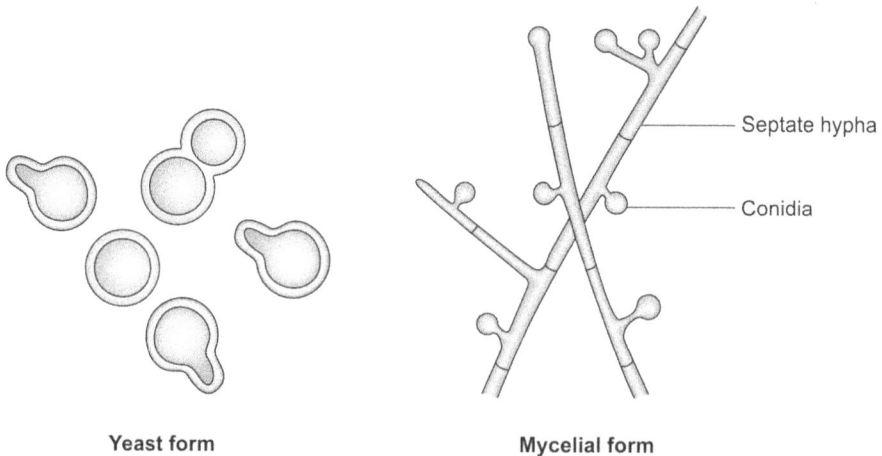

Fig. 52.1: *Blastomyces dermatitidis:* Yeast and mycelial forms.

2. Chronic pneumonia.
3. Disseminated diseases—case fatality is high in the generalized disease.
4. Cutaneous blastomycosis

2. Paracoccidioidomycosis

This is a chronic granulomatous disease of the skin, mucosa, lymph nodes, and internal organs.

Causative fungus: It caused by *Paracoccidioides brasiliensis,* a dimorphic fungus. It is called "South American blastomycosis".

Clinical Manifestations

In the usual case of chronic paracoccidioidomycosis, the yeasts spread from the lung to other organs, particularly the skin and mucocutaneous tissue, lymph nodes, spleen, liver, adrenals, and other sites. Many patients present with painful sores involving the oral mucosa.

Laboratory Diagnosis

1. **Specimens:** Sputum or pus, crusts and biopsies from granulomatous lesions.
2. **Direct microscopy:** Microscopy usually reveals numerous yeast cells with multiple buds, which is diagnostic **(Figs. 52.2A and B).**

3. **Culture:** *P. brasiliensis* grows in the mycelial phase in culture at 25–30°C, and in the yeast phase in tissue or at 37°C.

3. Coccidioidomycosis

This is primarily an infection of the lungs caused by *Coccidioides immitis,* a dimorphic fungus.

Morphology

The fungus is dimorphic, occurring in the tissue as yeast and in culture as the mycelial form. In culture and in soil *C. immitis* grows as a mold, producing large numbers of barrel-shaped arthrospores (4 × 6 µm diameter) which are highly infectious **(Figs. 52.3A and B).**

The yeast form is a spherule with a thick, doubly refractile wall and filled with endospores. Endospores are released by rupture of the spherule wall and develop to form new spherules **(Fig. 52.4).**

Clinical Features

1. An asymptomatic or self-limiting pulmonary illness.
2. A self-limited influenza-like illness called **valley fever, San Joaquin Valley fever, or desert rheumatism.**
3. Chronic progressive disseminated disease (coccidioidal granuloma).

4. Histoplasmosis

Histoplasmosis is an intracellular infection of the reticuloendothelial system caused by the dimorphic fungus *Histoplasma capsulatum.*

Pathogenesis

Infection is acquired by inhalation. Most infections are asymptomatic.

1. **Pulmonary infection:** The clinical picture closely resembles tuberculosis.
2. **Disseminated histoplasmosis:** The reticuloendothelial system is involved with resultant lymphadenopathy, hepatosplenomegaly, fever, anemia, and a high rate of fatality.
3. **Skin and mucosa:** Granulomatous and ulcerative lesions may develop on the skin and mucosa.

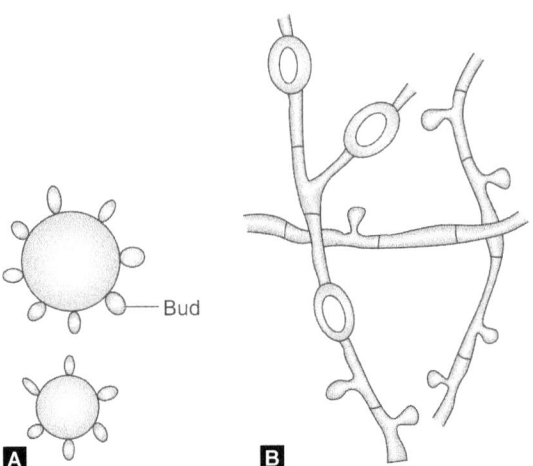

Figs. 52.2A and B: *Paracoccidioides brasiliensis.* (A) Yeast phase; (B) Mycelial phase.

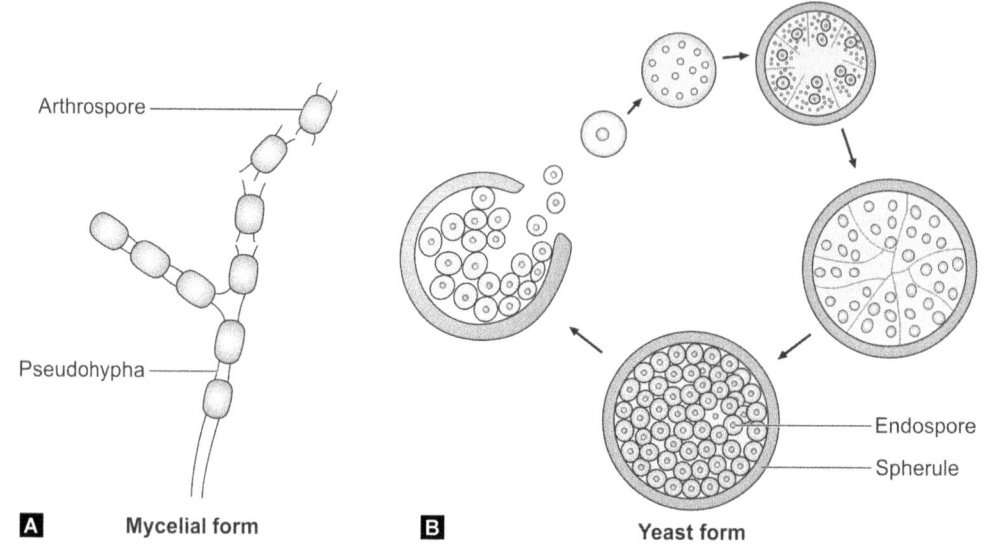

Figs. 52.3A and B: *Coccidioides immitis*: (A) Arthrospores formation; (B) Spherule formation with endospores.

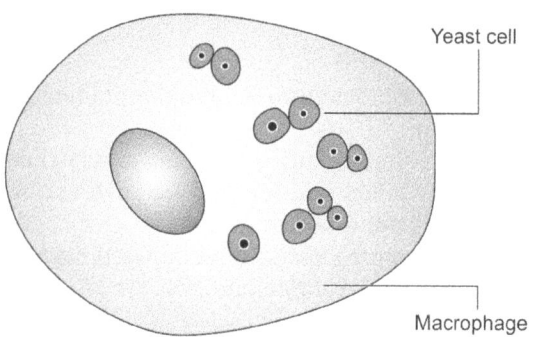

Fig. 52.4: *H. capsulatum*: Yeast cells in macrophage.

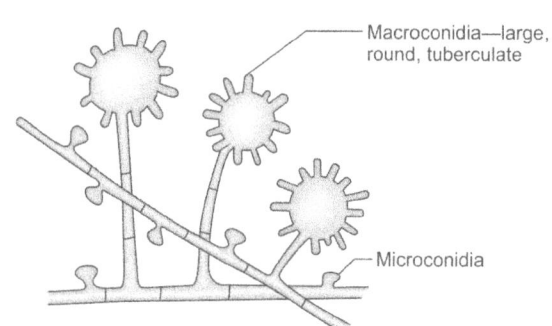

Fig. 52.5: *H. capsulatum*: Mycelial form.

4. **Oral manifestations:** The nodular, ulcerative or vegetative oral lesions may be present on the buccal mucosa, lips, gingiva, and tongue to palate.

Laboratory Diagnosis

1. **Specimens:** Blood films, bone marrow slides, and biopsy specimens may be examined microscopically.
2. **Culture:** The yeast phase cells is produced in culture at 37°C. On SDA, the mold colonies are white to tan fluffy with septate branching hyphae with two types of unicellular, asexual spores.
   a. Large round, **tuberculate macroconidia** (8–14 µm in diameter) are most prominent and are diagnostic.
   b. Small spores or microconidia are also present **(Fig. 52.5)**.
3. **Serological tests:** Agglutination, precipitation, and complement fixation. Tests for antigen detection by radioimmunoassay or ELISA are useful.
4. **Histoplasmin skin test:** The test is similar to tuberculin test but antigen used is histoplasmin.

KEY POINTS

- **Blastomycosis:** Blastomycosis is caused by *Blastomyces dermatitidis*.
- **Coccidioidomycosis** is caused by *Coccidioides immitis*, a dimorphic fungus.
- **Histoplasmosis:** Histoplasmosis is caused by an intracellular fungus *Histoplasma capsulatum*, a dimorphic fungus.

IMPORTANT QUESTION

1. Write short notes on:
   a. Dimorphic fungi
   b. Histoplasmosis

MULTIPLE CHOICE QUESTIONS

1. All the following statements are true for spherule of *Coccidioides immitis*, except:
   a. It is infective stage of the fungus
   b. It reproduces by endosporulation
   c. It contains endospores
   d. It is not found in culture
2. Which of the following fungi infects reticuloendothelial system?
   a. *Aspergillus fumigatus*
   b. *Histoplasma capsulatum*
   c. *Trichophyton rubrum*
   d. All of the above
3. The diagnostic form of *Histoplasma capsulatum* is:
   a. Arthrospore
   b. Spherule
   c. Macroconidia
   d. Microconidia

ANSWERS

1. a   2. b   3. c

Chapter 53: Opportunistic Mycoses

LEARNING OBJECTIVES

After reading and studying this chapter, you should be able to:
- Describe diseases caused by *Candida albicans*.
- Describe the following: Thrush or oral thrush; Germ tube test or Reynolds–Braude phenomenon
- Discuss laboratory diagnosis of candidiasis.
- List opportunistic fungi.
- Discuss cryptococcosis.
- Discuss laboratory diagnosis of *Cryptococcus neoformans*.
- Describe species of *Aspergillus*.
- Describe the following: Aspergillosis; mucormycosis; pneumocystosis.

OPPORTUNISTIC FUNGI

Patients with compromised host defenses are susceptible to ubiquitous fungi, are referred to as **opportunistic fungi**.

Causative Fungal Agents

A. Yeast and yeast-like fungi (*Cryptococcus, Candida spp., torulopsis*)
B. Filamentous fungi (*Aspergillus, Mucor, Absidia, Rhizopus, Cephalosporium, Fusarium, Penicillium, Geotrichum, Scopulariopsis*)
C. Others: *Pneumocystis carinii*.

YEAST-LIKE FUNGI

Candidiasis

Candidosis (candidiasis, moniliasis) is an infection of the skin, mucosa, and rarely of the internal organs, caused by a yeast-like fungus *Candida albicans*, and occasionally by other *Candida* species. Candidosis is an opportunistic endogenous infection, the most common predisposing factor being diabetes.

Morphology

In culture or tissue, candida species grow as oval, budding yeast cells (3-6 µm in size). They also form pseudohyphae **(Fig. 53.1)**.

Species of Candida

Important species of *Candida* found in man are: (i) *C. albicans*; (ii) *C. stellatoidea*; (iii) *C. tropicalis*; (iv) *C. krusei*; (v) *C. guilliermondii*.

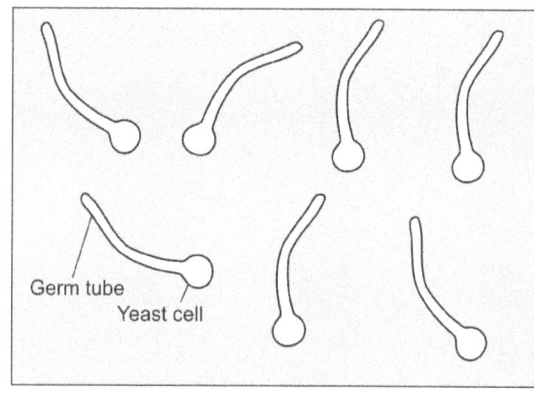

Fig. 53.1: *Candida albicans* showing germ tubes.

(vi) *C. parapsilosis*; (vii) *C. glabrata* (viii) *C. viswanathii*.

Pathogenesis

The risk factors associated with superficial candidiasis include acquired immunodeficiency syndrome (AIDS), pregnancy, diabetes, young or old age, birth control pills, and trauma (burns, maceration of the skin). Lesions caused by candida are as follows:

a. Mucocutaneous Lesions
- Oral thrush
- Vulvovaginitis
- Balanitis
- Conjunctivitis
- Keratitis

b. Skin and Nail Infections
i. *Intertriginous infection:* Intertriginous infection occurs in moist, warm parts of the body such as the axillae, groin, and intergluteal or inframammary folds.
ii. *Interdigital involvement:* Interdigital involvement between the fingers follows repeated prolonged immersion in water.
iii. *Onychomycosis:* Candidal invasion of the nails and around the nail plate causes onychomycosis. Paronychia and onychia are seen in occupations that lead to frequent immersion of the hands in water.
iv. *Napkin dermatitis:* In infants it may lead to napkin dermatitis.

c. Systemic Candidiasis
- *Intestinal candidosis:* It is a frequent sequel to oral antibiotic therapy and may present as diarrhea not responding to treatment.
- Bronchopulmonary candidosis
- Septicemia
- Endocarditis
- Meningitis
- Kidney infections
- Urinary tract infections

d. Oral Manifestations
Various manifestations of candidiasis are as follows:

- Thrush
- Chronic oral candidiasis
- Chronic mucocutaneous candidiasis
- Angular stomatitis (angular cheilitis)
- Circumoral candidal dermatitis

Thrush (*Pseudomembrane candidiasis*): The lesions are, soft, white slightly elevated plaques frequently occurring on the buccal mucosa of tongue, but may also be seen on the gingiva, palate and floor of the mouth. In severe cases, the entire oral cavity may be affected. Thrush is very common in patients with human immunodeficiency virus (HIV) infection or in cancer patents undergoing chemotherapy or radiotherapy. Infection may also be seen in neonates and infants due to incompletely developed immune system. It is also common in debilitated and chronically ill persons.

Laboratory Tests

Diagnosis can be established by microscopy and culture.

A. **Specimens:** Specimens include swabs and scrapings from superficial lesions, blood, spinal fluid, tissue biopsies, urine, exudates, and material from removed intravenous catheters.
B. **Direct microscopy:** Wet films or Gram stained smears from lesions or exudates show budding gram positive cells. Skin or nail scrapings are first placed in a drop of 10% potassium hydroxide (KOH) and calcofluor white.
C. **Culture:** Cultures are obtained on Sabouraud's dextrose agar (SDA) and on ordinary bacteriological culture media, e.g., blood agar at room temperature or at 37°C. Colonies are creamy white, smooth, and with a yeasty odor. Gram stained smear from colonies shows gram positive budding yeast cells.
D. **Identification:** *C. albicans* is identified by the production of germ tubes or chlamydospores. Other candida isolates are speciated with a battery of biochemical reactions.

1. **Germ tube test:** *C. albicans* has ability to form germ tubes within two hours when incubated in human serum at 37°C *(Reynolds-Braude phenomenon)*.
2. **Chlamydospores**
3. **Carbohydrate fermentation and carbohydrate assimilation tests**

E. **Serology** using a latex agglutination test or an enzyme immunoassay.

F. **Skin test**

CRYPTOCOCCOSIS

Cryptococcosis is subacute or chronic infection caused by the capsulate yeast *Cryptococcus neoformans*. It is most frequently recognized as a disease of the central nervous system (CNS), although the primary site of infection is the lungs.

Morphology

Microscopically, in culture or clinical material, *C. neoformans* is a spherical budding yeast (5–10 µm in diameter), surrounded by a thick polysaccharide capsule **(Fig. 53.2)**.

Serotypes

Adsorbed antisera have defined five serotypes (A-D and AD) and three varieties. *C. neoformans* var. *grubii* (serotype A), *C. neoformans* var. *neoformans* (serotype D), and *C. neoformans* var. *gattii* (serotype B or C).

Pathogenesis

Infection is usually acquired by inhalation. The primary pulmonary infection may be asymptomatic or may mimic an influenza-like respiratory infection, often resolving spontaneously. Pulmonary cryptococcosis may lead to a mild pneumonitis.

Cryptococcal meningitis is the most serious type of infection. It is often seen in AIDS. Lesions of the skin, mucosa, viscera, and bones may also occur. In its disseminated form, the disease may resemble tuberculosis. Visceral forms simulate tuberculosis and cancer clinically. Bones and joints may be involved. Cutaneous cryptococcosis varies from small ulcers to large granulomas.

Laboratory Diagnosis

A. **Specimens:** Specimens include spinal fluid, tissue, exudates, sputum, blood, and urine.
B. **Microscopic examination—India ink or nigrosine preparation:** Specimens are examined in wet mounts, both directly and after mixing with India ink. In unstained, wet preparations of CSF mixed with a drop of India ink or nigrosine, the capsule can be seen as a clear halo around the yeast cells **(Fig. 53.2)**.
C. **Culture:** On Sabouraud agar (without cycloheximide) cultured at 25–30°C and 37°C, colonies normally appear within 2–3 days. In culture, *C. neoformans* appears as smooth, mucoid, cream colored colonies. Cultures can be identified by growth at 37°C and detection of urease.
D. **Serological tests:** Cryptococcal capsular polysaccharide antigen can be detected in CSF and blood by latex agglutination and ELISA test.
E. **Animal inoculation test:** Intracerebral or intraperitoneal inoculation into mice leads to a fatal infection in case of *C. neoformans*. Capsulated budding yeast cells can be

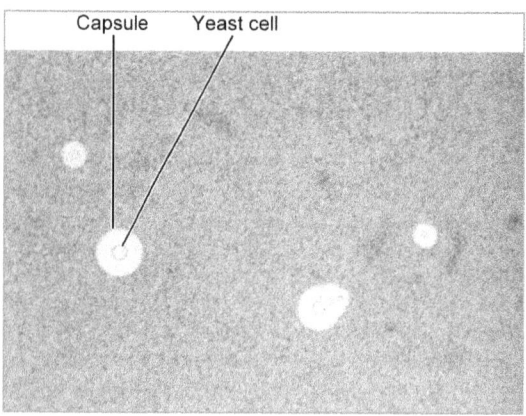

Fig. 53.2: *Cryptococcus neoformans:* India ink preparation of spinal fluid showing yeast cells surrounded by a large capsule.

demonstrated in the brain of the infected mice.

ASPERGILLOSIS

Aspergillosis is a spectrum of diseases that may be caused by a number of aspergillus species. The most important species are *A. fumigatus, A. niger, A. flavus, A. terreus,* and *A. nidulans.*

Pathogenesis

This mold produces abundant small conidia that are easily aerosolized. Following inhalation of these conidia, atopic individuals often develop severe allergic reactions to the conidial antigens. In immunocompromised patients the conidia may germinate to produce hyphae that invade the lungs and other tissues.
A. Localized infections—may involve the nasal sinuses, the ear canal, the cornea, or the nails.
B. Systemic aspergillosis
   1. **Pulmonary aspergillosis**
      a. Allergic asthma
      b. Bronchopulmonary aspergillosis
      c. Colonizing aspergillosis (Aspergilloma)
   2. **Invasive aspergillosis:** The fungus actively invades the lung tissue.
   3. **Endocarditis**
   4. **Paranasal granuloma**

Laboratory Diagnosis

A. **Specimens:** Sputum, other respiratory specimens, or lung biopsy tissue provide good specimens.
B. **Microscopic examination**: On direct examination of sputum with KOH or calcofluor white or in histologic sections, the fungus appears as nonpigmented septate mycelium, with characteristic dichotomous branching and an irregular outline.
In tissue sections *Aspergillus* species are best seen after staining with PAS or methenamine-silver.
C. **Culture**: *Aspergillus* species grow readily on Sabouraud's dextrose agar (SDA) without cycloheximide at 25–37°C. Colonies appear after 1–2 days.
Aspergillus fumigatus: The colonies of *A. fumigatus* are granular to cottony and usually have some shades of green, green-gray or green-brown pigmentation.
Aspergillus niger: The surface of the colonies of *A. niger* is covered by a dense aggregate of jet black conidia.
Lactophenol cotton blue preparation: Species are identified according to the morphology of their conidial structures. Asexual conidia are arranged in chains, carried on elongated cells called 'sterigmata', borne on the expanded ends (vesicles) of conidiophores **(Figs. 53.3A to D)**.
D. **Skin tests**
E. **Serological tests:** Immunodiffusion, counter immunoelectrophoresis (CIE), and ELISA
F. **Polymerase chain reaction (PCR)**

MUCORMYCOSES (ZYGOMYCOSIS, SYSTEMIC PHYCOMYCOSIS)

Mucormycosis is an opportunistic mycosis caused by a number of molds classified in the **order Mucorales of the class Zygomycetes.** The leading pathogens among this group of fungi are species of the genera *Rhizopus, Rhizomucor, Absidia, Cunninghamella,* and *Mucor.* These fungi are ubiquitous thermotolerant saprophytes.

PENICILLIOSIS

There are more than 150 known species of the genus *Penicillium*. Except for infections caused by *Penicillium marnefeii*, the role other species of *Penicillium* have in infections of the clinical entity penicilliosis is difficult to confirm **(Fig. 53.4)**.

Pathogenesis

It causes penicillosis, keratitis, otomycosis, and rarely deep infections. *Penicillium marneffei* causes serious disseminated disease with characteristic papular skin lesions in AIDS

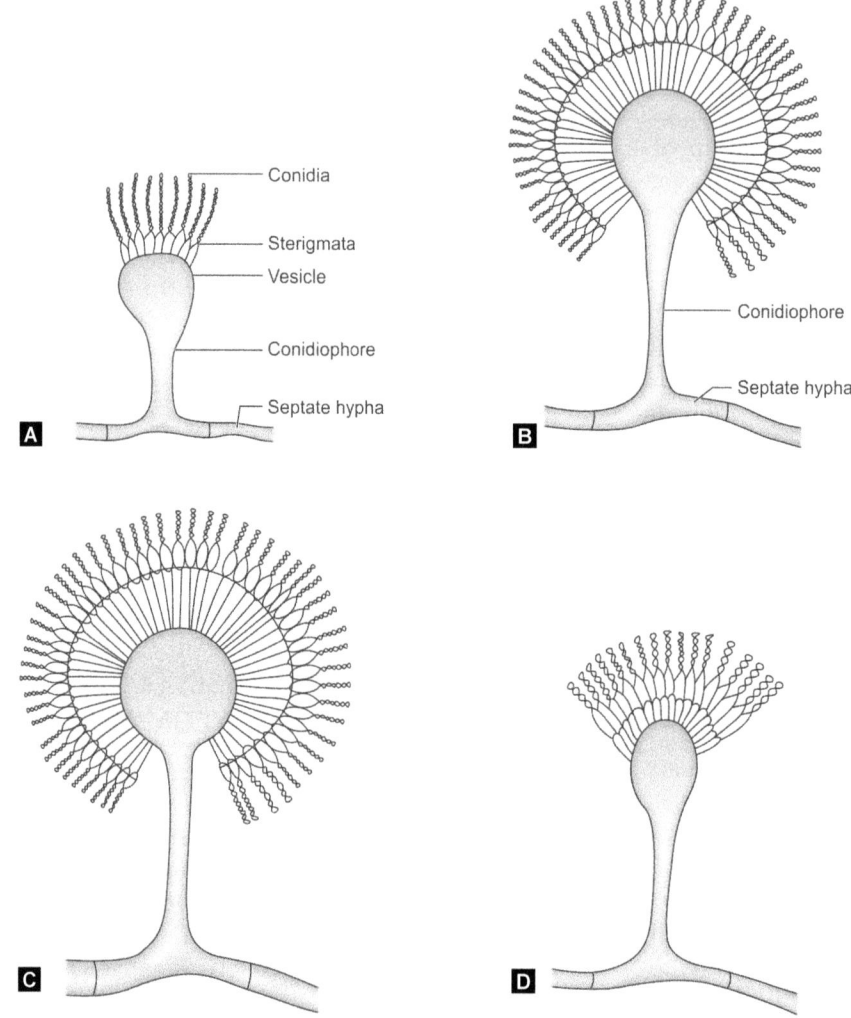

Figs. 53.3A to D: *Aspergillus* spp.: (A) *A. fumigatus*; (B) *A. flavus*; (C) *A. niger*; and (D) *A. terreus*.

patients in South-east Asia. Cutaneous lesions and subcutaneous abscesses have been reported.

PNEUMOCYSTOSIS

Pneumexystis jiroveci, previously known as *Pneumexystis carinii*, is the causative agent of *Pneumocystis carinii* pneumonia (PCP). Transmission of infection occurs by inhalation. PCP is the most common opportunistic infection in HIV-patients.

KEY POINTS

- Candidosis caused by a yeast-like fungus *Candida albicans*.
- Cryptococcosis is subacute or chronic infection caused by the capsulate yeast *Cryptococcus neoformans*.

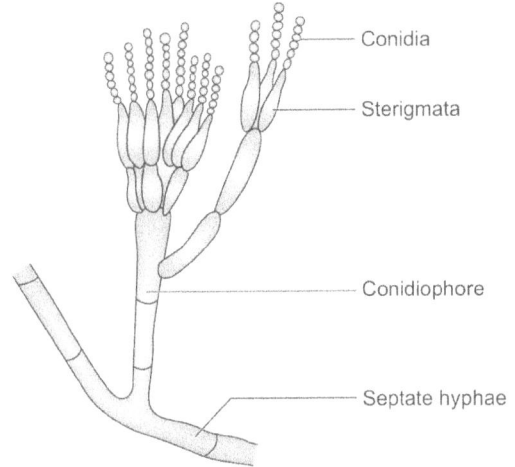

Fig. 53.4: Penicillium.

- **Aspergillosis:** The *species most* frequently involved in human infections are *A. fumigatus, A. flovus,* and *A. niger.*

IMPORTANT QUESTION

1. Write short notes on:
   a. Candidiasis, Candidosis, or Moniliasis
   b. Cryptococcosis
   c. Opportunistic systemic mycoses
   d. Aspergillosis
   e. Opportunistic fungi

MULTIPLE CHOICE QUESTIONS

1. Which of the following species of *Candida* is most frequently responsible for human infections?
   a. *Candida albicans*
   b. *C. krusei*
   c. *C. glabrata*
   d. *C. stellatoidea*

2. ***Candida albicans* can be differentiated from other species of candida by:**
   a. Germ tube test
   b. Chlamydospore formation on corn meal agar
   c. Carbohydrate fermentation and assimilation tests
   d. All of the above

3. Which of the following fungi is capsulated?
   a. *Aspergillus fumigatus*
   b. *Cryptococcus neoformans*
   c. *Candida albicans*
   d. None of the above

4. ***Cryptococcus neoformans* shows all the following features, *except*:**
   a. It assimilates inositol
   b. It assimilates lactose
   c. It produces urease
   d. It produces melanin

5. Which of the following fungi is/are associated with zygomycosis?
   a. *Mucor*
   b. *Rhizopus*
   c. *Absidia*
   d. All of the above

ANSWERS

1. a   2. d   3. b   4. c
5. d

Medical Parasitology

SECTION OUTLINE
54. Protozoology
55. Helminthology

Protozoology

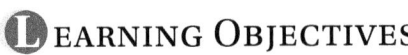

After reading and studying this chapter, you should be able to:
- Describe pathogenesis, clinical symptoms, and laboratory diagnosis of *Entamoeba histolytica* and *Giardia lamblia*.
- Discuss the life cycle and the laboratory diagnosis of kala-azar.
- Describe the life cycle of malarial parasite.
- Differentiate features of different plasmodia of man.
- Describe the following: Pernicious malaria; Blackwater fever; laboratory diagnosis of malaria.

INTRODUCTION

Medical parasitology: Medical parasitology deals with parasites, which infect and disease they produce in human beings.

Parasite: A parasite is a living organism which depends on a living host for its survival and derives nutrition from the host, without giving any benefit to the host.

Host: It is defined as an organism which harbors the parasite. Different types of host are as follows:
1. **Definitive host:** It is the host that harbors the adult stage of the parasite or where the parasite replicates sexually.
2. **Intermediate host:** It is the host that harbors the larval stages of the parasite or where the parasite replicates asexually.
3. **Reservoir host:** It is the host that harbors the parasite and acts as an important source of infection.

CLASSIFICATION OF PARASITES

Parasites are classified into protozoa and helminthes. A classification of medically important protozoa and helminthes is given in Table 54.1.

PROTOZOA

Table 54.1 lists the clinically significant members of these groups.

Table 54.1: Classification of medically important protozoa and helminths.

Group	Examples
A. Protozoa (unicellular)	
1. Amoebae	*Entamoeba histolytica* *E. coli* *E. gingivalis*
2. Flagellates	*Giardia lamblia* *Trichomonas vaginalis* *Leishmania* sp.
3. Sporozoa	*Plasmodium vivax* *P. falciparum* *Toxoplasma gondii*
4. Ciliates	*Balantidium coli*
B. Helminths (multicellular)	
1. Cestodes (tapeworms)	*Taenia* sp., *Echinococcus* sp.
2. Nematodes (roundworms)	Roundworm, hookworm, threadworm
3. Trematodes (flukes)	*Fasiola* sp., *Schistosoma* sp.

ENTAMOEBA HISTOLYTICA

Entamoeba histolytica is worldwide in distribution. It is more common in tropics and subtropical countries than in the temperate zone. It lives in the large intestine of man.

Morphology

Entamoeba histolytica occurs in three forms: trophozoite, precystic, and cyst stage (**Fig. 54.1**).

Trophozoite

Size ranges from 18 to 40 μm (average 20–30 μm) in diameter.

The cytoplasm of the trophozoite is divided into two portions—a clear outer *ectoplasm* and a granular *endoplasm*. Red blood cells, occasionally leukocytes and tissue debris are found inside the cytoplasm. Typical amoeboid motility is a crawling or gliding movement and not a free-swimming one.

The nucleus is spherical in shape, and varying in size from 4–6 μm. In stained preparations the nuclear structure shows: (1) **karyosome**, small dot-like, central in position, and surrounded by a clear halo, (2) **nuclear membrane,** delicate and lined with a single layer of uniformly distributed fine chromatin granules and (3) the space between the karyosome and the nuclear membrane is traversed by a fine thread of **linin network** having a spoke-like radial arrangement.

Precystic Stage

It is smaller in size, varying from **10 to 20 μm**. It is round or slightly ovoid with a blunt pseudopodium. The nuclear structure has same characteristics as of the trophozoite.

Cyst: It is round, 10–15 μm in diameter and is surrounded by a highly refractile membrane, called the cyst wall. A mature cyst is a quadrinucleate spherical body. Nuclear structure is similar to that of trophozoite. It starts as a uninucleate body but soon divides by binary fission and develops into two and then four nuclei. The early cyst (uninucleate and binucleate bodies) contains one to four chromatoid or chromidial bar and a glycogen mass. Chromatoid or chromidial bars do not

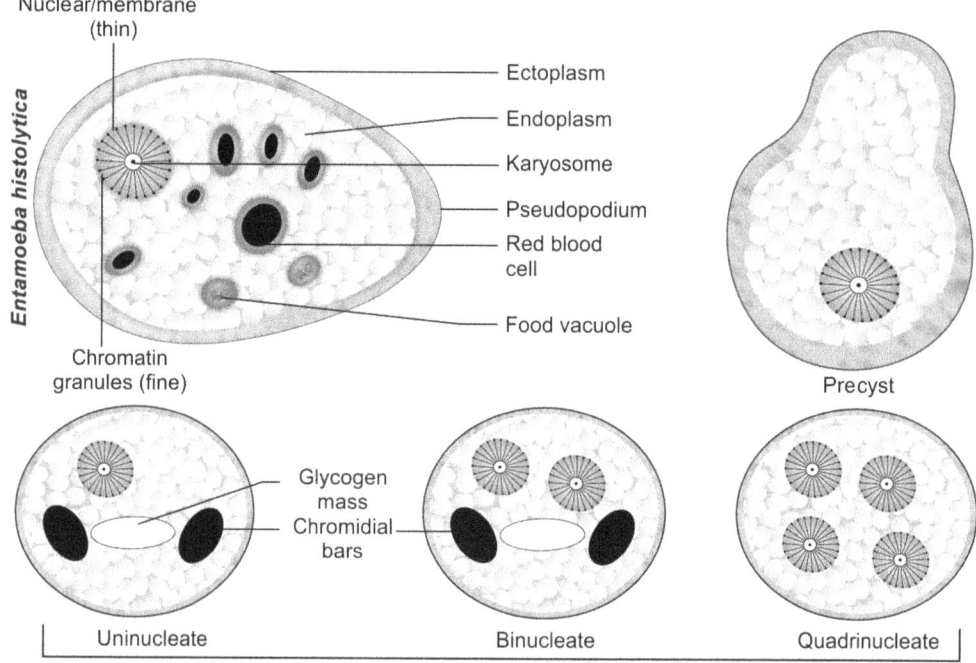

Fig. 54.1: Different morphological forms of *Entamoeba histolytica*.

stain with iodine but are seen as refractile oblong bars with rounded ends in preparations with normal saline and as black when stained with iron—hematoxylin. Glycogen mass stains brown with iodine. Both the glycogen mass and the chromidial bars gradually disappear as the cyst matures from uninucleate to the quadrinucleate stage.

Life Cycle

Entamoeba histolytica passes its life cycle (**Fig. 54.2**) only in one host, the man. The mature quadrinucleate cysts are the infective forms of the parasite. The cysts ingested in contaminated food or water pass through the stomach undamaged and enter the small intestine. The *excystation* occurs when the cyst reaches the cecum or the lower part of the ileum. When the reaction of the surrounding *medium* becomes alkaline, the cyst-wall is damaged by trypsin in the intestine, leading to *excystation*. During this process, the cytoplasm gets detached from the cyst wall and amoeboid movements appear, causing a tear in the cyst wall, through which cyst liberates a single amoeba with four nuclei, a *tetranucleate amoeba* which eventually produces eight *metacystic trophozoites* by the division of nuclei with successive fission of cytoplasm. The young amoebulae are actively motile and invade the tissues and ultimately lodge in the submucous tissue of the large gut, their normal habitat. Here, they grow and multiply by binary fission. The characteristic lesion of amebiasis is due to the trophozoite phase of the parasite. During growth, *E. histolytica* secretes a proteolytic enzyme which brings about destruction and necrosis of tissues leading to **flask-shaped ulcers**.

The tissue invading amoebae gradually recede from the dead tissues toward the margin of healthy ones and in this way the trophozoites of *E. histolytica*, entering into deeper layers and may sometimes actually find their way into the radicles of the portal vein to be carried away to the liver. Those parasites that remain in the intestinal wall may cause an attack of acute dysentery (ulcerative colitis) in which a large number of trophozoites are discharged along with the slough. In the liver, they multiply and produce amebic hepatitis and amebic liver abscess.

The lesions become quiescent and commence to heal after some time, when the effect of the parasite on the host is gradually toned down together with the concomitant increase in the tolerance of the host. A certain number of trophozoites are discharged into the lumen of the bowel and are transformed into small precystic forms from which the cysts are developed, which are passed in feces to repeat the cycle (**Fig. 54.2**).

Pathogenesis and Clinical Features

The term *"amebiasis"* is used clinically to denote all those conditions which are produced in the human host by infection with *E. histolytica*. The incubation period is from 1 to 4 months. Amebiasis can be classified as **intestinal (primary)** and **extraintestinal (metastatic) amebiasis.**

i. **Intestinal amebiasis**: The typical manifestation of intestinal amebiasis is *amebic dysentery*. The amoebae produce characteristic ulcerative lesions and profuse bloody diarrhea. The lesions may be generalized or localized (ileocecal region and sigmoidorectal region are involved).

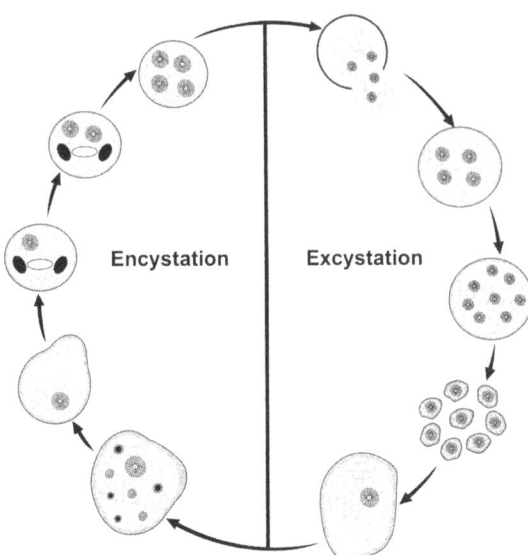

Fig. 54.2: Life cycle of *Entamoeba histolytica*.

ii. **Extraintestinal amebiasis:** Hepatic involvement is the most common extra-intestinal complication of amoebiasis. Hepatic invasion is multifocal, the right lobe being more affected. There is also an *enlargement of the liver is known as **amebic hepatitis**.* One or more of the lesions in the liver may extend peripherally to develop into *amebic abscesses*. The center of the abscess contains thick chocolate brown pus (**"anchovy sauce pus"**).

Involvement of distant organs is by haematogenous spread such as **the brain, spleen, adrenals, and kidneys**.

Pleuropulmonary amebiasis usually follows extension of hepatic abscess through the diaphragm.

Laboratory Diagnosis

Definitive diagnosis of amebiasis depends on the demonstration of *E. histolytica* in tissues or discharges from the lesions such as stool, pus of liver abscess and sputum.

Intestinal Amebiasis

A. **Examination of stool**

Acute amebic dysentery: The stool sample has to be inspected for macroscopic and microscopic features. The disease has to be differentiated from bacillary dysentery (Table 54.2).

a. **Macroscopic appearance:** The stool is copious, semiliquid, brownish black in color and contains foul smelling fecal

Table 54.2: Differences between amebic and bacillary dysentery.

Character	Amoebic dysentery	Bacillary dysentery
A. Clinical		
1. Onset	Slow	Acute
2. Fever	Absent	Present
3. Toxicity	Absent	Present
4. Abdominal tenderness	Localized	Generalized
5. Tenesmus	Absent	Present
B. Stool		
a. Macroscopic		
1. Number	6–8 motions a day	Over 10 motions a day
2. Amount	Copious	Small
3. Odor	Offensive	Odorless
4. Color	Dark red	Bright red
5. Reaction	Acidic	Alkaline
6. Consistency	Not adherent to container	Adherent to the container
b. Microscopic		
1. RBCs	In clumps, yellowish brown	Discrete, sometimes in clumps due to rouleaux formation, bright red
2. Pus cells	Few	Numerous
3. Macrophages	Few	Numerous, many of them contain RBCs hence may be mistaken for *Entamoeba histolytica*
4. Eosinophils	Present	Scarce
5. Charcot-Leyden crystals	Present	Absent
6. Pyknotic bodies	Present	Absent
7. Ghost cells	Absent	Present
8. Parasites	Trophozoites of *E. histolytica*	Absent
9. Bacteria	Many motile bacteria	Few or absent

material intermingled with blood and mucus. It is acid in reaction. It does not adhere to the container.
   b. **Microscopic appearance**: The cellular exudate is scanty and consists of a few pus cells, macrophages and epithelial cells. The red cells are clumped and yellowish or brownish red in color. **Charcot-Leyden crystals** are often present, they appear as diamond-shaped crystals, clear, and refractile.
   Demonstration of *E. histolytica*: In freshly passed motion unmixed with urine or antiseptics, actively motile trophozoites of *E. histolytica* can be demonstrated in unstained films.
B. **Blood examination** shows moderate leukocytosis.
C. **Serological tests:** Serology is usually negative in early cases and in the absence of deep invasion

Diagnosis of Hepatic Amebiasis (Amebic Liver Abscess)

1. **Diagnostic aspiration:** The aspirated "pus" may be examined for the demonstration of trophic forms of *E. histolytica*.
2. **Liver biopsy:** Trophozoite forms *E. histolytica* may be demonstrated in specimens of liver biopsy taken from cases of amebic hepatic abscess.
3. **Stool examination:** Cysts of *E. histolytica* are present in less than 15% cases of amebic liver abscess.
4. **Blood examination:** It shows leukocytosis.
5. **Serological tests (immunological diagnosis):** The various serological tests which may be used as immunodiagnostic methods are the indirect **hemagglutination (IHA), latex agglutination (LA), gel diffusion precipitation (GDP), counter-current immunoelectrophoresis (CIE), and enzyme-linked immunosorbent assay (ELISA)**.
6. **Intradermal test**.
7. **Radiological examination**. The right dome of the diaphragm is generally found to be situated at a higher level.

ENTAMOEBA COLI

Entamoeba coli is worldwide in distribution. It is a nonpathogenic commensal intestinal amoeba and lives in the lumen of large intestine. Its medical importance is that it has to be differentiated from *E. histolytica*. *Entamoeba coli* also exist mainly in two stages, i.e., trophozoite, and cyst and a transitory stage of precystic form.

Differences between *E. histolytica* and *E. coli* are shown in **Table 54.3**.

FLAGELLATES

Depending on their habitat, flagellates can be considered under two headings:
1. **Intestinal flagellates:** Found in the alimentary and urogenital tracts.
   Hemoflagellates—flagellates found in blood and tissues.

Table 54.3: Differential features of intestinal entamoebae.

Trophozoite	E. histolytica	E. coli
Size (μm)	20–30	20–40
Motility	Active	Sluggish
Cytoplasm	Clearly defined into ectoplasm and endoplasm	Differentiation into ectoplasm and endoplasm indistinct
Cytoplasmic inclusions	Red blood cells, leukocytes and tissue debris; no bacteria	Bacteria and other particles; no red blood cells
Nucleus	Not clearly visible in unstained films	Visible in unstained films
Karyosome	Small, central	Large, eccentric
Nuclear membrane	Delicate, with fine chromatin dots	Thick, with coarse chromatin granules

2. **Intestinal flagellates:** The flagellates of clinical significance include *Giardia lamblia (duodenalis), Dientamoeba fragilis,* and *Trichomonas vaginalis.*

GIARDIA LAMBLIA (GIARDIA INTESTINALIS)

Geographical distribution: It is worldwide in distribution.

Habitat: It lives in the duodenum and upper jejunum.

Morphology

Giardia has a simple life cycle, existing in the two phases—**trophozoite and cyst (Fig. 54.3).**

Trophozoite: It has been described variously as pyriform, heart-shaped or racket shaped. The vegetative form or *trophozoite* is rounded anteriorly and pointed posteriorly. Dorsal surface is convex and ventral surface is concave with a *sucking disk,* which occupies almost the entire anterior half of the body. The size of the trophozoite is 14 μm long and 7 μm broad. It is bilaterally symmetrical and all the organs of the body are paired. It possesses 2 *nuclei,* 4 pairs of *flagella,* and 2 sausage-shaped *parabasal bodies* lying transversely, posterior to the sucking disk.

Cyst: The cyst is oval in shape, 12 μm long and 8 μm broad. The young cyst contains two and the mature cyst four nuclei situated at one end or lie in pairs in opposite poles. The axostyles lie diagonally forming a dividing line within the cyst-wall. The remnants of the flagella and the margins of the sucking disc may he seen inside the cytoplasm.

Life Cycle

Infection of man is acquired by the ingestion of cysts in contaminated food and water. Within half an hour of ingestion, the cyst hatches out into two trophozoites, which multiply successively by binary fission and colonize in the duodenum. Encystment occurs in the large intestine when the conditions in the duodenum are unfavorable. The trophozoites as they pass down the colon develop into cysts.

Pathogenesis and Clinical Features

Infection with G. *lamblia (duodenalis)* is initiated by ingestion of cysts. It may cause a disturbance of intestinal function, leading to malabsorption of fat.

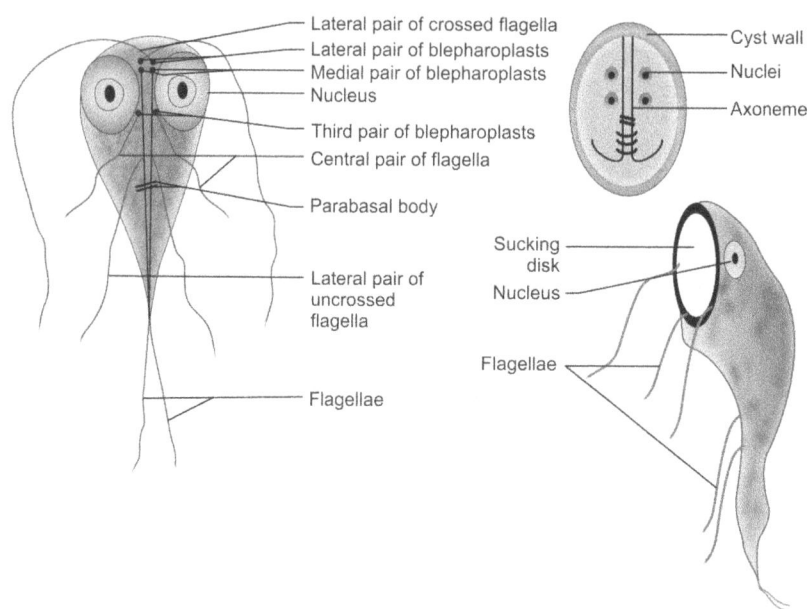

Fig. 54.3: Trophozoites and cyst of *Giardia lamblia.*

Infection with *Giardia* can be **asymptomatic**, can cause acute disease, or can develop into chronic recurrent diarrhea with malabsorption.

Ordinarily no clinical illness results, but in some it may lead to **mucus diarrhea, dull epigastric pain** and **flatulence**.

Chronic recurrent diarrhea is often accompanied by headache, lassitude, myalgia, and weight loss. The patients may suffer from malabsorption of fat, vitamins A and B_{12}, lactose, and xylose. Occasionally, giardia may colonize the gallbladder causing biliary colic and jaundice.

Laboratory Diagnosis

A. **Stool exemptions**: The diagnosis is confirmed by demonstrating the presence of *Giardia* in stool samples. The cysts and trophozoites can be found in diarrheal stools. Fresh (unfixed) stool samples can be examined in wet saline preparations for the presence of motile trophozoites.
B. **Duodenal aspiration:** If *Giardia* cannot be found in stool samples.

TRICHOMONAS

Trichomonas vaginalis is a member of the family Trichomonadidae.

The genus *Trichomonas* has been classified into three species according to their habitats:
i. *Trichomonas vaginalis* inhabiting the female genital tract; also found in the urinary tract of males and females is a sexually transmitted pathogen of the genitourinary tract.
ii. *Trichomonas tenax*—nonpathogenic inhabiting the oral cavity.
iii. *Trichomonas hominis* (8 µm) inhabiting the ileocecal region.

TRICHOMONAS VAGINALIS

Trichomonas vaginalis is the cause of urogenital infections.

Morphology and Life Cycle

Trichomonas vaginalis exits in only as the trophozoite phase and there being **no cystic phase**. The trophozoite is ovoid or pear-shaped, about 10–12 µm in length. The single **ovoid nucleus** is situated at the round anterior end and a cleft-like depression **(cystosome)** lies at its side. It has four anterior flagella and a fifth running along the outer margin of the undulating membrane, which is supported at its base by a rod-like structure, the *costa*.

The posterior end is pointed. The axostyle runs down the middle of the body and ends in the pointed tail-like extremity. The cytoplasm shows prominent granules, which are most numerous along side the axostyle and costa (**Fig. 54.4**).

Pathogenicity

Infection is often asymptomatic, particularly in the male. However, men occasionally experience urethritis, prostatitis, and other urinary tract problems. In females, it may produce severe pruritic vaginitis with an offensive, yellowish, often frothy discharge.

Laboratory Diagnosis

The trimomonad may be found in sedimented urine and vaginal secretions. Prostatic massage may sometimes be necessary for detection of the parasite in males.

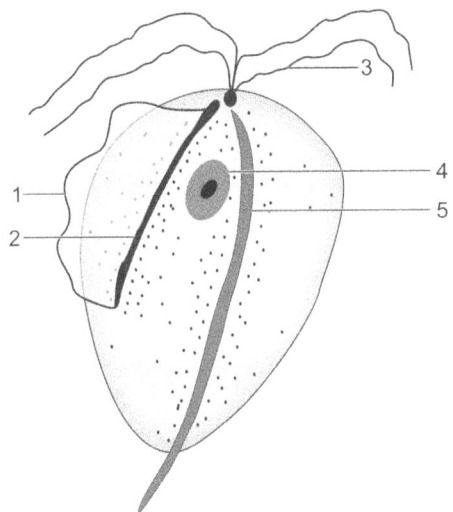

Fig. 54.4: *Trichomonas vaginalis* (1. Undulating membrane; 2. Costa; 3. Flagella; 4. Nucleus; 5. Axostyle).

HEMOFLAGELLATES

Blood- and tissue-dwelling protozoa—infect erythrocytes, reticuloendothelial cells, or the central nervous system. *Leishmania* and *Trypanosoma* are flagellates, and *Babesia*, *Plasmodium*, and *Toxoplasma* are sporozoans. Although *Pneumocystis* is traditionally considered to be a sporozoan, some investigators classify it as a yeast rather than a parasite.

LEISHMANIA DONOVANI

Leishmania donovani causes visceral leishmaniasis or kala-azar. It also causes the condition post-kala-azar dermal leishmaniasis (PKDL). It is a parasite of reticuloendothelial system. It is endemic in many places of India.

Morphology

The parasite exists in two forms **(Fig. 54.5)**:
1. Amastigote stage—in man and other mammals.
2. Promastigote stage—in the gut of insect (sandfly) and in artificial cultures.

Amastigote Stage (LD Body)

The habitat of the amastigote LD body is the reticuloendothelial system of vertebrate host (man, dog, hamster).

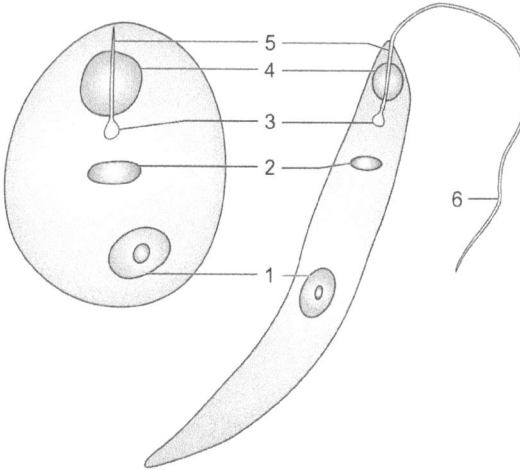

Fig. 54.5: Amastigote and promastigote forms of *Leishmania donovnii* (1. Nucleus; 2. Parabasal body; 3. Blepharoplast; 4. Vacuole; 5. Axoneme; 6. Flagellum).

Characteristics of amastigote stage are as follows:
 i. **Size and shape:** The *amastigote* form (LD body) is an ovoid or rounded cell, about 2–4 μm in size.
 ii. **Cell membrane**—delicate.
 iii. **Nucleus:** It is large oval or round and is stained red.
 iv. **Kinetoplast:** Lying at right angles to the nucleus is *kinetoplast*.
 v. **Parabasal body:** In well-stained preparations, the kinetoplast can be seen to consist of the *parabasal body* and a dot-like *blepharoplast*, with a delicate thread connecting the two.
 vi. **Axoneme:** The axoneme arising from the blepharoplast extends to the anterior tip of the cell.
 vii. **Vacuole:** Alongside the kinetoplast can be seen a clear unstained *vacuole*.

Promastigote Stage (Flagellar) Stage

Promastigote forms which develop in artificial cultures and insect vector (sandfly).
 i. **Shape and size:** *Promastigotes,* are initially short oval or pear-shaped forms, subsequently become long spindle-shaped cells, *15–25 μm* long, carrying a single *flagellum,* 15–30 in length.
 ii. **Cytoplasm and nucleus:** Stained films show pale blue cytoplasm, with a red nucleus in the center.
 iii. **Kinetoplast:** The *kinetoplast* lies transversely near the anterior end.
 iv. **Flagellum:** *Flagellum* may be of the same length as the body or even longer.

Life Cycle

The parasite has two stages **(Fig. 54.6)** in its life cycle:
1. The amastigote form, occurring in man (also in dog in some areas).
2. The promastigote form, occurring in sandfly.

The *amastigote form* resides in the cells of the reticuloendothelial system. They multiply by binary fission and goes on continuously till the cell becomes packed with the parasites.

Pathogenicity of *Leishmania donovani*

Incubation period: It generally varies from 3 to 6 months.

Clinical features: Infection with *L. donovani* produces the disease kala-azar or visceral leishmaniasis, characterized by *pyrexia, splenic enlargement, and lymphadenopathy* emaciation and anemia develop. The skin becomes dry, rough and darkly pigmented (hence, the name kala-azar). The hair becomes thin and brittle. Epistaxis and bleeding gums are common.

Laboratory Diagnosis

Methods employed in laboratory diagnosis are the following:

A. Direct Evidences

Demonstrate of the parasite *L. donovani* in materials obtained from patients. A parasitological diagnosis may be achieved in one of the following ways:

a. **Microscopical examination of a stained film:**
   i. **Peripheral blood:** The amastigotes are present in the peripheral blood by thick film method.
   ii. **Bone marrow biopsy:** The amastigote forms of parasite can readily be demonstrated in a stained film. The promastigote forms are demonstrated when the material obtained is cultured in Novy-MacNeal-Nicolle (NNN) medium.
   iii. **Spleen punctures:** When the organ is considerably enlarged, it is one of the most valuable methods for establishing the diagnosis. The amastigote forms are found in stained films and promastigote forms in culture. The only risk of spleen puncture is that bleeding might continue from the puncture wound in the soft and enlarged spleen, resulting in death.

b. **Blood culture:** Blood cultures are made on Novy-MacNeal-Nicolle (NNN) medium and the culture incubated at 22°C for 1–4 weeks. The parasite grows and promastigotes can be demonstrated.

c. **Animal inoculation:** Animal inoculation is not used for routine diagnosis.

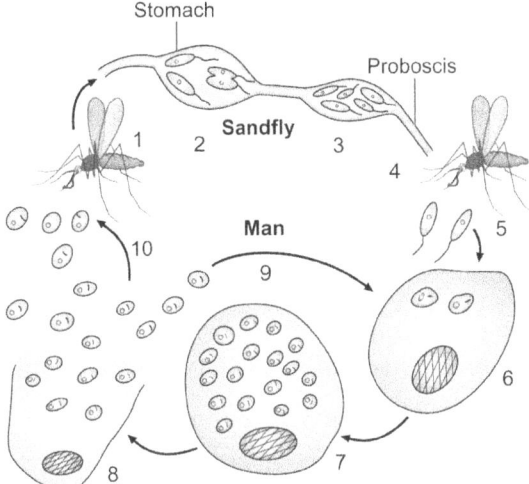

Fig. 54.6: Life cycle of *Leishmania donovnii*. (1. Sandfly feeding on infected person ingests amastigotes; 2. Transformation from amastigote to promastigote which multiplies by binary fission in the fly midgut; 3. Promastigote in pharynx; 4. Migrates to the fly proboscis and when sandfly bites; 5. Promastigotes are deposited in the skin; 6. They are phagocytosed by macrophages; 7. In which they multiply; 8. Macrophage ruptures and releases the amastigotes, some of which; 9. Invade other cells; 10. Amastigotes in peripheral blood and skin, are ingested by sandflies while feeding and repeat the cycle).

The host-cell is enlarged and eventually ruptures. The parasites are liberated into the circulation which are again either taken up by, or invade fresh cells and the cycle is repeated.

When a vector sandfly feeds on an infected person, the amastigotes present in peripheral blood and tissue fluids enter the insect along with its blood meal. The promastigotes multiply by longitudinal binary fission and reach enormous numbers. When the sandfly bites a person, the promastigotes get deposited in the puncture wound. They are phagocytozed by macrophage, in which they multiply, distending the cell. The macrophage ruptures, releasing the amastigotes, some of which are phagocytozed by other macrophages. Amastigotes in peripheral blood and skin are ingested by sandflies while feeding, to repeat the cycle.

Method of transmission: The species in Indian vector—*Phlebotomus argentipes*.

B. Indirect Evidences

They include the following:

i. **Blood count:** Blood examination shows a normocytic normochromic anemia, leukopenia, neutropenia, and thrombocytopenia. The proportion of leukocytes to erythrocytes is greatly altered.

ii. **Nonspecific serological tests.**
   a. **Aldehyde (formol gel) test:** The test depends upon an increase of serum gamma globulin. The aldehyde test is not positive till the disease is of at least 3 months' duration.
   b. **Antimony test:** This also depends upon a rise of serum gamma globulin. Antimony test is less reliable than the aldehyde test. It is not used nowadays.
   c. **Complement fixation test with WKK antigen:** The antigen originally used was prepared from human tubercle bacillus by Witebsky, Klingenstein and Kuhn (hence called the *WKK antigen*). The reaction is considered nonspecific in character, as the antigen used is prepared from human tubercle bacillus.

iii. **Specific serological tests:** These include complement fixation test (CFT), indirect fluorescent antibody test (IFA), counter immunoelectrophoresis, and ELISA tests. Molecular diagnosis (PCA and DNA method of detection) from various types of sample.

iv. **Leishmanin skin test.**

SPOROZOA

Malaria Parasites

Four species of *Plasmodia* cause malaria in man: *Plasmodium falciparum*, *Plasmodium malariae*, *Plasmodium ovale*, and *Plasmodium vivax*. In India, *P. vivax* and *P. falciparum* are very common but *P. ovale* does not occur.

Life Cycle and Morphology

The life cycle of malaria parasites comprises two stages—an *asexual phase* occurring in man and a *sexual phase* occurring in the mosquito (**Fig. 54.7**).

The Human Phase (Asexual Phase)

The sporozoite is the infective form of the malarial parasite. These sporozoites are present in the salivary gland of female anopheles mosquitoes. Man gets *infected* through the *bite* of the female *Anopheles* mosquito. The sporozoites pass into the bloodstream. Thus, human cycle starts and it comprises of following stages:
- Pre-erythrocytic schizogony
- Erythrocytic schizogony
- Gametogony
- Latent stage (hepatic)

i. Pre-erythrocytic Schizogony

Within an hour of being injected into the body by the mosquito, the sporozoites reach the liver and enter the hepatocytes to initiate the stage of pre-erythrocytic schizogony. The sporozoites, which are elongated spindle-shaped bodies become rounded inside the liver cells. They enlarge in size and undergo repeated nuclear division and develop into schizont. In 6–16 days, the schizont becomes mature and bursts, releasing thousands of merozoites.

The pre-erythrocytic cycle lasts for 8 days in *P. vivax*, 6 days in *P. falciparum*, 13–16 days in *P. malariae*, and 9 days in *P. ovale*. The release of merozoites from hepatocytes ends the exoerythrocytic cycle and begins the series of erythrocytic cycles.

ii. Erythrocytic Schizogony

The merozoites released by the pre-erythrocytic schizont invade the red blood cells. Inside the erythrocytes, the malarial parasites undergo erythrocytic schizogony. They pass through the stages of trophozoite, schizont, and merozoite (**Fig. 54.8**). The schizonts subsequently produce merozoites. The number of merozoites produced within each infected erythrocyte depends on the *Plasmodium* species and ranges from 6 to 36. The merozoites invade fresh erythrocytes in which they go through the same process of development.

In *P. falciparum* infection, erythrocytic schizonts aggregate in the capillaries of the brain and other internal organs, so that only ring forms

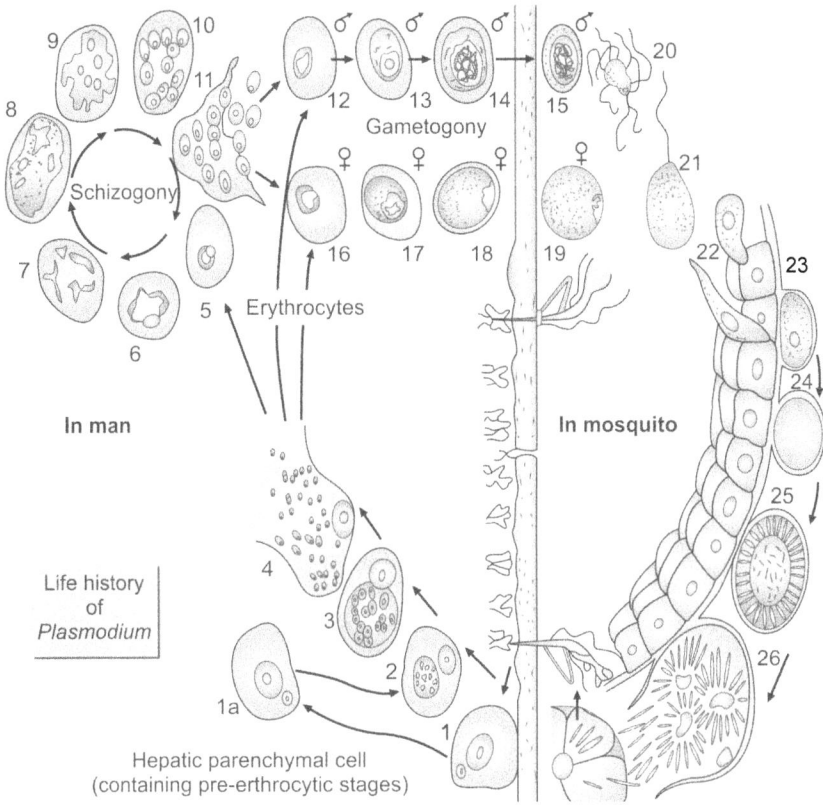

Fig. 54.7: Life history of malarial parasite [1–4. Pre-erythrocytic (or exoerythrocytic) asexual stages undergoing schizogony in liver; 1a. Hypnozoite (only in P. vivax and P. ovale among species infecting humans); 5–11. Erythrocytic asexual cycle; 12–15. Microgametocyte development; 16–19. Macrogametocyte development; 20. Exflagellation to produce microgametes; 21. Fertilization of macrogamete; 22. Ookinete penetrates cell (wall) of mosquito stomach; 23–25. Production of sporozoites within oocyst (sporogony); 26. Release of sporozoites, most reaching salivary glands of mosquito].

are found in the peripheral blood. Differential features of various plasmodia are shown in Table 54.4.

iii. Gametogony

Some merozoites that infect red cells do not proceed to become schizonts, but instead develop into sexually differentiated forms, the gametocytes—male and female gametes, which are called microgametocytes and macrogametocytes, respectively. In all species, the female (macrogametocyte) has cytoplasm staining dark blue with a small compact nucleus staining deep red. In the male (microgametocyte), the cytoplasm stains pale blue, light blue, or and the nucleus is larger, and diffuse (**Fig. 54.8**).

Latent Stage (Hepatic)

The initial tissue phase (*pre-erythrocytic* or *primary exo-erythrocytic phase*) disappears completely in P. vivax and P. ovale after establishment of blood infection. P. vivax and P. ovale generate an additional developmental form within hepatocytes. This form, known as a hypnozoite (meaning "sleeping animal"), is believed to be responsible for relapses of malaria. P. falciparum and P. malariae do not form hypnozoites and do not relapse.

Table 54.4: Differential features of different plasmodia of man.

Feature	P. vivax	P. falciparum	P. malariae	P. ovale
1. Forms in peripheral blood	Trophozoites, schizonts and gametocytes	Ring forms and gametocytes (crescent shaped)	Trophozoites, schizonts and gametocytes	Trophozoites, schizonts and gametocytes
2. Early trophozoite or ring form	2.5 mm in diameter, cytoplasm opposite the nucleus is thicker	1.25–1.5 mm in diameter, multiple rings in one red blood cell, form accole	Similar to that of P. vivax	Similar to that of P. vivax
3. Trophozoite	Irregular, amoeboid, vacuole present	Compact form, rarely amoeboid, pigments collect into a single mass	Band shaped, slightly amoeboid, vacuole inconspicuous	Compact, not amoeboid, vacuole inconspicuous
4. Schizont	9–10 mm in diameter, almost completely fills an enlarged erythrocyte	4.5–5.0 mm in diameter, fills two thirds of a normal size erythrocyte	6.5–7.0 mm in diameter, almost fills a normal size erythrocyte	6.2 mm in diameter, fills about three quarters of slightly enlarged erythrocyte
5. Merozoites	12–24 in number	18–24 in number	6–12 in number	6–12 in number
6. Gametocyte	Spherical, much large than a red blood cell	Crescentric (sickle-shaped), larger than a red blood cell	Round, size of a red blood cell	Round, size of a red blood cell
i. Female gametocyte (macro-gametocyte)	Spherical, larger than male gametocyte, cytoplasm stains deep blue, nucleus is small and compact	Sickle-shaped, longer, more slender, cytoplasm stains deep blue, nucleus is compact	Similar to that of P. vivax but smaller	Similar to that of P. vivax but smaller
ii. Male gametocyte (micro-gametocyte)	Spherical, smaller than female gametocyte, cytoplasm stains light blue or pale blue, nucleus is large and diffuse	Sickle-shaped, broader, shorter, cytoplasm stains light blue, nucleus is diffuse	Similar to that of P. vivax but smaller	Similar to that of P. vivax but smaller
7. Malarial pigments	Yellowish-brown	Dark-brown	Dark-brown	Dark yellowish-brown
8. Infected erythrocyte	Enlarged, pale, Schüffner's dots present	Size unaltered, Maurer's dots present	Normal size and no dots, Ziemann's dots on prolonged staining	Slightly enlarged, oval shaped and James' dots present
9. Age of the erythrocytes infected	Young	All ages (young and old)	Old	Young
10. Duration of erythrocytic schizongony	48 hours	≤48 hours	72 hours	48 hours

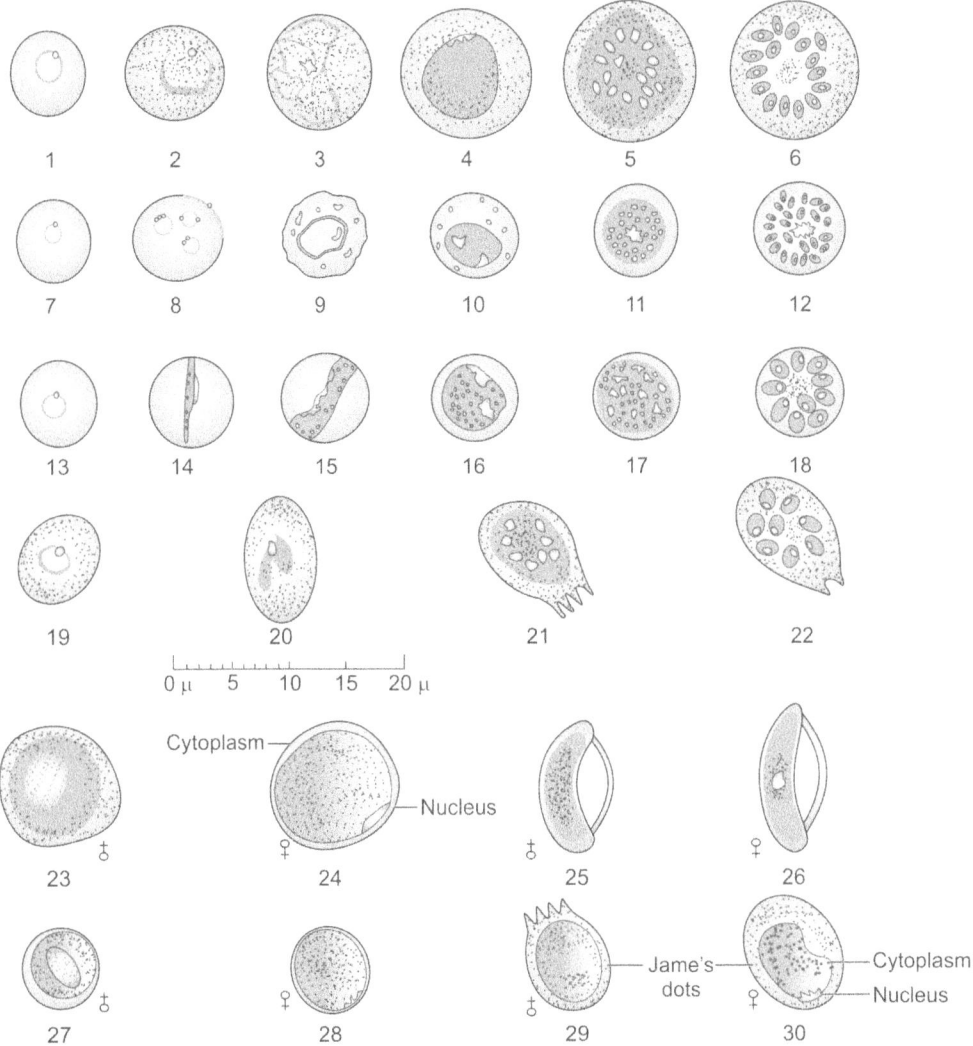

Fig. 54.8: Malarial parasites of man: Differential characters of erythrocytic phases [1–6 (*Plasmodium vivax*); 7–12 (*Plasmodium falciparum*); 13–18 (*Plasmodium malariae*); 19–22 (*Plasmodium ovale*); Gametocytes 23–24 (*Plasmodium vivax*); 25–26 (*Plasmodium falciparum*); 27–28 (*Plasmodium malariae*); 29–30 (*Plasmodium ovale*)]..

The Mosquito Phase (Sexual Cycle of Malarial Parasite)

When a female *Anopheles* mosquito ingests parasitized erythrocytes along with its blood meal, the asexual forms of malaria parasites are digested, but the gametocytes are set free in the stomach and undergo further development. Into the stomach of the mosquito, the male gametocyte divides into 5–8 nuclei, from each of which protrudes a long, actively motile, whip-like filaments which are the male gametes (*microgametes*) and then break free by the process called **exflagellation**. The female gametocyte does not divide, but undergoes a process of maturation to become the female gamete or *macrogamete*. It is fertilized by one of the microgametes to produce the *zygote*. The zygote, elongates and becomes a vermicular motile form called the **ookinete**. The ookinete develops into an **oocyst**. The oocyst matures, increasing in size and leads to the development within the oocyst of about a thousand sporozoites. The mature oocyst, ruptures, and the sporozoites enter the hemocoel. The sporozoites reach the salivary glands situated in the thorax of the mosquito, penetrate the acinar cells and enter the salivary ducts. The mosquito is now infective and when it feeds on man, the sporozoites are injected into the skin capillaries to initiate human infection.

Pathogenesis

Infection with the *Plasmodium* causes intermittent fever, which is known as **malaria**.
Incubation period: In *P. vivax, P. ovale,* and *P. falciparum* it is 10–14 days and in *P. malariae* it is 18 days to 6 weeks.

Clinical Features of Malaria

The typical picture of malaria consists of periodic bouts of fever with rigor, followed by anemia and splenomegaly.

Relapses of Malaria

In *P. vivax* and *P. ovale* infections, reactivation of hypnozoites leads to *relapses*.

Pernicious Malaria

The most serious and fatal type of malaria is malignant tertian (MT) malaria caused by *P. falciparum*. When not treated promptly and adequately, dangerous complications develop.

The term *pernicious malaria* has been applied to a complex of life-threatening complications that sometimes supervenes in acute falciparum malaria. These occur following heavy parasitization.
Clinical types: These may present in various forms—cerebral, algid and septicemic varieties.
1. **Cerebral malaria:** It is characterized by hyperpyrexia, coma, and paralysis.
2. **Algid malaria:** It resembles surgical shock, with cold clammy skin, peripheral circulatory failure and profound hypotension.
3. **Septicemic malaria.**

Blackwater Fever

A syndrome called *Blackwater fever* (malarial hemoglobinuria) is in falciparum malaria, particularly in patients who have experienced repeated infections and inadequate treatment with quinine. It is characterized by sudden intravascular hemolysis followed by fever and hemoglobinuria.

Immunity

Immunity is species-specific, stage-specific, and strain-specific and lasts only till malarial parasite infection remains active. This type of immunity is known as *premunition immunity*.

Laboratory Diagnosis

1. **Microscopical examination:** *A microscopical examination of a blood film* forms one of the most important diagnostic procedures in malaria. Two types of blood films are prepared for examination, the *thick* and the *thin* films. They can be made on separate slides, or more conveniently on the same slide.
Thick film: The drop of blood is touched with a clean dry slide, near one end. The blood on the slide is spread with the corner of another slide to produce a square or circular patch of moderate thickness. This is the thick film.
Thin film: The blood is spread evenly and thinly with the edge of a spreader slide and will consist of an unbroken smear of a single layer of red cells, ending in a tongue which stops a little short of the edge of the slide.
Combined thick and thin film on the same slide
Staining: Diluted Giemsa stain is applied over both thick and thin films. The rapid method commonly employed in India is the JSB stain, named after Jaswant Singh and Bhattacharji.
Smear examination: Thick films are best used as a screening procedure but species identification is difficult. Thin smear is examined for identifying the species of *Plasmodium*.

All asexual erythrocytic stages (ring forms, trophozoites, and schizonts) as well as gametocytes can be seen in peripheral blood in infection with *P. vivax, P. ovale,* and *P. malariae*, but in *P. falciparum* infection, only the ring form and gametocytes (crescent-shaped) can be seen. Multiple rings in an individual red blood cell with accole forms is diagnostic of *P. falciparum*.

2. **Cultural examination:** This is not required for diagnosis.
3. **Blood count:** This has very little importance in the diagnosis of malaria.
4. **Serological tests:** Immunoprecipitation tests, immunofluorescence, indirect hemagglutination (IHA), and ELISA are used for specific malaria antibodies.
5. **Molecular biologic approaches:** DNA probes and RNA probes.
6. **Other rapid diagnostic tests:** Dip stick or test strip with monoclonal antibodies against the target parasite antigens.

Treatment

The strategy of treatment is to cure the clinical disease with blood schizonticidal drugs such as chloroquine. Primaquine (a tissue schizonticidal drug should be administered in *P. vivax* and *P. ovale* because chloroquine does not destroy exo-erythocytic parasites. A combination of sulfadoxine and pyrimethamine (fansidar) or mefloquine is useful for *P. falciparum*.

KEY POINTS

- *Entamoeba histolytica* causes amebiasis which can be classified as intestinal (primary) and extraintestinal (metastatic) amebiasis.
- Infection with *Giardia lamblia* can be asymptomatic, can cause acute disease, or can develop into chronic recurrent diarrhea with malabsorption.
- *Trichomonas vaginalis* is a sexually transmitted pathogen of the genitourinary tract.
- Four species of *Plasmodia* cause malaria in *man*: *Plasmodium falciparum, Plasmodium malariae, Plasmodium ovale,* and *Plasmodium vivax*.
- Infection with the *Plasmodium* causes intermittent fever which is known as **malaria**.

IMPORTANT QUESTIONS

1. Describe the laboratory diagnosis of amebic dysentery.
2. Write short notes on:
    a. *Giardia lamblia*
    b. *Trichomonas vaginalis*.
3. Describe the life cycle and the laboratory diagnosis of kala-azar.
4. Describe the life cycle of *Plasmodium vivax* and the laboratory diagnosis of malaria caused by this parasite.
5. Describe briefly about:
    a. Pernicious malaria
    b. *Plasmodium falciparum*

MULTIPLE CHOICE QUESTIONS

1. Infective stage of *Entamoeba histolytica* is:
   a. Trophozoite
   b. Binucleate cyst
   c. Quadrinucleate cyst
   d. None of the above
2. Most common organ involved in extraintestinal amebiasis is:
   a. Liver
   b. Lung
   c. Brain
   d. Spleen
3. *Giardia lamblia* resides in:
   a. Duodenum and upper part of jejunum
   b. Cecum
   c. Colon
   d. Rectum
4. Amastigote form of *Leishmania donovani* resides in the:
   a. Cells of reticuloendothelial system
   b. Culture media
   c. Digestive tract of insect vector
   d. All of the above
5. Malaria infection can be transmitted by:
   a. Bite of infected female Anopheles mosquito
   b. Blood transfusion
   c. Vertical transmission through placental defect
   d. All of the above

ANSWERS

1. c   2. a   3. a   4. a
5. d.

Helminthology

LEARNING OBJECTIVES

After reading and studying this chapter, you should be able to:
- Describe *Cysticercus Cellulosae* or "Bladder Worm".
- Discuss the life cycle and the laboratory diagnosis of *Echinococcus granulosus*.
- Describe the life cycle of *Ascaris lumbricoides* and *Ancylostoma duodenale*.
- Describe the following: Hydatid cyst, *Wuchereria bancrofti*, Microfilaria.

INTRODUCTION

The helminths are a large group of parasitic worms that include cestodes (tapeworms), nematodes (roundworms), and trematodes (flukes).

CESTODES

Cestodes are members of the phylum Platyhelminthes and the class Cestoda. Commonly called **tapeworms**, the cestodes must pass through one or more hosts during their life cycle.

TAENIA SAGINATA

Common name: Beef tape worm,; the unarmed tapeworm of man.

Geographical distribution: *T. saginata* is worldwide in distribution, but the infection is not found in vegetarians and those who do not eat beef.

Habitat

Adult worm lives in the small intestine (upper jejunum) of man.

Morphology (Table 55.1)

Adult worm: It is white and semitransparent measuring 5-0 m in length but it may be up to 24 m.

The *scolex* ("head") measures 1-2 mm in diameter, is quadrate in outline and has four circular suckers (may be pigmented). The "head" is not provided with any rostellum or hooklets and moves against the peristaltic movement in the host's intestine.

The neck: The "neck" is fairly long and narrow (about 0.5 mm in width).

Proglottid (segments): The length of a mature segment is 3-4 times its breadth.

The number of proglottid is from 1.000 to 2.000.

Eggs (Fig. 55.1)

The eggs are liberated by the rupture of ripe proglottids.

The characteristics of the egg are as follows:
i. Spherical and brown in color (bile-stained).
ii. Measure 31–43 µm in diameter.
iii. The thin, outer transparent shell, when present, represents the remnant of the yolk mass; it causes the eggs to clump together.
iv. The inner embryophore is brown, thick-walled, and radially striated.
v. Contains an oncosphere (14–20 µm in diameter) with 3 pairs of hooklets.
vi. Does not float in saturated solution of common salt.

vii. Eggs are resistant and may remain viable for 8 weeks.
viii. Infective only to cattle.

TAENIA SOLIUM

Common name: The pork tapeworm; the armed tapeworm of man.
Geographical distribution: World-wide. The infection is common among those eating raw or insufficiently cooked "measly" pork. It is uncommon in Jews and Mohammedans who are not generally pork-eaters.
Habitat: Adult worm lives in the small intestine (upper jejunum).

Morphology (Table 55.1)

Adult worm: It measures about 2–3 m in length (Figs. 55.1A to C and Table 55.1).

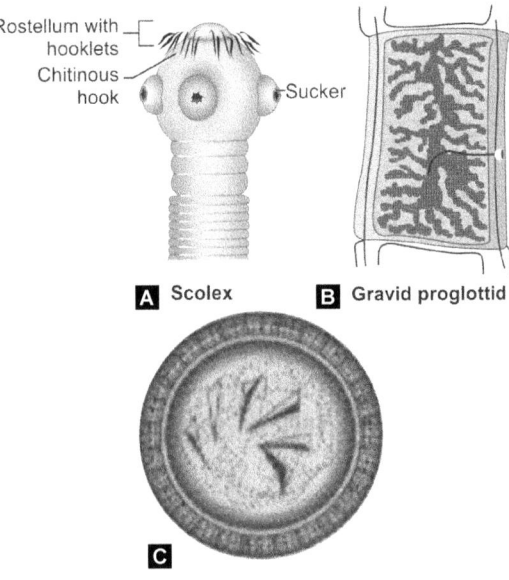

Figs. 55.1A to C: (A) The scolex; (B) Gravid proglottids; (C) Eggs of *Taenia solium*.

Table 55.1: Differentiating features of *Taenia saginata* and *Taenia solium*.		
	T. saginata	*T. solium*
1. Geographical distribution	Worldwide—who as a rule eat beef	Worldwide—in community eating pig meat
2. Habitat	Adult worm lives in the small intestine	Adult worm lives in the small intestine
Adult worms		
Length	5–10 meters	2–3 meters
Head	Large, quadrate; without rostellum and hooks; suckers may be pigmented	Small, globular; with rostellum and hooks; suckers not pigmented
Proglottides		
Number	1,000–2,000	Below 1,000
Expulsion	Expelled singly and may force anal sphincter	Expelled passively in chains of 5 or 6
Uterus	Lateral branches 15 to 30 on each side; thin and dichotomous	Lateral branches 5 to on each side; thick and dendritic
Vaginal sphincter	Present	Absent
Ovaries	Two in number, without any accessory lobe.	Two in number, with an accessory lobe
Testes	300–400 follicle	150–200 follicles
Intermediate host	Cattle (cow or buffalo)	Pig
Larval stage	*Cysticercus bovis* in the muscles of a cow or a buffalo (5–10 mm in breadth by 3–4 mm in length). It can live for about 8 months in the flesh of cattle. Does not occur in man	*Cysticercus cellulosae* in the muscles of the pig. Opalescent ellipsoidal body (8–10 mm in width by 5 mm in length). The long axis of the cyst lies parallel with the muscle fiber. A dense milk-white-spot at the side where the scolex with its hooks and suckers remains invaginated

The *scolex* ("head") measures 1 mm in diameter (about the size of a pin-head), is globular in outline and has four circular suckers. The "head" is provided with a rostellum armed with a double row of alternating large and small hooklets.

The "neck" is short, measuring from 5 to 10 mm in length.

Proglottids (segments): The total number is less than a thousand (800-900).

Mature segment measures 12 mm by 6 mm. The worm has a *life span* of as much as 25 years.

Eggs: The characteristics are the same as those for *T. saginata*. The eggs are infective to pig as well as to man.

Life Cycle of T. solium (Fig. 55.2)

1. The definitive host: Man
2. The intermediate host: Pig

The adult worm lives in the small intestine of man. The gravid segments pass passively out as short chains. The eggs escape from the ruptured wall of the uterus with the feces on the ground.

The oncospheres penetrate the intestinal wall, enter the mesenteric venules or lymphatics and are carried in systemic circulation to the different parts of the body. Usually, they travel *via* the portal vein and successively reach the following organs: the liver, the right side of the heart, lungs, the left side of the heart and the systemic circulation.

The naked oncospheres are filtered out from the circulating blood into the muscular tissues where they ultimately settle down and undergo further develop into the larval stage, *cysticercus cellulosae* in about 60-70 days.

Human beings are infected through the eating of undercooked beef containing the cysticercus cellulosae *(measly pork)*. Inside the alimentary canal of man, the scolex, on coming in contact with the bile, exvaginates and anchors to the gut-wall by means of its suckers and develops into an adult worm. The worm grows to sexual maturity and starts producing eggs, which are in their turn passed in the feces along with the gravid segments, thereby repeating the cycle.

Life Cycle of T. saginata (Fig. 55.2)

The life cycle is the same as described for *T. solium* except that:

Intermediate host: Cattle (cow or buffalo); human beings are infected through the eating of undercooked beef containing the cysticerci ("measly" beef).

Larval Stage of *T. solium*

Cysticercus cellulosae or 'Bladder Worm' (Fig. 55.3)

The larval stage of *T. solium* developing in the muscles of the pig is known as *Cysticercus cellulosae*. A mature cyst is an opalescent 'ellipsoidal body. The long axis of the cyst lies parallel with the muscle fiber. A dense milk-white spot can be seen at the side, where the scolex with its hooks and suckers remains invaginated. It contains a thick fluid, rich in protein and salt. It can only develop further when ingested by its definitive host, man.

Cysticercus bovis

This is the larval stage of *T. saginata* developing in the muscles of a cow or a buffalo and contains an unarmed scolex ("head" of the adult worm) invaginated at one side. The cysticerci can be seen on visual inspection as shiny white dots in the infected beef ("measly beef"). It can

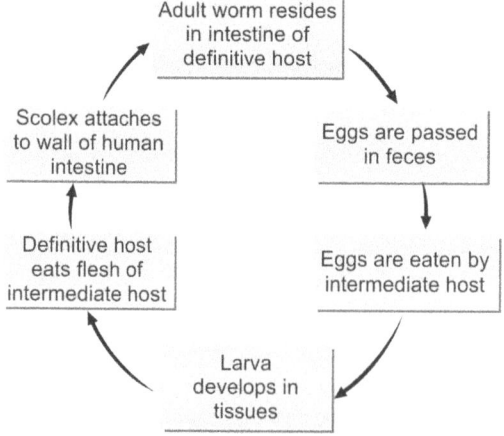

Fig. 55.2: The general cycle of tapeworm that infects humans.

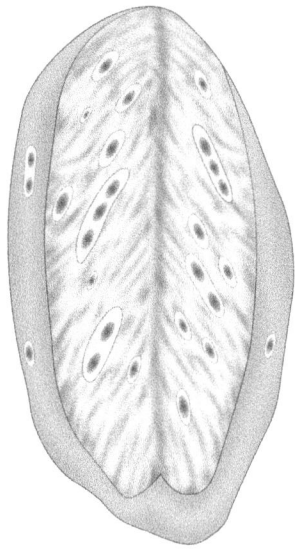

Fig. 55.3: *Cysticercus cellulosae.*

only develop further when ingested by man, its definitive host. *Cysticercus bovis* does not occur in man.

Mode of infection: By ingestion of undercooked meat of the intermediate hosts:
- In *T. saginata*: Beef containing *Cysticercus bovis*.
- In *T. solium*: Pork containing *Cysticercus cellulosae*.

Adult worms do not give rise to any symptom. Occasionally, they may be responsible for vague abdominal discomfort, chronic indigestion, anemia, and intestinal disorders.

Infection in Human Beings

Larval worms of *T. saginata* are not found in man but those of *T. solium* may occasionally be found.

Cysticercus' cellulosae: Man, occasionally serving as the larval host of *T. solium*, becomes infected in the same way as the pig.
i. By drinking contaminated water or by eating uncooked vegetables infected with eggs of *T. solium*.
ii. **Autoinfection:** In persons harboring the adult worm in the intestine, autoinfect himself either due to unclean and unhygienic personal habits by a reversal of peristaltic movements of the intestine whereby the gravid segments are thrown back to the stomach, equivalent to the swallowing of thousands of eggs.

Any organ or tissue may be involved, the most common being subcutaneous tissues and muscles. It may also affect the eyes, brain, and less often the heart, liver, lungs, abdominal cavity and spinal cord. The symptomatology depends on the site affected in brain.

Laboratory Diagnosis of Tapeworm Infection

Stool examination: A naked eye examination of the specimen should be made for segments of *Taenia* species. Infection with the adult worm is diagnosed by:

Demonstration of eggs: A microscopical examination of the stool for the eggs of the adult worm is carried out from the sample after concentrating.

Species diagnosis: The "head" and the gravid segment, when available, are the only means of establishing a species diagnosis. As the eggs of *T. saginata* cannot be differentiated from those of *T. solium*.

Diagnosis of Cysticercosis

This is based on the following:
i. **Biopsy examination of a subcutaneous nodule** containing cysticerci.
ii. **X-ray of skull and soft tissues (buttocks and thighs) may reveal calcified cysticerci.**
iii. **CT scan of brain**—for diagnosis of cerebral cysticercosis.
iv. MRI scan of brain
v. **Myelography**
vi. **Eosinophilia**
vii. **Serology**—indirect hemagglutination test. IFA and ELISA tests
viii. **Antigen detection:** ELISA test.
ix. A history of intestinal taeniasis often helps in the diagnosis.

Treatment

Praziquantel, niclosamide and mebendazole are useful in treatment of infection with the adult worm.

Prophylaxis

The preventive measures include the following:
1. Avoidance of eating raw or undercooked meat of the intermediate hosts.
2. Proper meat inspection in slaughther houses.
3. Proper sanitary control of sewage disposal and effective treatment of infected individual to prevent infection of the intermediate hosts.
4. It is important to detect and treat persons harboring adult worms as they can develop cysticercosis due to autoinfection.

GENUS *ECHINOCOCCUS*

Common names: The dog tapeworm; the hydatid worm.

Tapeworm belonging to the genus *Echinococcus* is *Echinococcus granulosus,* the *dog tapeworm* or the *hydatid worm.*

Geographical distribution: It is world-wide in distribution.

Habitat: Man harbors the larval form and *the adult worm* is found in the small intestine of dog and other canine animals.

Morphology

Adult worm (**Fig. 55.4**). It is a small tapeworm, measuring 3-6 mm in length. It comprises of a *scolex* ("head"), *neck* and *strobila* consisting of three *segments* (occasionally four). The first segment is immature, the second one is mature, and the last one (as well as the fourth one, when present) is gravid. The terminal segment is by far the biggest.

Scolex: The *scolex* bears four suckers and a protrusible rostellum with two circular rows of hooks.

Neck: The *"neck"* is short and thick.

Egg (Fig. 55.5): It is ovoid in shape and measures 32-36 µm in length by 25-32 µm in breadth. It contains a hexacanth embryo with three pairs of hooks. The egg is infective to man, cattle, sheep, and other herbivorous animals.

Larval form (Fig. 55.6): This is found within the hydatid cyst developing inside the intermediate hosts. It represents the structure of the *scolex* of the future adult worm and remains invaginated within a vesicular body. When it enters the definitive host, the *scolex* with four suckers and

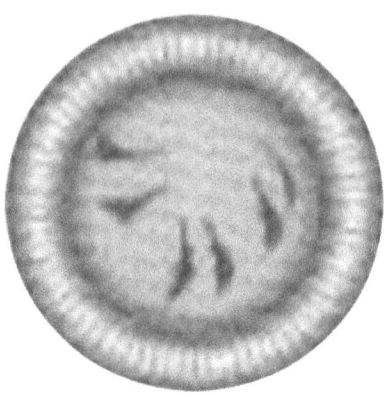

Fig. 55.5: Egg of *Echinococcus granulosus.*

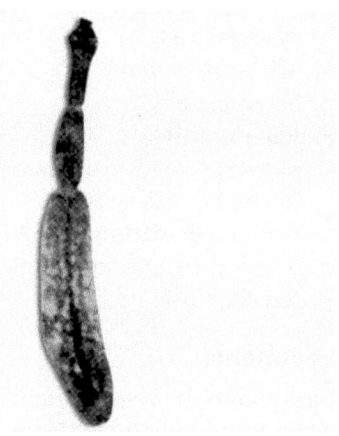

Fig. 55.4: *Echinococcus granulosus,* adult worm.

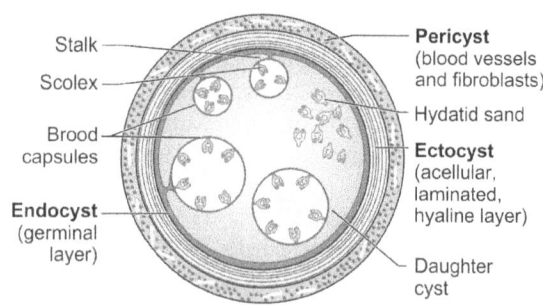

Fig. 55.6: Hydatid cyst.

rostellar hooklets, becomes evaginated and develops into an adult worm.

Life Cycle: The worm passes its life cycle (**Fig. 55.7**) in two hosts.

1. *Definitive hosts:* Dog, wolf, fox, and jackal. The dog is the optimum definitive host. The adult worm lives in the small intestine of these animals, which discharge a large number of eggs in their feces.
2. *Intermediate hosts:* Sheep, pig, cattle, horse, goat, and man. The sheep appears to be the optimum intermediate host. The larval stage is passed in these animals and man, giving rise to hydatid cyst.

The eggs are discharged in the feces of the definitive hosts (dog and allied animals) and are swallowed by the intermediate hosts, sheep and other domestic animals while grazing in the field, and also by man (particularly children) due to intimate handling of infected dogs.

In the duodenum, the egg shell disintegrates, setting free the hexacanth embryos which penetrate the intestinal wall and enter the radicles of the portal vein. The embryos are carried to the liver to be arrested in the sinusoidal

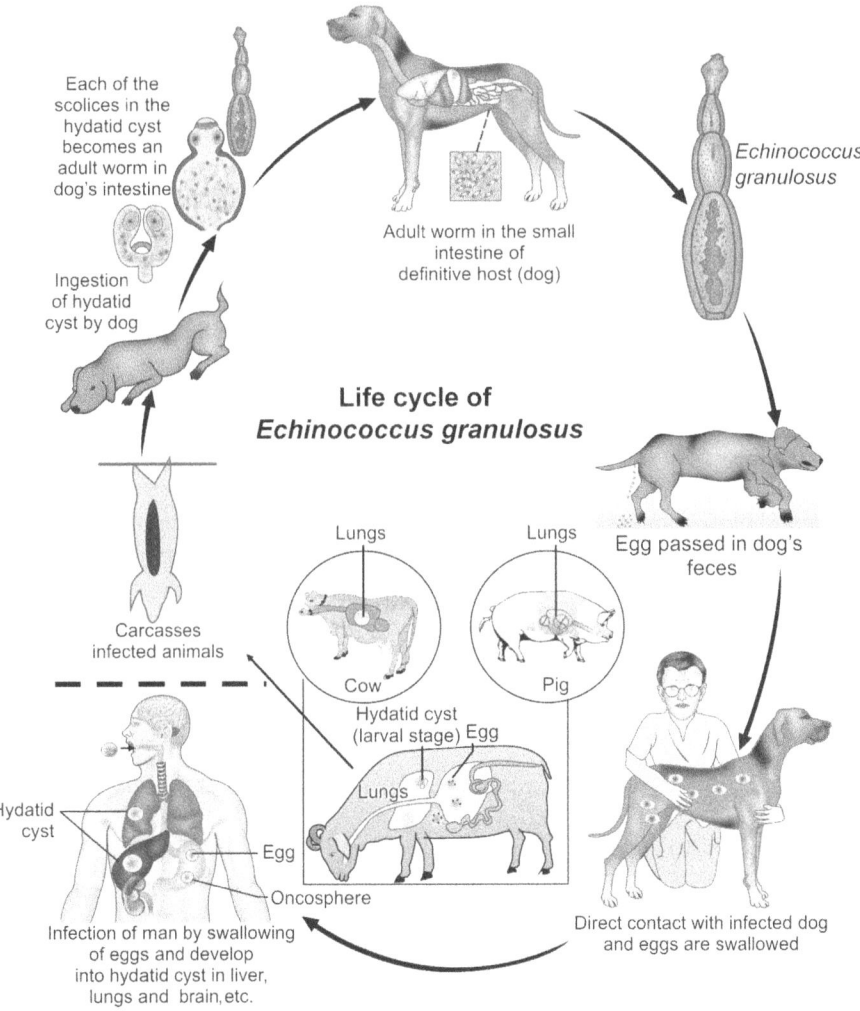

Fig. 55.7: Life cycle of *Echinococcus granulosus*.

capillaries. The liver acts as the first filter for the embryos, which get arrested in the sinusoidal capillaries. Some of the embryos may pass through the hepatic capillaries, enter the pulmonary circulation and filter out in the lungs so that lungs act as the second filter. A few of the embryos may pass the pulmonary capillaries, enter the general blood stream and lodge in the various organs and tissues, such as the spleen, kidneys, eye, brain or bones. Practically, all the organs of the domestic animals may be invaded but they are chiefly found in the liver and lungs.

Wherever the embryo settles, it forms a hydatid cyst, the young larva being transformed into a hollow bladder (*H. hydatis,* drop of water). From the inner side of the cyst, brood capsules with a number of scolices are developed. The cyst has a thick' opaque white outer *cuticle* or *laminated layer,* and a thin inner *germinal layer* containing nucleated cells. A hydatid cyst developing from a single egg (oncosphere) may contain thousands of scolices. When sheep or cattle harboring hydatid cysts die or are slaughtered, dogs may feed on the carcass or offal. Inside the intestine of dogs" the scolices develop into the adult worms that mature and produce eggs. Thus, the life cycle is repeated. When infection occurs in man, the cycle comes to a dead end, because the human hydatid cysts are unlikely to be eaten by dogs. The natural cycle is thus maintained by dog and sheep.

Pathogenicity

The larval worm of *E. granulosus* in man causes unilocular hydatid disease.

Mode of infection: The eggs in the dog's feces are ingested by man. This occurs in the following ways:
 i. *Direct contact:* By a direct contact with infected dogs
 ii. By allowing the dog to feed from the same dish
 iii. By taking uncooked vegetables contaminated with infected canine feces.

Infection is generally acquired in childhood when intimate contact with pet dogs is more likely.

Pathogenesis of hydatid cyst: The cyst-wall secreted by the embryo consists of two layers:
1. *Outer cuticular layer (ectocyst):* It is a laminated hyaline membrane (**Fig. 55.6**) thickness up to 1 mm and has the appearance of the white of a hard-boiled egg. It is elastic and when incised or ruptured curls on itself exposing the inner layer containing the brood capsules and daughter cysts.
2. *Inner or germinal layer (endocyst).* It is very thin containing nucleated cells embedded in a protoplasmic mass (**Fig. 55.6**).

Laboratory Diagnosis

This consists of the following:
1. *Casoni reaction:* An immediate hypersensitivity skin test introduced by Casoni.
   Principle: Immediate hypersensitivity
   Antigen—fresh sterile hydatid fluid from human cases (removed by operation) or from animals (obtained from slaughterhouse) is used as antigen (sterilized by Seitz or membrane filtration).
   Procedure: Intradermal injection of 0.2 mL of a fresh sterile hydatid fluid (sterilized by Seitz filter) produces within half an hour, in all positive cases, a large wheal (5 cm in diameter) with multiple pseudopodia; it fades in an hour. Sterile normal saline, 0.2 mL, is injected in the other arm for control. The test is very sensitive, but false positive reactions may appear in a number of other conditions.
2. *Blood examination:* Generalized eosinophilia (20–25%).
3. *Serological tests:* These include precipitation, complement fixation, bentonite flocculation, latex agglutination and ELISA. Indirect hemagglutination, immunofluorescence and immunoelectrophoresis have been widely used. (e) Molecular methods such as DNA probe and PCR.
4. *Exploratory cyst puncture:* Exploratory puncture of the cyst yields hydatid fluid and demonstration of scolices in the hydatid sand provides conclusive diagnosis. But this procedure is risky and not recommended

as it may cause escape of hydatid fluid and consequent anaphylaxis.
5. *Radiological examination:* Radiological examination ultrasonography and CT scan reveal the diagnosis in most cases.
6. IV pyelogram is helpful for detection of renal hydatid cyst.

NEMATODES

ASCARIS LUMBRICOIDES—THE COMMON ROUNDWORM

The round worm, *Ascaris lumbricoides* is the largest nematode parasite in the human intestine.

Geographical distribution: It is cosmopolitan, having a world-wide distribution, being especially prevalent in the tropics.

Habitat: The adult worm lives in the lumen of the small intestine (jejunum) of man.

Morphology

They are large cylindrical worms, with tapering ends, the anterior end being more pointed than the posterior. The mouth at the anterior end has three finely *denticulated* lips, one dorsal and two *ventrolateral*.

Male: Male worm measures about 15-25 cm in length 3-4 mm in diameter. The tail end of the male is curved ventrally in the form of a hook. Two curved copulatory spicules protrude from cloaca. The anus opens with the ejaculatory duct into the cloaca (**Fig. 55.8**).

Female: It is longer and stouter than the male. It measures 25-40 cm in length 5 mm diameter. Its posterior extremity is straight and conical. The anus is subterminal and opens directly on the ventral aspect in the form of a transverse slit. The vulva is situated on the midventral aspect and opens at the junction of the anterior and the middle-third of the body; at this section the worm is narrower and is called the **vulvar waist** or genital girdle. The genital tubules of the *gravid* worm contain an enormous number of eggs. A single worm lays up to 200,000 eggs per day.

Eggs: Two types of eggs are passed by the worms—*fertilized eggs and unfertilized eggs.*

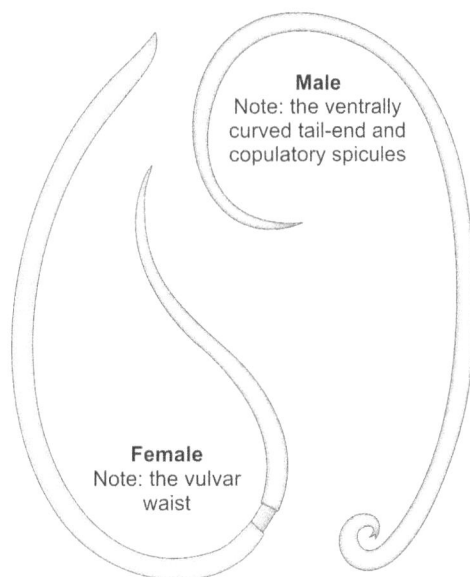

Fig. 55.8: *Ascaris lumbricoides*, adult worm.

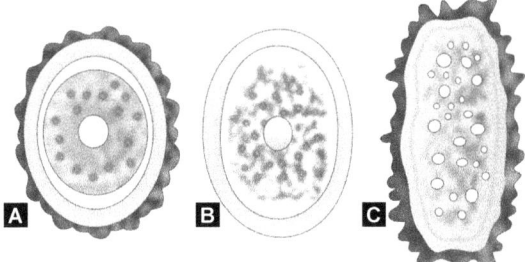

Fig. 55.9: Eggs of *Ascaris lumbricoides*: (A) Fertilized; (B) Decorticated; (C) Unfertilized.

The characteristics of a fertilized egg (**Fig. 55.9**) are as follows:
 i. Fertilized egg is round or oval in shape and measures 60–75 μm in length by 40–50 μm in breadth.
 ii. It is bile-stained and brownish (golden brown) in color.
 iii. It is surrounded by a thick, smooth translucent shell with an outer albuminous coat, which is thrown into rugosities or mammillations. This outer coat is sometimes lost (decorticated egg).
 iv. It contains a very large conspicuous, unsegmented ovum with a clear crescentic area at each pole.
 v. It floats in saturated solution of common salt.

The characteristics of this *unfertilized egg* (**Fig. 55.9**) are as follows:
i. It is narrower, longer (80 mm in length by 55 mm in breadth).
ii. It is brownish in color (bile stained).
iii. The shell is thinner with an irregular coating of albumin.
iv. The ovum is small atrophied.
v. It does not float in saturated salt solution used for concentration (heaviest of all helminthic eggs).

Life Cycle

The worm passes its life cycle in one host (**Fig. 55.10**) and no intermediate host is required. Man is the only known definitive host of *lumbricoides*. The various stages in the life cycle are described below:

Stage 1: *Eggs in feces—fertilized Ascaris* eggs are unsegmented when passed with the feces. They are not infective to man when freshly passed.

Stage 2: *Development in soil*—the development of the egg in soil usually takes from 10 to 40 days, during which time a rhabditiform larva is developed from the unsegmented ovum and undergoes first molting within the egg-shell. The ripe egg containing the coiled-up embryo is infective to man.

Stage 3: *Infection by ingestion and liberation of Larvae*—infection with food, drink, or raw vegetables occurs by ingestion when the egg containing the infective rhabditiform larva is swallowed. The embryonated eggs pass down to the duodenum and the rhabditiform larvae are liberated in the upper part of the small intestine.

Stage 4: *Migration through the lungs*—the larvae liberated in the small intestine burrow their way through the mucous membrane of the small intestine and are carried by the portal circulation to the liver. They pass out of the liver and via right heart enter the pulmonary circulation. They grow much bigger and increase in length in the lungs and molt twice.

Stage 5: *Re-entry into the stomach and the small Intestine*—after development in the lungs, the larvae pierce the lung capillaries and reach the alveoli. From the lung alveoli the larvae crawl up the bronchi and trachea, are propelled into the larynx and pharynx and are swallowed. They pass down the esophagus to the stomach and localize in the upper part of the small intestine (their normal abode) where they mature. Another molting occurs. They become sexually mature and the gravid females start laying eggs, to repeat the cycle. The adult worm has a life span of 12-20 months.

Mode of Infection

Infection is effected by *swallowing* ripe Ascaris eggs (embryonated eggs) with raw vegetables cultivated on a soil fertilized by infected human excreta.
- *Infecting agent:* Embryonated egg.
- *Migration of larvae:* Through lungs.
- *Portal of entry:* Alimentary canal.
- *Site of Location:* Small intestine.

Pathogenicity and Clinical Features

Infection of *A. lumbricoides* in man is known as ascariasis. The symptoms attributed to Ascaris infection, may be divided into two groups: (a) those produced by the migrating larvae and (b) those produced by the adult worms.

a. Symptoms due to the Migrating Larvae

Larvae in the lungs: *Ascaris Pneumonia (Loeffler's Syndrome)*.

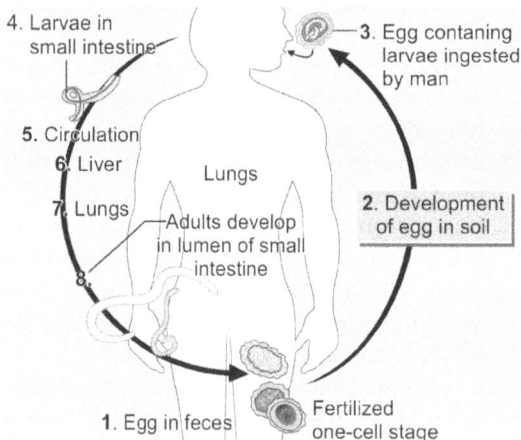

Fig. 55.10: Life cycle of *Ascaris lumbricoides*.

Larvae in general circulation: Disturbances have been reported due to their presence in the brain, spinal cord, heart and kidneys.

b. Symptoms due to the Adult Worms

Clinical manifestations due to *adult worm* vary from asymptomatic infection to severe and even fatal consequences. The pathological effects, when present, are caused by:
 a. **Spoliative action:** Patients have loss of appetite and are often listless.
 b. **Toxic action**
 c. **Mechanical effects**

Laboratory Diagnosis

A. Direct Evidences

 a. **Finding of adult worms:**
   i. In the stool or vomit.
   ii. *X-ray diagnosis:* Diagnosis may often be made by barium contrast radiography of the abdomen.
 b. **Finding of eggs:**
   i. *In the stool:* The most important method for the diagnosis of ascariasis is the demonstration of eggs in feces by a *direct microscopical examination* of a saline emulsion of the stool. Concentration by *floatation method* may be employed for the detection of eggs in the stool.
   ii. *In the bile:* It may reveal *Ascaris* eggs.

B. Indirect Evidences

 i. **Blood examination:** Eosinophilia suggests associated strongyloidiasis or toxocariasis.
 ii. **Skin test:** A skin test with ascaris antigen gives a positive result, but is unreliable and not used for diagnosis.
 iii. **Serological tests** are useful in diagnosis of extraintestinal ascariasis (Loeffler's syndrome).

ANCYLOSTOMA DUODENALE

- **Common name:** Old world hookworm.
- **Geographical distribution:** It is found in certain areas in Brazil, a part of India, most of China, and throughout Southeast Asia, Indonesia, and the islands of the South and the Southwest Pacific.

Habitat: The adult worm lives in the small intestine of man, mostly in the jejunum, less often in the duodenum and rarely in the ileum.

Morphology

Adult worm: *Ancylostoma* adults are small, grayish white or pinkish.

The anterior end of the worm is bent slightly dorsally and is in the same direction as the general body curvature. This cervical curvature gave it *the name hookworm.*

Buccal capsule: The mouth is well developed and is not at the tip but directed toward the dorsal surface. The large and prominent *buccal capsule* is lined with a hard chitin-like substance and is provided with 6 teeth, 4 hook-like on the ventral surface, and 2 knob-like (triangular plates) on the dorsal surface **(Fig. 55.11)**.

Male Worm

The male worm is provided with a prominent copulatory bursa posteriorly **(Fig. 55.11)**.

Copulatory bursa: This consists of three lobes: (1) dorsal and (2) lateral. Each lobe is supported by chitinous rays; the dorsal lobe contains 3

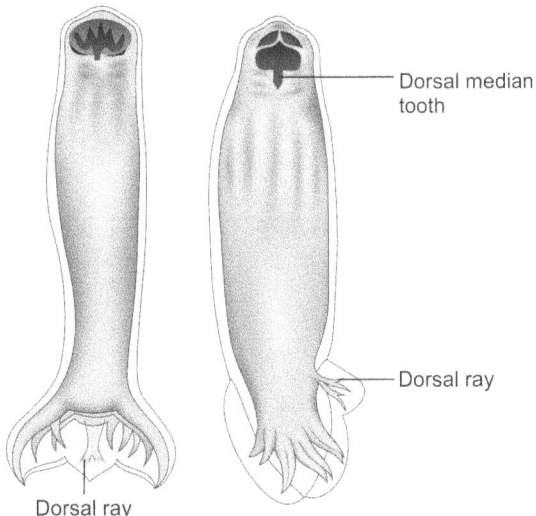

Fig. 55.11: Hookworm adult worm.

(1 single dorsal ray and 2 externodorsal rays); the two lateral lobes contain 10 (3 pairs of lateral rays and 2 pairs of ventral rays). Total number of rays are 13.

Female Worm

Differences between Male and Females

The sexes are easily differentiated by their sizes, the shape of the tail (posterior end) and the position of the genital opening **(Table 55.2)**. The worm assumes a Y-shaped figure during copulation due to the position of the genital opening.

Distinctive features of the egg **(Fig. 55.12)** are as follows:
  i. Regularly oval or elliptical in shape, measuring 65 µm in length by 40 µm in breadth.
 ii. Colorless (not bile-stained).
iii. Surrounded by a thin transparent hyaline shell-membrane.
 iv. Contains a segmented ovum usually with 4 blastomeres when passed in feces.
  v. Has a clear space between the egg shell and the segmented ovum.
 vi. Floats in saturated solution of common salt.

Life Cycle

Man is the only definitive host for *A. duodenale*. No intermediate host is required.

The life cycle of hookworms is presented in **Figure 55.13**. The following are the various stages of the life cycle.

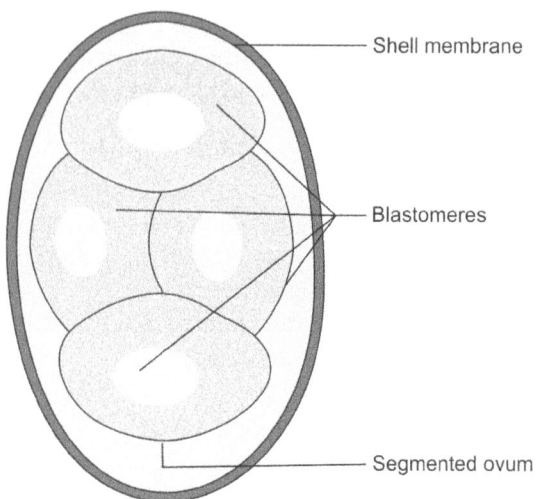

Fig. 55.12: Egg of hookworm.

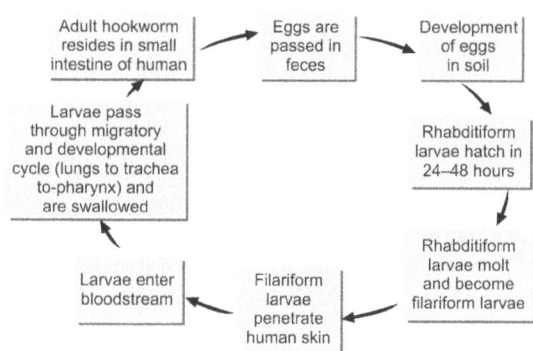

Fig. 55.13: Life cycle of hookworm.

Stage 1: *Passage of eggs from the infected host*—hookworm eggs, containing segmented ova with 4 blastomeres, are passed out in the feces of the human host.

Stage 2: *Development in soil*—from each egg a feeding larva called *rhabditiform larva* hatches out in the soil. The rhabditiform larva molts twice, and becomes a *filariform larva* the infective stage of the parasite.

Stage 3: *Entrance into a new host*—the filariform larvae are infective to man. When a person walks barefooted on soil containing filariform larva, they penetrates the skin and enters a migratory phase.

Table 55.2: Differences between male and female Ancylostoma adults.

	Male	Female
1. Size	Smaller; about 8 mm in length	Longer than male; about 12.5 mm in length
2. Posterior end	Expanded in an umbrella-like fashion (copulatory bursa)	Tapering; no expanded bursa
3. Genital opening	Posteriorly opens with the cloaca	At the junction of posterior and middle third of the body

Stage 4: *Migratory phase*—on reaching the subcutaneous tissues, the larvae enter into migratory phase that takes it to the lymphatics or small venules. They pass through the lymph-vascular system into the venous circulation and are carried *via* the right heart into the pulmonary capillaries, where they break through the capillary walls and enter into the alveolar spaces. They then migrate on to the bronchi, trachea and larynx, crawl over the epiglottis to the back of the pharynx and are ultimately swallowed. During migration or on entering the esophagus, a third molting takes place.

Stage 5: *Localization and laying of eggs*—the growing larvae settle down in the small intestine, undergo a fourth molting and develop into adolescent worms.

The adults live in the small intestine, where they attach to the mucosa via their buccal cavity and suck juices from host tissues.

They are sexually mature and the fertilized females begin to lay eggs in the feces. The cycle is thus repeated.

Pathogenicity

The worm causes hookworm disease or sancylostomiasis in man.
- **Infecting agent:** Filariform larva.
- **Portal of entry:** Skin.

Those produced by the larval forms while entering the skin of the host.
1. **Ancylostome dermatitis or ground itch:** In penetrating the skin, the larvae may cause an allergic reaction known as ground itch. It occurs at the site of entry.
2. **Creeping eruption (cutaneous larva migrans):** It is a condition in which the filariform larvae wander about through the skin in an aimless manner for several weeks and months, producing a reddish itchy papule along the path traversed by the larvae (termed "larva migrans"). Humans can be infected with the filariform larvae of hookworms that normally infect other animals.
   Causes: This is particularly seen with those species of parasites which are not adapted to man.
3. Signs of pneumonitis are due to allergic reactions to the larvae and to the damage caused when larvae break out of capillaries and move into the lung. A marked eosinophilia occurs at this stage.

Clinical Features of Hookworm Infection

Findings may include iron deficiency anemia, pica, poor appetite, nausea, vomiting, diarrhea or constipation, rapid pulse, and cardiac hypertrophy.

Infection may also occur by the accidental drinking of water contaminated with filariform larvae. Infection by this method is not common.

Laboratory Diagnosis

This consists of the following:

A. Direct Methods

Examination of Stool
a. **Macroscopic examination:** *A macroscopic* examination of stool is necessary to find the adult worms.
b. **Microscopical examination:** A direct *microscopical* examination of stool may easily demonstrate the presence of characteristic hookworm eggs. Concentration techniques may be needed to locate the eggs when small numbers are present.

Egg of *A. duodenale* or *N. americanus* cannot be differentiated by morphology of eggs. Thus, a specific diagnosis can be made by studying the morphology of adult worms or the mature infective filariform larvae for hookworm anemia.

B. Indirect Methods

i. **Blood examination:** This is carried out to ascertain the nature of anemia and the presence of eosinophilia.
ii. **Stool examination:** It may show occult blood and Charcot-Leyden crystals in a majority of cases of hookworm disease.

NECATOR AMERICANUS

Common name: The American hookworm or the New World hookworm.

The life cycle, general morphology, pathogenicity, and diagnosis are the same as described for *A. duodenale*.

VISCERAL LARVA MIGRANS

The life cycle of most nematodes parasitizing man include larva migration through various tissues and organs of the body. Sometimes the larva appears to lose their way and wander aimlessly. This condition is called larva migrans. Larva migrans can be classified depending on whether the larval migration takes place in the skin (*cutaneus larva migrans*) or in deeper tissues *Visceral larva migrans*.

Visceral larva migrans: This condition is caused by the migration of larvae of nonhuman species of nematodes that infect by the oral route. The most common cause is dog ascarid (*Toxocara canis*) less often cat ascarid (*Toxocara cati*). The infective eggs present the soil are ingested and the larvae hatch in the small intestine, penetrate the gut wall and migrate to the liver. They may remain in the liver or migrate to other organs, such as lungs, brain, or eyes. In man, they induce granulomatous lesions, which cause local damage. Fever, hepatomegaly, pneumonitis, hyperglobulinemia and pica are common findings. Marked leukocytosis occurs, with high eosinophilia.

Diagnosis can be made by serological tests, such as passive hemagglutination, bentonite flocculation, and microprecipitation for diagnosis of toxocariasis. Deworming of household pets helps in prevention by limiting the contamination of soil.

ENTEROBIUS VERMICULARIS

Common name: Threadworm, Pinworm, Seatworm

Geographical distribution: It is worldwide in distribution in both temperate and tropical areas.

Habitat: Adult worms live in the cecum and vermiform appendix and adjacent parts of the ascending colon.

Morphology

Adult Worm

It is small and white in color, more or less spindle-shaped. It resembles a short piece of thread.

Cervical alae: At the anterior extremity both male and female worm possess a pair of wing-like expansions, *known as cervical alae*. The esophagus is dilated posteriorly into a conspicuous globular bulb (a doublebulb esophagus), a characteristic feature of this worm.

Male: It measures 2–4 mm in length and 0.1–0.2 mm across its girth. The posterior third of the body is curved and sharply truncated. Usually dies after fertilizing the female.

Female: It measures 8–12 mm in length and 0.3–0.5 mm across its thickest part. Its posterior third extremity is straight and drawn out into a long, tapering and finely pointed tail.

Eggs: The general characteristics of the *egg* (**Fig. 55.14**) are as follows:
 i. Colorless, i.e., not bile-stained.
 ii. Plano-convex in shape, i.e., flattened on one side (the ventral side) and convex on the other (the dorsal side).

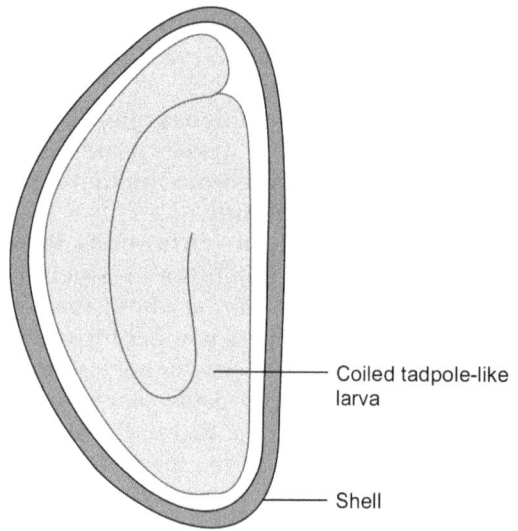

Fig. 55.14: Egg of *Enterobius vermicularis*.

iii. Measures 50–60 µm in length by 30 µm in breadth.
iv. Surrounded by a transparent shell.
v. Contains a coiled tadpole-like larva.
vi. Floats in saturated solution of common salt.

Life Cycle

No intermediate host is required and is completed in a single host (**Fig. 55.15**).

The male fertilizes the female and dies. The gravid female then migrates from the small intestine down to the caecum and colon to the rectum. At night, when the host is in bed, the worm comes out through the anus and crawls about on the perianal and perineal skin and deposit the eggs and these eggs are subsequently transferred to food and swallowed by the patient himself or the infection may occur direct from anus-to-mouth, a very common habit with children. A type of autoinfection described as "retrofection" involves hatching of the embryonated eggs after their deposition in the perianal area and subsequent migration back into the rectum and large intestine.

Infection occurs by ingestion of these eggs. Children are the usual victims and familial infection is common. The egg-shells are dissolved by digestive juices and the larvae escape in the small intestine where they develop into adolescent worms. The cycle is then repeated.

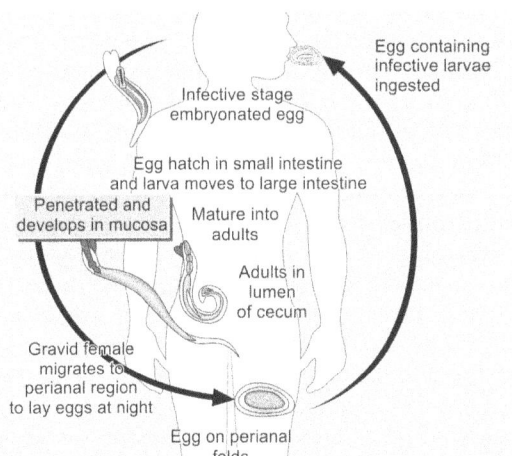

Fig. 55.15: Life cycle *Enterobius vermicularis*.

Pathogenesis

Infection of *E. vermicularis* in man is known as enterobiasis. The significant pathology is the irritation caused by the gravid females around the anus. In most cases, clinical manifestations represent an allergic reaction to pinworm secretions and excretions, which produce intense perianal itching. Attachment of the adult worms to the intestinal wall may produce some inflammation. The migrating females often enter into the female genital tract and female urethra, causing inflammation. These worms may even enter into the peritoneal cavity through the Fallopian tubes.

Clinical Features

1. Pruritus periani and an eczematous condition round the anus and perineum.
2. Salpingitis
3. Nocturnal enuresis (frequency of micturition).

Laboratory Diagnosis

This depends upon (i) the finding of adult worm and (ii) demonstration of eggs.

1. **Detection of adult worms:** The worms are often discovered by the patient himself or by the parents of the children. Adult worms may be detected in the perianal region or on the surfaces of the stools.
2. **Demonstration of eggs:** Eggs are generally demonstrated in the scrapings from the perianal skin by a NIH swab (**Fig. 55.16**). The swab is taken immediately after the patient wakes up in the morning. Eggs can also be recovered from under the finger-nails and the washings from garments. Eggs are present in the feces only in a small proportion of patients; microscopical examination of stool for eggs of *E. vermicularis* may occasionally be successful.

WUCHERERIA BANCROFTI

Elephantiasis is caused most commonly by *Wuchereria bancrofti*. The parasite is largely

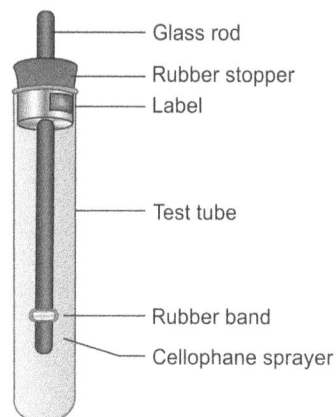

Fig. 55.16: NIH swab.

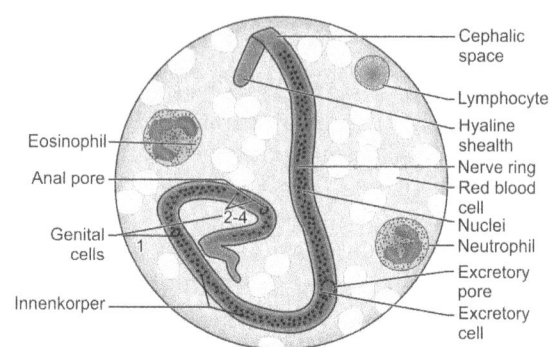

Fig. 55.17: Morphology of *Microfilaria bancrofti*. 1 and 2-4, G-cells (so called "genital cells").

confined to the tropics and subtropics, occurring in India. In India, it is distributed chiefly along the sea-coast and along the banks of big rivers (except Indus).

Habitat: Adult worms are found in the lymphatic vessels and lymph nodes of man only.

Morphology

Adult Worms

The adult worms are long hair-like, transparent and often creamy-white in color. They are filiform in shape and both ends are tapering.

The *female* is larger (8–10 cm in length by 0.2–0.3 mm in thickness) than male (2.5–4 cm in length by 0.1 mm in thickness). The tail-end of male is curved ventrally and contains two spicules of unequal length while tail-end of female is narrow and abruptly pointed. Males and females remain coiled together usually in the abdominal and inguinal lymphatic and in the testicular tissues and can only be separated with difficulty. The females are really ovoviviparous (laying eggs with well developed embryos). The *life span* of the adult worms is long, probably 5–10 years.

Embryos (Microfilariae)

When unstained, the microfilaria has a colorless and transparent body with blunt head and rather pointed tail measuring about 290 μm in length by 6–7 μm in breadth and is covered by a hyaline sheath.

The sheath is much longer than the larval body so that the larva can move forwards and backwards within it.

Somatic cells or nuclei: Appear as granules in the central axis of the body and extend from the head to the tail end. These granules do not extend up to the tip of the tail and helps in the identification of the species as a distinguishing feature of *M. bancrofti* (**Fig. 55.17**).

Life Cycle

W. bancrofti passes its life cycle (**Fig. 55.18**) in two hosts: *man (definitive host)* and *mosquito (intermediate host)*.

Adult forms of *Wuchereria* live in the lymph nodes of humans and can survive for 4–5 years. The male fertilizes female. The gravid females give birth to microfilariae, and these organisms circulate in the blood. These microfilariae are ingested by female mosquitoes when they take a blood meal. During their developmental cycle in the mosquito, the microfilariae increase in length and become infective to man. Mosquitos belonging to the genus *Culex, Aedes* and *Anopheles* mosquitoes act as intermediate hosts for *Wuchereria*. When the infected mosquito bites a human being, the *larvae* are deposited on the skin near the site of puncture. The larvae either enter through the puncture wound, and begin to grow into adult forms and become sexually mature. The male fertilizes the female and the gravid females give birth to larvae. The embryos are capable of living in the peripheral

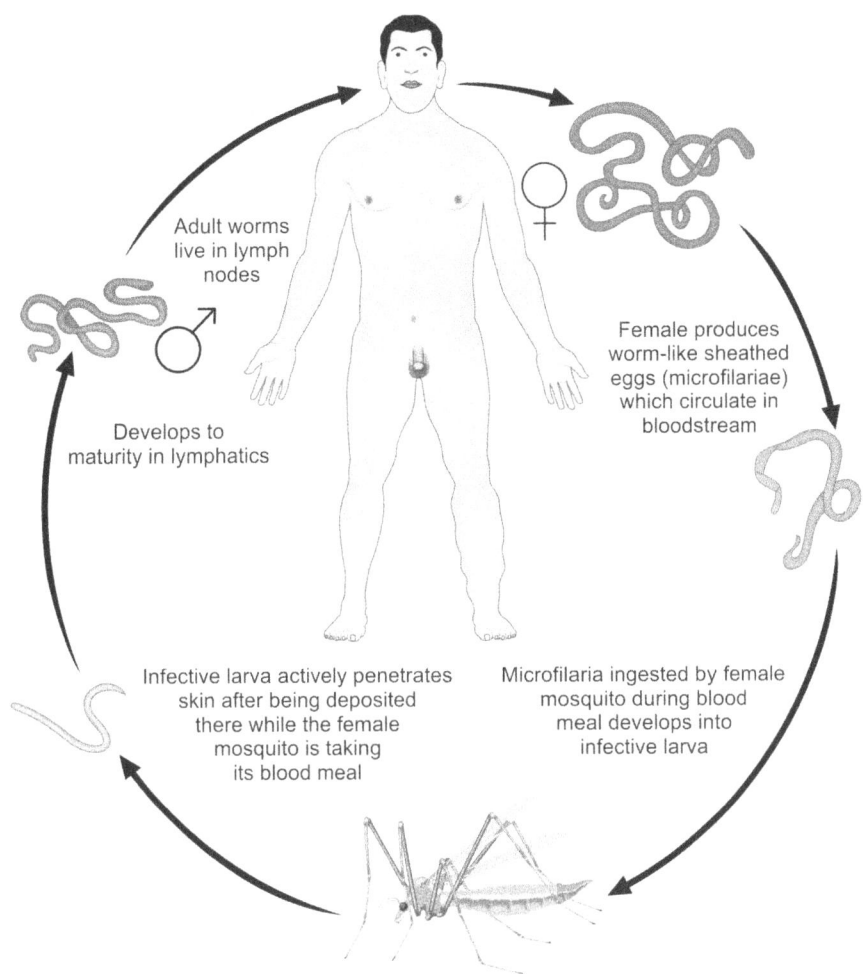

Fig. 55.18: Life cycle *Wuchereria bancrofti*

blood for a circulation, thus completing the cycle. They then enter through the puncture wound or penetrate through the skin on their own reach the lymphatic channels, settle down at some spot (inguinal, scrotal or abdominal lymphatics) subsequently taken up by the female culicine mosquitoes during their blood-meal.

Pathogenicity and Clinical Features

Infection with this parasite is called wuchereriasis (commonly called "filariasis").

i. **The disease is of two types:** Classical filariasis the characteristic manifestations of filariasis due to obstruction of lymph vessels and nodes. The essential features are lymphagiovarix, lymphorrhagia, or chylorrhagia, hydrocele, lymphedema, and elephantiasis.

ii. **Occult filariasis:** This term is applied to clinical conditions not directly due to lymphatic involvement, but due to hypersensitivity reactions to filarial antigens. The best studied syndrome is tropical pulmonary eosinophilia is probably due to the accumulation of microfilariae in lung tissues. Patients with tropical pulmonary eosinophilia typically have persistent eosinophilia and high titers of IgE antibody. Blood eosinophil count is above 3,000 per cmm and may even go up to 50,000 or more. Microfilariae are not usually detectable in blood.

Laboratory Diagnosis

A. Direct Evidence

i. **Detection of microfilariae:** In the peripheral blood, chylous urine, exudate of lymph varix and in the hydrocele fluid. The microfilariae appear in blood at night. In India, night blood samples are collected between 10 PM and 4 AM.
ii. **Demonstration of the adult worm:** Demonstration of the adult worm in biopsy specimens and the calcified worm may be seen on X-ray examination.

B. Indirect Evidences

i. Skin test with filarial antigen
ii. Blood examination—shows eosinophilia (5–15%).
iii. Serological tests—such as complement fixation test, indirect hemagglutination, indirect fluorescent antibody, immunodiffusion and immunoenzyme tests.

TREMATODES

The trematodes, more commonly called flukes, are so named on account of their conspicuous suckers are parasites of intestinal tract, bile ducts, lungs or blood of man.

Most trematodes are leaf-shaped unsegmented flat worms and oval in shape called flukes. Most are hermaphroditic except schistosomes which are unisexual.

Eggs are operculated or lid at one end, except those of schistosomes and can develop only in water. Trematodes pass their life cycle in two different hosts.

Classification of Trematodes

1. **Intestinal trematodes (intestinal flukes):** *Fasciola*.
2. **Hepatic trematodes (liver flukes):** *Fasciola hepatica*
3. **Lung trematodes (lung flukes):** *Paragonimus westermani*
4. **Blood trematodes (blood flukes):** *Scistosoma haematobium, Scistosoma mansoni, Scistosoma japonicum*

KEY POINTS

- The larval stage of *T. solium* developing in the muscles of the pig is known as *Cysticercus cellulosae.*
- *Cysticercus bovis:* This is the larval stage of *T. saginata* developing in the muscles of a cow or a buffalo.
- *Echinococcus granulosus* causes *unilocular echinococcosis* or *hydatid disease* in man.
- Infection of *A. lumbricoides* in man is known as ascariasis.
- The adult worm lives in the small intestine of man, mostly in the jejunum.
- Mode of infection: This occurs when man walks bare-foot on the fecally contaminated soil.
- Infection of *E. vermicularis* in man is known as enterobiasis.
- Infection with *Wuchereria bancrofti* is called wuchereriasis (commonly called "filariasis").

IMPORTANT QUESTIONS

1. Write short notes on:
    a. Differences between *Taenia solium* and *Taenia saginata*
    b. *Cysticercus cellulosae*
    c. Hydatid cyst
2. Describe the life cycle of *Echinococcus granulosus* and the laboratory diagnosis of hydatid cyst.
3. Name the various hookworms. Describe the life cycle of *Ancylostoma duodenale.*
4. Write short notes on:
    a. Life cycle of *Ascaris lumbricoides*
    b. *Enterobius vermicularis*
    c. Larva migrans
    d. NIH swab
    e. Microfilaria
    f. *Wuchereria bancrofti*

MULTIPLE CHOICE QUESTIONS

1. Raw or undercooked pork may act as a source of infection for:
   a. *Taenia solium*
   b. *Taenia saginata*
   c. *Diphyllobothrium latum*
   d. *Ancylostoma duodenale*
   e. *Toxoplasma gondii*
2. Which of the following parasites is transmitted by dog?
   a. *Echinococcus granulosus*
   b. *Hymenolepis nana*
   c. *Taenia solium*
   d. *Diphyllobothrium latum*
3. Blood-sucking insects may transmit:
   a. *Ancylostoma duodenale*
   b. *Ascaris lumbricoides*
   c. *Wuchereria bancrofti*
   d. *Strongyloides stercoralis*

ANSWERS

1. a   2. a   3. c

Miscellaneous

SECTION OUTLINE
56. Infective Syndrome
57. Laboratory Control of Antimicrobial Therapy
58. Normal Microbial Flora of the Human Body
59. Antimicrobial Chemotherapy
60. Immunoprophylaxis
61. Vehicles, Vectors and Rodents
62. Pathogenesis and Common Diseases

CHAPTER 56

Infective Syndrome*

LEARNING OBJECTIVES

After reading and studying this chapter, you should be able to:
- List causative organisms of meningitis.
- Discuss the laboratory diagnosis of acute pyogenic meningitis.
- List causative organisms of urinary tract infection.
- Discuss the laboratory diagnosis of urinary tract infection.
- Describe the following: Sore throat; diarrhea; dysentery; food poisoning sexually transmitted diseases (STDs); pyrexia of unknown origin (PUO).

MENINGITIS

Meningitis is an inflammation of the membranes surrounding the brain and spinal cord. It may be caused by bacteria, viruses, fungi or protozoa. Most cases of meningitis fall into one of two categories: **purulent meningitis (acute pyogenic meningitis)** and **aseptic meningitis**. The causative agents of these types are given in **Table 56.1**.

Purulent Meningitis (Acute Pyogenic Meningitis)

Laboratory Diagnosis

A. **Collection of specimens:** The principal specimen to be examined is of cerebrospinal fluid (CSF) collected by lumbar puncture under strict aseptic conditions. It should not be kept in a refrigerator, which tends to kill *Haemophilus* (*H*). *influenzae*. If delay for a few hours is unavoidable, the specimen is best kept in an incubator at 37°C.

B. **Laboratory examination of CSF for cells and microorganisms:**
  1. Naked eye examination
  2. Cell count (Table 56.2)

Table 56.1: Causative agents of purulent and aseptic meningitis.

Purulent meningitis	Aseptic meningitis
• Neisseria meningitidis	A. Viruses
• Streptococcus pneumoniae	Enteroviruses (echoviruses, polioviruses, coxsackieviruses)
• Haemophilus influenzae	
• Escherichia coli	
• Group B streptococci	➤ Mumps
• Pseudomonas	➤ Herpes simplex
• Salmonellae	➤ Varicella-zoster
• Staphylococcus aureus	➤ Measles
• Staphylococcus epidermidis	➤ Adenoviruses
	➤ Arboviruses
• Listeria monocytogenes	B. Spiral bacteria
• Klebsiella spp.	C. Other bacteria
• Anaerobic cocci	D. Fungi
• Bacteroides	E. Protozoa
In neonates and infants	
• Escherichia coli	
• Group B streptococci	
• Pseudomonas	
• Salmonellae	
• Staph. aureus	
• H. influenzae	
• Listeria monocytogenes	
• Streptococcus pneumoniae	
• Klebsiella spp.	

---

*This chapter was contributed by Dr Sourabh Kumar, Demonstrator, Department of Pathology, Government Medical College, Chandigarh-160047.

Table 56.2: Typical CSF findings in different types of meningitis.

Characteristic	Normal CSF	Acute pyogenic meningitis	CSF in Tuberculous meningitis	Viral meningitis
I. Pressure	Normal	Highly increased	Moderately increased	Slightly increased
II. Direct examination				
a. Cell count				
1. Total cell (per cu. mm)	1–3	1,000–20,000	50–500	10–500
2. Predominant	Lymphocytes	Neutrophils (90–95%)	Lymphocytes (90%)	Lymphocytes
b. Biochemical analysis				
1. Total proteins (mg%)	30–45	100–600 (highly increased)	80–120 (moderately increased)	60–80 (slightly increased)
2. Sugars (mg%)	40–80	Diminished or absent (10–20)	Diminished (30–50)	Normal
III. Bacteriological examination				
a. Microscopy				
1. Gram staining	Nil	Gram-negative cocci, Gram-positive cocci, Gram-negative bacilli or Gram-positive bacilli may be found depending upon the causative agent responsible.	–	–
2. Ziehl-Neelsen staining	Nil	Nil		–
b. Culture	Nil	According to the causative agent, specific organism may grow on appropriate media	Acid-fast bacilli (AFB) may be found M. tuberculosis may grow on LJ media	Viruses may be grown on cell cultures

(CSF: cerebrospinal fluid; LJ: Löwenstein–Jensen)

3. **Gram film of CSF:** After taking some CSF for the cell count, the remainder should be centrifuged to deposit any cells and bacteria and a film of the deposit should be stained by Gram's method.
   The supernatant from the centrifuged CSF should be tested for its content of glucose and protein.
4. **Culture**
   i. **CSF culture:** Immediately after centrifugation of the CSF and the removal of some of the deposit for the Gram film, the remainder of the deposit should be seeded heavily on to culture media and **a-tube** of cooked-meat broth. If the plate cultures remain free from growth, and turbidity develops in the cooked-meat broth, the broth should be filmed and subcultured.
   ii. **Blood culture:** Blood culture is particularly useful in meningitis.
5. **Biochemical tests:** The supernate from the centrifuged CSF should be tested for its content of glucose and protein **(Table 56.2)**.
6. **Antigen detection:** The supernatant part of CSF contains antigen.
7. **Agglutination:** The isolated organisms may be grouped by agglutination with appropriate antisera.
8. **Demonstration of bacterial endotoxin.**

Aseptic Meningitis

The great majority of cases are due to viruses (viral meningitis). A few cases with CSF findings resembling those of viral meningitis are caused by leptospires, fungi *(Cryptococcus neoformans* or *Candida albicans)* and amoebae *(Naegleria* or *Hartmanella).*

Laboratory Diagnosis

Cerebrospinal fluid (CSF) is used for:

Cell count and biochemical tests, microscopy, culture and other tests according to suspected causative agents (viruses, fungi or protozoa).

Tuberculous Meningitis

When a tuberculous infection is suspected, the centrifuged deposit of the *CSF* should be examined in an auramine or Ziehl-Neelsen stained film for acidfast bacilli and cultured on one or two slopes of Löwenstein-Jensen medium.

URINARY TRACT INFECTIONS

Urinary tract infection (UTI) may be defined as the presence of bacteria undergoing multiplication in urine within the urinary drainage system. Micro-organisms causing UTI are shown in **Table 56.3**.

Laboratory Diagnosis

(For details *refer* Chapter 28.)

SORE THROAT

Sore throat is essentially an acute tonsillitis or pharyngitis. It is characterized by redness and edema of mucosa, exudation of tonsils, pseudomembrane formation, edema of uvula, gray coating of tongue and enlargement of cervical lymph nodes. Causative agents of sore throat are given in **Table 56.4**.

Pseudomembrane formation: *Corynebacterium diphtheriae, Candida albicans,* β-hemolytic group A *Streptococcus, Treponema vincentii* and *Leptotrichia buccalis* may lead to pseudomembrane formation.

Table 56.3: Causes of urinary tract infection.

A. **Gram-negative bacilli**
   Gram-negative bacilli are by far the most common infecting agents.
   1. *Escherichia coli* causes approximately 80% of acute infections in patients without catheters
   2. *Proteus mirabilis*
   3. *Klebsiella*
   4. *Enterobacter* (occasionally)
   5. *Serratia*
   6. *Pseudomonas aeruginosa*
B. **Gram-positive cocci—lesser role in UTIs**
   1. *Staphylococcus saprophyticus* (10–15%)
   2. *S. epidermidis* (1–5%)
   3. *S. aureus* (1–5%)
   4. *Enterococcus* spp. (1–5%)
C. **Other organisms which may occasionally cause UTI**
   1. *Mycobacterium tuberculosis*
   2. *Enterobacter*
   3. *Citrobacter*
   4. *Salmonellae*
   5. *Streptococcus pyogenes*
   6. *S. agalactiae*
   7. *Gardnerella vaginalis*
D. **Fungus**
   Candida albicans may cause UTI in diabetics and immunocompromised patients.

Table 56.4: Causative agents of sore throat.

A. **Bacteria**
   - *Streptococcus* β-hemolytic group A and occasionally groups C and G
   - *Corynebacterium diphtheriae*
   - *Haemophilus influenzae*
   - *Bordetella pertussis*
   - *Neisseria gonorrhoeae*
   - *Treponema vincentii*
   - *Leptotrichia buccalis*
B. **Fungi**
   - *Candida albicans*
C. **Viruses**
   - Epstein–Barr virus
   - Adenoviruses
   - Coxsackievirus A

Laboratory Diagnosis

For laboratory diagnosis, refer to the respective chapters.

DIARRHEA

Infective diarrhea may be caused by viruses, bacteria, protozoa and Fungi **(Table 56.5)**.

Table 56.5: Causative agents of infective diarrhea.

A. **Bacteria**
- Vibrio cholerae
- V. parahaemolyticus
- Escherichia coli (ETEC, EPEC)
- Salmonella enteritidis
- S. typhimurium
- Other Salmonella spp.
- Campylobacter spp.
- Yersinia enterocolitica
- Shigella spp.
- Clostridium perfringens
- C. difficile
- Staphylococcus aureus
- Bacillus cereus
- Aeromonas hydrophila
- Plesiomonas shigelloides

B. **Viruses**
- Rotavirus
- Astrovirus
- Calicivirus
- Norwalk virus
- Adenovirus

C. **Protozoa**
- Entamoeba histolytica
- Giardia lamblia
- Cryptosporidium parvum
- Isospora belli

D. **Cestodes**
- Hymenolepis nana

E. **Nematodes**
- Trichuris trichiura
- Strongyloides stercoralis
- Ascaris lumbricoides
- Hookworms

F. **Trematodes**
- Schistosoma mansoni

(EPEC: enteropathogenic *E. coli*; ETEC: enterotoxigenic *E. coli*)

Laboratory Diagnosis

For laboratory diagnosis, refer to the respective chapters.

DYSENTERY

Dysentery results from "enteroinvasive" microorganisms **(Table 56.6)** that penetrate through the mucosa and cause inflammation of the intestinal wall.

Laboratory Diagnosis

For laboratory diagnosis, refer to the respective chapters.

Table 56.6: Microorganisms causing dysentery.

A. **Bacteria**
- Shigella dysenteriae
- Shigella flexneri
- Shigella boydii
- Shigella sonnei
- Escherichia coli (EIEC, EPEC, EHEC)

B. **Protozoa**
- Entamoeba histolytica
- Balantidium coli

(EIEC: enteroinvasive *Escherichia coli*; EPEC: enteropathogenic *E. coli*; EHEC: enterohemorrhagic *Escherichia coli*)

Table 56.7: Causative agents of food poisoning.

1. **Infective type**
   - Salmonella typhimurium
   - Salmonella Enteritidis
   - Salmonella Heidelberg
   - Salmonella Indiana
   - Salmonella Newport
   - Salmonella Dublin
   - Vibrio parahaemolyticus
   - Campylobacter jejuni

2. **Toxic type**
   - Staphylococcus aureus
   - Bacillus cereus
   - Clostridium botulinum

3. **Infective-toxic type**
   - Clostridium perfringens

FOOD POISONING

It is of three types **(Table 56.7)**:

A. **Infective type:** In this type, multiplication of bacteria occurs in vivo when infective doses of microorganisms are ingested with food. Incubation period is generally 8–24 hours. The typical example of this type of food poisoning is by *Salmonellae*.

B. **Toxic type:** In this type, the disease follows ingestion of food with preformed toxin. Incubation period is short (2–6 hours). Example is staphylococcal food poisoning.

C. **Infective-toxic type:** In this type, bacteria release the toxin in the bowel. The incubation period is 6–12 hours. The typical example is *Clostridium (Cl). perfringens* food poisoning.

Laboratory Diagnosis

For laboratory diagnosis, refer to the respective chapters.

SEXUALLY TRANSMITTED DISEASES

The sexually transmitted diseases (STDs) are a group of communicable diseases which are transmitted predominantly or entirely by sexual contact. The causative organisms include a wide range of bacterial, viral. Protozoal and fungal agents. STD may present as genital ulcers, genital discharge without any genital lesion or only as systemic manifestations **(Table 56.8)**.

Table 56.8: Organisms causing sexually transmitted diseases.

STDs	Organisms
A. **Painless genital ulcers**	
➢ Syphilis	*Treponema pallidum*
➢ Lymphogranuloma venereum (LGV)	*Chlamydia trachomatis*
➢ Donovanosis	*Calymmatobacterium granulomatis*
B. **Painful genital ulcers**	
➢ Chancroid	*Haemophilus ducreyi*
➢ Herpes genitalis	Herpes simplex viruses (HSV) type 2 and 1
C. **Urethral discharge**	
➢ Gonorrhea	*Neisseria gonorrhoeae*
➢ Nongonococcal urethritis (NGU)	*Chlamydia trachomatis* (types D–K) *Ureaplasma urealyticum Mycoplasma genitalium Mycoplasma hominis*
D. Vaginal discharge	
➢ Gonorrhea	*Neisseria gonorrhoeae*
➢ NGU	*Chlamydia trachomatis*
➢ Trichomoniasis	*Mycoplasma hominis*
➢ Vaginitis	*Trichomonas vaginalis*
➢ Vulvovaginal candidiasis	*Gardnerella vaginalis Mobiluncus* spp. *Candida albicans*
E. **Genital warts**	Human papillomaviruses
F. **No genital lesions but only systemic manifestations**	HIV-1 and HIV-2 Hepatitis B virus (HBV) Hepatitis C virus (HCV)
G. **Miscellaneous**	Group B streptococci Molluscum contagiosum virus *Cytomegalovirus Phthirus pubis Sarcoptes scabei Shigella* spp. *Campylobacter* spp. *Giardia lamblia Entamoeba histolytica*

Table 56.9: Causes of PUO.

Infective causes

a. **Bacterial**
   ➢ Urinary tract infections
   ➢ Lung, subdiaphragmatic, appendix and other deep abscesses
   ➢ Septicemia associated with cryptic abscesses, pneumonia, pyelonephritis, biliary tract infection, infective endocarditis and immunodeficiencies; enteric fever
   ➢ Tuberculosis
   ➢ Brucellosis

b. **Parasitic**
   ➢ Malaria
   ➢ Hepatic amebiasis
   ➢ Leishmaniasis
   ➢ Trypanosomiasis
   ➢ Toxoplasmosis
   ➢ Filariasis

c. **Viral**
   ➢ EBV infection
   ➢ CMV infection
   ➢ HIV infection
   ➢ Rubella and other infectious fevers without typical rash

(EBV: Epstein-Barr virus; CMV: cytomegalovirus; HIV: human immunodeficiency virus; PUO: pyrexia of unknown origin)

PYREXIA OF UNKNOWN ORIGIN

Pyrexia of unknown origin (PUO) may be defined (a) any febrile illness (body temperature greater than 38°C) on several occasions, (b) duration of fever of more than 3 weeks, and (c) failure to reach a diagnosis despite 1 week of inpatient investigation. It is also known as **"fever of unknown origin" (FUO)**.

Causes of PUO

Infection is the most common cause of PUO. However, there are important noninfectious causes of fever. The causes of PUO are given in **Table 56.9**.

Laboratory Diagnosis of PUO

Tests should first be done for the more likely infections and then, if these are negative, tests for the less likely should be done.

KEY POINTS

- Most cases of meningitis fall into one of two categories: Purulent meningitis and aseptic meningitis.
- For specimen collection various methods are used.
- Diarrhea is defined as the passage of loose, liquid or watery stools.
- Dysentery results from "enteroinvasive" micro-organisms.
- Sore throat is essentially an acute tonsillitis or pharyngitis.
- Food poisoning is of three types: **(A) Infective type, (B) Toxic type, and (C) Infective-toxic type.**
- The causes of PUO include *infections (bacterial, parasitic and viral).*

IMPORTANT QUESTIONS

1. Name various organisms causing meningitis. Discuss the laboratory diagnosis of acute pyogenic meningitis.
2. Name various organisms causing urinary tract infection. Discuss the laboratory diagnosis of this condition.
3. Name various organisms causing sore throat. How will you diagnose it in the laboratory?
4. Enumerate the etiological agents of dysentery. Discuss in detail the laboratory diagnosis of dysentery.
5. Name various organisms causing food poisoning. Describe briefly the laboratory diagnosis of this condition.
6. Name various organisms causing sexually transmitted diseases. Discuss the laboratory diagnosis of syphilis.
7. Define and enumerate the causes of pyrexia of unknown origin (PUO). Discuss the laboratory diagnosis of PUO.

MULTIPLE CHOICE QUESTIONS

1. Which of the following agent's cause/s aseptic meningitis?
   a. Herpes simplex
   b. Enteroviruses
   c. Arboviruses
   d. All of the above
2. Which of the following bacteria is the most common cause of UTI?
   a. *E. coli*
   b. *Ps. aeruginosa*
   c. *Staph. aureus*
   d. *Staph. saprophyticus*
3. Which of the following organisms may lead to pseudomembrane formation in throat?
   a. *C. diphtheriae*
   b. *Strep. pyogenes*
   c. *Candida albicans*
   d. All of the above
4. Which of the following agents can cause diarrhea?
   a. Rotavirus
   b. *Vibrio cholerae*
   c. *S. typhimurium*
   d. All of the above
5. Which of the following agents can cause dysentery?
   a. Enteroinvasive *Escherichia coli* (EIEC)
   b. *Shigella dysenteriae*
   c. *Entamoeba histolytica*
   d. All of the above
6. Which of the following bacteria can cause infective type of food poisoning?
   a. *S. enteritidis*
   b. *Clostridium botulinum*
   c. *Staph. aureus*
   d. All of the above
7. Ulcer/s is/are painless in which of the following sexually transmitted diseases?
   a. Syphilis
   b. Chancroid
   c. Herpes genitalis
   d. All of the above
8. Genital ulcer is painful in:
   a. Syphilis
   b. Chancroid
   c. Lymphogranuloma venereum
   d. Donovanosis
9. Which of the following conditions can result in PUO?
   a. Urinary tract infection
   b. Enteric fever
   c. Malaria
   d. All of the above

ANSWERS

1. d   2. e   3. d   4. d
5. d   6. d   7. a   8. b
9. d

CHAPTER 57

Laboratory Control of Antimicrobial Therapy

LEARNING OBJECTIVES

After reading and studying this chapter, you should be able to:
- List different methods of antibiotic sensitivity testing.
- Describe disk diffusion methods.
- Explain Stokes disk diffusion method and its reporting.
- Differentiate between Stokes disk diffusion and modified Stokes disk diffusion method.

INTRODUCTION

As strains of most pathogenic organisms differ from one another within their species in their antibiotic sensitivities, sensitivity tests are required as a routine.

ANTIBIOTIC SENSITIVITY TESTS

Antibiotic sensitivity tests are of two types:
A. **Diffusion methods**
   1. Kirby-Bauer disk diffusion method
   2. Stokes disk diffusion method
B. **Dilution methods**
   1. Broth dilution method
   2. Agar dilution method

A. Diffusion Methods

Here the drug is allowed to diffuse through a solid medium so that a gradient is established, the concentration being highest near the site of application of the drug and decreasing with distance (**Fig. 57.1**). The test bacterium is seeded on the medium and its sensitivity to the drug determined from the inhibition of its growth.

Medium: Mueller-Hinton broth and agar may be used for testing aerobic and facultative anaerobic isolates.

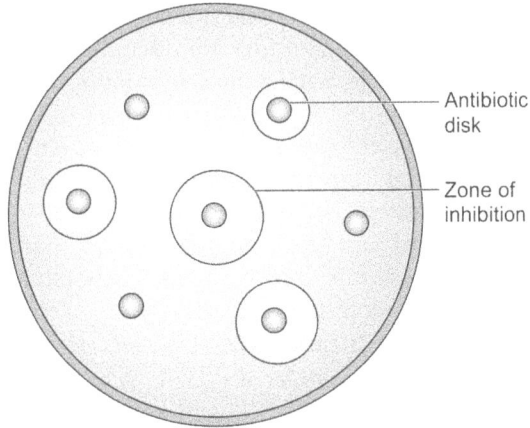

Fig. 57.1: Kirby-Bauer disk diffusion method.

Antibiotic disks: Commercially prepared antibiotic disks 6 mm in diameter or disks prepared locally in the laboratory are used.

1. Kirby-Bauer Disk Diffusion Method

A. **Preparation of inoculum (growth method):** Inoculate the dried surface of a Mueller-Hinton agar plate.
B. **Testing of antibiotics:** The appropriate antimicrobial-impregnated disks are placed on the surface of the agar (**Fig. 57.1**). The plates are then incubated at 35°C for 16–18 hours.

C. **Interpretation:** The interpretation of zone size into susceptible, moderately susceptible or resistant is based on the interpretation chart.

2. Stokes Disk Diffusion Method

The test organism is inoculated on central one-third and control on upper and lower thirds of the plate. However, in modified Stokes disk diffusion method, the test organism is inoculated in the upper and lower thirds and control on central one-third. A uninoculated gap should separate the test and control areas on which antibiotic disks are applied **(Fig. 57.2)**. Plates should be incubated in air at 35–37°C overnight (ideally, for 16–18 hours).

Reading and reporting results: Measure the inhibition zones of the control strain, i.e., the distance in millimeters from the edge of the disk to the zone edge. Each zone size is interpreted as follows:
1. **Sensitive:** The zone size of the test strain is larger than, equal to or not more than 3 mm smaller than that of the control strain.
2. **Intermediate:** The zone size of the test strain is at least 2 mm, but also 3 mm smaller than that of the control strain.
3. **Resistant:** The zone size of the test strain is smaller than 2 mm.

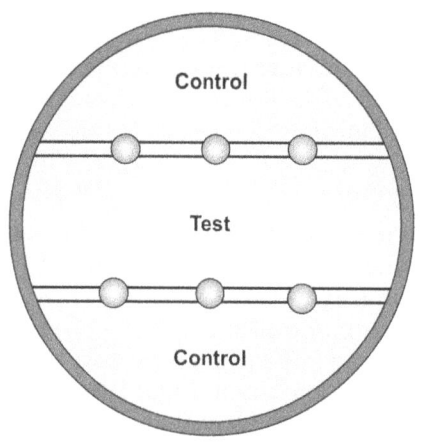

Fig. 57.2: Stokes disk diffusion method.

Epsilometer or E-test

The E-test, a modification of the disk diffusion test, utilizes a strip impregnated with a gradient of concentrations of an antimicrobial drug. Multiple strips, each containing a different drug, are placed on the surface of an agar medium that has been uniformly inoculated with the test organism. Each strip contains a gradient of an antibiotic and is labeled with a scale of minimal inhibitory concentration (MIC) values. The MIC is determined by reading a number of the numerical scale printed on the strip at the point where the bacterial growth intersects it.

B. Dilution Methods

Dilution tests may be done by the tube dilution or agar dilution methods.

1. Broth Dilution Method

Serial dilutions of the drug in Mueller-Hinton broth are taken in tubes and a standardized suspension of the test bacterium inoculated. An organism of known sensitivity should also be titrated. Incubate at 35–37°C for 16–18 hours and read the results. Incubate at 30°C for determination of *minimum inhibitory concentration* (MIC).

MIC is the lowest concentration of antimicrobial agent at which there is no visible growth. For determination of minimum bactericidal concentration (MBC), subculture from each tube showing no growth over a quarter of a nutrient medium free from antimicrobial agent. Incubate and examine them for growth. The tube containing lowest concentration of the antimicrobial agent that fails to yield growth, on subculture, is the MBC of the antimicrobial agent for the test strain. MIC inhibits the bacterial growth while MBC kills the bacterium.

2. Agar Dilution Method

Here, serial dilutions of the drug are prepared in agar (Mueller–Hinton agar) and poured into plates. The "agar dilution" method is more convenient when several strains are to be tested at the same time.

KEY POINTS

- Antibiotic susceptibility tests are of two types: Diffusion tests and dilution tests.
- Diffusion tests consists of Kirby-Bauer and Stokes' disk method.

IMPORTANT QUESTION

1. Write short notes on:
   a. Disk diffusion test
   b. Kirby-Bauer disk diffusion method
   c. Stokes disk diffusion method

MULTIPLE CHOICE QUESTIONS

1. Which of the following media is most suitable for antibiotic sensitivity testing?
   a. Mueller-Hinton medium
   b. Nutrient agar
   c. Blood agar
   d. MacConkey agar
2. The pH of the medium for antibiotic sensitivity testing should be:
   a. 6.0–6.2
   b. 6.8–7.0
   c. 7.2–7.4
   d. 7.6–7.8
3. Addition of 5% salt in the medium is done when testing antibiotic susceptibility of:
   a. Methicillin resistant staphylococci
   b. Pneumococci
   c. Coliforms
   d. Nonfermenting gram-negative bacilli

ANSWERS

1. a   2. c   3. a

Normal Microbial Flora of the Human Body

LEARNING OBJECTIVES

After reading and studying this chapter, you should be able to:
- Describe role of normal flora in human body.
- List of organisms present as normal flora in normal flora of upper respiratory tract and gastrointestinal tract.

INTRODUCTION

The term **"normal microbial flora"** denotes the population of microorganisms that inhabit the skin and mucous membranes of healthy normal persons.

NORMAL FLORA OF THE SKIN

The predominant resident microorganisms of the skin are aerobic and anaerobic diphtheroid bacilli (e.g., *Corynebacterium, Propionibacterium*); nonhemolytic aerobic and anaerobic staphylococci *[Staphylococcus epidermidis*, occasionally *Staphylococcus* (*S*) *aureus*, and *Peptostreptococcus* species]; gram-positive, aerobic, spore-forming bacilli that are ubiquitous in air, water, and soil; alpha hemolytic streptococci (viridans streptococci) and enterococci (*Enterococcus* species); and gram-negative coliform bacilli and *Acinetobacter*. Fungi and yeasts are often present in skin folds; acid-fast, nonpathogenic mycobacteria occur in areas rich in sebaceous secretions (genitalia, external ear). Hair frequently harbors *Staph. aureus* and forms a reservoir for cross infection.

NORMAL FLORA OF THE CONJUNCTIVA

The predominant organisms of the conjunctiva are diphtheroids (*Corynebacterium xerosis.*), *S. epidermidis,* and nonhemolytic streptococci. Neisseriae and gram-negative bacilli resembling hemophili (*Moraxella* species) are also frequently present. The conjunctival flora is normally held in check by the flow of tears, which contain antibacterial lysozyme.

NORMAL FLORA OF THE NOSE, NASOPHARYNX AND ACCESSORY SINUSES

The floor of the nose harbors *corynebacteria, staphylococci, and streptococci Haemophilus* species and *Moraxella lacunata* may also be seen.

The nasopharynx of the infant is sterile at birth but, within 2–3 days after birth, acquires the common commensal flora and the pathogenic flora carried by the mother and the attendants. Certain gram-negative organisms from the intestinal tract such as *Pseudomonas aeruginosa, E. coli,* paracolons and *Proteus* are also occasionally found in normal persons. After penicillin therapy, they may be the predominant flora.

NORMAL FLORA OF THE MOUTH

The mucous membranes of the mouth and pharynx are often sterile at birth but may be contaminated by passage through the birth canal. Within 4–12 hours after birth, viridans streptococci become established as the most prominent members of the resident flora and remain so for life. They probably originate in the respiratory tracts of the mother and attendants. Early in life, aerobic and anaerobic staphylococci, gram-negative diplococci (Neissetiae, *Moraxella catarrhalis*), diphtheroids, and occasional lactobacilli are added. When teeth begin to erupt, the anaerobic spirochetes, *Prevotella* species (especially *P. melaninogenica*), *Fusobacterium* species, rothia species, and *Capnocytophaga* species establish themselves, along with some anaerobic vibrios and lactobacilli. Yeasts (*Candida* species) occur in the mouth.

NORMAL FLORA OF THE UPPER RESPIRATORY TRACT

Within 12 hours after birth alpha hemolytic streptococci are found in the upper respiratory tract and become the dominant organisms of the oropharynx and remain so for life. Small bronchi and alveoli are normally sterile. In the pharynx and trachea, flora similar to that of the mouth establish themselves. The predominant organisms in the upper respiratory tract, particularly the pharynx, are nonhemolytic.

NORMAL FLORA OF THE GASTROINTESTINAL TRACT

At birth: At birth the intestine is sterile, but organisms are soon introduced with food. In all cases, within 4–24 hours of birth an intestinal flora is established partly from below and partly by invasion from above.

Breastfed children: In breastfed children the intestine contains lactobacilli *(L. bifidus)*, enterococci, colon bacilli and staphylococci. In artificially fed (bottle fed) children intestine contains *L acidophilus* and colon bacilli and in part by enterococci, gram-positive aerobic and anaerobic bacilli.

Normal adult: Because of the low pH of the stomach, it is virtually sterile except soon after eating. The stomach's acidity keeps the number of microorganisms at a minimum.

As the pH of intestinal contents becomes alkaline, the resident flora gradually. In the adult duodenum, there are 10^3–10^6 bacteria per gram of contents; in the jejunum and ileum, 10^5–10^8 bacteria per gram; and in the cecum and transverse colon, 10^8–10^{10} bacteria per gram. In the upper intestine, lactobacilli and enterococci predominate, but in the lower ileum and cecum, the flora is fecal. In the sigmoid colon and rectum, there are about 10^{11} bacteria per gram of contents, constituting 10–30% of the fecal mass.

In the normal adult colon, 96–99% of the resident bacterial flora consists of anaerobes: *Bacteroides* species, especially *B. fragilis*; *Fusobacterium* species; anaerobic lactobacilli, e.g., bifidobacteria; clostridia (*C. perfringens*, 10^3–10^5/g); and anaerobic gram-positive cocci (*Peptostreptococcus* species). Only 1–4% are facultative aerobes.

NORMAL FLORA OF THE GENITOURINARY TRACT

Mycobacterium smegmatis, a harmless commensal, is found in the smegma of the genitalia of both men and women. From apparently normal men, aerobic and anaerobic bacteria can be cultured from a high proportion, including lactobacilli, *Garnerella vaginalis*, alpha hemolytic streptococci and *Bacteroids species*. *Chlamydial trachomatis* and *Ureaplasma urealyticum* may also be present. The female urethra is either sterile or contains a few gram-positive cocci.

Female vaginal area: The female vaginal area has an acid pH between puberty and menopause, but the secretions are alkaline at other times.

At birth: At birth the vagina is sterile. In the first 24 hours it is invaded by micrococci, enterococci and diphtheroids. In 2–3 days, the maternal estrin induces glycogen deposition in the vaginal epithelium. This facilitates the growth of a lactobacillus (Doderlien's bacillus) which produces acid from glycogen, and the flora for a few weeks is similar to that of the adult. After the passively transferred estrin has been eliminated in the urine, the glycogen disappears, along with

Doderlien's bacillus and the pH of the vagina becomes alkaline. This brings about a change in the flora to micrococci, alpha and nonhemolytic streptococci, coliforms and diphtheroids.

At puberty: At puberty, the glycogen reappears and the pH changes to acid due to the metabolic activity of Doderlien's bacilli, *E. coli* and yeasts. This appears to be an important mechanism in preventing the establishment of other, possibly harmful microorganisms in the vagina. During pregnancy there is an increase in *Staphylococcus epidermidis,* Doderlien's bacilli, and yeasts. After menopause, lactobacilli again diminish in number and a mixed flora returns and the flora resembles that found before puberty.

KEY POINT

- The term "normal microbial flora" denotes the population of microorganisms that inhabit the skin and mucous membrane of normal healthy individuals.

IMPORTANT QUESTIONS

1. What is normal microbial flora of the human body? Write briefly on role of normal flora in human body.
2. Write short notes on:
   a. Normal bacterial flora.
   b. Normal flora in the mouth and upper respiratory tract.
   c. Normal flora of the genitourinary tract.

MULTIPLE CHOICE QUESTIONS

1. The majority of normal bacteria flora are present in:
   a. Conjunctiva
   b. Skin
   c. Nasopharynx
   d. Large intestine
2. Which bacteria is responsible for producing acidic pH in adult vagina?
   a. *Lactobacillus*
   b. *Bacteroides* species
   c. Diphtheroids
   d. *Gardnerella vaginalis*

ANSWERS

1. d   2. a

Antimicrobial Chemotherapy

LEARNING OBJECTIVES

After reading and studying this chapter, you should be able to:
- Describe mechanism of action of antibacterial drugs.
- Describe mechanism of drug resistance.
- List cephalosporins of first, second, third, and fourth generation.

INTRODUCTION

Antimicrobial Agent

Antimicrobial agent is a chemical substance inhibiting the growth or causing the death of a microorganism.

Antibiotic

Antibiotic as originally defined was a chemical substance produced by various species of microorganisms that was capable of inhibiting the growth or causing death of other microorganisms in low concentration. However, with the advent of synthetic methods, this definition has been modified.

Chemotherapeutic Agents

Chemotherapeutic agents are the chemical substances used to kill or inhibit the growth of microorganisms already established in the tissues of the body. Nowadays, the term *antibiotic* is used loosely to describe agents (mainly, but not exclusively, antibacterial agents) used to treat systemic infection.

Antimicrobial agent (AMA): It would be more meaningful to use the term **antimicrobial agent (AMA)** to designate synthetic as well as naturally obtained drugs that attenuate microorganisms.

Antiseptics or disinfectants: Antimicrobial substances that are too toxic to be used other than in topical therapy or for environmental decontamination are referred to as *antiseptics* or *disinfectants*.

ANTIBACTERIAL AGENTS

The principal types of antibacterial agents are listed in **Table 59.1**. These have been grouped according to their site of action.

MECHANISMS OF ACTION OF ANTIBACTERIAL DRUGS

Mechanisms of action' of antibacterial agents can be placed under the headings:
1. Inhibition of bacterial cell wall synthesis
2. Inhibition of bacterial cytoplasmic membrane function
3. Inhibition of bacterial nucleic acid synthesis
4. Inhibition of bacterial protein synthesis

1. Inhibiton of Bacterial Cell Wall Synthesis

The antibiotics which inhibit cell wall synthesis are β-lactam antibiotics (penicillins and cephalosporins), glycopeptides, bacitracin, cycloserine, fosfomycin and isoniazid.

β-Lactam Agents

This group includes penicillins, cephalosporins and other compounds that feature a β-lactam ring in their structure.

Table 59.1: Mechanisms of antibacterial drug action.

1. **Inhibitors of bacterial cell wall synthesis**
   - Penicillins
   - Cephalosporins
   - Vancomycin
   - Bacitracin
   - Cycloserine
   - Fosfomycin
2. **Inhibitors of bacterial cytoplasmic membrane function**
   - Polymyxins
   - Gramicidin
   - Tyrocidine
3. **Inhibition of bacterial nucleic acid synthesis**
   - Quinolones
   - Rifamycins
   - Nitroimidazoles
   - Nitrofurans
   - Novobiocin
4. **Inhibition of bacterial protein synthesis**
   - Aminoglycosides
   - Chloramphenicol
   - Tetracyclines
   - Macrolides
   - Lincosamides
   - Fusidic acid
   - Streptogramins
   - Mupirocins
5. **Metabolic antagonism**
   - Sulfonamides
   - Trimethoprim
   - Dapsone
   - Isoniazid

Penicillins

Each member of the family of penicillins shares a common basic structure. Penicillins are a group of antimicrobial substances, all of which possess a common chemical nucleus (6-aminopenicillanic acid) which contains a β-lactam ring essential to their biologic activity.

Resistance to Penicillin
Resistance to penicillin may be due to:
i. **Production of penicillin-destroying enzymes (β-lactamases)**
ii. Impermeability of cell envelope.
iii. Alteration or lack of penicillin receptors.
iv. Failure of activation of autolytic enzymes in the cell wall, e.g., in staphylococci.
v. Cell-wall deficient (L) forms or mycoplasmas, which do not synthesize peptidoglycan.

Cephalosporins

Cephalosporins are a family of antibiotics originally isolated in 1948 from the fungus *Cephalosporium,* and their β-lactam structure is very similar to that of the penicillins. They are grouped as the first-, second-, third-, and fourth generation cephalosporins. These include cephalexin and cephradine (first generation), cefaclor and cefprozil (second generation), cefixime and ceftibuten (third generation), and cefepime (fourth generation). The later generations are generally more effective against gram-negative bacteria and are less susceptible to destruction by β-lactamases.

Other β-Lactam Antibiotics

Various agents with diverse properties share the structural feature of a β-lactam ring with penicillins and cephalosporins. Two other groups of β-lactam drugs, **carbapenems** and **monobactams**, are very resistant to β-lactamases.

Glycopeptides

Two glycopeptides, vancomycin and teicoplanin, are in clinical use. They are mainly used in serious infections with staphylococci and enterococci that are resistant to other drugs.

2. Inhibition of Bacterial Cytoplasmic Membrane Function

Only polymyxins have been regularly used systemically among membrane active agents used in human medicine. Two members of the family are in therapeutic use: polymyxin B and colistin (polymyxin E).

Polymyxin B and colistin (polymyxin E) exhibit potent antipseudomonal activity, but toxicity has limited their usefulness, except in topical preparations and bowel decontamination regimens.

3. Inhibitors of Nucleic Acid Synthesis

Quinolones

The quinolones are synthetic drugs that contain the 4-quinolone ring. The first quinolone, nalidixic acid was synthesized in 1962. **Nalidixic acid and its early congeners** are narrow-spectrum agents active only against gram-negative bacteria.

Newer quinolones such as ciprofloxacin, norfloxacin, ofloxacin, pefloxacin and lomefloxacin are broad spectrum quinolones. These have been successfully used in a wide variety of infections, but resistance is becoming more prevalent.

Rifamycins

This group of antibiotics is characterized by excellent activity against mycobacteria, although other bacteria are also susceptible. Staphylococci in particular are exquisitely sensitive. Rifampicin and rifabutin are most widely used.

Nitroimidazoles

The representative of the group most commonly used clinically is metronidazole, but similar derivatives include tinidazole, ornidazole and nimorazole. They are primarily antiprotozoal agents, but they exhibit potent activity against anaerobic bacteria.

Nitrofurans

These include:

Nitrofurantoin—an agent used exclusively in urinary tract infection.

Furazolidone—is used in enteric infections.

Novobiocin

It is quite active against staphylococci and streptococci, but is no longer favored because of problems of resistance and toxicity. *Staphylococcus saprophyticus* is novobiocin resistant.

4. Inhibition of Bacterial Protein Synthesis

Several types of antibacterial drugs inhibit prokaryotic protein synthesis. Of these, only the aminoglycosides are bactericidal; the others are all bacteriostatic. Two classes of drugs that have recently been approved for use are the oxazolidinones and the streptogramins. A synergistic combination of two streptogramins is bacteriocidal against some organisms.

Chloramphenicol: Use of chloramphenicol has been limited to typhoid fever, meningitis and a few other clinical indications.

Tetracyclines: Tetracyclines are broad-spectrum agents with important activity against chlamydiae, rickettsiae, mycoplasmas and, surprisingly, malaria parasites, as well as most conventional.

Metabolic Antagonism

Sulfonamides and diaminapyrimidines: They are now little used alone, but the combination of sulfamethoxazole with trimethoprim (co-trimoxazole) is still widely used.

RESISTANCE TO ANTIMICROBIAL DRUGS

The spread of drug-resistant pathogens is one of the most serious threats to the successful treatment of microbial disease.

Mechanisms of Drug Resistance

The most common mechanisms of acquired antimicrobial resistance are:

1. **Drug-inactivating enzymes**
   Penicillinase: The best-known example is the hydrolysis of the β-lactam ring of many penicillins by the enzyme penicillinase.
2. **Alteration in the target molecule:**
   Examples: Alterations in the penicillin-binding proteins prevent β-lactam drugs from binding to them.
3. **Decreased uptake of the drug**
   4. **Increased elimination of the drug**

KEY POINTS

- **Antibiotic** as originally defined was a chemical substance produced by various species of microorganisms that was capable of inhibiting the growth or causing death of other microorganisms in low concentration.
- **Chemotherapeutic agents** are the chemical substances used to kill or inhibit the growth of microorganisms already established in the tissues of the body.

IMPORTANT QUESTIONS

1. Define the terms antimicrobial agent, chemotherapeutic agent and antibiotic. Name various mechanisms of action of antibiotics giving examples.
2. Write short notes on:
   a. Cephalosporins
   b. Quinolones

MULTIPLE CHOICE QUESTIONS

1. Which of the following antibiotics act/s by inhibiting cell wall synthesis?
   a. Penicillins
   b. Vancomycin
   c. Bacitracin
   d. All of the above
2. Which of the following antibiotics acts by inhibiting cytoplasmic membrane?
   a. Polymyxin
   b. Thyrocidine
   c. Gramicidin
   d. All of the above
3. Which antibiotic/s act/s by inhibiting bacterial nucleic acid synthesis?
   a. Quinolones
   b. Novobiocin
   c. Nitrofurans
   d. All of the above
4. Which of the following antibiotics act/s by inhibiting bacterial protein synthesis?
   a. Aminoglycosides
   b. Tetracycline
   c. Macrolides
   d. All of the above
5. Which antibiotic/s act/s as metabolic antagonists for their action?
   a. Sulfones
   b. Trimethoprim
   c. Isoniazid
   d. All of the above
6. What is the genetic basis of drug resistance in *Mycobacterium tuberculosis*?
   a. Transformation
   b. Transduction
   c. Mutation
   d. Conjugation
7. *Staphylococcus aureus* acquire drug resistance by:
   a. Transformation
   b. Transduction
   c. Mutation
   d. Conjugation

ANSWERS

1. d   2. d   3. d   4. d
5. d   6. c   7. b

Immunoprophylaxis

LEARNING OBJECTIVES

After reading and studying this chapter, you should be able to:
- List of immunizing agents.
- Describe vaccines types and classification, storage and handling, cold chain.
- Discuss immunization schedule.
- Describe National Immunization Schedule.

INTRODUCTION

An important contribution of microbiology to medicine has been immunization, which is one of the most effective methods of controlling infectious diseases.

IMMUNIZING AGENTS

The immunizing agents may be classified as:
A. Vaccines
B. Immunoglobulins

Vaccines

A vaccine is a preparation from an infectious agent that is administered to humans and other animals to induce protective immunity against a given disease. There are two types of vaccines that induce **active** immunity: those that contain **live virus** whose pathogenicity has been **attenuated** and those that contain **killed virus.** An *attenuated* virus is one that is unable to cause disease, but retains its antigenicity and can induce protection.

Types of Vaccines

a. **Live vaccines:** Live vaccines (e.g., BCG vaccine for tuberculosis, measles, and oral polio) are prepared from live (generally attenuated) organisms. These organisms have been passed repeatedly in the laboratory in tissue culture or chick embryos and have lost their capacity to induce full blown disease but retain their immunogenicity. In general, live vaccines are more potent immunizing agents than killed vaccines.

b. **Inactivated or killed vaccines:** Organisms killed by heat or chemicals, when infected into the body stimulate active immunity. They are usually safe but generally less efficacious than live vaccines. Killed vaccines usually require a primary series of 2 or 3 doses of vaccine to produce an adequate antibody response, and in most cases "booster" injections are required. Killed vaccines are usually administered by subcutaneous or intramuscular route.

Examples of vaccines:
1. **Bacterial vaccines:** Active immunity is induced by vaccines prepared from bacteria or their products. Bacterial vaccines are composed of capsular polysaccharides, inactivated protein exotoxins (toxoids), and killed bacteria. There are three major types of inactivated bacterial vaccines: **Toxoid** (inactivated toxins), **inactivated (killed)** bacteria, and surface components of the bacteria, such

as **capsule or protein subunits.** Most antibacterial vaccines protect against the pathogenic action of toxins.

Certain organisms produce exotoxins, e.g., diphtheria and tetanus bacilli. The toxins produced by these organisms are detoxicated and used in the preparation of vaccines. In general, toxoid preparations are highly efficacious and safe immunizing agents.

Vaccines against *Haemophilus (H). influenzae* B, *Neisseria meningitidis, Salmonella typhi,* and *Streptococcus pneumoniae* (23 strains) are prepared from capsular polysaccharides.

2. **Viral vaccines**

   Inactivated viral vaccines: These are available for **polio** (injectable polio vaccine-Salk)**, hepatitis A, influenza, and rabies,** among other viruses

   Subunit vaccine: Consist of the **bacterial or viral components** that elicit a protective immune response, e.g., **two viral** subunit vaccines **hepatitis B virus (HBV) vaccine** and the **human papilloma virus (HPV) vaccine** contain purified viral antigens

c. **DNA vaccines**

   Future directions for vaccination
   1. **Hybrid virus vaccines**
   2. **Genetically engineered subunit vaccines:** Influenza, rabies, herpes simplex virus subunit vaccines
   3. **Peptide subunit vaccines**
   4. **Adjuvants** in addition to alum are being developed to enhance the immunogenicity.
   5. **DNA vaccines**
   6. **Reverse vaccinology**: A new approach, termed *reverse vaccinology*, was used to develop a vaccine for *Neisseria meningitidis* B.

THE COLD CHAIN

The "cold chain" is a system of storage and transport of vaccines at low temperature from the manufacturer to the actual vaccination site. The cold chain system is necessary because vaccine failure may occur due to failure to store and transport under strict temperature controls. The success of national immunization program is highly dependent on supply chain system for delivery of vaccines and equipment, with a functional system that meets 6 rights of supply chain. The right vaccine in the right quantity at the right place at the right time in the right condition (no temperature breaks in cold chain) and at the right cost.

Cold Chain Equipment

The cold chain equipment used in Universal Immunization Program are classified as follows:
A. Storage-electrical, solar, nonelectrical
B. Transportation

Transportation: Refrigerated vaccine van; insulated vaccine van; cold box vaccine carrier.

Correct Storage and Use of Diluents

Only use the diluents supplied and packaged by the manufacturer with the vaccine, since the diluent is specifically designed for the needs of that vaccine, with respect to volume, pH level and chemical properties.

Store the diluents, between +2 and +8°C in the ice-lined refrigerator (ILR). If there are constraints of space, then store diluents outside the cold chain. However, remember to cool diluents for at least 24 hours before use to ensure that vaccines and diluents are at +2° to +8°C when being reconstituted. Otherwise, it can lead to thermal shock, i.e., the death of some or all the essential live organisms in the vaccine. Store the diluents and droppers with the vaccines in the vaccine carrier during transportation. Diluents should not come in direct contact with the ice pack.

IMMUNIZATION

Immunization is of three types: **Active immunization, passive immunization** and **combined passive and active immunization.**

A. Active Immunization

Active immunization is the protection of susceptible humans from communicable diseases by the administration of vaccines (vaccination).

Universal Immunization Program (UIP)

In May 1974, the World Health Organization (WHO) officially launched a global immunization program, known as **Expanded Program on Immunization (EPI)** to protect all children of the world against six vaccine-preventable diseases, namely—diphtheria, whooping cough, tetanus, polio, tuberculosis, and measles by the year 2000. EPI was launched in India in January 1978. The Program is now called **Universal Child Immunization.** The Indian version, the **Universal Immunization Program,** was launched on November 19, 1985.

Immunization Schedules

1. **National Immunization Schedule**
   The National Immunization Schedule is given in **Table 60.1**. The first visit may be made when the infant is 6 weeks old; the second and third visits, at intervals of 1–2 months. Oral polio vaccine may be given

Table 60.1: National Immunization Schedule (NIS) for infants, children and pregnant women (India).

Vaccine	Due age	Maximum age	Dose	Diluent	Route	Site
For pregnant women						
TT-1	Early in pregnancy		0.5 mL	No	Intramuscular	Upper arm
TT-2*	4 weeks after TT-1		0.5 mL	No	Intramuscular	Upper arm
TT-booster*	If received TT doses in a pregnancy within the last 3 years		0.5 mL	No	Intramuscular	Upper arm
For infants						
Bacillus Calmette-Guerin (BCG)	At birth	Till one year of age	(0.05 mL until 1 month) 0.1 mL beyond age 1 month	Yes Manufacturer supplied diluent (sodium chloride)	Intradermal	Upper arm (left)
Hepatitis B Birth dose	At birth	Within 24 hours	0.5 mL	No	Intramuscular	Anterolateral side of mid-thigh (left)
bOPV-0	At birth	Within the first 15 days	2 drops	–	Oral	Oral
bOPV-1, 2 and 3	At 6, 10 and 14 weeks	Till 5 years of age	2 drops	–	Oral	Oral
Pentavalent 1, 2 and 3** (Diphtheria + Pertusis + Tetanus + Hepatitis B + Hib)	At 6, 10 and 14 weeks**	1 year of age	0.5 mL	No	Intramuscular	Anterolateral side of mid-thigh (left)
Fractional inactivate polio vaccine (IPV)	At 6 and 14 weeks	1 year of age	0.1 mL	No	Intradermal	Upper arm (right)

(Contd...)

(Contd...)

Vaccine	Due age	Maximum age	Dose	Diluent	Route	Site
Rotavirus+ (where applicable)	At 6, 10 and 14 weeks	1 year of age	5 drops	No	Oral	Oral
Pneumococcal conjugate vaccine (PCV)—where applicable	At 6 and 14 weeks At 9 completed months booster	1 years of age	0.5 mL	No	Intramuscular	Anterolateral side of mid-thigh (right)
Measles/rubella 1st dose##	At 9 completed months-12 months	5 years of age	0.5 mL	Yes Manufacturer supplied diluent (sterile water)	Subcutaneous	Upper arm (right)
Japanese encephalitis-1 (when applicable)	At 9–12 months	15 years of age	0.5 mL	Yes Manufacturer supplied diluent (phosphate buffer solution)	Subcutaneous	Upper arm (left)
Vitamin A 1st dose	At 9 months	5 years of age	1 mL	–	Oral	Oral
For children			(1 lakh IU)			
DPT booster-1	16–24 months	7 years of age	0.5 mL	No	Intramuscular	Anterolateral side of mid-thigh (left)
Measles/Rubella 2nd dose##	16–24 months	5 years of age	0.5 mL	Yes Manufacturer supplied diluent (sterile water)	Subcutaneous	Upper arm (right)
bOPV booster	16–24 months	5 years of age	2 drops	No	Oral	Oral
Japanese encephalitis-2@ (when applicable)	16–24 months*	Till 15 years of age	0.5 mL	Yes Manufacturer supplied diluent (phosphate buffer solution)	Subcutaneous	Upper arm (left)
Vitamin A$ (2nd to 9th dose)	At 16 months. Then one dose every 6 months	Up to the age of 5 years	2 mL (2 lakh IU)	–	Oral	Oral

(Contd...)

(Contd...)

Vaccine	Due age	Maximum age	Dose	Diluent	Route	Site
DPT booster-2	5–6 years	7 years of age	0.5 mL	No	Intramuscular	Upper arm
Tetanus toxoid (TT)	10 years and 16 years	16 years	0.5 mL	No	Intramuscular	Upper arm

*Give TT-2 or booster doses before 36 weeks of pregnancy. However, give these even if more than 36 weeks have passed. Give TT to a woman in labor, if she has not previously received TT.
** Pentavalent vaccine is introduced in place of DPT and Hep B 1, 2 and 3.
+ Rotavirus vaccine is being introduced in phases.
MR vaccine introduced in phases replacing measles vaccine in the UIP schedule. If first does delayed beyond 12 months ensure minimum 1 month gap between 2 MR doses.
@ JE vaccine has been introduced in selected endemic districts. If first dose is delayed beyond 12 months ensure minimum 3 months gap between 2 JE doses.
$ The 2nd to 9th doses of vitamin A can be administered to children 1–5 years old during biannual rounds, in collaboration with ICDS.

Note:
- Human papilloma virus (HPV) vaccine—presently not in schedule.
- Tetanus diphtheria (Td) to replace TT—to be added in schedule.

concurrently with oral polio vaccine (OPV). Bacillus Calmette–Guérin (BCG) can be given with any of the three doses but the site for the injection should be different. The schedule also covers immunization of women during pregnancy against tetanus.

2. **WHO Expanded Program on Immunization (EPI) schedule**
The purpose is to assist health planners to develop an appropriate country specific immunization schedule based on local conditions.

B. Passive Immunization

Passive immunization is used when it is considered necessary to protect a patient at short notice and for a limited period. Antitoxic, antibacterial or antiviral antibodies in human (homologous) or animal (heterologous) serum are injected to give temporary protection.

Preparations for passive immunization: Three types of preparations are available for passive immunization:
1. Normal human immunoglobulin,
2. Specific (hyperimmune) human immunoglobulin, and
3. Antisera or antitoxins

1. **Normal human immunoglobulin:** Normal human Ig is used to prevent measles in highly susceptible individuals and to provide temporary protection against hepatitis A infection
2. **Specific human immunoglobulin:** These preparations are made from the plasma of patients who have recently recovered from an infection or are obtained from individuals who have been immunized against a specific infection. They, therefore, have a high antibody content against an individual infection and provide immediate protection, e.g., specific human Igs are used for passive immunization against tetanus [human tetanus immunoglobulin (HTIG)], hepatitis B (HBIG), and rabies (HRIG).
3. **Antisera:** The term *antiserum* is applied to materials prepared in animals. Originally, passive immunization was achieved by the administration of antisera or antitoxins prepared from nonhuman sources such as horses.

The current trend is in favor of using immunoglobulins wherever possible.

C. Combined Passive and Active Immunization

In some diseases (e.g., tetanus, diphtheria, and rabies) passive immunization is often undertaken in conjunction with inactivated vaccine products, to provide both immediate (but temporary) passive immunity and slowly developing active immunity. If the injections are given at separate sites, the immune response to the active agent, may or may not be impaired by immunoglobulin.

KEY POINT

- Immunoprophylaxis is the prevention of disease by the production of active or passive immunity.

IMPORTANT QUESTIONS

1. Define vaccine, its type and classification.
2. Discuss cold chain and discuss the methods of safe storage and handling of vaccines.
3. Write short notes on:
   a. Live attenuated vaccines
   b. Killed vaccines
   c. Toxoids

MULTIPLE CHOICE QUESTIONS

1. Which of the following vaccines is/are killed vaccines?
   a. Cholera vaccine
   b. Pertussis vaccine
   c. Japanese encephalitis vaccine
   d. All of the above
2. An example of killed inactivated vaccine is:
   a. MMR vaccine
   b. Influenza vaccines
   c. Oral polio vaccine
   d. BCG vaccine
3. An example of live attenuated vaccine is:
   a. Hepatitis B vaccine
   b. Rocky Mountain spotted fever vaccine
   c. Yellow fever vaccine
   d. Rabies vaccine
4. Which of the following vaccines is/are subunit vaccine/s?
   a. Hepatitis B vaccine (plasma derived)
   b. Vi typhoid fever vaccine
   c. Meningococcal vaccine
   d. All of the above
5. Toxoid is used for active immunization against:
   a. Pertussis
   b. Diphtheria
   c. Typhoid fever
   d. Tuberculosis
6. Specific immunoglobulins are available for passive immunization against:
   a. Tetanus
   b. Rabies
   c. Hepatitis B
   d. All of the above
7. Combined passive and active immunization is available against all the diseases, *except*:
   a. Poliomyelitis
   b. Tetanus
   c. Rabies
   d. Diphtheria

ANSWERS

1. d   2. b   3. c   4. d
5. b   6. d   7. a

CHAPTER 61: Vehicles, Vectors and Rodents

LEARNING OBJECTIVES

After reading and studying this chapter, you should be able to:
- Discuss the role of vehicles and vectors in transmission of infectious agents.
- Describe the following: water-borne diseases; diseases transmitted by blood and blood products; diseases transmitted by rodents.

VEHICLES AND VECTORS

The agents of transmission that bring the microorganism from the reservoir to the host may be a living entity, in which case they are called *vectors*, or they may be a nonliving entity referred to as a *vehicle or fomite*.

Modes of transmission: The human host may acquire microbial agents by various means referred to as the **modes of transmission**: The mode of transmission is:
A. **Direct:** Transmitted by direct contact between reservoir and host
B. **Indirect:** Transmitted to host (human host) via **intervening agent(s)**, such as vectors.

VEHICLE-BORNE

Vehicle-borne transmission implies transmission of the infectious agent through the agency of water, food, ice, blood, serum plasma or other biological products, such as tissues and organs. Of these water and food are the most frequent vehicles of transmission, because they are used by everyone.

A. **Diseases transmitted by water and food:**
- Acute diarrheas
- Typhoid fever
- Cholera
- Poliomyelitis
- Hepatitis A virus infection
- Food poisoning
- Intestinal parasitic infestation

B. **Diseases transmitted by blood:**
- **Viruses**
  - Hepatitis B
  - Human immunodeficiency viruses (HIV)
  - Human T cell lymphotropic viruses
  - Infectious mononucleosis
  - Cytomegalovirus
- **Bacteria**
  - Syphilis
  - Brucellosis
- **Parasites**
  - Malaria
  - Trypanosomiasis (Chaga's disease)
  - *Trypanosoma cruzi*

VECTOR-BORNE

Vector is defined as an arthropod or any living carrier (e.g., snail) that transports an infectious agent to a susceptible individual. Transmission by a vector may be mechanical or biological.

Definitive Host

The host in which the sexual cycle of the agent occurs is called the definitive host, e.g., mosquito is the definitive host in malaria.

Intermediate Host

The host in which the asexual cycle of the agent occurs is called the intermediate host, e.g., mosquito in filaria and cyclops in guinea-worm disease.

Infestation

By infestation is meant the lodgment, development, and reproduction of arthropods on the surface of the body or in the clothing, e.g., louse infestation.

RODENTS

Rats and mice are part of man's environment and they act as sources or reservoirs of some important communicable diseases, such as plague and typhus fever.

Classification

Rodents may be classified into two distinct groups:
1. **Domestic rodents:** The rodents of chief public health concern are those that live in close association with man, namely the black rat *(Rattus rattus)* and the Norway rat (*R. norvegicus*) and the house mouse *(Mus musculus).*
   a. **Black rat *(Rattus rattus)*:** *Rattus rattus* is a domestic animal whose area of movement is usually restricted. It readily infests ships, and therefore its public health importance is considerable. *Rattus rattus* is also a good climber and infestation generally occurs in the roofs of houses, though in some places it does burrow.
   b. **Norway rat (*R. norvegicus*):** *R. norvegicus* is a semidomestic animal which frequents sewers, drains as well as houses.
2. **Wild rodents:** The common wild rodents in India are *Tatera indica, Bandicota bengalensis varius (Gunomys kok), B. indica, Millardia meltada, M. gleadowi* and *Mus. booduga.*

Rodents and Disease

A number of diseases are associated with rodents. Broadly these are:
1. **Bacterial:** Plague, tularemia, salmonellosis
2. **Viral:** Lassa fever, hemorrhagic fever, encephalitis
3. **Rickettsial:** Scrub typhus, murine typhus, rickettsial pox
4. **Parasitic:** Hymenolepis diminuta, leishmaniasis, amebiasis, trichinosis, Chagas disease
5. **Others:** Rat bite fever, leptospirosis, histoplasmosis, ring worm, etc.

Mode of Transmission

1. **Direct:** The mode of transmission may be directly through rat bite (e.g., rat bite fever).
2. **Contamination:** Some may be through contamination of food or water (e.g., salmonellosis, leptospirosis).
3. **Rat fleas:** Some may be through rat fleas (e.g., plague and typhus).

Antirodent Measures

1. **Sanitation measures:** Sound environmental sanitation is the most effective weapon in deratization campaign.
2. **Trapping:** Trapping of rats is a simple operation. The captured rats must be destroyed which may be done by drowning them in water.
3. **Rodenticides:** Rodenticides are of two main types—single dose (acute) and multiple-dose (cumulative) which requires repeated feedings over a period of 3 more days.
4. **Fumigation:** Fumigation is an effective method of destroying, both rats and rat fleas.
5. **Chemosterilants:** A chemosterilant is a chemical that can cause temporary or permanent sterility in either sex or both sexes. Rodent chemosterilants are still in the experimental stage.

KEY POINTS

- Transmission of the infectious disease occurs by four main routes: airborne, contact, vehicle, and vector-borne.
- **Rodents:** Rodents may be classified into two distinct groups:
  1. **Domestic rodents**
  2. **Wild rodents**

IMPORTANT QUESTIONS

1. Discuss the role of vehicles and vectors in transmission of infectious agents.
2. Write short notes on:
   a. Water-borne diseases
   b. Diseases transmitted by blood and blood products
   c. Diseases transmitted arthropods as vectors
   d. Diseases transmitted by rodents

MULTIPLE CHOICE QUESTIONS

1. All diseases can be transmitted by water and food, *except*:
   a. Cholera
   b. Poliomyelitis
   c. Hepatitis A virus infection
   d. Hepatitis C virus infection
2. Which of the following diseases can be transmitted by blood?
   a. Hepatitis
   b. HIV infection
   c. Syphilis
   d. All of the above

ANSWERS

1. d   2. d

Pathogenesis and Common Diseases

LEARNING OBJECTIVES

After reading and studying this chapter, you should be able to:
- List human diseases caused by bacteria, viruses, fungi and parasites.

COMMON DISEASES CAUSED BY DIFFERENT MICROORGANISMS

Infectious Agent

Pathogenic microorganisms are infectious agents. These pathogens vary among bacteria, viruses, fungi, and parasites. All these microorganisms require food for growth and a suitable environment to live. The strength of the microorganism, the number of microorganisms present, the effectiveness of a person's immune system, and the length of exposure to the microorganisms determine a pathogen's ability to produce disease.

HUMAN DISEASES CAUSED BY BACTERIA

Knowing the type of organism is important to the treatment of the patient. With many diseases, proper diagnosis and treatment are not possible until the specific microorganism causing the illness has been identified **(Table 62.1)**.

Table 62.1: Human diseases caused by bacteria.		
Type	**Species**	**Disease**
Gram-positive cocci	Staphylococcus aureus	**Cutaneous infections:** Folliculitis, boils, carbuncles, impetigo, and purulent abscesses. These cutaneous infections can progress to **deeper abscesses** involving other organ systems and progress to septicemia and bacteremia. **Toxin-induced diseases:** Food poisoning, scalded skin syndrome (SSS), toxic shock syndrome (TSS) **Other systemic diseases:** Bacteremia include pneumonia, empyema, septic arthritis, osteomyelitis, acute endocarditis, and catheter-related bacteremia.

	Streptococcus pyogenes	A. **Respiratory infection**
		   1. Streptococcal pharyngitis
		   2. Scarlet fever
		B. **Pyogenic cutaneous infections**—impetigo, erysipelas, cellulitis, necrotizing fasciitis involving deep subcutaneous tissues
		Streptococcal toxic shock syndrome.
		Nonsuppurtive sequelae: Rheumatic fever and acute glomerulo-nephritis.

(Contd...)

(Contd...)

Type	Species	Disease
	Streptococcus pneumoniae	Pneumonia, meningitis, sinusitis and otitis media, bacteremia, and endocarditis
Gram-negative cocci	Neisseria meningitis	Meningitis, meningoencephalitis, bacteremia, pneumonia, arthritis, urethritis
	Neisseria gonorrhoeae	Urethritis, cervicitis, salpingitis, pelvic inflammatory disease, proctitis, bacteremia, arthritis, conjunctivitis, and pharyngitis
Gram-positive bacilli	C. diphtheriae	• Diphtheria occurs in Two forms **(respiratory and cutaneous)**. • A tough gray to white pseudomembrane, may appear on the tonsils and then spread downward into the larynx and trachea. • **Systemic effects** involving the **kidneys, heart, and nervous system.** • In **cutaneous diphtheria,** systemic complications are less common. **Complications:** 1. **Asphyxia** 2. **Acute circulatory failure** 3. **Postdiphtheritic paralysis** 4. **Septic, such as pneumonia and otitis media**
	Bacillus anthracis	Emetic (vomiting) and diarrheal forms of gastroenteritis; ocular infection, other opportunistic infections.
	Clostridium perfringens	1. Soft tissue infections (cellulitis, suppurative myositis, myonecrosis) 2. Food poisoning 3. Septicemia
	Clostridium tetani	Tetanus
	Clostridium botulinum	**Botulism:** It is of three types—foodborne botulism, wound botulism, and infant botulism
	Clostridium difficile	1. A symptomatic colonization 2. Antibiotic-associated diarrhea (AAD) 3. Pseudomembranous colitis
Gram-negative rods	Escherichia coli	1. **Urinary tract infection**; limited to bladder (cystitis) or can spread to kidneys (pyelonephritis) or prostate (prostatitis) 2. **Diarrhea:** EHEC is an important cause of hemorrhagic colitis (HC) and hemolytic uremic syndrome (HUS) in the United States 3. **Pyogenic infections:** Neonatal meningitis 4. **Bacteremia**
	Klebsiella pneumoniae	Primary community-acquired pnuemonia, nosocomial infections, urinary tract infections, wound infections, bacteremia and meningitis and rarely diarrhea
	Proteus spp.	Urinary tract infections, wound infections, pneumonia
	Shigella dysenteriae	• Bacillary dysentery (Shigellosis) • Hemolytic colitis and hemolytic uremic syndrome (HUS)
	Salmonella spp.	• Asymptomatic colonization (primarily with *S. typhi* and *S. paratyphi*). • Enteric fever also called typhoid fever (*S. typhi*) or paratyphoid fever (*S. paratyphi*). • Enteritis—characterized by fever, nausea, vomiting, bloody or nonbloody diarrhea, and abdominal cramps • Bacteremia

(Contd...)

(Contd...)

Type	Species	Disease
	Vibrio cholerae	Cholera
	Campylobacter spp.	**Zoonotic infection**; gastroenteritis, septicemia, meningitis, spontaneous abortion, proctitis, Guillain–Barre syndrome, septicemia and is disseminated to multiple organs
	Helicobacter pylori	Gastritis, peptic ulcers, gastric adenocarcinoma
	Pseudomonas aeruginosa	A. **Community infections:** 1. Otitis externa and varicose ulcers 2. Corneal infections 3. Jacuzzi rash or whirlpool rash; Jacuzzi rash or whirlpool rash 4. Industrial eye injuries B. **Hospital infections:** 1. Localized lesions 2. Septicemia and endocarditis 3. Ecthyma gangrenosum and many other types of skin lesions 4. Infection of the nail bed 5. Infantile diarrhea and sepsis 6. Shanghai fever 7. Other infections: Gastrointestinal tract, central nervous system, and musculoskeletal system P. aeruginosa is regularly a cause of nosocomial pneumonia, nosocomial urinary tract infections, surgical site infections, infections of severe burns and infections of patients undergoing either chemotherapy for neoplastic diseases or **antibiotic therapy.**
	Burkholderia cepacia	Respiratory tract infections, particularly in patients with cystic fibrosis; urinary tract infections; septic arthritis; peritonitis; septicemia; opportunistic infections
	Burkholderia pseudomallei	Asymptomatic colonization; cutaneous infection with regional lymphadenitis, fever, and malaise; pulmonary disease ranging from bronchitis to necrotizing pneumonia
	Burkholderia mallei	Glanders in livestock
	Legionella pneumophilia	Legionnaire's disease, a life-threatening multifocal pneumonia; Pontiac fever, a self-limited, febrile, flu-like illness
	Yersinia pestis Pasteurella multocida	Plague 1. Local abscess at the site of a cat or dog bite 2. Infarctions of the respiratory system 3. Meningitis or cerebral abscess
	Francisella tularensis	Tularemia (rabbit fever)
	Haemophilus influenzae Haemophilus ducreyi	Meningitis, epiglottitis, cellulitis, arthritis, otitis, sinusitis, lower respiratory tract disease, conjunctivitis
	Haemophilus influenzae biogroup aegyptius	Purulent conjunctivitis and Brazilian purpuric fever (BPF).
	Haemophillus ducreyi	Sexually transmitted disease (STD) *chancroid or soft sore*
	Bordetella pertussis	Whooping cough
	Brucella melitensis	Brucellosis
	Mycobacterium tuberculosis	**Pulmonary tuberculosis** **Complications** include miliary tuberculosis, disseminated tuberculosis, tubercular meningitis, tuberculosis of the skin, tuberculosis of the middle ear and ocular structures

(Contd...)

(Contd...)

Type	Species	Disease
	Atypical mycobacteria	(A) Localized lymphadenitis; (B) Skin lesions following traumatic inoculation of bacteria; (C) Tuberculosis-like pulmonary lesions; (D) Disseminated disease
	Mycobacterium leprae	Leprosy
	Spirochetes	
	Treponema pallidum	Syphilis
	Borrelia recurrentis	Relapsing fever
	Borrelia burgdorferi	Lyme disease
	Leptospira interrogans-Leptospirosis	Leptospirosis
	Mycoplasma Ureaplasma	*Mycoplasma pneumonia:* Primary atypical pneumonia
	Actinomycetes	Actinomycosis
	Miscellaneous bacteria	
	Listeria monocytogenes	Septicemia and meningitis are the most common forms of listeriosis. Intrauterine infection of the fetus may result in abortion, stillbirth, premature delivery, or acute-onset disseminated infection in the newborn infant (including the form known as granulomatosis infantisepticum). Asymptomatic infection of the female genital tract may cause infertility. Meningitis or septicemia may occur in neonates.
	Erysipelothrix rhusiopathiae	Three forms of human infection—(1) **erysipeloid**, (2) **generalized cutaneous form** and (3) **septicemia**
	Alcaligenes faecalis	Urinary tract infection, infantile gastroenteritis, and typhoid-like fever in humans
	Chromobacterium violaceum	Intestinal and genitourinary infections and septicemic illnesses with pneumonia
	Flavobacterium meningosepticum	Opportunistic infections, neonatal meningitis in premature infants and pneumonia in immunocompromised hosts
	Calymmatobacterium (donovania) granulomatis	Granuloma inguinale, a sexually transmitted disease
	Acinetobacter species	Nosocomial infections
	Streptobacillus moniliformis and *Spirillum minus*	Rat bite fever
	Eikenella corrodens	In the settings of a human bite wound or fistfight injury. Other infections are endocarditis, sinusitis, meningitis, brain abscesses, pneumonia, and lung abscesses.
	Cardiobacterium hominis	Endocarditis
	Capnocytophaga species	Severe periodontal disease in juveniles, bacteremia and severe systemic disease in immunocompromised patients
	Gardnerella vaginalis	Bacterial vaginosis

(Contd...)

(Contd...)

Type	Species	Disease
	Rickettsiaceae and Bartonellaceae	Rickettsia rickettsiae—rocky mountain spotted fever
	Chlamydia and Chlamydophila	Trachoma
	Chlamydia trachomatis	Ornithosis (Psittacosis)
	Chlamydia psittaci Chlamydophila pneumoniae	Pneumonia

Human Diseases Caused by Fungi

Fungal (mycotic) infections are among the most common diseases found in humans.

Mycotic infections are diseases caused by yeasts and molds. Some are superficial, involving the skin and the mucous membranes. Most frequently, the infections involve the external layers of the skin, the hair, and the nails and are commonly referred to as ringworm (dermatomycosis). Other common sites include men's beards (barber's itch), the feet (athlete's foot), and around the nails. Domestic pets sometimes have ringworm infection and are frequently the source of infection for humans (**Table 62.2**).

Fungi also invade the deeper tissues of the body at times. Most of these infections produce no signs or symptoms; however, some become serious and potentially fatal, especially in a patient who is severely immunocompromised, such as coccidioidomycosis (valley fever) and histoplasmosis (a systemic fungal respiratory disease).

Mycoses (Fungus Infections)

Infection caused by fungus is known as mycosis (Plural: mycoses). Classification of fungal disease according to primary sites of infections is given in **Table 62.2**.

Table 62.2: Classification of fungal disease according to primary sites of infections.

Type of mycosis	Caustive fungal agents	Mycosis
A. Superficial	Malassezia species	Pityriasis versicolor
	Hortaea werneckii	Tinea nigra
	Trichosporon species	White piedra
	Piedraia hortae	Black piedra
B. Cutaneous	Microsporum species, trichophyton species, and Epidermophyton floccosum	Dermatophytosis
	Candida albicans and other candida species	Candidiasis of skin, mucosa, or nails
C. Subcutaneous	Sporothrix schenckii	Sporotrichosis
	Phialophora verrucosa, Fonsecaea pedrosoi, others	Chromoblastomycosis
	Pseudallesheria boydii, Madurella mycetomatis, others	Mycetoma
	Exophiala, bipolaris, exserohilum, and others	Phaeohyphomycosis
D. Systemic (primary, endemic)	Coccidioides immitis, C. posadasii	Coccidioidomycosis
	Histoplasma capsulatum	Histoplasmosis
	Blastomyces dermatitidis	Blastomycosis
	Paracoccidioies brasiliensis	Paracoccidioidomycosis
E. Opportunistic	Candida albicans and other candida species	Systemic candidiasis
	Cryptococcus neoformans	Cryptococcosis
	Aspergillus fumigatus and other aspergillus species	Aspergillosis
	Species of Rhizopus, Absidia, Mucor, and other zygomycetes	Mucomycosis (zygomycosis)
	Penicillium marneffei	Penicilliosis

Human Diseases Caused by Parasites (Tables 62.3 and 62.4)

Table 62.3: Human diseases caused by parasites.

Phylum	Pathogen	Disease
Rhizopoda	Acanthamoeba species	Amoebic keratitis
	Entamoeba histolytica	Amoebic dysentery
	Naegleria fowleri	Microencephalitis
Mastigophora (flagellata)	Giardia lamblia (G. intestinalis)	Giardiasis
	Trichomonas vaginalis	Protozoal vaginitis
	Trypanosoma brucei	African sleeping sickness
	Trypanosoma cruzi	Chaga's disease
Ciliophora (ciliata)	Balantidium coli	Balantidial dysentery

Table 62.4: Human diseases caused by helminths.

Phylum	Pathogen	Disease
Platyhelminthes	Paragonimus westermanni (lung fluke)	Paragonimiasis
	Schistosoma sp. (blood flukes)	Schistosomiasis
	Clonorchis sinensis (Chinese liver fluke)	Clonorchiasis
	Taenia saginata (beef tapeworm)	Taeniasis
	Taenia solium (pork tapeworm)	Taeniasis
	Hymenolepsis nana (dwarf tapeworm)	Hymenolepasis
	Diphyllobothrium latum (fish tapeworm)	Diphyllobothriasis
	Echinococcus granulosus (dog tapeworm)	Echinococcosis
	Fasciola hepatica (sheep liver fluke)	Fascioliasis
Nematoda (roundworms)	Strongyloides stercoralis (threadworm)	Strongyloidiasis
	Ascaris lumbricoides (roundworm)	Ascariasis
	Necator americanus (hookworm)	New world hookworm disease
	Ancylostoma duodenale	Old world hookworm disease (hookworm)
	Enterobius vermicularis (pinworm)	Pinworm feotalism
	Trichuris trichiura (whipworm)	Trichuriasis
	Trichinella spiralis (trichinaworm)	Trichinosis
	Wuchereria bancrofti	Elephantiasis or bancroftian filariasis
	Dirofilaria immitis (heartworm)	Filariasis

Viruses

The human diseases caused by DNA viruses are listed in **Table 62.5** and the RNA viruses are listed in **Table 62.6**.

Table 62.5: Human diseases caused by DNA viruses.

Family	Viruses	Disease
1. Poxviridae family	Smallpox virus	Smallpox
2. Herpesviridae	Herpesviruses	HSV-1 causes acute herpetic gingivostomatitis, acute herpetic pharyngotonsillitis, herpes labialis, herpes encephalitis, eczema herpeticum, and herpetic whitlow. HSV-2 causes genital herpes, neonatal infection, and aseptic meningitis. **Varicella Zoster Virus (VZV)** causes chickenpox (varicella) and herpes zoster or shingles, two distinct clinical entities in humans.

(Contd...)

(Contd...)

Family	Viruses	Disease
	Cytomegalovirus	Mononucleosis syndrome in immunocompetent hosts. Congenital CMV infection, acquired CMV infection, CMV infection in immunocompromised patients, and CMV infection in immunocompetent adult hosts. CMV generally causes subclinical infection
	Epstein-Barr Virus	Infectious mononucleosis, Burkitt's lymphoma, Hodgkin's disease, and nasopharyngeal carcinoma.

3. Adenoviridae		A. Respiratory diseases
		  1. Pharyngitis
		  2. Pneumonia
		  3. Acute respiratory diseases (ARD)
		B. Eye infections
		  1. Pharyngoconjunctival fever
		  2. Epidemic keratoconjunctivitis (EKC)
		  3. Acute follicular conjunctivitis
		C. Diarrhea
		D. Mesenteric adenitis and intussusception in children

4. Papovaviridae family	Papovaviruses: Papillomavirus	Papillomaviruses cause several different kinds of warts in humans, including cutaneous warts, genital warts, respiratory papillomatosis, oral papillomas, and cancer.
	Polyomavirus	There is to date no documented association with any naturally occurring tumor of man
5. Parvoviridae	1. Parvoviruses	None pathogenic in humans
	2. Dependovirus	None pathogenic in humans
	3. Erythrovirus	Respiratory infection with an erythematous maculopapular rash [erythema infectiosum (slapped cheek disease), joint disease, aplastic crisis in children with chronic hemolytic anemia (sickle cell disease), nonimmune fetal hydrops following infection during pregnancy and persistent anemia in immunodeficients
6. Hepadnaviridae family	Hepatitis type B virus	**Hepatitis B (serum hepatitis)**

Table 62.6: Human diseases caused by RNA viruses.

Family	Viruses	Disease
Picornaviridae	Poliovirus	**Polio**
	Coxsackievirus	Herpangina (vesicular pharyngitis), aseptic meningitis, hand-foot-and-mouth disease, respiratory infections, epidemic myalgia or Bornholm disease, myocardial and pericardial infections, Juvenile diabetes, neonatal infections, chronic fatigue syndrome
	Echoviruses	1. Aseptic meningitis 2. Respiratory illnesses in children 3. Infantile diarrhea 4. Occasionally, conjunctivitis, muscle weakness, and spasm
	Hepatitis A virus	Hepatitis (infectious hepatitis)
	Rhinovirus	• Common cold • Upper respiratory tract infections

(Contd...)

(Contd...)

Family	Viruses	Disease
Orthomyxoviridae	Influenza virus types A, B, and C	Influenza
Paramyxoviridae	Parainfluenza virus	Respiratory tract syndromes ranging from a **mild cold-like upper respiratory tract infection** (coryza, pharyngitis, mild bronchitis, wheezing, and fever) to **bronchiolitis and pneumonia**
	Measles virus	Measles, atypical measles, and subacute sclerosing panencephalitis (SSPE)
	Mumps virus	Mumps
	Respiratory syncytial virus	Common cold to pneumonia
Togaviridae	Rubella virus	Rubella
	Western, eastern, and Venezuelan equine encephalitis virus	Encephalitis in horses and humans
	Ross River virus	Epidemic polyarthritis
	Sindbis virus	No association with human diseases
	Semliki Forest virus	No association with human disease
Flaviviridae	Yellow fever virus	Yellow fever
	Dengue virus	Dengue fever
	St. Louis encephalitis virus	Mild febrile illness to frank encephalitis
	Hepatitis C virus	Acute hepatitis; chronic persistent infection; severe rapid progression to cirrhosis
Bunyaviridae	California encephalitis virus	Encephalitis, aseptic meningitis and fever
	LaCrosse virus	Encephalitis, aseptic meningitis and fever
	Sandfly fever virus	Pappataci fever (three day fever)
	Crimean Congo hemorrhagic fever virus	Fever, myalgia, (muscle ache), dizziness, neck pain and stiffness, backache, headache, sore eyes and photophobia (sensitivity to light). There may be nausea, vomiting, diarrhea, abdominal pain and sore throat early on, followed by sharp mood swings and confusion
	Hanta virus	Hemorrhagic fever with renal syndrome
Arenaviridae	Lymphocytic choriomeningitis virus	Lymphocytic choriomeningitis
	Lassa fever virus	Lassa fever
	Tacaribe group of Arenavirus complex (Junin, Guanarito Machupo, and Sabia viruses)	South American hemorrhagic fever
Rhabdoviridae	Rabies virus	Rabies
Reoviridae	Rotavirus	Diarrhea in infants and children
	Colorado tick fever virus	Mountain fever or tick fever
Coronaviridae	Coronavirus	Common colds, gastroenteritis in infants; severe acute respiratory syndrome (SARS)

(Contd...)

(Contd...)

Family	Viruses	Disease
Retroviridae	Human T-cell leukemia virus types I	Adult T-cell leukemia/lymphoma
	Human immunodeficiency virus-1 and 2	Acquired immunodeficiency syndrome (AIDS)
Caliciviridae	Norwalk virus	Epidemic viral gastroenteritis in adults
	Hepevirus-Hepatitis E virus	Acute hepatitis including jaundice, chronic hepatitis cirrhosis, hepatocellular carcinoma
Filoviridae	Ebola virus	Hemorrhagic fever
	Marburg virus	Hemorrhagic fever

The families of RNA viruses and some important members are described in **Table 62.7**.

Table 62.7: Families of RNA viruses and some important members.

Family	Members
Picornaviridae	Rhinoviruses, *poliovirus*, echoviruses, coxsackievirus, hepatitis A virus
Orthomyxoviridae	*Influenza virus* types A, B, and C
Paramyxoviridae	Parainfluenza virus, Sendai virus, *measles virus*, mumps virus, respiratory syncytial virus
Togaviridae	*Rubella virus*; western, eastern, and venezuelan equine encephalitis virus; Ross River virus; Sindbis virus; Semliki forest virus
Flaviviridae	*Yellow fever virus*, dengue virus, St. Louis encephalitis virus, hepatitis C virus
Bunyaviridae	*California encephalitis virus*, La Crosse virus, sandfly fever virus, hemorrhagic fever virus, Hanta virus
Arenaviridae	*Lassa fever virus*, Tacaribe virus complex, Gunin and Machupo viruses), lymphocytic choriomeningitis virus
Rhabdoviridae	*Rabies virus*, vesicular stomatitis virus, *Ebola virus*, Marburg virus
Reoviridae	*Rotavirus*, Colorado tick fever virus
Coronaviridae	Coronavirus
Retroviridae	Human T-cell leukemia virus types I and II, *human immunodeficiency virus*, animal oncoviruses
Caliciviridae	Norwalk virus, Delta agent
Filoviridae	*Ebola virus*, Marburg virus

KEY POINT

Pathogenic microorganisms are infectious agents. These pathogens vary among bacteria, viruses, yeasts, fungi, and protozoa. Human infections caused by gram-positive and gram-negative cocci and gram-positive and gram-negative bacilli. Mycotic infections are diseases caused by yeasts and molds. Human diseases caused by parasites, such as protozoa, helminths and by virus (DNA viruses and RNA viruses).

IMPORTANT QUESTIONS

1. Name various diseases caused by gram-positive cocci.
2. Name various diseases caused by gram-negative cocci.
3. Name various diseases caused by gram-positive bacilli.
4. Name various diseases caused by gram-negative bacilli.
5. Name various diseases caused by prozoa and helminths.
6. Name various diseases caused by DNA viruses.
7. Name various diseases caused by RNA viruses.

SECTION 8: Infection Control and Safety

SECTION OUTLINE
63. Healthcare-associated Infections
64. Isolation Precautions and Use of Personal Protective Equipment
65. Hand Hygiene
66. Sterilization and Disinfection
67. Specimen Collection (Review)
68. Biomedical Waste Management
69. Antibiotic Stewardship
70. Patient Safety Indicators
71. Incidents and Adverse Events
72. International Patient Safety Goals
73. Safety Protocols
74. Employee Safety Indicators
75. Healthcare Worker Immunization and management of Occupational Exposure

CHAPTER 63: Healthcare-associated Infections

LEARNING OBJECTIVES

After reading and studying this chapter, you should be able to:
- Define healthcare-associated infections. Enumerate organisms causing it.
- Describe routes of transmission of hospital-associated infections.
- Discuss diagnosis and control of hospital-associated infections.
- Describe prevention of urinary tract infection (UTI).
- Describe prevention of surgical site infection (SSI).
- Describe prevention of ventilator-associated events (VAE).
- Discuss prevention of central line-associated blood-stream infection (CLABSI).
- Discuss infection control committee.
- Discuss infection control team.

INTRODUCTION

- **Healthcare-associated infections (HAIs)** include those with hospital onset and those with community onset in patients with previous healthcare encounters. Hospital-onset HAIs manifest 48 hours or more after admission to a hospital, within 30 days of discharge from a healthcare facility or if a patient visited an outpatient medical facility within the past 6–12 months.
- Community-associated infections are defined as infections manifesting and diagnosed within 48 hours of admission in patients without any previous encounter with healthcare.

HAI has replaced old confusing terms such as *hospital infection, hospital-acquired infection* or *nosocomial infection*.

SOURCES OF INFECTIONS

A. Exogenous

Exogenous source may be another person in the hospital *(cross-infection)* or a contaminated item of equipment or building service *(environmental infection)*.

1. **Contact with other patients and staff:** Patients and hospital personnel suffering from infection, or asymptomatic carriers are the most important sources.
2. **Environmental sources:** These include inanimate objects, air, water and food in the hospital.
   Inanimate objects: Equipment, materials, such as sanitary installation (bed pans, urinals), lights, table, blankets, medical equipment (endoscopes, catheters, needles, spatula and other instruments), floors, food and water (contaminated by kitchen or other hospital staff or visitor).

B. Endogenous

The infecting organism are derived from the patient's own skin, gastrointestinal or upper respiratory flora.

ROUTES OF TRANSMISSION

Routes of HAI transmission are by: **Contact, airborne transmission, vehicle transmission** (Table 63.1).

Table 63.1: Routes of transmission.

1. Contact transmission

	i. Direct-contact	Involves a direct surface-to-body contact and physical transfer of microorganisms between a susceptible host and an infected or colonised person
	ii. Indirect-contact	Involves contact of a susceptible host with an intermediate object, usually inanimate, such as contaminated instruments, needles, or dressings, or contaminated gloves that are not changed between patients
	iii. Droplet transmission	**Droplet transmission** occurs when droplets are generated from a human reservoir, mainly during coughing, sneezing, or talking, or during the performance of certain procedures, such as bronchoscopy. Transmission occurs when droplets containing pathogens from the infected person are propelled a short distance (<1 meter) through the air and deposited on the host
2. Air-borne transmission		Air-borne transmission occurs by dissemination of air-borne droplet nuclei (small-particles,<5 μm in size of evaporated droplets containing microorganisms) that remain suspended in the air for long periods of time or dust particles containing an infectious agent. Droplet nuclei, dust particles, or skin squamous containing microorganisms are transmitted by air currents. Microorganisms transmitted in this manner include Mycobacterium tuberculosis and rubeola (measles) and varicella (chickenpox) viruses
3. Vehicle transmission		**Vehicle transmission** applies to microorganisms transmitted through contaminated items, such as food, water, medications, medical devices and equipment, toys, and biological products, such as blood, tissues or organs
4. Vector-borne transmission		Vector-borne transmission occurs when vectors, such as mosquitoes, flies, rats, and other vermin, transmit microorganisms

MICROORGANISMS CAUSING HEALTHCARE-ASSOCIATED INFECTIONS (HAIS)

A. **'ESKAPE' pathogens:** ESKAPE pathogens are responsible for majority of nosocomial infections. They are referred to as **'ESKAPE' pathogens**, which is an acronym for:
- *Enterococcus faecium*
- *Staphylococcus aureus*
- *Klebsiella pneumoniae*
- *Acinetobacter baumannii*
- *Pseudomonas aeruginosa*
- *Enterobacter* species

B. **Other infections**
- *Escherichia coli*
- *Mycobactrium tuberculosis*—nosocomially acquired
- *Legionella pnemophila*
- *Candida albicans*
- *Clostridium difficile* diarrhea
- SARS-CoV-2 (COVID-19)

C. **Blood borne infections** transmitted through contaminated blood or blood products, such as HIV, hepatitis A virus (HAV) and hepatitis C virus (HCV).

TYPES OF HEALTH CARE-ASSOCIATED INFECTIONS

1. Catheter-associated urinary tract infections (CAUTI)
2. **Ventilator-associated pneumonia (VAP)**
3. **Central line-associated bloodstream infection (CLABSI)**
4. Surgical site infections (SSIs)

1. Catheter-associated Urinary Tract Infections (CAUTI)

Urinary Tract Infection

Most hospital-acquired infections of the urinary tracts are associated with urethral catheterization.

Causative Organisms

Escherichia coli, Klebsiella, Proteus, Pseudomonas and enterococci, *Candida* spp., and other fungi cause the remainder of the infections.

Risk Factors

Advanced age, female gender, severe underlying disease, and the placement of indwelling urinary catheters.

2. Ventilator-associated Pneumonia (VAP)

Ventilator-associated pneumonia (VAP) defined as a new pneumonia occurring >48 hours after endotracheal intubation, is a common and serious hospital-acquired infection. It occurs in up to 20% of patients receiving mechanical ventilation, and is associated with increased antibiotic use, length of hospitalization, and healthcare costs.

Causative Organisms

Staphylococcus aureus, Klebsiella, Enterobacter, Serratia, Proteus, Escherichia coli, Pseudomonas aeruginosa, Acinetobacter, Legionella pneumophila, Respiratory viruses.

Risk Factors

Advanced age, chronic lung disease, large-volume aspiration, chest surgery, hospitalization in intensive care units, and intubation or attachment to a mechanical ventilator (which controls breathing).

3. Central Line-associated Bloodstream Infection (CLABSI)

A central line-associated bloodstream infection (CLABSI) is defined as a laboratory-confirmed bloodstream infection not related to an infection at another site that develops within 48 hours of central line placement. A central line-associated bloodstream infection is a serious infection that occurs when microbes enter the bloodstream through a central line.

Causative Organisms

Gram-positive organisms (coagulase-negative staphylococci; enterococci and *Staphylococcus aureus*), gram-negative bacteria (*Klebsiella; Enterobacter; Pseudomonas; E. coli; Acinetobacter*), *Candida* species, and others.

Risk Factors

Host factors (severity of illness, lack of skin integrity, type of immunosuppression), factors related to the device (catheter insertion and maintenance processes, type and size of catheter, number of lumens, insertion site) and finally factors related to the function of catheter, and the duration of placement.

4. Surgical Site Infections (SSIs)

Surgical site infections (SSIs) are infections of the incision or organ or space that occur after surgery. The incidence of postoperative infection is higher in elderly patients. Most wound infections manifest within a week of surgery.

Causative Organisms

Gram-positive organisms (*S. aureus*, coagulase-negative staphylococci, and enterococci), gram-negative rods (*Pseudomonas aeruginosa, Escherichia coli, Proteus*); *Candida* spp.

Risk Factors

Patient factors (age, tobacco use, diabetes, and malnutrition) and procedure-specific risk factors (emergency surgery and the degree of bacterial contamination of the surgical wound at the time of the procedure). Inappropriate timing of prophylactic antimicrobial agents.

DIAGNOSIS AND CONTROL OF HOSPITAL INFECTION

The most important steps in preventing nosocomial infections are to first recognize their occurrence and then establish policies to prevent their development. Hospital infection may occur sporadically or as outbreaks.

Etiological Diagnosis

Etiological diagnosis is by the routine bacteriological methods of smear, culture, identification and sensitivity testing. When an outbreak occurs, the source should be identified and eliminated. This requires the sampling of possible sources of infection such as hospital personnel, inanimate objects, water, air or food. Typing of isolate-phage, bacteriocin, antibiogram or biotyping—from cases and sites may indicate a causal connection. Obvious examples of sources of hospital outbreaks are nasal carriage of staphylococci by surgeons or *Pseudomonas* growing in hand lotions. Carriers should be suitably treated.

The cause of infection may be a defective autoclave or improper techniques such as boiling infusion sets in ward sterilizers. A careful analysis of the pattern of infection may often reveal the source.

INFECTION CONTROL POLICY

There will normally be two parts:

1. Infection Control Committee (ICC)

Every hospital should have an infection control committee (ICC) with responsibilities that include the production and implementation of a disinfection policy. The committee will consist of a medical microbiologist who will usually serve as chairman, a physician, a surgeon, nurse teachers, nurse representatives for surgery, obstetrics, gynecology and medicine, and sterile service manager. Where hospitals obtain disinfectants through their purchasing department then the purchasing officer should be invited to attend relevant meetings. The ICC should meet regularly to formulate and update policy for the whole hospital matters having implications for infection control and to manage outbreaks of nosocomial infection.

2. Infection Control Team

An infection control team of workers, headed by the **infection control doctor** (usually the microbiologists), to take up day-to-day responsibility for this policy. The functions of this team include **surveillance and control of infection and monitoring of hygiene practices,** advising the infection control committee on matters of policy relating to the prevention of infection and the education of all staff in the microbiologically safe performance of procedures. **The *infection control nurse*** is a key member of this team. Close working links between the microbiology laboratory, infection control nurse and the different clinical specialties and support services (including sterile services, laundry, pharmacy and engineering) are important to establish and maintain the infection control policy, and to ensure that it is rationally based and that the recommended procedures are practicable.

PREVENTION OF HOSPITAL-ASSOCIATED INFECTIONS

1. Standard/universal precautions
2. Precautions for prevention of transmission of infection
3. Bundles in infection

1. Standard (Routine) Precautions

Standard precautions should be applied to the care of all patients. This includes limiting healthcare worker contact with all secretions or biological fluids; skin lesions, mucous membranes, and blood or body fluids. Healthcare workers must wear gloves for each contact which may lead to contamination, and also gown, mask and eye protection where contamination of clothes or the face is anticipated.

2. Transmission Precautions

It is the disease-specific and categories approach to isolation into new transmission categories to be taken based on the route of transmission of organisms like contact precautions, air-borne precautions, etc. These precautions are designed for specific patients with highly transmissible pathogens (*See* Chapter 64 for detail).

3. Bundles in Infection

Care "bundles" are simple sets of evidence-based practices that, when implemented collectively, improve the reliability of their delivery and improve patient outcomes. Care bundles include a set of evidence-based measures that, when implemented together, have shown to improve patient care and have a greater impact than that of the isolated implementation of individual measures.

Specific Care Bundles

Specific care bundles include bundles for the prevention of central line-associated bloodstream infections (CLABSI), bundle for the prevention of catheter-associated urinary tract infections (CAUTI), bundle for the prevention of ventilator-associated pneumonia (VAP), and bundle for the prevention of surgical site infection.

1. Bundles for the Prevention of Central Line-associated Bloodstream Infections (CLABSI)

Central lines are used commonly in intensive care units (ICUs) and in non-ICU populations such as dialysis units, intraoperatively, and oncology patients. CLABSI prevention bundles include the following components:

1. **Insertion bundle:**
   a. **Maximal sterile barrier precautions** (surgical mask, sterile gloves, cap, sterile gown, and large sterile drape).
   b. **Skin cleaning with alcohol-based chlorhexidine** (rather than iodine).
   c. **Avoidance of the femoral vein** for central venous access in adult patients; use of subclavian rather than jugular veins.
   d. Dedicated staff for central line insertion, and competency.
   e. Standardized insertion packs.
   f. Availability of insertion guidelines (including indications for central line use) and use of checklists with trained observers.
   g. Use of ultrasound guidance for insertion of internal jugular lines.

2. **Maintenance bundle:**
   a. **Daily review of central line necessity.**
   b. **Prompt removal of unnecessary lines.**
   c. **Disinfection prior to manipulation of the line.**
   d. **Daily chlorhexidine washes** (in ICU, patients >2 months).
   e. Disinfect catheter hubs, ports, connectors, etc., before using the catheter.
   f. Change dressings and disinfect site with alcohol-based chlorhexidine every 5–7 days (change earlier if soiled).
   g. Replace administration sets within 96 hours (immediately if used for blood products or lipids).
   h. Ensure appropriate nurse-to-patient ratio in ICU (1:2 or 1:1).

2. Bundle for the Prevention of Catheter-associated Urinary Tract Infections (CAUTI)

CAUTI is defined as a urinary tract infection (significant bacteriuria plus symptoms and/or signs attributable to the urinary tract with no other identifiable source) in a patient with current urinary tract catheterization or who has been catheterized in the past 48 hours. There are a number of strategies with varying levels of evidence to prevent CAUTI before and after placement of urinary catheters. These generally include appropriate use, aseptic insertion and maintenance, early removal, and hand hygiene. Recently, a large study in the United States demonstrated that a simple intervention comprising three components reduced catheter use and CAUTI rates in non-ICU acute care settings:
   a. Avoiding the use of urinary catheters by considering alternative methods for urine collection.
   b. Using an aseptic technique for insertion and proper maintenance after insertion.
   c. Daily assessment of the presence and need for indwelling urinary catheters.

3. Bundle for the Prevention of Ventilator Associated Pneumonia (VAP)

The following bundle of ventilator care processes have been shown to substantially reduce VAP

rates, and are recommended in international guidelines:
  a. Elevate the head of the bed to between 30 and 45 degrees.
  b. Daily "sedation interruption" and daily assessment of readiness to extubate.
  c. Daily oral care with chlorhexidine.
  d. Prophylaxis for peptic ulcer disease.

Other components of the VAP bundle may include:
  a. Utilization of endotracheal tubes with subglottic secretion drainage (only for patients ventilated for longer than 24 hours).
  b. Initiation of safe enteral nutrition within 24–48 hours of ICU admission.

4. Bundle for the Prevention of Surgical Site Infection (SSI)
The following evidence-based interventions should be provided as part of a bundle of care to prevent SSI:
  a. Administration of parenteral antibiotic prophylaxis.
     - Antibiotic prophylaxis should be administered within 60 minutes prior to incision, including for cesarean section.
     - Re-dosing is recommended for prolonged procedures and in patients with major blood loss or excessive burns.
  b. Patients should be washed with soap or an antiseptic agent within a night prior to surgery.
  c. Avoid hair removal: Use electric clippers if necessary.
  d. Use alcohol-based disinfectant for skin preparation in the operating room.
  e. Maintain intraoperative glycemic control with target blood glucose levels <200 mg/dL (in patients with and without diabetes).
  f. Maintain perioperative normothermia.
  g. Administer increased fraction of inspired oxygen during surgery and after extubation in the immediate postoperative period in patients with normal pulmonary function.

KEY POINTS

- **Healthcare-associated infections (HAIs)** include those with hospital onset and those with community onset in patients with previous healthcare encounters.
- Sources of infections:
  A. **Exogenous:** Exogenous source may be another person in the hospital *(cross-infection)* or a contaminated item of equipment or building service *(environmental infection)*.
  B. **Endogenous:** The infecting organism are derived from the patient's own skin, gastrointestinal or upper respiratory flora.
- Types of **healthcare-associated infections:**
  1. Catheter-associated urinary tract infections (CAUTI)
  2. Ventilator-associated pneumonia (VAP)
  3. Central line-associated bloodstream infection (CLABSI)
  4. Surgical site infections (SSIs)
- **Diagnosis and control of hospital infection:** The most important steps in' preventing nosocomial infections are to first recognize their occurrence and then establish policies to prevent their development. Hospital infection may occur sporadically or as outbreaks.
- **Infection control policy:** There will normally be two parts:
  1. **Infection control committee (ICC)**
  2. **Infection control team**
- **Prevention of hospital associated infections:**
  1. Standard/universal precautions
  2. Precautions for prevention of transmission of infection
  3. **Bundles in infection:** Care "bundles" are simple sets of evidence-based practices that, when implemented collectively, improve the reliability of their delivery and improve patient outcomes.
  Specific care bundles include bundles for the prevention of central line-associated bloodstream infections (CLABSI), bundle for the prevention of catheter-associated urinary tract infections (CAUTI), bundle for the prevention of ventilator-associated pneumonia (VAP), and bundle for the prevention of surgical site infection.

IMPORTANT QUESTIONS

1. Define health care-associated infections. Enumerate organisms causing it.
2. Write short notes on:
   a. Routes of transmission of hospital-associated infections
   b. Diagnosis and control of hospital-associated infections
   c. Prevention of urinary tract infection (UTI)
   d. Prevention of surgical site infection (SSI)
   e. Prevention of ventilator-associated events (VAE)
   f. Prevention of central line-associated bloodstream infection (CLABSI)
   g. Infection control committee
   h. Infection control team

MULTIPLE CHOICE QUESTIONS

1. Bacteria that are most commonly transmitted by direct hand contact, causing nosocomial infection are:
   a. *Escherichia coli*
   b. *Enterococcus* species
   c. *Staphylococcus aureus*
   d. *Clostridium perfringens*
2. **Hospital-associated respiratory infections are caused by the which of the following bacteria?**
   a. *Staphylococcus aureus*
   b. *Klebsiella*
   c. *Enterobacter*
   d. All of the above
3. **The pathogen that is transmitted by air in a hospital is:**
   a. Hepatitis A virus
   b. *Legionella* species
   c. *Shigella* species
   d. Human immunodeficiency virus
4. **The control of hospital-acquired infection is the main responsibility of:**
   a. Medical superintendent of hospital
   b. Head of department of medicine
   c. Head of department of microbiology
   d. Hospital infection control committee

ANSWERS

1. c   2. d   3. b   4. d

Isolation Precautions and Use of Personal Protective Equipment

CHAPTER 64

LEARNING OBJECTIVES

After reading and studying this chapter, you should be able to:
- Describe standard precautions in health care.
- Types of precautions and patients requiring those precautions.
- Discuss standard precautions and transmission-based precautions. Describe infection prevention and control for home and hospital settings. Discuss Personal Protective Equipment (PPE) and its use.

ISOLATION TECHNIQUE

Isolation guidelines contain two tiers of approach:

A. Standard Precautions

Standard precautions are to be followed for all patients, irrespective of their infection status. These are to be used to avoid contact with blood, body fluids, secretions and excretions regardless of whether contaminated grossly with blood or not; nonintact skin; and mucous membrane. They are the basic level of infection control precautions which are to be used, as a minimum, in the care of all patients.

B. Transmission Precautions

The second tier condenses the disease-specific and categories approach to isolation into new transmission categories to be taken based on the route of transmission of organisms like contact precautions, airborne precautions, etc. These precautions are designed for specific patients with highly transmissible pathogens (**Table 64.1**).

STANDARD PRECAUTIONS IN HEALTH CARE

Background

Standard precautions are meant to reduce the risk of transmission of bloodborne and other pathogens from both recognized and unrecognized sources.

They are the basic level of infection control precautions which are to be used, as a minimum, in the care of all patients.

Hand hygiene is a major component of standard precautions and one of the most effective methods to prevent transmission of pathogens associated with health care. In addition to hand hygiene, the use of **personal protective equipment** should be guided by **risk assessment** and the extent of contact anticipated with blood and body fluids, or pathogens.

In addition to practices carried out by health workers when providing care, all individuals (including patients and visitors) should comply with infection control practices in healthcare settings. The control of spread of pathogens from the source is key to avoid transmission. Among source control measures, **respiratory hygiene/cough etiquette**, developed during the severe acute respiratory syndrome (SARS) outbreak, is now considered as part of standard precautions.

Worldwide escalation of the use of standard precautions would reduce unnecessary risks associated with health care. Promotion of an **institutional safety climate** helps to improve conformity with recommended measures and thus subsequent risk reduction. Provision of

Chapter 64: Isolation Precautions and Use of Personal Protective Equipment

Table 64.1: Types of precautions and patients requiring those precautions.

Type of precaution	Specific etiologic agents	Infection control measure to be undertaken by hospital
STANDARD PRECAUTIONS (TIER 1)	–	Use standard precautions for the care of all patients. This general mandate is necessary because it is sometimes not known if the patient is colonized or infected with certain pathogenic microorganisms. Barrier precautions reduce the need to handle sharps.
TRANSMISSION PRECAUTIONS (TIER 2) Airborne precautions	In addition to standard precautions, use airborne precautions for patients known or suspected to have serious illnesses transmitted by airborne droplet nuclei. Examples of such illnesses include the following: • Measles • Varicella (including disseminated zoster) • Tuberculosis • Smallpox	• Patient in private room that has monitored negative air pressure, 6–12 air changes per hour, and appropriate discharge of air outdoors or monitored HEPA filtration of room air before air is circulated to other areas of the hospital or cohorting of patients—that is, placing patients with the same infection in the same room, if private rooms are not available • Health care workers (HCWs) to wear respiratory protection when entering room of patient with known or suspected tuberculosis and, if not immune, for patients with measles or varicella as well • Transport patients out of their room only after placement of a surgical mask
Droplet precautions	• Invasive *Haemophilus influenzae* type b infection, including meningitis, pneumonia, epiglottitis, and sepsis • Invasive *Neisseria meningitidis* infection, including meningitis, pneumonia, and sepsis • Diphtheria (pharyngeal) • *Mycoplasma pneumoniae* • Pertussis • Pneumonic plague • Streptococcal pharyngitis, pneumonia, or scarlet fever in infants and young children • Adenovirus • Influenza virus • Mumps • Parvovirus B_{19} • Rubella • Tuberculosis caused by *Mycobacterium tuberculosis*	• Place patient in private room without special air handling or ventilation or cohort patients • HCWs should wear mask when working within 3 feet of patient • Transfer patients out of their room only after placement of a surgical mask.
Tuberculosis (TB) isolation	Tuberculosis caused by *Mycobacterium tuberculosis*	• TB isolation should be practiced for all patients with known or suspected TB. [Suspected TB is defined by agency policy and generally means any patient with a positive acid-fast bacillus (AFB) smear, with a cavitating lesion seen on chest X-ray study, or identified as high risk by a screening tool] • Isolation is mandatory in a single-patient room designated as negative-pressure airflow and having at least 6–12 air exchanges per hour. It is necessary to vent room air to the outside and, to maintain negative pressure, to close the door

(Contd...)

(Contd...)

Type of precaution	Specific etiologic agents	Infection control measure to be undertaken by hospital
		• It is obligatory for health care workers to wear an N-95 or higher particulate respirator mask when entering an AFB isolation room (check agency's policy for type of mask) • It is obligatory for health care workers to be fit-tested* before using a respirator for the first time. This ensures that the type and the size of the respirator is appropriate for the individual • It is obligatory for health care workers to fit-check† the respirator's fit before each use • Respirator is permitted to be reused and stored according to manufacturer's recommendations and agency policy

Contact precautions	• Gastrointestinal, respiratory, skin, or wound infections or colonization with multidrug-resistant bacteria
	• Enteric infections with a low infectious dose or prolonged environmental survival, including the following:
	  a. Clostridium difficile
	  b. Diapered or incontinent patients with the following:
	    1. *Escherichia coli* O157:H7
	    2. *Shigella*
	    3. Hepatitis A
	    4. *Rotavirus*
	• Respiratory syncytial virus, parainfluenza virus, and enteroviral infections in infants and young children
	• Skin infections that are highly contagious or that tend to occur on dry skin, including the following:
	  a. Diphtheria (cutaneous)
	  b. Herpes simplex virus (neonatal or mucocutaneous)
	  c. Impetigo
	  d. Major (noncontaminated) abscesses, cellulitis, or decubitus ulcers
	  e. Pediculosis
	  f. Scabies
	  g. Staphylococcal furunculosis in infants and young children
		In addition to standard precautions, use contact precautions for patients known or suspected to have serious illnesses easily transmitted by direct patient contact or by contact with items in the patient's environment. Examples of such illnesses include the following:
		Gastrointestinal, respiratory, skin, or wound infections or colonization with multidrug-resistant bacteria judged by the infection prevention and control committee, and current state, regional, and national recommendations, to be of special clinical and epidemiologic significance

(Contd...)

(Contd...)

Type of precaution	Specific etiologic agents	Infection control measure to be undertaken by hospital
	h. Methicillin-resistant *Staphylococcus aureus* (MRSA) i. Vancomycin-resistant enterococci (VRE) j. Extended-spectrum beta-lactamase (ESBL) (necessitates 9 months of contact precautions). This enzyme attaches to the cell wall of *E. coli* and some Klebsiella organisms, which in turn makes the organisms multidrug-resistant. Once treatment is completed, the enzyme is still found in the feces for up to 9 months k. Zoster (disseminated or in the immunocompromised host) l. Viral or hemorrhagic conjunctivitis m. Viral hemorrhagic infections (Ebola, Lassa, or Marburg)	
Immuno-compromised patients		Immunocompromised patients vary in their susceptibility to healthcare-associated infections depending on the severity and the duration of immunosuppression. They are generally at increased risk for bacterial, fungal, parasitic, and viral infections from both endogenous and exogenous sources In general, the use of standard precautions for all patients and transmission-based precautions for specified patients reduces the acquisition by these patients of institutionally acquired organisms from other patients and environments. Leukopenic patients will sometimes require additional protective measures, other than standard precautions. In such instances, the physician or infection preventionist instructs nursing staff as to the necessary protective measures (e.g., masks, private room). They place an isolation sign on the door, which lists the additional protective measures that staff and visitors are required to follow for the safety of the patient
Monitoring of isolation		Transmission-based isolation practices are monitored on an ongoing basis by the infection preventionist

*****Fit test:** Procedure to determine adequate fit of respirator, usually by qualitative measure (wearers are exposed to a concentrated saccharin solution and asked if they can detect taste while wearing respirator).

†**Fit-chek:** Procedure in which worker uses negative pressure to see if mask is properly sealed to face.

adequate staff and supplies, together with leadership and education of health workers, patients, and visitors, are critical for an enhanced safety climate in healthcare settings.

Important Advice

- Promotion of a safety climate is a cornerstone of prevention of transmission of pathogens in health care.
- Standard precautions should be the minimum level of precautions used when providing care for all patients.
- Risk assessment is critical. Assess all health-care activities to determine the personal protection that is indicated.
- Implement source control measures for all persons with respiratory symptoms through promotion of respiratory hygiene and cough etiquette.

Checklist

Health Policy

- Promote a safety climate.
- Develop policies which facilitate the implementation of infection control measures.

Hand Hygiene

- Perform hand hygiene by means of hand rubbing or hand washing.
- Perform hand washing with soap and water if hands are visibly soiled, or exposure to spore-forming organisms is proven or strongly suspected, or after using the restroom. Otherwise, if resources permit, perform hand rubbing with an alcohol-based preparation.
- Ensure availability of handwashing facilities with clean running water.
- Ensure availability of hand hygiene products (clean water, soap, single use clean towels, alcohol-based hand rub). Alcohol-based hand rubs should ideally be available at the point of care.

Personal Protective Equipment (PPE)

- Assess the risk of exposure to body substances or contaminated surfaces BEFORE any health-care activity. **Make this a routine!**
- Select PPE based on the assessment of risk:
  - Clean nonsterile gloves
  - Clean, nonsterile fluid-resistant gown
  - Mask and eye protection or a face shield

Respiratory Hygiene and Cough Etiquette

- Education of health workers, patients and visitors.
- Covering mouth and nose when coughing or sneezing.
- Hand hygiene after contact with respiratory secretions.
- Spatial separation of persons with acute febrile respiratory symptoms.

STANDARD PRECAUTIONS

Key Elements at a Glance

1. **Hand hygiene**[1]
   Summary technique:
   - Hand washing (40–60 sec): Wet hands and apply soap; rub all surfaces; rinse hands and dry thoroughly with a single use towel; use towel to turn off faucet.
   - Hand rubbing (20–30 sec): Apply enough product to cover all areas of the hands; rub hands until dry.

   Summary indications:
   - Before and after any direct patient contact and between patients, whether or not gloves are worn.
   - Immediately after gloves are removed.
   - Before handling an invasive device.
   - After touching blood, body fluids, secretions, excretions, nonintact skin, and contaminated items, even if gloves are worn.
   - During patient care, when moving from a contaminated to a clean body site of the patient.

---

1. For more details, see: WHO Guidelines on Hand Hygiene in Health Care (Advanced draft), at: http://www.who.int/patientsafety/information_centre/ghhad_download/en/index.html.

- After contact with inanimate objects in the immediate vicinity of the patient.
2. **Gloves**
   - Wear when touching blood, body fluids, secretions, excretions, mucous membranes, nonintact skin.
   - Change between tasks and procedures on the same patient after contact with potentially infectious material.
   - Remove after use, before touching non-contaminated items and surfaces, and before going to another patient. Perform hand hygiene immediately after removal.
3. **Facial protection (eyes, nose, and mouth)**
   - Wear (1) a surgical or procedure mask and eye protection (eye visor, goggles) or (2) a face shield to protect mucous membranes of the eyes, nose, and mouth during activities that are likely to generate splashes or sprays of blood, body fluids, secretions, and excretions.
4. **Gown**
   - Wear to protect skin and prevent soiling of clothing during activities that are likely to generate splashes or sprays of blood, body fluids, secretions, or excretions.
   - Remove soiled gown as soon as possible, and perform hand hygiene.
5. **Prevention of needle stick injuries from other sharp instruments**[2]
   Use care when:
   - Handling needles, scalpels, and other sharp instruments or devices
   - Cleaning used instruments
   - Disposing of used needles and other sharp instruments.
6. **Respiratory hygiene and cough etiquette**
   Persons with respiratory symptoms should apply source control measures:
   - Cover their nose and mouth when coughing/sneezing with tissue or mask, dispose of used tissues and masks, and perform hand hygiene after contact with respiratory secretions

Health care facilities should:
- Place acute febrile respiratory symptomatic patients at least 1 meter (3 feet) away from others in common waiting areas, if possible.
- Postvisual alerts at the entrance to health-care facilities instructing persons with respiratory symptoms to practise respiratory hygiene/cough etiquette.
- Consider making hand hygiene resources, tissues and masks available in common areas and areas used for the evaluation of patients with respiratory illnesses.

7. **Environmental cleaning**
   Use adequate procedures for the routine cleaning and disinfection of environmental and other frequently touched surfaces.
8. **Linens**
   Handle, transport, and process used linen in a manner which:
   - Prevents skin and mucous membrane exposures and contamination of clothing.
   - Avoids transfer of pathogens to other patients and or the environment.
9. **Waste disposal**
   - Ensure safe waste management.
   - Treat waste contaminated with blood body fluids, secretions and excretions as clinical waste, in accordance with local regulations.
   - Human tissues and laboratory waste that is directly associated with specimen processing should also be treated as clinical waste.
   - Discard single use items properly.
10. **Patient care equipment**
    - Handle equipment soiled with blood, body fluids, secretions, and excretions in a manner that prevents skin and mucous membrane exposures, contamination of clothing, and transfer of pathogens to other patients or the environment.
    - Clean, disinfect, and reprocess reusable equipment appropriately before use with another patient.

---

2. The SIGN Alliance at: http://www.who.int/injection_safety/sign/en/

PERSONAL PROTECTIVE EQUIPMENT

Personal protective equipment (PPE) refers to a variety of barriers used either alone or in combination to protect health care workers from contact with transmissible pathogens. These include single-use disposable gloves, aprons and long-sleeved gowns as well as facial protection for eyes, nose and mouth. Facial protection, footwear and hair cover or cap.

For PPE to be protective and considered appropriate, blood and body fluids must not be able to penetrate the PPE material. The equipment must be accessible to the employee and must be worn whenever there is the potential for exposure to infectious material; it must be removed before leaving the work area and must be placed in an area designated for PPE. Ensure sufficient supplies of appropriate PPE. HCWs should be trained on the use of PPE as part of the infection prevention and control (IPC) training.

PPE should be removed prior to leaving the isolation room and discarded into appropriate health care waste stream. PPE should be put on and taken off in correct sequence and disposed in accordance with the Biomedical Waste Management and Handing Rules 2016, and 2018. Hand hygiene should always be the final step following removal and disposal of PPE. All respirators should be fit-tested for each individual so that each person is assured that his or hers is working properly. Males must have their facial hair to achieve a tight fit.

Uses
- Healthcare workers (HCWs) who provide direct care to patients and who may come in contact with blood, body fluids, excretions, and secretions.
- Support staff including cleaners, and laundry staff in situations where they may have contact with blood, body fluids, secretions, and excretions.
- Laboratory staff, who handle patient specimens
- Family members who provide care to patients and are in a situation where they may have contact with blood, body fluids, secretions and excretions.
- Healthcare workers (HCWs) in a hemodialysis unit, because of the high risk of transmission of blood-borne infections during the various activities associated with hemodialysis and handling of equipment; and
- Patients in a hemodialysis unit, in the form of a barrier over clothing during cannulation and decannulation, central line connection, disconnection/dressing change.

1. **Gloves:** In addition to wearing gloves as outlined in standard precautions, gloves should be worn on entering an isolation room or cohort area and for all interactions that involve contact with the patient or items in close proximity to the patient (such as medical equipment, bed rails, etc.) (**Box 64.1**). Again, hands must be washed after the removal of gloves. Gloves should

---

Box 64.1: Hand hygiene and medical glove use.

Hand Hygiene: Why, How and When?
- The use of gloves does not replace the need for cleaning your heads.
- Hand hygiene must be performed when appropriate regardless of the indication for glove use.
- Remove gloves to perform hand hygiene, when an indication occurs while wearing gloves.
- Discard gloves after each task and clean your hands—gloves may carry germs.
- Wear gloves only when indicated according to standard and contact precautions (see examples in the pyramid below)—otherwise they become a major risk for germ transmission.

The glove pyramid—to aid decision making on when to wear (and not wear) gloves (**Fig. 64.1**)
Gloves must be worn according to STANDARD and contact precautions. The pyramid details some clinical example in which gloves are not indicated, and others in which clean or sterile gloves are indicated. Hand hygiene should be performed when appropriate regardless of indications for glove use.

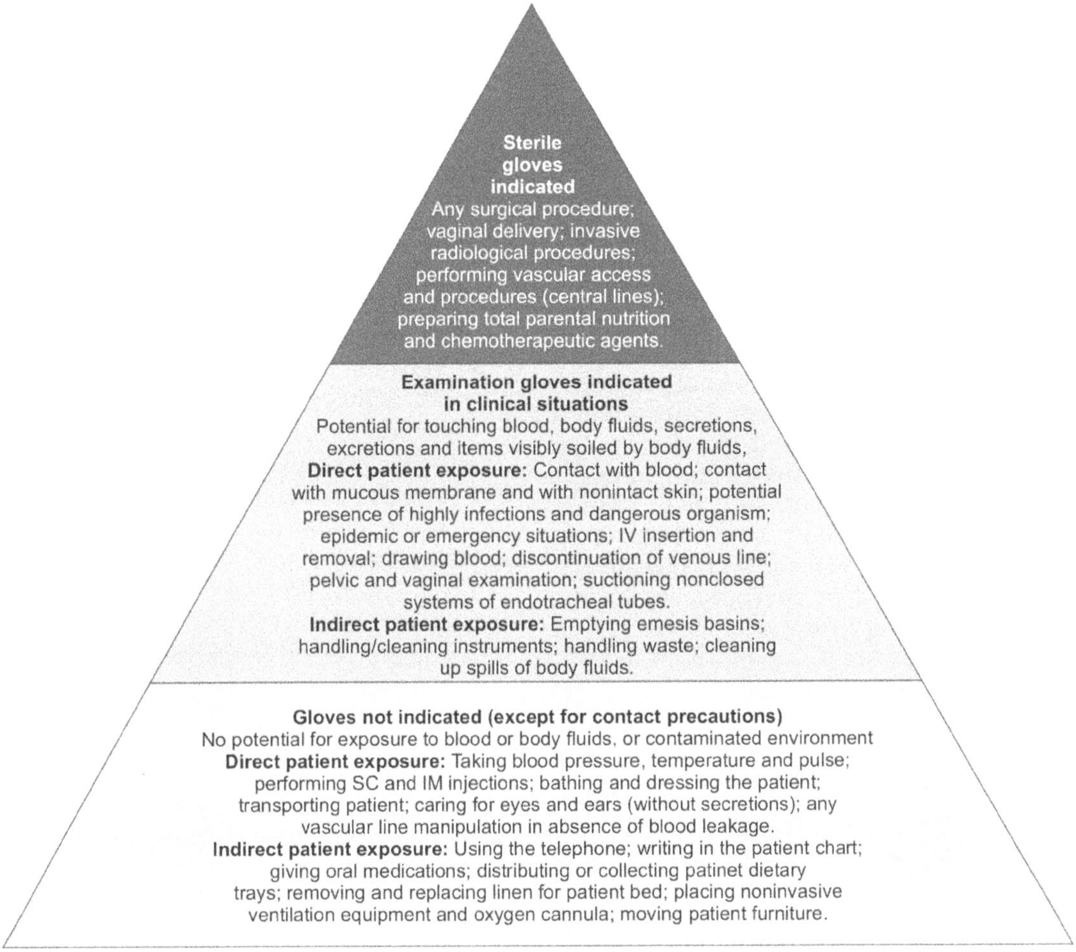

Fig. 64.1: The glove pyramid.
(SC: subcutaneous; IM: intramuscular)

Sterile gloves indicated
Any surgical procedure; vaginal delivery; invasive radiological procedures; performing vascular access and procedures (central lines); preparing total parental nutrition and chemotherapeutic agents.

Examination gloves indicated in clinical situations
Potential for touching blood, body fluids, secretions, excretions and items visibly soiled by body fluids,
Direct patient exposure: Contact with blood; contact with mucous membrane and with nonintact skin; potential presence of highly infections and dangerous organism; epidemic or emergency situations; IV insertion and removal; drawing blood; discontinuation of venous line; pelvic and vaginal examination; suctioning nonclosed systems of endotracheal tubes.
Indirect patient exposure: Emptying emesis basins; handling/cleaning instruments; handling waste; cleaning up spills of body fluids.

Gloves not indicated (except for contact precautions)
No potential for exposure to blood or body fluids, or contaminated environment
Direct patient exposure: Taking blood pressure, temperature and pulse; performing SC and IM injections; bathing and dressing the patient; transporting patient; caring for eyes and ears (without secretions); any vascular line manipulation in absence of blood leakage.
Indirect patient exposure: Using the telephone; writing in the patient chart; giving oral medications; distributing or collecting patinet dietary trays; removing and replacing linen for patient bed; placing noninvasive ventilation equipment and oxygen cannula; moving patient furniture.

be removed in the following circumstances:
- After body fluid exposure risk
- Before leaving the patient's environment (room or cohort bed space). Gloves must be discarded between patients and must never be washed for reuse, as microorganisms cannot be reliably removed from glove surfaces and glove integrity may be compromised. It may be necessary to change gloves and perform hand hygiene during the care of a single patient in order to prevent cross-contamination of different body sites or before touching noncontaminated areas in the patient's environment. Gloves do not preclude the need for hand hygiene and this should always be performed after glove removal.

2. **Aprons and gowns:** A disposable plastic apron and gloves should be donned before entering the room/cohort bed space of a patient infected or colonized with a multidrug resistant organisms (MDRO). PPE should be changed between each patient in a cohort area and should be removed and discarded into

appropriate health care waste stream prior to leaving the patient's room/bed space, in order to prevent contamination of noncontaminated areas. Hands should be decontaminated after PPE removal.

3. **Aprons versus long-sleeved gowns:** Aprons/long-sleeved gowns should be worn when contact with the patient and environment is anticipated. Healthcare workers should consider selecting long-sleeved gowns in preference to aprons if the level of anticipated environmental exposure may result in contamination of unprotected sleeves or arms when wearing an apron; or in situations where close physical contact with the patient is anticipated (e.g., pediatric setting, assistance with body care). Where extensive exposure to blood and body fluids is anticipated, fluid repellent gowns may be more appropriate and situations should be risk-assessed on an individual basis.

4. **Facial protection**
   Indications: Usual facial protection includes a medical/ surgical mask (triple-layer surgical mask) and eye protection (face shield or goggles), to protect the conjunctivae and the mucous membranes of the nose, eyes and mouth during activities that are likely to generate splashes or sprays of blood, body fluids, secretions or excretions. Eye protection should also be used while providing care to patients with respiratory symptoms, such as coughing and sneezing, since sprays of secretions may occur.
   Face masks and eye protection should be worn in accordance with standard precautions when performing splash-generating procedures, such as wound irrigation, oral suctioning, intubation, when caring for patients with open tracheostomies, where there is potential for projectile secretions and where there is evidence of transmission of MDRO from heavily colonized sites, such as an extensive burn wound. Masks are not otherwise recommended for health care workers carrying out routine care. Face masks should be single-use disposable and fluid resistant. Personal spectacles and contact lenses are not considered to provide adequate eye protection.

5. **Footwear**
   - A closed footwear, which can be easily cleaned and disinfected, must be used whenever work processes or environments could cause foot injuries or spillage of blood or body fluids.
   - Personal footwear should be changed when entering clean areas, such as OTs, labor rooms, ICU.
   - Shoe covers may be used over street shoes to protect clean areas from soil and dirt brought in by shoes.

6. **Hair covers**
   Long hair must be secured with a rubber band and hair cover worn to protect the hair and to protect the patient from falling hair.

KEY POINTS

Standard precautions are meant to reduce the risk of transmission of blood borne and other pathogens from both recognized and unrecognized sources of infections. They are the basic level of infection control precautions which are to be used, as a minimum, in the care of all patients.

Isolation technique
- **Standard precautions:** The first contains precautions designed to **care for all patients** in health care facilities regardless of their diagnosis or presumed infectiousness.
- **Transmission precautions:** The second tier condenses the **disease-specific and categories** approach to isolation into new **transmission categories**: airborne, droplet, and contact precautions.

Personal Protective Equipment
Personal protective equipment (PPE) refers to a variety of barriers used either alone or in combination to protect health care workers from contact with transmissible pathogens. These include single-use disposable gloves, aprons and long-sleeved gowns as well as facial protection for eyes, nose and mouth. Facial protection, footwear and hair cover or cap.

IMPORTANT QUESTION

1. Write briefly on:
   a. Standard precautions in health care
   b. Healthcare facility for standard precautions
   c. Types of precautions and patients requiring those precautions
   d. Infection prevention and control for home and hospice settings
   e. Personal protective equipment (PPE) and its use

MULTIPLE CHOICE QUESTIONS

1. **Standard precautions are followed for:**
   a. All patients irrespective of their infection status.
   b. Only for patients to avoid contact with blood.
   c. For contaminated equipment and articles.
   d. Patients with only recognized sources of infection.

2. **Transmission precautions are meant for:**
   a. Disease-specific approach to isolation.
   b. Disease-specific and categories approach to isolation.
   c. All of the above
   d. None of the above.

3. **PPE should be used by:**
   a. Health care workers who provide direct care to patients.
   b. Laboratory staff, who handle patient specimens.
   c. Health care workers in a hemodialysis unit.
   d. All of the above

ANSWERS

1. a   2. b   3. d

Hand Hygiene

LEARNING OBJECTIVES

After reading and studying this chapter, you should be able to:
- Discuss hand hygiene.
- Describe types of hand hygiene.
- Discuss hand washing and use of alcohol hand rub.
- Describe moments of hand hygiene.
- Discuss WHO hand hygiene promotion.

INTRODUCTION

Hand hygiene is the single most important measure for prevention of infection. Hands can become contaminated with infectious agents through contact with a patient, patient surroundings, the environment, or other health care workers (HCWs). Hand hygiene removes dust/soil, organic material and transient micro-organisms from the skin and reduces the risk of cross-contamination.

Any action of hygienic hand antisepsis in order to reduce transient microbial flora (generally performed either by hand rubbing with an **alcohol-based formulation** or **handwashing with plain or antimicrobial soap and water).**

Hand hygiene is the single most important and basic preventive technique for interrupting the infectious process. **Box 65.1** indicates when it is essential to initiate hand hygiene. Performing hand hygiene will provide the necessary protection before you care for a patient.

HAND HYGIENE: WHY, HOW AND WHEN?

Why?
- Thousands of people die every day around the world from infections acquired while receiving health care.

> **Box 65.1:** Essential hand hygiene.
>
> **Hand hygiene is essential:**
> - When hands are visibly soiled
> - Before and after caring for a patient
> - After contact with organic material, such as feces, wound drainage, and mucus
> - In preparation for an invasive procedure, such as suctioning, catheterization, or injections
> - Before changing a dressing or having contact with open wounds
> - Before preparing and administering medications
> - After removing disposable gloves or handling contaminated equipment
> - Before and after using the toilet
> - Before and after eating
> - At the beginning and end of the shift

- Hands are the main pathways of germ transmission during health care.
- Hand hygiene is therefore the most important measure to avoid the transmission of harmful germs and prevent healthcare-associated infections.
- This brochure explains how and when to practice hand hygiene.

Who?
- Any healthcare worker, caregiver or person involved in direct or indirect patient care

needs to be concerned about hand hygiene and should be able to perform it correctly and at the right time.

How?

- Clean your hands by **rubbing them with an alcohol-based formulation**, as the preferred mean for routine hygienic hand antisepsis if hands are not visibly soiled. It is faster, more effective, and better tolerated by your hands than washing with soap and water.
- **Wash your hands with soap and water** when hands are visibly dirty or visibly soiled with blood or other body fluids or after using the toilet.
- If exposure to potential spore-forming pathogens is strongly suspected or proven, including outbreaks of *Clostridium difficile*, hand washing with soap and water is the preferred means.

HAND WASH

To effectively clean hands soiled with dirt or organic matter, or if you have handled a contaminated article, soap or detergents that contain antiseptic and water are required **(Fig. 65.1)**.

HAND RUB

Use alcohol-based hand rubs (ABHR), when hands are not visibly soiled or tap and running water is not available **(Fig. 65.2)**.

Surgical Hand Scrub

Hand scrubbing with an antiseptic agent before beginning a surgical procedure reduces the number of microorganisms, and inhibits the growth of microorganisms on hands under the gloves. Chlorhexidine or povidone-iodine-containing soaps are the most commonly used products for surgical hand scrub. The antimicrobial efficacy of alcohol-based formulations is superior to that of all other currently available methods of preoperative surgical hand preparation **(Fig. 65.3)**.

IMPROVING THE IMPLEMENTATION OF HAND HYGIENE

Hand hygiene can be improved through a multimodal strategy suggested by WHO. The key components are:

- **System change:** Ensuring that the necessary infrastructure is in place to allow healthcare workers (HCWs) to practice hand hygiene. This has two essential elements:
  - Access to a safe, continuous water supply as well as to soap and towels.
  - Readily accessible alcohol-based hand rub at the point of care.
- **Training/education:** Providing regular training on the importance of hand hygiene, based on the "My 5 moments for hand hygiene" approach (**Fig. 65.4**), and the correct steps for hand rubbing and handwashing, to all HCWs.
- **Evaluation and feedback:** Monitoring hand hygiene practices and infrastructure, along with related perceptions and knowledge among HCWs, while providing performance and results feedback to staff.
- **Reminders at the workplace:** Prompting and reminding HCWs about the importance of hand hygiene and about the appropriate indications and procedures for performing it.
- **Institutional safety climate:** Creating an environment and perceptions that facilitate raising awareness about patient safety issues while guaranteeing improvement of hand hygiene as a high priority at all levels.

YOUR 5 MOMENTS FOR HAND HYGIENE (FIG. 65.4)

1. Before Touching a Patient

WHY? To protect the patient against colonization and, in some cases, against exogenous infection, by harmful germs carried on your hands.
WHEN? Clean your hands before touching a patient when approaching him/her.*

---

*Note: Hand hygiene must be performed in all indications described regardless of whether gloves are used or not

Hand hygiene technique with soap and water
Duration of the entire procedure: 40–60 seconds

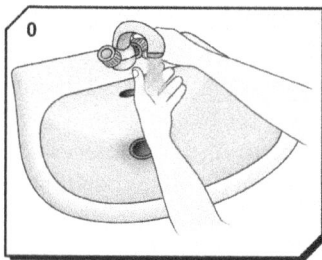
0
Wet hands with water

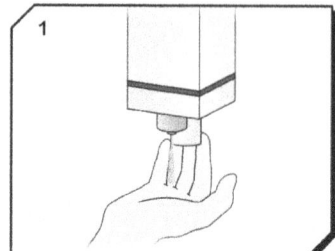
1
Apply enough soap to cover all hand surfaces

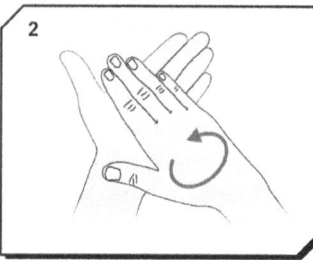
2
Rub hands palm to palm

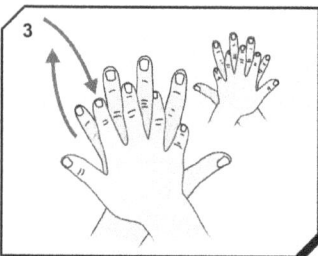
3
Right palm over left dorsum with interlaced fingers and vice versa

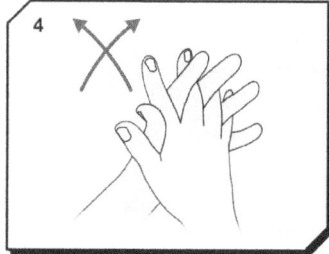
4
Palm to palm with fingers interlaced

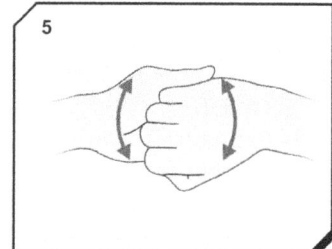
5
Backs of fingers to opposing palms with fingers interlocked

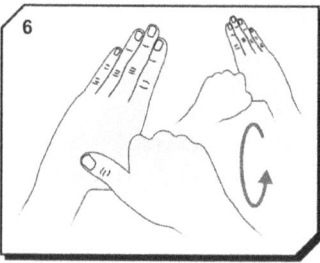
6
Rotational rubbing of left thumb clasped in right palm and vice versa

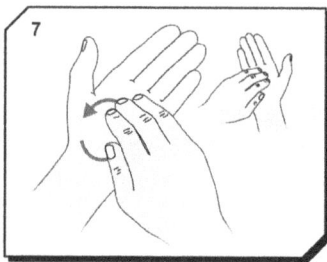
7
Rotational rubbing, backward and forward with clasped fingers of right hand in left palm and vice versa

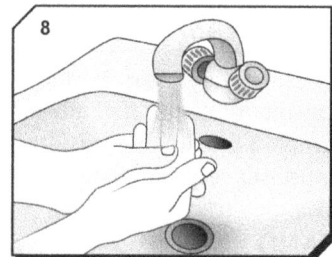
8
Rinse hands with water

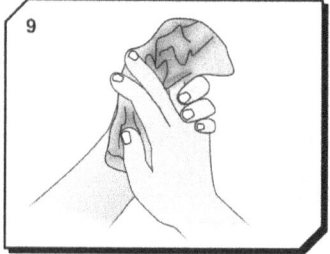
9
Dry hands thoroughly with a single use towel

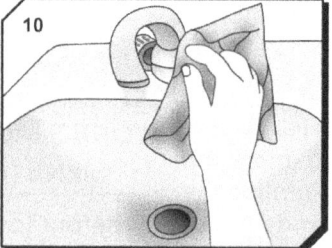
10
Use towel to turn off faucet

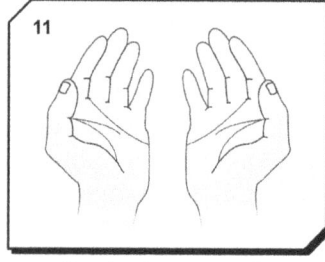
11
Your hands are now safe

Hand care
- Take care of your hands by regularly using a protective hand cream or lotion, at least daily.
- Do not routinely wash hands with soap and water immediately before or after using an alcohol-based handrub.
- Do not use hot water to rinse your hands.
- After handrubbing or handwashing, let your hands dry completely before putting on gloves.

Please remember
- Do not wear artificial fingernails or extenders when in direct contact with patients.
- Keep natural nails short.

Fig. 65.1: How to hand wash?

Hand hygiene technique with alcohol-based formulation

Duration of the entire procedure: 20–30 seconds

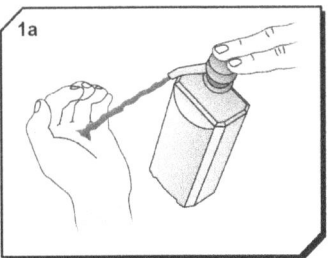
Apply a palmful of the product in a cupped hand, covering all surfaces

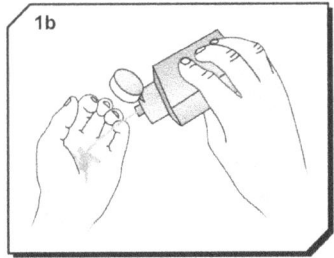

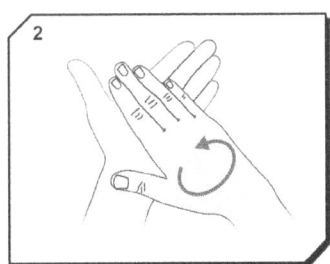
Rub hands palm to palm

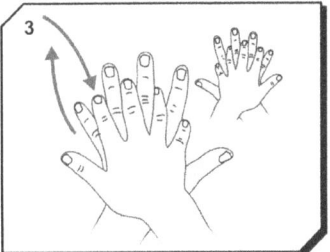
Right palm over left dorsum with interlaced fingers and vice versa

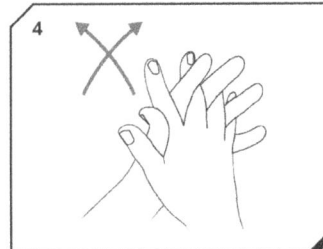
Palm to palm with fingers interlaced

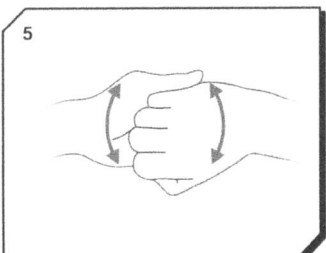
Backs of fingers to opposing palms with fingers interlocked

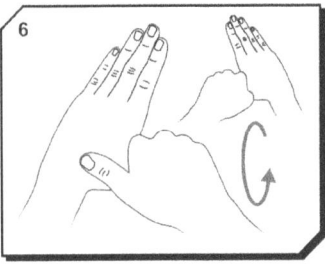
Rotational rubbing of left thumb clasped in right palm and vice versa

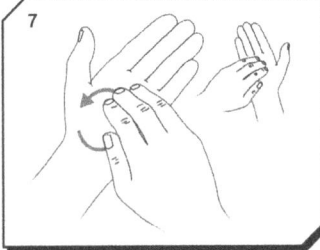
Rotational rubbing, backward and forward with clasped fingers of right hand in left palm and vice versa

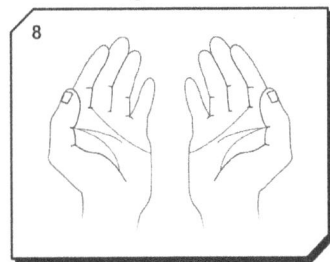
Once dry, your hands are safe

Fig. 65.2: How to hand rub?

Situations when moment 1 applies:
a. *Before shaking hands, before stroking a child's forehead*
b. *Before assisting a patient in personal care activities:* To move, to take a bath, to eat, to get dressed, etc.
c. *Before delivering care and other noninvasive treatment:* Applying oxygen mask, giving a massage.
d. *Before performing a physical noninvasive examination:* Taking pulse, blood pressure, chest auscultation, recording ECG.

2. Before Clean/Aseptic Procedure

WHY? To protect the patient against infection with harmful germs, including his/her own germs, entering his/her body.

WHEN? Clean your hands immediately before accessing a critical site with infectious risk for the patient (e.g., a mucous membrane, nonintact skin, an invasive medical device)*

Situations when moment 2 applies:
a. Before brushing the patient's teeth, instilling eye drops, performing a digital vaginal or

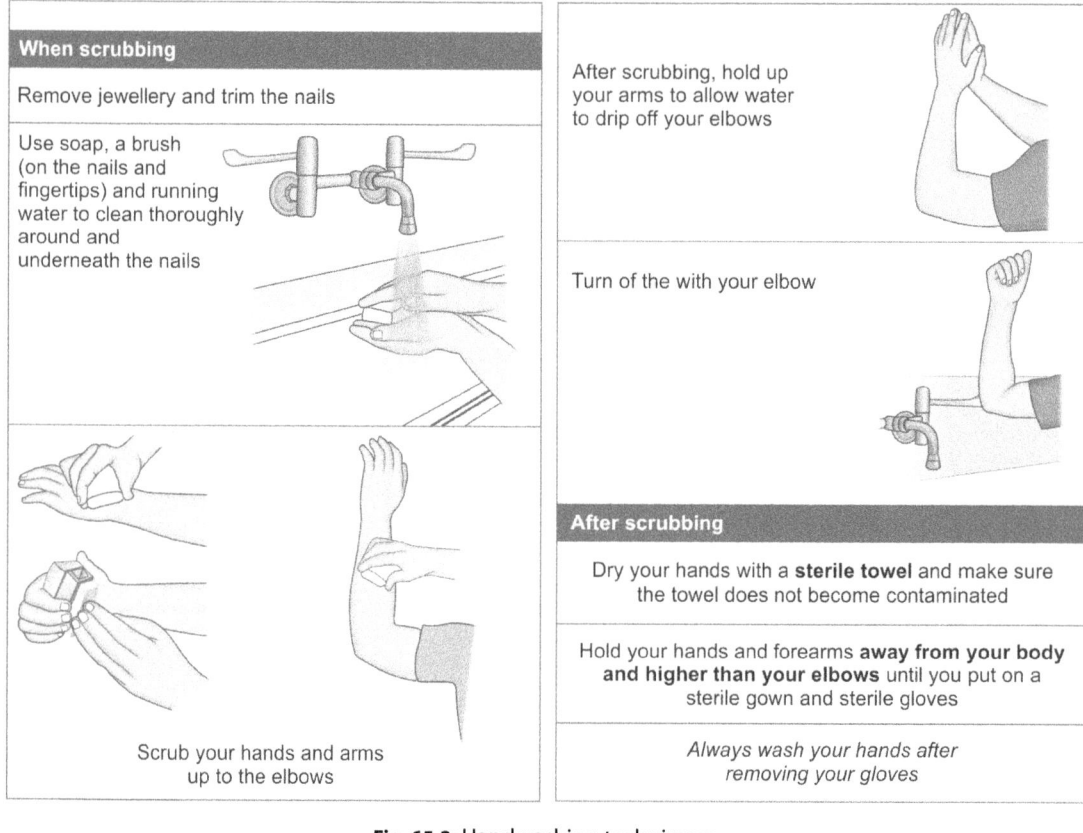

Fig. 65.3: Handwashing techniques.

rectal examination, examining mouth, nose, ear with or without an instrument, inserting a suppository/pessary, suctioning mucous.
b. Before dressing a wound with or without instrument, applying ointment on vesicle, making a percutaneous injection/puncture.
c. Before inserting an invasive medical device (nasal cannula, nasogastric tube, endotracheal tube, urinary probe, percutaneous catheter, drainage), disrupting/opening any circuit of an invasive medical device (for food, medication, draining, suctioning, monitoring purposes).
d. Before preparing food, medications, pharmaceutical products, sterile material

3. After Body Fluid Exposure Risk

WHY? To protect you from colonization or infection with patient's harmful germs and to protect the health-care environment from germ spread.

WHEN? Clean your hands as soon as the task involving an exposure risk to body fluids has ended (and after glove removal).*

Situations when moment 3 applies:
a. When the contact with a mucous membrane and with nonintact skin ends.
b. After a percutaneous injection or puncture; after inserting an invasive medical device (vascular access, catheter, tube, drain, etc); after disrupting and opening an invasive circuit
c. After removing an invasive medical device
d. After removing any form of material offering protection (napkin, dressing, gauze, sanitary towel, etc).
e. After handling a sample containing organic matter, after clearing excreta and any other

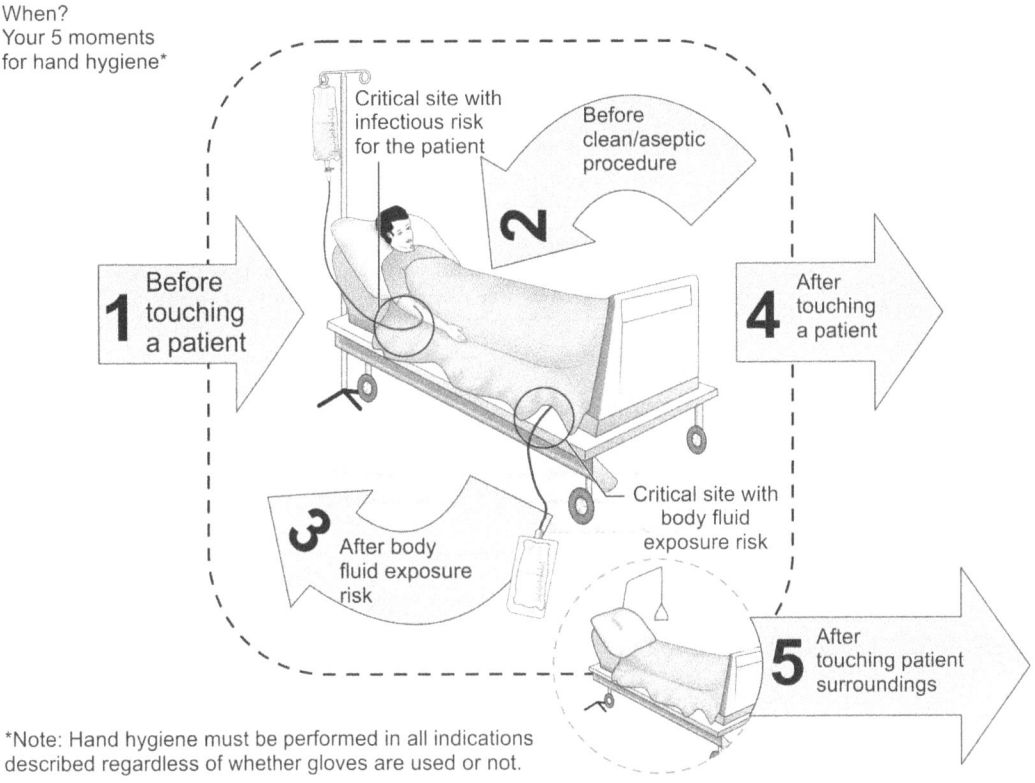

Fig. 65.4: Your 5 moments for hand hygiene.

body fluid, after cleaning any contaminated surface and soiled material (soiled bed linen, dentures, instruments, urinal, bedpan, lavatories, etc).

4. After Touching a Patient

WHY? To protect you from colonization with patient germs and to protect the health-care environment from germ spread.

WHEN? Clean your hands when leaving the patient's side, after having touched the patient*

Situations when moment 4 applies, If they correspond to the last contact with the patient before leaving him/her:

a. After shaking hands, stroking a child's forehead
b. After you have assisted the patient in personal care activities: To move, to bath, to eat, to dress, etc.
c. After delivering care and other noninvasive treatment: Changing bed linen as the patient is in, applying oxygen mask, giving a massage
d. After performing a physical noninvasive examination: Taking pulse, blood pressure, chest auscultation, recording ECG.

5. After Touching Patient Surroundings

WHY? To protect you from colonization with patient germs that may be present on surfaces/objects in patient surroundings and to protect the health-care environment against germ spread.

WHEN? Clean your hands after touching any object or furniture when living the patient surroundings, without having touched the patient.*

***Note:** Hand hygiene must be performed in all indications described regardless of whether gloves are used or not

This Moment 5 applies in the following situations if they correspond to the last contact with the patient surroundings, without having touched the patient:
a. After an activity involving physical contact with the patients immediate environment: changing bed linen with the patient out of the bed, holding a bed trail, clearing a bedside table.
b. After a care activity: adjusting perfusion speed, clearing a monitoring alarm.
c. After other contacts with surfaces or inanimate objects (note—ideally try to avoid these unnecessary activities): leaning against a bed, leaning against a night table/bedside table.

Hand care	Actions to prevent skin irritation
Hand hygiene	Any action of hygienic hand antisepsis in order to reduce transient microbial flora (generally performed either by handrubbing with an alcohol-based formulation or handwashing with plain or antimicrobial soap and water)
Indication for hand hygiene	Moment during health care when hand hygiene must be performed to prevent harmful germ transmission and/or infection
Invasive medical device	Any medical device that enters the body either through a body opening or through a skin or mucous membrane breaking

Glossary

Alcohol-based formulation	An alcohol-containing preparation (liquid, gel or foam) designed for application to the hands for hygienic hand antisepsis
Body fluids	Blood; excretions like urine, feces, vomit; meconium; lochia; secretions like saliva, tears, sperm, colostrum, milk, mucous secretions, wax, vernix; exudates and transudates like lymphatic, pleural fluid cerebrospinal fluid, ascitis fluid, articular fluid, pus (except sweat); organic samples like tissues, cells, organ, bone marrow, placenta
Clean/aseptic procedure	Any care activity that implies a direct or indirect contact with a mucous membrane, nonintact skin, an invasive medial device. During such a procedure no germs should be transmitted
Critical site	Critical sites are associated with risk of infection. They either correspond to body sites or medical devices that have to be protected against harmful germs (called critical sites with risk of infection for the patient), or body sites or medical devices that potentially lead to hand exposure to body fluids and bloodborne pathogens (called critical sites with body fluid exposure risk)

KEY POINTS

- **Hand hygiene:** Any action of hygienic hand antisepsis in order to reduce transient microbial flora (generally performed either by hand rubbing with an **alcohol-based formulation** or **handwashing with plain or antimicrobial soap and water).**
- Hand hygiene is the single most important and basic preventive technique for interrupting the infectious process.
- To effectively clean hands soiled with dirt or organic matter, or if you have handled a contaminated article, soap or detergents that contain antiseptic and water are required. The standard is to wash for **15–30 seconds** using hospital approved soap, running hands under warm water (both cold and very hot water increase the risk of drying and chapping the skin). All forms of health care–associated infections can result from improper hand hygiene and use of contaminated equipment.

IMPORTANT QUESTION

1. Write short notes on:
   a. Hand hygiene
   b. Types of hand hygiene
   c. Handwashing and use of alcohol hand rub
   d. Moments of hand hygiene

MULTIPLE CHOICE QUESTIONS

1. **Hand washing is essential:**
   a. When hands are visibly soiled
   b. Before and after caring for a patient
   c. After contact with organic material
   d. All of the above
2. **Indications for hand washing with soap and water are:**
   a. When there is visibly heavy contamination
   b. After using toilet
   c. Before and after having food
   d. All of the above

ANSWERS

1. d   2. d

CHAPTER 66

Sterilization and Disinfection

LEARNING OBJECTIVES

After reading and studying this chapter, you should be able to:
- Classify and describe the different methods of sterilization and disinfection.
- Discuss the application of the different methods in the laboratory, in clinical and surgical practice.
- Choose the most appropriate method of sterilization and disinfection to be used in specific situations in the laboratory, in clinical and surgical practice.
- Describe the following: Aseptic techniques Spaulding's classification; environment cleaning; equipment cleaning.

INTRODUCTION

Sterilization: Sterilization is defined as the process by which an article, surface, or medium is freed of all living microorganisms either in the vegetative or spore state.

Disinfection: Disinfection is the killing, inhibition, or removal of microorganisms that may cause disease.

Antiseptics: Antiseptics are chemical agents applied to tissue to prevent infection by killing or inhibiting pathogen growth; they also reduce the total microbial population.

Cleaning: The removal of visible soil (e.g., organic and inorganic material) from objects and surfaces and normally is accomplished manually or mechanically using water with detergents or enzymatic products.

METHODS OF STERILIZATION AND DISINFECTION (BOX 66.1)

A. Physical agents
B. Chemical agents

A. Physical Agents

1. **Sunlight:** Sunlight has appreciable bactericidal activity and plays an important role in the spontaneous sterilization that occurs under natural conditions. It is a natural method of sterilization in cases of water in tanks, rivers, and lakes.
2. **Drying:** Drying in air has a deleterious effect on many bacteria.
3. **Heat:** Heat is the most reliable and universally applicable method of sterilization. Either **dry or moist heat** may be applied.

Mechanism of Action

Dry heat: The lethal effect of dry heat, or desiccation in general, is usually due to **protein denaturation, oxidative damage,** and **toxic effects of elevated levels of electrolytes**.

Moist heat: Kills microorganisms by **coagulation and denaturation of their enzymes** and structural proteins.

Dry Heat Sterilization

i. **Red heat:** Inoculating wires loops and points of forceps are sterilized by holding them almost vertically in a Bunsen flame until red hot.
ii. **Flaming:** Scalpel blades, glass slides, mouth of culture tubes and bottles are exposed to a flame for a few seconds.

> **Box 66.1:** Methods of sterilization and disinfection.

A. Physical agents
1. **Heat**
   ➢ **Dry heat:**
      - Incineration—at temperature of 870–980°C
      - Red heat
      - Flaming
      - Hot air sterilizer
      - Microwave ovens
   ➢ **Moist heat:**
      - At temperature below 100°C: Pasteurization, vaccine production, inspissation, water bath
      - At a temperature of 100°C: Boiling steaming, tyndallization
      - At temperature above 100°C: Autoclave
2. **Filtration:** 0.22–0.45 μm pore size; high efficiency particle air (HEPA)
3. **Radiation:**
   i. **Nonionizing:** Infrared and ultra violet rays are of nonionizing type
   ii. **Ionizing radiation:** These include X-rays, γ (gamma) rays, and cosmic rays
4. **Ultrasonic and sonic vibrations:** Variable exposure to 254-nm wavelength

B. Chemical agents
1. **Surface-active disinfectants:** Quaternary ammonium compounds (quats) and soap
2. **Phenol and phenolics:** Cresol, chlorhexidine, chloroxylenol and hexachlorophene
3. Biguanide (chlorhexidine)
4. Halogens
5. **Alcohols:** Ethyl alcohol (ethanol) and isopropyl alcohol
6. Heavy metal derivatives mercury, silver, arsenic, zinc, and copper
7. **Chemical food preservatives:** Organic acids nitrate/nitrites
8. **Aldehydes:** Formaldehyde, glutaraldehyde, orthophthaldehyde
9. **Chemical sterilization:**
   ➢ Ethylene oxide and other gaseous sterilants
   ➢ Plasma sterilization
   ➢ Supercritical fluids
10. Peroxygens and other forms of oxygen—hydrogen peroxide, peracetic acid (peroxyacetic acid, or PAA), ozone (O_3)

iii. **Incineration:** By this method, infective material is reduced to ashes, such as pathological waste materials, surgical dressings, contaminated material, animal carcasses and other clinical waste are safely destroyed by incineration.

iv. **Hot air oven:** Hot air sterilizer is the most widely used method of sterilization by dry heat. It is used to process materials which can withstand high temperatures for length of time needed for sterilization by dry heat, but which are likely to be affected by contact with steam. Hot air oven is electrically heated, with heating. It should be fitted with a fan to provide forced air circulation throughout the oven chamber, a temperature indicator, a control thermostat and timer, open mesh shelving and adequate wall insulation.

Preparation of Load
1. **No overloading:** It must **not be overloaded** and the individual articles or packs of the load are positioned to allow free circulation of hot air between and around the item.
2. **Articles:** Should be thoroughly **clean and dry.**
3. **Glassware:** Should be perfectly **dry before being placed in the oven.**
4. **Test tubes and flasks:** Should be **wrapped in paper.**
5. **Rubber materials,** except silicon rubber, will not withstand the sterilizing temperature.

6. **Cotton plugs:** May get charred at 180°C.
7. **Heat-sensitive materials:** Dry heat sterilization is slow and not suitable for heat-sensitive materials like many plastic and rubber items.

Sterilizing Cycle
The sterilization hold time—is set to **160°C for 2 hours or 170°C for 1 hour, or 180°C for 30 minutes**.

Uses of Hot Air Oven
It is a method of choice for sterilization of:
1. **Glassware**—such as tubes, flasks, measuring cylinders, all-glass syringes, glass petri dishes and glass pipettes.
2. **Metal instruments**—such as forceps, scissors, and scalpels.
3. **Nonaqueous materials and powders, oils and greases** in sealed containers and swab sticks packed in test tubes.

Sterilization Controls
A. **Biological control:** An envelope containing a filter paper strip impregnated with spores of *Bacillus subtilis* subsp. *niger* is inserted into suitable packs. No growth of *Bacillus subtilis* subsp *niger* indicates proper sterilization.
B. **Chemical indicator:** A chemical indicator, such as **Browne's tubes No. 3** containing red solution is inserted in each load and a color change from red to green is observed which indicates proper sterilization.
C. **Thermocouples**: Thermocouples may also be used periodically.

Moist Heat (Box 66.1)
Moist heat is divided into three forms:
A. At temperature below 100°C
B. At a temperature of 100°C
C. At temperature above 100°C

A. At a Temperature Below 100°C
Pasteurization of milk: Disinfection by moist heat at temperature below 100°C is termed **pasteurization.** Milk can be pasteurized in two ways. The temperature is employed either **63°C for 30 minutes** (holder **method**) or **72°C for 15–20 seconds** (the **flash method**) followed by **rapid cooling to 13°C or lower.**

i. **Vaccine preparation**
ii. **Inspissation:** Media, such as Lowenstein-Jensen and Loeffler's serum are rendered sterile by heating at 80–85°C for half an hour on three successive days (**fractional sterilization**). This process is called **inspissation** and instrument used is called *inspissator.*
iii. **Water bath**

B. Temperature at 100°C
a. **Boiling:** Boiling at 100°C for 10–30 minutes kills all vegetative spores and some bacterial spores. Sporing bacteria require prolonged periods of boiling. Therefore, it is not recommended for sterilization of instruments for surgical procedures.
b. **Steam at atmospheric pressure at 100°C for 90 minutes**
This can be provided by the traditional Koch and Arnold steamer (or by the multipurpose autoclave).
c. **Tyndallization:** An exposure of steam at 100°C for **20** minutes on three successive days is called **tyndallization or intermittent sterilization.** This is a fractional method of sterilization. The instrument commonly used is Koch and Arnold steamer.

Principle: Vegetative cells and some spores are killed during the first heating and that the more resistant spores subsequently germinate and are killed during either the second or the third heating. Though generally adequate, this method may fail with spores of certain anaerobes and thermophiles.

Uses: This method is useful in sterilizing heat-sensitive culture media containing, such materials as carbohydrates, egg or serum, which are damaged by higher temperature of autoclave.

C. Moist Heat at Temperature Above 100°C
Steam under pressure: Steam above 100°C or saturated steam is more efficient sterilizing agent than hot air.

Autoclave

Autoclaving is the process of sterilization by saturated steam under high pressure above 100°C. Steam sterilization is carried out in a pressure chamber called an **autoclave** (a device somewhat like a fancy pressure cooker).

Principle of Autoclave

The principle of the autoclave or steam sterilizer is that water boils when its vapor pressure equals that of the surrounding atmosphere. When pressure inside a closed vessel increases, the temperature at which water boils also increases. Saturated steam has penetrative power and is a better sterilizing agent than dry heat.

Various Components of Autoclave

In its simplest form, the laboratory autoclave consists of a **vertical or horizontal cylinder of gunmetal or stainless steel**, in a supporting sheet iron case. **The lid or door** is fastened by screw clamps and made airtight by a suitable washer. The autoclave has on its lid or upper side a discharge tap for air and steam, a pressure gauge and a safety valve that can be set to blow off at any desired pressure. Heating is done by gas or electricity. The domestic pressure cooker serves as a miniature autoclave and may be used for sterilizing small articles in clinics and similar establishments.

Types of steam sterilizers: Several types of steam sterilizers are available. Even the domestic pressure cooker can be used as a sterilizer.

Procedure

1. **Water:** Sufficient water is put in the cylinder.
2. **Lid:** The lid is screwed tight with the discharge tap open and the safety valve is adjusted to the required pressure.
3. **Air removal:** The steam-air mixture is allowed to escape freely till all the air has been displaced.
4. The discharge tap is now closed.
5. **Holding period:** The steam pressure rises inside and when it reaches the desired set level (15 psi), the safety valve opens and the excess steam escapes. From this point, the holding period (15 minutes) is calculated.
6. **Autoclave cooling:** When the holding period is over, the heater is turned off and the autoclave allowed to cool.
7. **Air entry in the autoclave:** The discharge tap is opened slowly and air is allowed to enter the autoclave.
8. **Removal of articles:** The lid is now opened and the sterilized articles removed.

Note: Temperature: 121°C.

Chamber pressure: 15 psi (per square inch)—these conditions are generally used. However, sterilization can also be done at higher temperatures, at 126°C (20 lbs/square inch) for 10 minutes or at 133°C (30 lbs/square inch) for 3 minutes.

Uses

i. For sterilizing culture media and other laboratory supplies, aqueous solutions, rubber material, dressing materials, gowns, dressing, linen, gloves, instruments and pharmaceutical products.
ii. For all materials that are water containing, permeable or wettable and not liable to be damaged by the process.
iii. Particularly useful for materials which cannot withstand the higher temperature of hot air oven.

Sterilization Controls

A. **Biological control (bacterial spores):** An envelope containing a filter paper strip impregnated with 10^6 spores of *Bacillus stearothermophilus* is placed with the load in the coolest and least accessible part of the autoclave chamber. No growth of *B. stearothermophilus* after sterilization is over and indicates proper sterilization.
B. **Chemical control:** A Browne's tube containing red solution changes to green when exposed to temperature of 121°C for 15 minutes in autoclave. It indicates proper sterilization.
C. **Autoclave tapes**
D. **Thermocouples:** May also be used which records the temperature by a potentiometer.

Filtration

Filtration is the principal method used in the laboratory for the sterilization of heat labile materials, e.g., sera, solutions of sugars or antibiotics used for preparation of culture media.

Uses of Filtration
1. **Heat sensitive solutions:** For sterilization of pharmaceuticals, ophthalmic solutions, culture media, oils, antibiotics, and other heat sensitive solutions.
2. **For separation of bacteriophages and bacterial toxins from bacteria.**
3. **Isolation of organisms which are scanty in fluids.**
4. **Concentration of bacteria from liquids.**
5. **For virus isolation.**

Types of Filters
  i. **Earthware filters:** These are manufactured in several different grades of porosity. The fluid to be sterilized is forced by suction or pressure from inside to outside or vice versa.
  ii. **Asbestos filters (Seitz filter):** They are made up of a disk of asbestos (magnesium trisilicate). It is supported on a perforated metal disk within a metal funnel. Filter disk is discarded after use.
  iii. **Sintered Glass filters:** They are prepared by size grading powdered glass followed by heating. The pore size can be controlled by the general particle size of the glass powder.
  iv. **Membrane filters:** Membrane filters consist of a variety of polymeric materials such as cellulose nitrate, cellulose diacetate, polycarbonate, and polyester. They are manufactured as disks from 13 to 293 mm diameter and with porosities from 0.015 to 12 mm.
  v. **Syringe filters**
  vi. **Vacuum and "in-line" filters**
  vii. **Pressure filtration**
  viii. **Air filters**

Radiation

Two types of radiations are used:
  i. Nonionizing
  ii. Ionizing

i. Nonionizing
Infrared and ultra violet rays are of nonionizing type. The effectiveness of UV light as a lethal and mutagenic agent is closely correlated with its wavelength. It is most effectively absorbed by DNA and this infers with DNA replication. Ultraviolet radiation can be produced artificially by mercury vapor lamps.

Practical Applications
1. **To disinfect drinking water.**
2. **Disinfection of enclosed areas**—such as entryways, hospital wards, operating theaters, laboratories and in ventilated safety cabinets in which dangerous microorganisms are being handled.

ii. Ionizing Radiation
These include X-rays, γ (gamma) rays, and cosmic rays. These have very high penetrative power and are highly lethal to all cells including bacteria. Ionizing radiations damage the DNA by various mechanisms.

Applications
  i. **For sterilization in pharmacy and medicine.**
  ii. **Sterilization of packaged disposable articles**—such as plastic syringes, intravenous lines, catheters and gloves that are unable to withstand heat.
  Cold sterilization: Since there is no appreciable increase in temperature in this method it is known as **cold sterilization.**
  iii. **Use for antibiotics, hormones, sutures, and vaccines** and to prevent food spoilage.

Disinfection

Disinfection is used to destroy microorganisms. However, it does not destroy spores. The solutions used are called **disinfectants**, or possibly bactericidal solutions (the suffix "-cidal" is derived from a Latin word meaning "to kill"). These solutions are too strong for human skin to tolerate and are used only on inanimate objects. If a disinfectant solution comes in contact with human tissue, the tissue will feel "slippery." This is the first step of tissue breakdown. When using a disinfectant solution, use clean gloves to protect your skin (Skill 12-10).

B. Chemical Agents

Germicidal chemicals can be used to disinfect and, in some cases, sterilize **(Table 66.1)**.

Mechanisms of Action

The main modes of action are:
A. **Agents that damage the cell membrane**
 1. Surface active disinfectants
 2. Phenolic compounds
 3. Alcohols
B. **Agents that denature proteins**
 1. Acids and alkalies
 2. Alcohols
C. **Agents that modify functional groups of proteins and nucleic acids**.
 1. Heavy metals and their compounds
 2. Oxidizing agents
    – Halogens
    – Hydrogen peroxide
 3. Dyes
    – Aniline dyes
    – Acridine dyes

Table 66.1: Chemical agents used in sterilization and disinfection.

Chemical agent	Use
Surface-Active Agents	
1. Soaps and acid anionic detergents	Skin degerming and removal of debris
2. Acid-anionic detergents	Sanitizers in dairy and food-processing industries
3. Cationic detergents (quaternary ammonium compounds)	Antiseptic for skin, instruments, utensils, and rubber goods
Phenol and Phenolics	
1. Phenol	Rarely used
2. Phenolics	Environmental surfaces, instruments, skin surfaces, and mucous membranes
3. Bisphenols	Disinfectant hand soaps and skin lotions
Alcohols	• Skin antiseptics • Thermometers and other instruments
Organic acids	Sorbic acid and benzoic acid effective at low pH; parabens much used in cosmetics, shampoos; calcium propionate used in bread
Heavy metals and their compounds	Silver nitrate may be used to prevent gonorrheal ophthalmia neonatorum; mercurochrome disinfects skin and mucous membranes; copper sulfate is an algicide
Halogens	• Iodine is an effective antiseptic available as a tincture and an iodophor; • Chlorine gas is used to disinfect water • Chlorine compounds are used to disinfect dairy equipment, eating utensils, household items, and glassware
Peroxygens (oxidizing agents)	Contaminated surfaces; some deep wounds, in which they are very effective against oxygen-sensitive anaerobes
Aldehydes	Glutaraldehyde (Cidex) is less irritating than formaldehyde and is used for disinfection of medical equipment.
Gaseous sterilants	Excellent sterilizing agent, especially for objects that would be damaged by heat

4. Alkylating agents
   - Aldehydes: Formaldehyde, glutaraldehyde
   - Ethylene oxide

A. Agents that Damage the Cell Membrane

1. Surface-active agents

Substances that alter the energy relationships at interfaces, producing a reduction of surface or interfacial tension, are referred to as **surface-active agents or surfactants**.

Classification: These surfactants are classified into cationic, anionic, nonionic and ampholytic (amphoteric). Of these, the cationic and anionic compounds have been the most useful antibacterial agents.

   a. **Cationic agents: Quaternary ammonium compounds (quats)** include cetrimide (cetavalon), benzalkonium chloride (Zephiran, a brand name) and cetylpyridinium chloride (Cepacol, a brand name).
   b. **Anionic agents:** These include soap and fatty acids.
   c. **Ampholytic (amphoteric) compounds** known as "**Tego**" compounds.

2. Phenols and phenolics

Phenol derivatives: Certain phenol derivatives, such as **cresol, chlorhexidine, chloroxylenol** and **hexachlorophane** are commonly used as antiseptics.
   i. **Cresols:** Cresols is sold under the trade names of *Lysol* and *Creolin*. "**White fluids**" such as Lysol are most commonly used for sterilization of infected glass wares, cleaning floors, disinfection of excreta.
   ii. **Chlorhexidine: Savlon (chlorhexidine and cetrimide)** is widely used in wounds, preoperative disinfection of skin, as bladder irrigant, etc. However, contact with the eyes can cause damage.
   iii. **Chloroxylenol:** It is an active ingredient of Dettol.
   iv. **Hexachlorophene:** Used for surgical and hospital microbial control procedures.

B. Agents that Denature Proteins

Alcohols

Ethyl alcohol (ethanol) and **isopropyl alcohol** are the most frequently used. They must be used at a concentration of 60–70% in water to be effective. They are most frequently used as skin disinfectants and act by **denaturing bacterial proteins**.

C. Agents that Modify Functional Groups of Proteins and Nucleic Acids

1. Heavy metals

For many years the ions of heavy metals, such as **mercury, silver, arsenic, zinc and copper** were used as germicides.

2. Oxidizing agents

The most useful antimicrobial agents in this group are the **halogens** and **hydrogen peroxide**.
   i. **Halogens: Chlorine** and **iodine** are among our most useful disinfectants.
      a. **Iodine**: Iodine compounds are the most effective halogens available for disinfection.
         Uses
         i. **Skin disinfectant**
         ii. **Iodophors** Povidone-iodine (**betadine**) for wounds and *Wescodyne* for skin and laboratory disinfection are some popular brands.
      b. **Chlorine:** In addition to **chlorine** itself, there are three types of chlorine compound **hypochlorites** and **inorganic, and organic chloramines**. The disinfectant action of all chlorine compounds is due to the liberation of free chlorine.
         Uses: The usual disinfectant for water supplies, swimming pools, dairy and food industries.
      c. **Hypochlorites: Bleaching powder or hypochlorite solution** is the most widely used for human immunodeficiency virus (HIV) infected material.
         Chloramines are used as antiseptics for dressing wounds.

ii. **Hydrogen peroxide:** It is used to disinfect plastic implants, contact lenses, and surgical prostheses.

3. Dyes
Aniline dyes and **acridine dyes** are two groups of dyes which are used extensively as skin and wound antiseptic. Both are **bacteriostatic in high dilution** but are of low bactericidal activity.
i. Aniline dyes—**brilliant green, malachite green and crystal violet.**
ii. Acridine dyes—are **proflavine, acriflavine, euflavine and aminacrine.**

4. Alkylating agents
The lethal effects of aldehydes (formaldehyde and glutaraldehyde) and ethylene dioxide result from their alkylating action on proteins.

Aldehydes
i. **Formaldehyde:** Formaldehyde is employed in the liquid and vapor states. Exposure of skin or mucus membranes to formaldehyde can be toxic and the gas is irritant and toxic when inhaled.

Uses
a. **Formalin:**
   i. Used for preserving fresh tissues.
   ii. Formalin has been used to inactivate viruses in the **preparation of vaccines**.
b. **Formaldehyde:**
   i. It is used to preserve anatomical specimens
   ii. For destroying anthrax spores in hair
   iii. As an antiseptic mouthwash
   iv. For the disinfection of membranes in dialysis equipment
   v. A preservative in hair shampoos
c. **Formaldehyde gas:**
   i. Used for sterilizing instruments, heat sensitive catheters and for fumigating wards, sick rooms and laboratories.
   ii. Clothing, bedding, furniture and books can be satisfactorily disinfected under properly controlled conditions.
ii. **Glutaraldehyde:** This has an action similar to formaldehyde. It is used as 2% buffered solution. It can be used for delicate instruments having lenses. It is available commercially as "cidex".

Uses
a. **Cold sterilant:** It has been used increasingly as a **cold sterilant** for **surgical instruments,** such as **cystoscopes, endoscopes, and bronchoscope.**
b. Used safely to sterilize corrugated rubber anesthetic tubes and face masks, plastic endotracheal tubes, metal instruments, and polythene tubing.

Vapor-phase Disinfectants
Ethylene Oxide
It is highly inflammable and, in concentrations in air >3%, highly explosive.

Uses
a. **Sterilization of articles liable to be damaged by heat:** It is especially used for sterilizing heart-lung machines, respirators, sutures, dental equipment, books, and clothing.
b. **Sterilization of a wide range of materials—** such as glass, metal and paper surfaces, clothing, plastics, soil, some foods, and tobacco.

Formaldehyde Gas
It is used for fumigation of complex heat-sensitive equipment, including anesthetic machine and baby incubators and for periodic decontamination of laboratory safety cabinets.

Beta-propiolactone (BPL)
This destroys microorganisms more readily than ethylene oxide but does not penetrate materials well and may be carcinogenic.

Use: In the liquid form it has been used to sterilize vaccines and sera.

Categories of disinfectant (Box 66.2)

Disinfection Guidelines
1. Surfaces and items to disinfect floors, door knobs, window handles, buttons, switches, furniture surfaces, telephones, intercoms, trash cans, sinks, toilets, bath tubs, faucets, shower heads, floor drains, ventilators, computers, keyboards, fans, etc.

> **Box 66.2:** Categories of disinfectant.

1. **High-level disinfection:** A germicide that kills all microbial pathogens except large numbers of bacterial spores. High-level disinfection can generally approach sterilization in effectiveness, whereas spore forms can survive intermediate-level disinfection, and many microbes can remain viable when exposed to low-level disinfection. High-level disinfectants are used for items involved with invasive procedures that cannot withstand sterilization procedures (e.g., certain types of endoscopes, surgical instruments with plastic or other components that cannot be autoclaved).
   Examples:
   - Treatment with moist heat
   - Use of liquids, such as glutaraldehyde, hydrogen peroxide, peracetic acid, chlorine dioxide, and other chlorine compounds.
2. **Intermediate-level disinfectants:** A germicide that kills all microbial pathogens except bacterial endospores. Intermediate-level disinfectants are used to clean surfaces or instruments in which contamination with bacterial spores and other highly resilient organisms is unlikely. These include flexible fiberoptic endoscopes, laryngoscopes, vaginal specula, anesthesia breathing circuits, and other items. These have been referred to as semicritical instruments and devices.
   Examples: Alcohols, iodophor compounds, phenolic compounds
3. **Low-level disinfectants:** A germicide that kills most vegetative bacteria and lipid-enveloped and medium-size viruses. Low-level disinfectants are used to treat noncritical instruments and devices, such as blood pressure cuffs, electrocardiogram electrodes, and stethoscopes. They do not penetrate through mucosal surfaces or into sterile tissues although, these items come into contact with patients.
   Example: Quaternary ammonium compounds.

2. **Tools and equipment:** Alcohol or bleach (0.05% sodium hypochlorite), towels, rubber gloves and masks.
3. **Disinfection procedures:**
   a. Start with wiping clean the less soiled surfaces.
   b. Towels should be soaked in bleach before use.
   c. Rinse articles and surfaces with water and wipe dry 10 minutes after disinfection.
   d. Diluted bleach can be used to disinfect toilets.
   e. Do not flush large amounts or highly concentrated bleach down the toilet to keep sewage treatment plant running smoothly. Wear a mask and rubber gloves while using bleach.

Chemical Sterilization

Sterilization with liquid chemicals is possible, but even sporicidal chemicals, such as glutaraldehyde are usually not considered to be practical sterilants. However, the gaseous chemosterilants are frequently used as substitutes for physical sterilization processes. Their application requires a closed chamber similar to a steam autoclave. Probably the most familiar example is *ethylene oxide*:

1. ***Ethylene oxide:*** Ethylene oxide kills all microbes and endospores but requires a lengthy exposure period of several hours. It is toxic and explosive in its pure form, so it is usually mixed with a nonflammable gas, such as carbon dioxide. Larger hospitals often are able to sterilize even mattresses in special ethylene oxide sterilizers.
2. ***Chlorine dioxide*** is a short-lived gas has been used to fumigate enclosed building areas contaminated with endospores of anthrax.
3. ***Plasmas:*** Plasma is a state of matter in which a gas is excited, in this case by an electromagnetic field, to make a mixture of nuclei with assorted electrical charges and free electrons. *Plasma sterilization* is a reliable method to sterilizing metal or plastic surgical instruments used for many newer procedures in arthroscopic or laparoscopic surgery.

Table 66.2: List of the recommended concentrations of disinfectants commonly used in the hospitals.

Disinfectant	Concentration
Betadine (iodophor)	2%
Bleaching powder (calcium hypochlorite)	14 g in 1 L of water
Dettol (chloroxylenol)	4%
Ethyl alcohol	70%
Glutaraldehyde	2%
Lysol	2.5%
Savlon (chlorhexidine and cetrimide)	2%, 5%
Sodium hypochlorite	1%, 0.1%

4. **Peroxygens and other forms of oxygen:** Peroxygens are a group of oxidizing agents that includes hydrogen peroxide and peracetic acid.
   i. **Hydrogen peroxide**—is an antiseptic found in many household medicine cabinets and in hospital supply rooms. The food industry is increasing its use of hydrogen peroxide for aseptic packaging. Hydrogen peroxide is used to disinfect plastic implants, contact lenses and surgical prosthesis.
   ii. **Peracetic acid (peroxyacetic acid or PAA):** It is one of the most effective liquid chemical sporicides available and can be used as a sterilant. Its mode of action is similar to that of hydrogen peroxide.

Applications: Disinfection of food-processing and medical equipment, especially endoscopes.

List of the recommended concetrations of disinfectants commonly used in the hospitals (**Table 66.2**).

CLEANING

Cleaning is the removal of foreign materials, such as soil and organic material, from objects. Generally, cleaning involves use of water and mechanical action with or without detergents. When an object comes in contact with infectious or potentially infectious material, the object is contaminated. If the object is disposable, it is usually discarded unless formal policies and procedures are in place for reprocessing the object. It is necessary to thoroughly clean reusable objects and then either disinfect or sterilize them before reuse.

Environmental Cleaning

The term "environmental cleaning" refers broadly to the organized processes employed by hospitals for cleaning, disinfecting, and monitoring. Environmental cleaning (EC) is a fundamental principle of preventing infection in the hospital setting. Both porous surfaces (e.g., mattresses) and nonporous surfaces (e.g., bed rails) in patient rooms are highly susceptible to bacterial contamination with dangerous pathogens, including *Clostridium difficile*, and antibiotic-resistant organisms, such as methicillin-resistant *Staphylococcus aureus* (MRSA), vancomycin-resistant *enterococci* (VRE), and multiple species of *Acinetobacter* (*Acinetobacter* spp). Hard, nonporous surfaces, which include common items, such as furniture, bed rails, and medical equipment, as well as fixed spaces such as floors and bathroom facilities, form part of the environmental reservoir that can lead to significant microbial contamination. Appropriate cleaning of these surfaces is an important part of an overall strategy to reduce the risk of health-care-associated infections (HAIs).

A wide variety of cleaning agents and disinfection technologies are commercially available, each with potential benefits and disadvantages. Additionally, hospitals often monitor the quality of room cleaning and disinfection to ensure that surfaces have been treated appropriately. Several monitoring strategies exist, which range from simple visual inspection, to microbiologic testing of surface contamination, to technologic innovations that measure the adequacy of surface cleaning. As the variety of options for cleaning, disinfecting, and monitoring grow, hospitals are faced with many choices, but limited evidence exists on the comparative effectiveness of these interventions, especially related to HAI rates within the hospital.

Equipment Cleaning

When cleaning equipment that is soiled by organic material, such as blood, fecal matter, mucus, or pus, put on a mask and protective eyewear or goggles (or a face shield) and waterproof gloves. These barriers provide protection from infectious organisms (as discussed earlier). You will need a stiff bristled brush and detergent or soap for cleaning. The following steps ensure that an object is clean:

1. Rinse a contaminated object or article with cold running water to remove organic material. Hot water causes the protein in organic material to coagulate and stick to objects, making removal difficult.
2. After rinsing, wash the object with soap and warm water. Soap or detergent reduces the surface tension of water and emulsifies dirt and remaining material. Rinse the object thoroughly to remove the emulsified dirt.
3. Use a brush to remove dirt or material in grooves or seams. Friction dislodges contaminated material for easy removal. Open any hinged items for cleaning.
4. Rinse the object in warm water.
5. Dry the object and prepare it for disinfection or sterilization if indicated by the intended use of the item.
6. Consider the brush, the gloves, and the sink in which the equipment is cleaned contaminated and make sure it is cleaned and dried per hospital protocol.

ASEPSIS

Asepsis is absence of pathogenic microorganisms. It is divided into two categories—medical and surgical:

1. **Medical asepsis (clean technique):** It consists of techniques that inhibit the growth and spread of pathogenic microorganisms. Medical asepsis is also known as **clean technique** and is used in many daily activities. They include hand washing, bathing, cleaning environment, gloving, gowning, wearing masks, hair and shoe covers, disinfecting articles and use of antiseptics changing patients' bed linen. You follow principles of medical asepsis in the home, for instance, with the common practice of washing your hands before preparing food.
2. **Surgical asepsis (sterile technique):** It destroys all microorganisms and their **spores** (the reproductive cell of some microorganisms, such as fungi or protozoa). Surgical asepsis is known as **sterile technique** and is used in specialized areas or skills, such as care of surgical wounds, urinary catheter insertion, invasive procedures, and surgery.

SPAULDING'S CLASSIFICATION

Spaulding's classification was proposed by Earle H. Spaulding in 1939, and it is the guideline that should determine the disinfection or sterilization method that should be chosen according to the medical instrument (**Table 66.3**).

Critical items: Instruments that touch places where no single microorganism should exist are critical items, e.g., a surgical instrument. These must be sterilized unconditionally.

Semicritical items: Instruments that contact incised skin or mucous membranes are semicritical items, e.g., endoscopes and anesthesia equipment. These should undergo high-level disinfection.

Noncritical items: Instruments that touch intact skin are noncritical items, e.g., fomites. These require low-level disinfection.

KEY POINTS

- Sterilization is the process by which an article, surface, or medium is freed of all living microorganisms either in the vegetative or spore state
- Disinfection is the killing, inhibition, or removal of microorganisms that may cause disease.
- Cleaning is the removal of foreign materials, such as soil and organic material, from objects.
- The term "environmental cleaning" refers broadly to the organized processes employed by hospitals for cleaning, disinfecting, and monitoring.

Table 66.3: Spaulding's classification of medical equipment/devices and required level of processing/reprocessing.

Classification	Definition	Level of processing/reprocessing	Examples
Critical Equipment/device	Equipment/device that enters sterile tissues, including the vascular system	Cleaning followed by sterilization	• Surgical instruments • Implants • Biopsy instruments • Foot care equipment • Eye and dental equipment
Semicritical Equipment/device	Equipment/device that comes in contact with non-intact skin or mucous membranes but does not penetrate them	• Cleaning followed by high-level • Disinfection (as a minimum) • Sterilization is preferred	• Respiratory therapy equipment • Anesthesia equipment • Tonometer
Noncritical Equipment/device	Equipment/device that touches only intact skin and not mucous membranes, or does not directly touch the client/patient/resident	• Cleaning followed by low-level • Disinfection (in some cases, cleaning alone is acceptable)	• ECG machines • Oximeters • Bedpans, urinals, commodes

- Methods of sterilization and disinfection:
  - Physical agents: Heat (dry heat, moist heat); filtration, radiation, ultrasonic and sonic vibrations.
  - Chemical agents
- When cleaning equipment that is soiled by organic material, such as blood, fecal matter, mucus, or pus, put on a mask and protective eyewear or goggles (or a face shield) and waterproof gloves.

Chemical agents that damage the cell membrane:
1. **Surface-active agents**
   a. Cationic agents
   b. Anionic agents
   c. Ampholytic (amphoteric) agents: Phenol derivatives: Certain phenol derivatives such as **cresol, chlorhexidine, chloroxylenol** and **hexachlorophene** are commonly used as antiseptics.
2. **Alcohols:** Ethyl alcohol (ethanol) and isopropyl alcohol are the most frequently used.
3. **Heavy metals:** Mercuric chloride, silver nitrate
4. **Oxidizing agents:**
   i. **Halogens**
      a. **Iodine**
      b. **Chlorine**
      c. **Hypochlorites**
   ii. **Hydrogen peroxide**
5. **Dyes:** Aniline dyes and acridine dyes are two groups of dyes which are used extensively as skin and wound antiseptic

6. **Alkylating agents:** The lethal effects of aldehydes (formaldehyde and glutaraldehyde) and ethylene dioxide result from their alkylating action on proteins.
7. **Vapor-phase disinfectants:**
   a. Ethylene oxide
   b. Formaldehyde gas
   c. Beta-propiolactone (BPL)

IMPORTANT QUESTIONS

1. Define sterilization and disinfection. Classify the various agents used in sterilization.
2. Define the terms sterilization, disinfection and cleaning. Name various agents used for sterilization and disinfection.
3. Define sterilization. Classify the methods of sterilization.
4. Write short notes on:
   a. Spaulding's classification
   b. Environment cleaning
   c. Equipment cleaning
5. Name various types of disinfectants and discuss the role of halogens in chemical disinfection.
6. Give an account of testing antimicrobial potency of disinfectants and antiseptics.
7. Write short notes on:
   a. Phenols as disinfectants
   b. Halogens as disinfectants

c. Aldehydes as disinfectants
d. Alcohols as disinfectants
e. Vapour-phase disinfectants or gaseous sterilization
f. Surface active disinfectants
g. Quaternary ammonium compounds
h. Oxidizing agents

MULTIPLE CHOICE QUESTIONS

1. The holder method of pasteurization is not effective against:
   a. *Escherichia coli*
   b. *Coxiella burnetii*
   c. *Staphylococcus aureus*
   d. *Salmonella typhi*
2. The bacterial spore that is most frequently used as indicator of sterilization by hot-air oven is:
   a. *Bacillus subtilis*
   b. *Clostridium tetani*
   c. *Bacillus pumilus*
   d. *Bacillus globigii*
3. Which of the following does not kill endospores?
   a. Autoclaving
   b. Hot air sterilization
   c. Pasteurization
   d. None of the above
4. Sterilization at 100°C for 20 minutes on three successive days is known as:
   a. Tyndallization
   b. Inspissation
   c. Pasteurization
   d. Vaccine bath
5. Which bacterial spores are used as sterilization control in autoclave?
   a. *Bacillus cereus*
   b. *Bacillus stearothermophilus*
   c. *Clostridium perfringens*
   d. *Pseudomonas aeruginosa*
6. Autoclave is not useful for sterilization of:
   a. Disposable plastic petri dishes
   b. Surgical dressings
   c. Metallic instruments
   d. Liquid paraffin
7. Which of the following is most effective for sterilizing mattresses and petri dishes?
   a. Chlorine
   b. Autoclaving
   c. Ethylene oxide
   d. Glutaraldehyde
8. Which one of these disinfectants does not act by disrupting the plasma membrane?
   a. Phenolics
   b. Ethylene oxide
   c. Halogens
   d. Phenol
9. Ionizing radiation can be used for sterilization of:
   a. Plastic syringes
   b. Gloves
   c. Catheters
   d. All of the above
10. The most widely used disinfectant for human immunodeficiency virus (HIV) infected material is:
    a. Phenol
    b. Lysol
    c. Hypochlorite solution
    d. Silver nitrate
11. Glutaraldehyde is used as a cold sterilant for sterilization of:
    a. Cystoscopes
    b. Endoscopes
    c. Bronchoscope
    d. All of the above
12. All the following statements are true for ethylene oxide, *except*:
    a. It diffuses through many types of porous materials.
    b. It is used for sterilizing heart-lung machines, respirators, books, and clothing.
    c. It is used for sterilizing glass, metal and paper surfaces, clothing, plastics, and some foods.
    d. It is suitable for fumigating rooms.
13. Which test is used to simulate the natural conditions under which the disinfectants are used in the hospitals?
    a. Kelsey–Sykes capacity test
    b. Rideal–Walker test
    c. In-use test
    d. Chick–Martin test

ANSWERS

1. b   2. a   3. c   4. a
5. b   6. d   7. c   8. c
9. d   10. c   11. d   12. d
13. a

CHAPTER 67

Specimen Collection (Review)

LEARNING OBJECTIVES

After reading and studying this chapter, you should be able to:
- Discuss the appropriate method of collection of samples in the performance of laboratory tests in the detection of microbial agents causing infectious diseases.
- Demonstrate the appropriate method of collection of samples in the performance of laboratory tests in the detection of microbial agents causing infectious diseases.
- Demonstrate respect for patient samples sent to the laboratory for performance of laboratory tests in the detection of microbial agents causing infectious diseases.
- Discuss confidentiality pertaining to patient identity in laboratory.
- Choose the appropriate laboratory test in the diagnosis of the infectious disease.
- Demonstrate confidentiality pertaining to patient identity in laboratory results.
- Choose and interpret the results of the laboratory tests used in diagnosis of the infectious diseases.

INTRODUCTION

Diagnostic medical microbiology is concerned with the etiologic diagnosis of infection.

SPECIMENS

In clinical microbiology, a clinical specimen (hereafter, specimen) represents a portion or quantity of human material that is tested, examined, or studied to determine the presence or absence of particular microorganisms. Samples for microbiological examination need to be carefully collected. It is essential to use sterile containers which are leak-proof and able to withstand transportation through the post if necessary. It is essential to use sterile containers. Safety for the patients, hospital, and laboratory staff is very important. Special precautions required for "high-risk" specimens need to be defined by the laboratory and hospital management.

UNIVERSAL PRECAUTIONS

Concerns about transmission of the hepatitis B virus (HBV) and human immunodeficiency virus (HIV) led to the introduction of "universal precautions", to minimize the infections in medical laboratory workers and health care personnel. These universal precautions include:

1. Assume that all specimens/patients are potentially infectious for HIV and other blood borne pathogens.
2. All blood specimens or body fluids should be placed in a leak-proof impervious bags for transportation to the laboratory.
3. Use gloves while handling blood and body fluid specimens and other objects exposed to them. If there is a likelihood of spattering, use face masks with glasses or goggles.
4. Wear laboratory coats or gowns while working in the laboratory. Wrap-around gowns should be preferred. These should not be taken outside.

5. Never pipette by mouth. Mechanical pipetting devices should be used.
6. Decontaminate the laboratory work surfaces with an appropriate disinfectant after the spillage of blood or other body fluids and when the procedures are completed.
7. Limit use of needles and syringes to situations for which there are no other alternatives.
8. Biological safety hoods should be used for laboratory work.
9. All the potentially contaminated materials of the laboratory should be decontaminated before disposal or reprocessing.
10. Always wash hands after completing laboratory work and remove all protective clothings before leaving the laboratory.

COLLECTION OF SPECIMENS

Specimens may be collected by several methods using aseptic technique.

A. Infections of Wounds and Other Tissues

Pus or *exudate* is often submitted on a swab for laboratory investigation. Whenever possible, pus or exudate should be submitted in a small screw-capped bottle, a firmly stoppered tube or syringe, or a sealed capillary tube. Fragments of excised tissue removed at wound toilet, or curettings from infected sinuses and other tissues, should be sent in a sterile container without fixative.

B. Upper Respiratory, Ear and Eye Infections

1. An adequate view of the throat should be ensured by good lighting and the use of a disposable wooden spatula to pull outward and so depress the tongue.
2. **Oral cavity:** The most common method used to collect specimens from the anterior nares or throat is the sterile swab.
   Anterior nares: If pus is present, collect this on swabs. If no pus is present, moisten swabs and then swab the anterior nares.
   Throat: For bacteriological sampling: A plain, albumen-coated or charcoal-coated cotton-wool swab should be used to collect as much exudate as possible from the tonsils, posterior pharyngeal wall and any other area that is inflamed or bears exudate. The swab should be replaced in its tube with care not to soil the rim. If it cannot be delivered to the laboratory within about 1 hour, it should be placed in a refrigerator at 4°C until delivery or, preferably, it should be submitted in a tube of transport medium for bacteriological specimens.
3. **Nasopharyngeal swabs: Pernasal swab**—collection of nasopharyngeal secretion by a *pernasal* swab in charcoal transport medium for the diagnosis of whooping cough.
   Postnasal swab: A postnasal swab, may be used for the detection of potential pathogens carried in the nasopharynx of healthy persons, e.g., *Meningococcus*.
4. **The glottis and epiglottis:** Swabs are firmly rubbed over inflamed and ulcerated areas.
5. **Paranasal sinuses:** If pus is present in these sinuses, it is collected on swabs or aspirated with a syringe and needle.

C. From the Gastrointestinal Tract

Feces and rectal swabs are the most readily available specimens.

1. **Feces:** Feces is collected in a container which is a 25 mL screwcapped, wide-mouthed, glass or plastic bottle.
2. **Fresh feces** may be collected by inserting well and twisted around several times a soft rubber catheter into the rectum. Transmit the specimen quickly to the laboratory.
3. **In suspected parasitic infestations:** For examination for parasites, a small sample may be taken from a morning stool microscopic examination for eggs and adult parasites. The sample is placed in a preservative (polyvinyl alcohol, buffered glycerol, saline, or formalin) for microscopic examination for eggs and adult parasites.

D. From the Lower Respiratory Tract

Sputum: Sputum is the most common specimen collected in suspected cases of lower respiratory tract infections. A morning sample is best.

Sputum is collected in specially designed sputum cups.

Stomach aspiration: In cases such as tuberculosis in which there is little sputum, stomach aspiration may be necessary.

E. Urinary Tract Infections

After the patient has cleansed the urethral meatus (opening), a small container is used to collect the urine. Instruct the patient to collect a **midstream sample**. A urine sample may be stored under refrigeration (4–6°C) for up to 24 hours.

F. From the Genital Tract

1. **Genital infections in women**
   High vaginal swab: The specimen generally collected for the diagnosis of vaginitis, vaginosis or uterine sepsis.
2. **In** suspected infections due to *Neisseria gonorrhoeae*
   In women: An *endocervical swab* must be collected for examination for gonococci. **Rectal and pharyngeal swabs** should also be considered. Swabs for culture should be placed in tubes of Amies' transport medium for delivery to the laboratory.
3. **Collection of specimens in men**
   i. **Urethral discharge:** Urethral discharge milked from the urethra may be expressed directly on to slides for examination in Gram-stained films for gonococci. Discharge collected in an inoculating loop should, if possible, be inoculated immediately on to warmed plates of heated-blood agar and selective medium for the culture of gonococci. If specimens have to be transported to the laboratory for the preparation of films and inoculation into culture, as much exudate as possible should be collected on a swab and the swab at once plunged into a tube of Amies' transport medium.
   ii. **Massage of the prostate per rectum:** When **prostatitis** is suspected and there is no spontaneous discharge from the urethra, massage of the prostate *per rectum* may express some exudate for examination.
4. **In suspected infections due to *Treponema pallidum*:** The examination of a chancre requires the careful collection of exudate and its preparation for darkground microscopy. A specimen of clotted venous blood should be collected for serological examination.
5. **In suspected infections due to trichomonas:** For examination for trichomonas, further, special specimens should be collected from the vagina and cervix, including a swab placed in clear trichomonas transport medium for microscopy and possibly culture.

G. From the Central Nervous System

The principal specimen to be examined is of cerebrospinal fluid (CSF) collected by lumbar puncture. Only 3–5 mL of fluid should be collected. The specimen must be dispatched to the laboratory as quickly as possible, for delay may result in the death of delicate pathogens, such as meningococci, and the disintegration of leukocytes. It should not be kept in a refrigerator, which tends to kill *Haemophilus* (*H*). *influenzae*. If delay for a few hours is unavoidable, the specimen is best kept in an incubator at 37°C.

H. From the Bloodstream

With precautions to avoid touching and recontaminating the venepuncture site, take the sample of blood. Inoculate the required volume into each blood culture bottle.

I. From Wound or Abscess

Touch a sterile swab to the pus, replace the swab in its container, and properly label the container. Pus, if present in a large amount, should preferably be collected in a bottle.

J. Fluid from Pleural and Peritoneal Cavities

Specimens have to be collected from these sites as carefully as are CSF and blood specimens.

These sites may be involved in acute (pyogenic) or in chronic (tuberculous) disease processes.

K. Ear Infections

Swabs are taken from the external auditory meatus mainly in three suspected conditions, acute otitis media, chronic suppurative otitis media, and otitis externa.

TRANSPORT OF SPECIMENS

Speed in transporting the specimen to the clinical laboratory after it has been obtained from the patient is of prime importance. Cerebrospinal fluid (CSF) should be examined immediately transported to the laboratory within 15 minutes. Special treatment is required for specimens when the microorganism is thought to be anaerobic. Microbiological specimens may be transported to the laboratory by various means.

HEALTH AND SAFETY PRECAUTIONS

- Observe universal precautions when collecting specimens.
- Follow proper blood collection techniques to minimize the risk of transmitting infectious diseases to clinical staff, and wear gloves when appropriate.
- Dispose of syringes and needles in a puncture-resistant, autoclavable discard container. A new sterile syringe and needle must be used for each patient.
- For transport to a microbiology laboratory, place the specimen in a container that can be securely sealed.
- Remove gloves and discard in an autoclavable container.
- Wash hands with antibacterial soap and water immediately after removing gloves.
- In the event of a needle-stick injury or other skin puncture or wound, wash the wound liberally with soap and water. Encourage bleeding.
- Report a needle-stick injury, any other skin puncture, or any contamination of the hands or body with CSF to the supervisor and appropriate health officials immediately as prophylactic treatment of the personnel performing the procedure may be indicated.

KEY POINT

Collection: Specimens may be collected by several methods using aseptic technique from various infections.

IMPORTANT QUESTIONS

1. How can clinical specimens be taken from a patient with various infectious diseases? Give specific examples of procedures used.
2. Write short notes on:
   a. Universal precautions
   b. Health and safety precautions

MULTIPLE CHOICE QUESTIONS

1. Clinical specimens are collected:
   a. By using sterile containers which are leak-proof
   b. By using aseptic technique
   c. All of the above
   d. None of the above
2. For urinary tract infections:
   a. Collect a midstream sample of urine
   b. No need to cleanse the urethral meatus (opening)
   c. Any container can be used
   d. Never store under refrigeration

ANSWERS

1. c   2. a

Biomedical Waste Management

LEARNING OBJECTIVES

After reading and studying this chapter, you should be able to:
- Define and classify hospital waste.
- Describe various methods of treatment of hospital waste.
- Describe laws related to hospital waste management.
- Describe laundry management process and infection control and prevention.

INTRODUCTION

Hospitals regularly generate waste which may be a potential health hazard to health care workers, the general public and the environment. Therefore, adequate management and disposal of waste is essential.

Agents which are associated with laboratory acquired infections: Most common agents which are associated with laboratory acquired infections include hepatitis B virus, *Coccidioides immitis*, *Bacillus anthracis*, *Brucella* species, *Mycobacterium tuberculosis*, *Francisella tularensis* and *Shigella* species.

DEFINITION OF BIOMEDICAL WASTE

According to Biomedical waste (Management and Handling) Rules, 1998 of India, "Biomedical waste" means any waste, which is generated during the diagnosis, treatment or immunization of human beings or animals or in research activities pertaining thereto or in the production or testing of biologicals.

Between 75 and 90% of the waste produced by the health care providers is **nonrisk or "general"** health care waste, comparable to domestic waste. The remaining 10–25% health care waste is regarded as **hazardous** and may create a variety of health risk.

Infectious wastes include all those medical wastes, which have the potential to transmit viral, bacterial or parasitic diseases. It includes both human and animal infectious waste and waste generated in laboratories, and veterinary practice. Infectious waste is hazardous in nature. Any waste with a potential to pose a threat to human health and life is called **hazardous waste**.

Noninfectious hazardous waste may be chemical (toxic, corrosive, inflammable, reactive and otherwise injurious), radioactive, and pharmacolocal (surplus or time expired drugs).

CATEGORIES OF BIOMEDICAL WASTE

The categories and types of biomedical waste are given in **Box 68.1**.

Box 68.1: Categories of biomedical waste and types of waste.

- **Yellow:** For human anatomical waste, animal anatomical waste, soiled waste, expired or discarded medicines, chemical waste, chemical liquid waste, discarded contaminated beddings and microbiology, biotechnology and other clinical waste
- **Red:** For contaminated plastic waste
- **White (Translucent):** For **waste sharps including metals**
- **Blue:** For **(a) Glassware; (b) Metallic body implants**

WASTE SEGREGATION

The biomedical waste should be segregated into containers/bags at the point of generation of the waste.

Collection bags: The biomedical waste should be segregated into containers/bags at the point of generation of the waste. Solid waste is collected in leak-resistant heavy-duty bags. Colored bags made of nonchlorinated plastic with biohazard sign and labels mentioning date and details of waste are to be used. The bags are tied tightly after they are three-fourths full. Waste should be segregated in bags of different colors to facilitate appropriate treatment and disposal **(Table 68.1)**.

Types of bags or containers used for biomedical waste **(Table 68.1)**.
A. Yellow Bags
B. Red Bags
C. White (Translucent)
D. Blue

Treatment and Disposal Technologies for Healthcare Waste (Table 68.1)

Waste Treatment

Following techniques are in use for treatment of infected material:
1. Incineration
2. Chemical disinfection

TABLE 68.1: Biomedical wastes categories and their segregation, collection, treatment, processing and disposal options.

		Part-I	
Category (1)	Type of waste (2)	Type of bag or container to be used (3)	Treatment and disposal options (4)
Yellow	a. **Human anatomical waste:** Human tissues, organs, body parts and fetus below the viability period (as per the Medical Termination of Pregnancy Act 1971, amended from time to time)	Yellow colored nonchlorinated plastic bags	Incineration or plasma pyrolysis or deep burial*
	b. **Animal anatomical waste:** Experimental animal carcasses, body parts, organs, tissues, including the waste generated from animals used in experiments or testing in veterinary hospitals or colleges or animal houses		
	c. **Soiled waste:** Items contaminated with blood, body fluids, such as dressings, plaster casts, cotton swabs and bags containing residual or discarded blood and blood components		Incineration or plasma pyrolysis or deep burial* In absence of above facilities, autoclaving or microwaving/hydroclaving followed by shredding or mutilation or combination of sterilization and shredding. Treated waste to be sent for energy recovery.

(Contd...)

*Disposal by deep burial is permitted only in rural or remote areas where there is no access to common biomedical waste treatment facility. This will be carried out with prior approval from the prescribed authority and as per the Standards specified in Schedule-III. The deep burial facility shall be located as per the provisions and guidelines issued by Central Pollution Control Board from time to time.

(Contd...)

Category	Type of waste	Type of bag or container to be used	Treatment and disposal options
	d. **Expired or discarded medicines:** Pharmaceutical waste like antibiotics, cytotoxic drugs including all items contaminated with cytotoxic drugs along with glass or plastic ampoules, vials etc.	Yellow colored nonchlorinated plastic bags or containers	Expired cytotoxic drugs and items contaminated with cytotoxic drugs to be returned back to the manufacturer or supplier for incineration at temperature >1,200°C or to common biomedical waste treatment facility or hazardous waste treatment, storage and disposal facility for incineration at >1,200°C or encapsulation or plasma pyrolysis at >1,200°C. All other discarded medicines shall be either sent back to manufacturer or disposed by incineration
	e. **Chemical waste:** Chemicals used in production of biological and used or discarded disinfectants	Yellow colored containers or nonchlorinated plastic bags	Disposed of by incineration or plasma pyrolysis or encapsulation in hazardous waste treatment, storage and disposal facility
	f. **Chemical liquid waste :** Liquid waste generated due to use of chemicals in production of biological and used or discarded disinfectants, silver X-ray film developing liquid, discarded formalin, infected secretions, aspirated body fluids, liquid from laboratories and floor washings, cleaning, house-keeping and disinfecting activities, etc.	Separate collection system leading to effluent treatment system	After resource recovery, the chemical liquid waste shall be pretreated before mixing with other wastewater. The combined discharge shall conform to the discharge norms given in Schedule-III.
	g. Discarded linen, mattresses, beddings contaminated with blood or bodyfluid	Nonchlorinated yellow plastic bags or suitable packing material	Nonchlorinated chemical disinfection followed by incineration or plasma Pyrolysis or for energy recovery
	h. **Microbiology, biotechnology and other clinical laboratory waste:** Blood bags, laboratory cultures, stocks or specimens of microorganisms, live or attenuated vaccines, human and animal cell cultures used in research, industrial laboratories, production of biological, residual toxins, dishes and devices used for cultures	Autoclave safe plastic bags or containers	In absence of above facilities, shredding or mutilation or combination of sterilization and shredding. Treated waste to be sent for energy recovery or incineration or plasma pyrolysis Pretreat to sterilize with nonchlorinated chemicals on-site as per National AIDS Control Organization or World Health Organization guidelines thereafter for incineration

(Contd...)

(Contd...)

Category	Type of waste	Type of bag or container to be used	Treatment and disposal options
Red	**Contaminated waste (recyclable):** Wastes generated from disposable items, such as tubing, bottles, intravenous tubes and sets, catheters, urine bags, syringes (without needles and fixed needle syringes) and vacutainers with their needles cut) and gloves	Red colored non-chlorinated plastic bags or containers	Autoclaving or microwaving/hydroclaving followed by shredding or mutilation or combination of sterilization and shredding. Treated waste to be sent to registered or authorized recyclers or for energy recovery or plastics to diesel or fuel oil or for road making, whichever is possible. Plastic waste should not be sent to landfill sites.
White (translucent)	**Waste sharps including metals:** Needles, syringes with fixed needles, needles from needle tip cutter or burner, scalpels, blades, or any other contaminated sharp object that may cause puncture and cuts. This includes both used, discarded and contaminated metal sharps	Puncture proof, leak proof, tamper proof containers	Autoclaving or dry heat sterilization followed by shredding or mutilation or encapsulation in metal container or cement concrete; combination of shredding cum autoclaving; and sent for final disposal to iron foundries (having consent to operate from the State Pollution Control Boards or Pollution Control Committees) or sanitary landfill or designated concrete waste sharp pit
Blue	a. **Glassware:** Broken or discarded and contaminated glass including medicine vials and ampoules except those contaminated with cytotoxic wastes	Cardboard boxes with blue colored marking	Disinfection (by soaking the washed glass waste after cleaning with detergent and sodium hypochlorite treatment) or through autoclaving or microwaving or hydroclaving and then sent for recycling
	b. **Metallic body implants**	Cardboard boxes with blue colored marking	

Part -II

1. All plastic bags shall be as per BIS standards as and when published, till then the prevailing Plastic Waste Management Rules shall be applicable.
2. Chemical treatment using at least 10% sodium hypochlorite having 30% residual chlorine for 20 minutes any other equivalent chemical reagent that should demonstrate $Log_{10}4$ reduction efficiency for microorganisms as given in Schedule-III.
3. Mutilation or shredding must be to an extent to prevent unauthorized reuse.
4. There will be no chemical pretreatment before incineration, except for microbiological, lab and highly infectious waste.
5. Incineration ash (ash from incineration of any biomedical waste) shall be disposed through hazardous waste treatment, storage and disposal facility, if toxic or hazardous constituents are present beyond the prescribed limits as given in the Hazardous Waste (Management, Handling and Trans-boundary Movement) Rules, 2008 or as revised from time to time.

(Contd...)

(Contd...)

6. Dead fetus below the viability period (as per the Medical Termination of Pregnancy Act 1971, amended from time to time) can be considered as human anatomical waste. Such waste should be handed over to the operator of common bio-medical waste treatment and disposal facility in yellow bag with a copy of the official Medical Termination of Pregnancy certificate from the Obstetrician or the Medical Superintendent of hospital or health care establishment.
7. Cytotoxic drug vials shall not be handed over to unauthorized person under any circumstances. These shall be sent back to the manufactures for necessary disposal at a single point. As a second option, these may be sent for incineration at common bio-medical waste treatment and disposal facility or TSDFs or plasma pyrolys is at temperature >1,200°C.
8. Residual or discarded chemical wastes, used or discarded disinfectants and chemical sludge can be disposed at hazardous waste treatment, storage and disposal facility. In such case, the waste should be sent to hazardous waste treatment, storage and disposal facility through operator of common bio-medical waste treatment and disposal facility only.
9. On-site pretreatment of laboratory waste, microbiological waste, blood samples, blood bags should be disinfected or sterilized as per the Guidelines of World Health Organization or National AIDS Control Organization and then given to the common bio-medical waste treatment and disposal facility.
10. Installation of in-house incinerator is not allowed. However in case there is no common biomedical facility nearby, the same may be installed by the occupier after taking authorization from the State Pollution Control Board.
11. Syringes should be either mutilated or needles should be cut and or stored in tamper proof, leak proof and puncture proof containers for sharps storage. Wherever the occupier is not linked to a disposal facility it shall be the responsibility of the occupier to sterilize and dispose in the manner prescribed.
12. Bio-medical waste generated in households during health care activities shall be segregated as per these rules and handed over in separate bags or containers to municipal waste collectors. Urban local bodies shall have tie up with the common bio-medical waste treatment and disposal facility to pickup this waste from the Material Recovery Facility (MRF) or from the house hold directly, for final disposal in the manner as prescribed in this Schedule.

3. Wet and dry thermal treatment
4. Microwave irradiation
5. Land disposal
6. Inertization

1. Incineration

Incineration is a high temperature dry oxidation process that reduces organic and combustible waste to inorganic incombustible matter and results in a very significant reduction of waste-volume and weight. This is a safe method of treating large solid infectious waste, particularly anatomy waste and amputated limbs, animal carcasses and the like. The incinerator subjects them to very high heat, converting them to ash, which would be only about a tenth of original volume. However, it is expensive and is generally used only by very large establishments.

Types of incinerators

Three basic kinds of incineration technology are of interest for treating health care waste:

a. Double-chamber pyrolytic incinerators which may be especially designed to burn infectious health care waste.
b. Single-chamber furnaces with static grate, which should be used only if pyrolytic incinerators are not affordable
c. Rotary kilns operating at high temperatures, capable of causing decomposition of genotoxic substances and heat-resistant chemicals.

Double chambered incineration

Incinerators should be installed at appropriate location, to avoid nuisance to patients and neighborhood. An incinerator should consist of two chambers, primary and secondary. The temperature of primary chamber should be 750–850°C while the temperature in the secondary chamber should be 1,000–1,100°C. Waste is burnt in one chamber (primary chamber) at 800°C. Combustion of gases emitted from the first chamber, occurs in the second or secondary chamber which has a high temperature of 1,000°C. The negative pressure is maintained inside the incinerator by the system, thereby forcing the end-gases out of the chimney.

The chimneys of incinerators should be 30 meters high and combustion efficiency (CE) of the incinerator should be at least 99%. **It is computed as follows:**

Advantage of incinerator
The incinerator has an advantage of dealing with all pathological and cytotoxic wastes. Body parts, animal waste, microbiological waste and soiled dressings can be treated with this technique.

Disadvantages of incinerator
1. It generates highly toxic gases [e.g., dioxins and furans, if polyvinyl chloride (PVC) plastics are present].
2. It adversely affects the health of the community.
3. Recycling and reprocessing of materials cannot be done.
4. Burning of plastic waste or sharps is also not recommended.

2. Chemical Disinfection

Chemicals are added to waste to kill or inactivate the pathogens it contains. This is very useful method for many items, particularly in small places. Chemical disinfection is most suitable for treating liquid waste, such as blood, urine, stools or hospital sewage. However, solid wastes including microbiological cultures, sharps, etc., may also be disinfected chemically with certain limitations.

3. Wet and Dry Thermal Treatment

Wet thermal treatment
Wet thermal treatment or steam disinfection is based on exposure of shredded infectious waste to high temperature, high pressure steam, and is similar to the autoclave sterilization process. The process is inappropriate for the treatment of anatomical waste and animal carcasses, and will not efficiently treat chemical and pharmaceutical waste.

Screw-feed technology
Screw-feed technology is the basis of a nonburn, dry thermal disinfection process in which waste is shredded and heated in a rotating auger. The waste is reduced by 80% in volume and by 20–35% in weight. This process is suitable for treating infectious waste and sharps, but it should not be used to process pathological, cytotoxic or radioactive waste.

4. Microwave Irradiation

This is another useful method of sterilization of small volume waste at the point of generation. Most microorganisms are destroyed by the action of microwave of a frequency of about 2,450 MHz and a wavelength of 12.24 cm. The water contained within the waste is rapidly heated by the microwaves and the infectious components are destroyed by heat conduction. This cannot be used for animal or human body parts, metal items or toxic or radioactive material.

The efficiency of the microwave disinfection should be checked routinely through bacteriological and virological tests.

5. Land Disposal

If a municipality or medical authority genuinely lacks the means to treat waste before disposal, the use of a land fill has to be regarded as an acceptable disposal route. There are two types of disposal land-**open dumps** and **sanitary landfills**. Health care waste should not be deposited on or around open dumps. The risk of either people or animals coming into contact with infectious pathogens is obvious.

6. Inertization

The process of "inertization" involves mixing waste with cement and other substances before disposal, in order to minimize the risk of toxic substances contained in the wastes migrating into the surface water or ground water. A typical proportion of the mixture is: 65% pharmaceutical waste, 15% lime, 15% cement and 5% water. A homogeneous mass is formed and cubes or pellets are produced on site and then transported to suitable storage sites.

BIOMEDICAL WASTE MANAGEMENT IN INDIA

National legislation is the basis for improving health care waste disposal practices in any country. It establishes legal control, and permits the national agency responsible for the disposal of health care waste, usually the Ministry of Health, to apply pressure for their implementation. The Ministry of Environment may also be involved. There should be a clear designation of responsibilities before the law is enacted.

The United Nations Conference on the Environment and Development (UNCED) in 1992, recommended the following measures:
a. Prevent and minimize waste production
b. Reuse or recycle the waste to the extent possible
c. Treat waste by safe and environmentally sound methods, and
d. Dispose off the final residue by landfill in confined and carefully designed sites

Biomedical waste (Management and Handling) Rule 1998, prescribed by the Ministry of Environment and Forests, Government of India, came into force on 28th July 1998. This rule applies to those who generate, collect, receive, store, dispose, treat or handle biomedical waste in any manner. **Table 68.1** shows the categories of biomedical waste, types of waste, and treatment and disposal options under rule 1998. The Act is superseded by Biomedical Waste Management rules 2016. **Table 68.1** shows the categories of biomedical waste, types of waste and treatment and disposal options under rule 2016. The 2016 rules have been amended in 2018 and 2019.

The biomedical waste should be segregated into containers bags at the point of generation of the waste. The color coding and the type of containers used for disposal of waste are as shown in **Table 68.1**.

Waste Management Program

All laboratories should develop waste management program according to the specific needs of the individual laboratory. The policies and procedures should be incorporated in the laboratory's operating manuals. Emphasis should be on waste minimization (by reducing waste, reuse, and recycling), proper segregation, and health and safety of the workers. All personnel generating, collecting, transporting, and storing infectious waste must be trained under the program.

Biosafety

Biosafety can be defined as a group of practices and procedures designed to provide safe environment for individuals who work with potentially hazardous biological materials in laboratory environments. The primary goal of biosafety to reduce or eliminate exposures to these agents through the use of containment:
- Safety organization
- Safety codes
- Hazards groups
- Containment level

Biomedical Waste Handlers

- Immunize all health care workers (HCWs) and others, involved in handling of biomedical waste for protection against diseases including hepatitis B and tetanus which are likely to be transmitted by handling of biomedical waste, in a manner as prescribed in the National Immunization Policy or the guidelines of the Ministry of Health and Family Welfare issued from time to time.
- Ensure occupational safety of all HCWs and others involved in handling of biomedical waste by providing appropriate and adequate personal protective equipment (PPE).
- Conduct health check-up at the time of induction and at least once in a year for all HCWs and others involved in handling of biomedical waste and maintain the records for the same.

LAUNDRY MANAGEMENT PROCESS AND INFECTION CONTROL AND PREVENTION

Laundry in a health care facility may include bed sheets and blankets, towels, personal clothing, patient apparel, uniforms, scrub suits, gowns, and drapes for surgical procedures. Although, contaminated textiles and fabrics in health care facilities can be a source of substantial numbers of pathogenic microorganisms, reports of health care associated diseases linked to contaminated fabrics are so few in number that the overall risk of disease transmission during the laundry process likely is negligible. When the incidence of such events are evaluated in the context of the volume of items laundered in health care settings, existing control measures (e.g., standard precautions) are effective in reducing the risk of disease transmission to patients and staff. Therefore, use of current control measures should be continued to minimize the contribution of contaminated laundry to the incidence of health care associated infections.

The control measures of the guideline are based on principles of hygiene, common sense, and consensus guidance; they pertain to laundry services utilized by health care facilities, either inhouse or contract, rather than to laundry done in the home. The purpose of the laundry portion of the standard is to protect the worker from exposure to potentially infectious materials during collection, handling, and sorting of contaminated textiles through the use of personal protective equipment, proper work practices, containment, labeling, hazard communication, and ergonomics. Laundry facility is usually partitioned into two separate areas—a **"dirty" area** for receiving and handling the soiled laundry and **a "clean" area** for processing the washed items. To minimize the potential for recontaminating cleaned laundry with aerosolized contaminated lint, areas receiving contaminated textiles should be at negative air pressure relative to the clean areas. Laundry areas should have handwashing facilities readily available to workers. Laundry workers should wear appropriate personal protective equipment (e.g., gloves and protective garments) while sorting soiled fabrics and textiles. Laundry equipment should be used and maintained according to the manufacturer's instructions to prevent microbial contamination of the system. Damp textiles should not be left in machines overnight.

KEY POINTS

- **Biomedical waste (BMW)** means any waste, which is generated during the diagnosis, treatment or immunization of human beings or animals or in research activities pertaining thereto or in the production or testing of biologicals.
- **Waste segregation:** Waste should be segregated in bags of different colors to facilitate appropriate treatment and disposal.
- There are various techniques of biomedical wastes. These include incineration, autoclaving, microwaving, hydroclaving, plasma torch, and chemical treatment.

IMPORTANT QUESTIONS

1. Describe various techniques used for the treatment and disposal of hospital waste.
2. Write short notes on:
   a. Segregation of waste
   b. Hospital waste management of biomedical waste

MULTIPLE CHOICE QUESTIONS

1. Categories of waste for contaminated plastic waste is:
   a. Yellow
   b. Red
   c. White translucent
   d. Blue
2. All is true about Incineration, *except*:
   a. It is a high temperature dry oxidation process
   b. This is a safe method of treating large solid infectious waste
   c. The incinerator subjects them to very high heat, converting them to ash
   d. It is cheap and is generally used only by very large establishments
3. Chemical disinfection is recommended for treatment of:
   a. Laboratory glassware
   b. Liquid waste such as blood, urine, stools or hospital sewage
   c. Laundry in a health care facility
   d. For distinction of gloves

ANSWERS

1. b   2. d   3. b

Antibiotic Stewardship

LEARNING OBJECTIVES

After reading and studying this chapter, you should be able to:
- Describe Antimicrobial stewardship (AMS).
- Discuss antimicrobial resistance (AMR).
- Describe multidrug-resistant organisms (MDRO).
- Infection control measures for multidrug-resistant organisms (MDRO).

ANTIMICROBIAL STEWARDSHIP

Antimicrobial stewardship (AMS) has been defined as "the optimal selection, dosage, and duration of antimicrobial treatment that results in the best clinical outcome for the treatment or prevention of infection, with minimal toxicity to the patient and minimal impact on subsequent resistance."

GOAL OF ANTIMICROBIAL STEWARDSHIP

The goal of antimicrobial stewardship is 3-fold.
1. To work with healthcare practitioners to help each patient receive the most appropriate antimicrobial with the correct dose and duration.
2. To prevent antimicrobial overuse, misuse, and abuse.
3. To minimize the development of resistance.

NEED OF ANTIMICROBIAL STEWARDSHIP

At present, the multifaceted etiology of antibiotic resistance has many factors which are at play. These include inadequate regulations and usage imprecisions, awareness deficiency in best practices which steers undue or inept use of antibiotics, use of antibiotics as a poultry and livestock growth promoter rather than to control infection, and online marketing which made the unrestricted availability of low-grade antibiotics very accessible.

IMPLEMENTING AN ANTIMICROBIAL STEWARDSHIP (AMS) PROGRAM

Implementing AMS programs is a strategy for changing this behavior over time.

1. Leadership

Leadership with dedicate necessary human, financial and information technology resource is important for implementation of AMS program. Early involvement of thought leaders from hospital administration and the various practitioner groups will improve acceptance and implementation.

2. Antimicrobial Stewardship Team

Establish a multidisciplinary antibiotic management team to draft policy. The group developing the antibiotic policy should be a multidisciplinary group with 6-10 members with expertise and experience in different subjects. Usually infectious diseases, internal medicine, surgery, pediatrics, clinical microbiology, pharmacology and hospital pharmacy. At least one member should have the skills to conduct literature and systematic reviews.

3. Infrastructure Support

The support of microbiology laboratory for antimicrobial susceptibility testing according to the latest guidelines of the Clinical and Laboratory Standard Institute (CLSI) are followed and are of utmost importance. The newer rapid molecular diagnostic tests are designed to help clinicians de-escalate earlier in the antibiotic course. Biomarkers, such as procalcitonin and C-reactive protein (CRP) and molecular methods, such as multiplex PCR must be available.

Hospital information system including laboratory information and manpower for supporting the program must be available.

4. Antimicrobial Policy

To develop an antibiotic policy each hospital shall establish a multidisciplinary antibiotic management team (AMT). The team's functions should include developing a hospital antimicrobial policy, monitoring the implementation of the antibiotic policy, receiving feedback, assessing outcome and discussing with clinicians, conducting a revision of the policy every year based on the experience of prescribers and antimicrobial susceptibility profiles, and setting audit targets.

5. Stewardship Strategies

There are two major approaches to antimicrobial stewardship, with the most successful programs generally implementing a combination of both.
  i. The front-end or preprescription approach
  ii. The back-end or postprescription approach

i. The Front-end or Preprescription Approach

The front-end or preprescription approach to stewardship uses restrictive prescriptive authority. Certain antimicrobials are considered restricted and require prior authorization for use by all except a select group of clinicians. Clinicians without authority to prescribe the drug in question must contact the designated antimicrobial steward and obtain approval to order the antimicrobial.

ii. The Back-end or Postprescription Approach

The back-end or postprescription approach to stewardship uses prospective review and feedback. The antimicrobial steward reviews current antibiotic orders and provides clinicians with recommendations to continue, adjust, change, or discontinue the therapy based on the available microbiology results and clinical features of the case. Studies of programs that use this approach have shown decreased antimicrobial use, decreased number of new prescriptions of antimicrobials, and improved clinician satisfaction.

6. Education and Training

Once the facility has outlined the competencies required for the different staff groups, it needs to develop a training delivery plan, in other words, identify a leader, teachers and participants, and make a time plan. The opportunity to use real-world clinical opportunities for training (e.g., ward rounds, clinical case discussions) should be emphasized. In addition, those in training should be encouraged to access external training opportunities, including available e-learning options.

MONITORING OF ANTIMICROBIAL STEWARDSHIP PROGRAM

A. Process Measures/Indicators of Antimicrobial Use

Process indicators are often used as a proxy measure of improvement, e.g., that antibiotic prescribing practices are moving in the right direction.
  1. **Documented indication for antibiotic use:** Tracking the types and acceptance of recommendations from prospective **audit and feedback** interventions, which can identify areas where more education or

additional focused interventions might be useful.
2. **Prescription compliance:** Compliance with current guidelines for surgical prophylaxis (antibiotics):
   - Culture taken before antibiotic.
   - Modification of the empirical antibiotics according to antibiotic susceptibility test.
   - Surgeries with prophylaxis administered within 60 minutes prior to surgery
   - Surgical prophylaxis stopped within 24 hours after surgery
3. **Administrative compliance:**
   - Correct administration of antibiotics such as dose, frequency and route.
   - Number of regimens switched to oral route
   - Compliance with current guidelines for surgical prophylaxis (antibiotics).

B. Outcome Measures/Indicators Related to Antimicrobial Use

   i. Antimicrobial use
   ii. Antibiotic resistance.
   iii. Clinical outcome indicator
   iv. Financial impact.

i. Antimicrobial Use

   a. **Defined daily dose (DDD):** It is the assumed average maintenance dose per day for a drug used for its main identification in adults.
   b. **Days of therapy (DOTs):** Number of days that a patient is on antibiotic regardless of dose.

ii. Antibiotic Resistance

Monitoring resistance at the patient has also been shown to be useful.

iii. Clinical Outcome Indicator

   a. **Morbidity:** It may be observed by length of stay in hospital.
   b. **Mortality:** Number of deaths during hospitalization or mortality at a specific time point after admission.

iv. Financial Impact

Stewardship programs can achieve significant cost savings, particularly drug cost savings. It can be analysed by calculating the cost of antimicrobial per patient day or per year or per admission.

RATIONAL USE OF ANTIBIOTICS

Rational use of antibiotics is extremely important as injudicious use can adversely affect the patient, cause emergence of antibiotic resistance and increase the cost of health care. Taking everything into account, it is important for the clinician to implement the "7D's of optimal antibiotic therapy: right Drug, right Dose, appropriate Direction (route of administration), De-escalation to pathogen directed therapy, and right Duration of therapy, watch for and consider Drug to drug interaction, always evaluate for possible immune Deficiency" to optimize antibiotic use in clinical settings.

1. Evaluate the Infection by Clinical Diagnosis

The majority of infections seen in general practice are of viral origin and antibiotics can neither treat viral infections nor prevent secondary bacterial infections in these patients.

2. Select an Appropriate Antibiotic Therapy

Definitive Therapy

When the etiology of the infection is known, the clinician should proceed with definitive therapy.

Empirical Therapy

A common approach can be prescribing a broad-spectrum antibiotic agent as initial empiric therapy.

Prophylactic Therapy

Antibiotic prophylaxis should be prescribed to susceptible patients to prevent specific infections that can cause definite detrimental effects.

3. Criteria for Choosing an Antibiotic Drug

Once the etiology of an infection is known, the clinician should recommend a most narrow spectrum antibiotic which is cost-effective and least toxic for the shortest duration possible.

4. Efficacy

Narrow Spectrum or Broad Spectrum

- Monotherapy or combination therapy
- To achieve synergistic effect against the infection
- Combination therapy also shortens the course of antibiotic therapy
- To prevent the development of bacterial resistance with long-term therapy
- Efficacy at the site of infection and tissue penetration
- Bactericidal versus bacteriostatic therapy

5. Dosage, Route of Administration and Duration

Oral/enteral route of administration should be preferred in patients with mild-to-moderate infections. Clinicians should reserve intravenous antibiotics for severe infection or for certain sites. Antibiotic treatment should generally be continued for a maximum of 5 days or a shorter period if this is clinically appropriate.

6. Patient Factors

The clinician should consider the age of the patient, immune status, pregnancy and lactation, associated conditions like renal and hepatic function, epilepsy, etc., while choosing the antibacterial agent.

7. Monitoring Response to Therapy

Response to therapy depends on the nature and sensitivity of the agent, specificity of the drug, bioavailability and dosage. Longer the doubling time of the organism, longer the time it takes to respond.

Since non-compliance is also one of the causes for treatment failure, the clinician should ensure patient adherence to the therapy. Treatment should be continued until all pathogens are eliminated from the tissues or until the infection has been sufficiently controlled for the normal host defences to eradicate it.

ANTIMICROBIAL RESISTANCE (AMR)

Antimicrobial resistance (AMR) poses a serious global threat of growing concern to human, animal, and environment health. This is due to the emergence, spread, and persistence of **multidrug-resistant (MDR)** bacteria exist across the animal, human, and environment triangle or niche and there is interlinked sharing of these pathogens in this triad.

Causes of Antibiotic Resistance

At present, the multifaceted etiology of antibiotic resistance has many factors which are at play. These include inadequate regulations and usage imprecisions, awareness deficiency in best practices which steers undue or inept use of antibiotics, use of antibiotics as a poultry and livestock growth promoter rather than to control infection, and online marketing which made the unrestricted availability of low-grade antibiotics very accessible.

Mechanism of Antimicrobial Resistance

Resistance to antibiotics is conveniently divided into mechanisms that are intrinsic or acquired resistance.

A. Intrinsic Mechanisms of Resistance

Intrinsic resistance is the innate ability of a bacterial species to resist the activity of a particular antimicrobial agent through inherent structural or functional characteristics, allowing tolerance of a particular drug or antimicrobial class. For example, some gram-negative bacteria are intrinsically resistant to the activity of macrolides. Alternatively, a bacterium may lack the target of the drug altogether.

B. Acquired Mechanisms of Resistance

Acquired mechanisms of resistance are caused by changes in the usual genetic makeup of a microorganism and by the results of altered cellular physiology and structure. The gene changes or exchanges that result from acquired resistance are usually caused by genetic mutation(s), acquisition of genes from other organisms via gene transfer mechanisms, or a combination of mutational and gene transfer events.

Global Action Plan to Control the Menace of Antibiotic Resistance

The global burden of AMR has no signs of receding, rather it piles up the pressure on human and veterinary medicine. The spread and sharing of AMR can be contained by the rational use of antibiotics, infection control, immunization, promoting good practices in food supply, and control of person-to-person spread by screening, treatment, awareness, and education. At the national, regional, and global levels, the tracking, bio-surveillance, and response and prevention strategies of AMR and MDR pathogens may help to control the "global resistome."

METHICILLIN-RESISTANT STAPHYLOCOCCUS AUREUS (MRSA)

Staphylococcus aureus is considered as the most notorious superbug. It is a nasal commensal of humans and can cause common skin infections. Penicillin-resistant strains require treatment with penicillinase resistant penicillins, such as nafcillin or oxacillin. Although methicillin is no longer used, isolates that are resistant to nafcillin or oxacillin have been traditionally termed **methicillin-resistant staphylococci**, e.g., **methicillin-resistant *Staphylococcus aureus* (MRSA)**; **methicillin-resistant *Staphylococcus epidermidis* (MRSE)**; **community associated methicillin-resistant *Staphylococcus aureus* (CA-MRSA)**; **healthcare–associated community-onset methicillin-resistant *Staphylococcus aureus* (HACO-MRSA)**.

MRSA Infections

Whether hospital-associated methicillin resistant *Staphylococcus aureus* (HA-MRSA), HACO-MRSA, or CA-MRSA—are costly and pose a serious threat to health institutions.

MRSA Prevention

Control of MRSA requires strict adherence to infection control practices, including barrier protection, contact isolation, and handwashing compliance. A number of prevention strategies are recommended to avoid becoming infected with MRSA.

1. Prevention in the Hospital

In the hospital, MRSA is commonly spread to patients from the hands of healthcare workers. To minimize this risk, to ensure that anyone who comes in contact with the patient washes their hands or uses an alcohol-based hand sanitizer before and after touching the patient. Patients with active infection should also wash their hands frequently. Hospitalized patients who are colonized or infected with MRSA should be placed on "contact precautions." This means that healthcare workers entering the patient's room must wear gloves and a clean cover gown to prevent contamination of their clothing.

2. Prevention in the Community

- Keep hands clean by washing thoroughly with soap and water.
- Alcohol-based hand sanitizers are a good alternative for disinfecting hands if a sink is not available.
- Keep cuts and scrapes clean, dry, and covered with a bandage until healed.
- Avoid touching other people's wounds or bandages.
- Avoid sharing personal items such as towels, washcloths, razors, clothing, or uniforms. Other items that should not be shared include brushes, combs, and makeup.

3. Care for Family Members of Infected Person

Careful preventive measures, including washing hands, keeping wounds covered, washing bed sheets and towels, and avoiding shared personal items, are recommended in these situations.

4. Basic Infection Prevention Measures

There are a number of other measures that may help to prevent the spread of infections, including infection with MRSA.

MULTIDRUG RESISTANT ORGANISMS (MDRO)

Infections caused by bacterial organisms resistant to most available antibiotics, called **multidrug resistant organisms (MDRO)**.

Examples are:
1. Multidrug resistant organisms (MDROs): Gram-negative bacteria (e.g., *Eschericha coli, Pseudomonas, Klebsiella, Enterobacter, Acinetobacter*) resistant to first line antibiotic agents and/or carrying certain resistance traits (e.g., ESBL = extended spectrum beta-lactamase, KPC = *Klebsiella pneumonia* carbapenemase)
2. Methicillin-resistant *Staphylococcus aureus* (MRSA).
3. Vancomycin-intermediate *Staphylococcus aureus* (VRSA).
4. Vancomycin-resistant *Staphylococcus aureus* (VRSA)
5. Vancomycin-resistant enterococci (VRE).
6. New Delhi metallo-beta-lactamase-1 (NDM-1).

Infection Control Measures for the Control of Multidrug-resistant Organisms (MDRO) in the Healthcare Setting

When MDRO are introduced into a healthcare setting, a number of factors aid the transmission and persistence of resistant strains in the environment.

1. Standard and Contact Precautions

Standard Precautions are extremely important in limiting the spread of all transmissible pathogens.
Contact precautions: In addition to standard precautions, should be routinely implemented in all acute healthcare facilities for any patient known to be infected with or colonised with an MDRO.

2. Hand Hygiene

Hands should be decontaminated by washing with an antiseptic soap or waterless antiseptic agent such as a 70% alcohol hand rub preparation.

Hand hygiene should always be performed before donning and after removal of gloves. The importance of hand hygiene should be reinforced in an outbreak setting.

3. Patient Placement and Priority for Isolation

Patients colonised or infected with an MDRO should be placed in individual single rooms with en-suite toilet facilities. When a sufficient number of single rooms is not available, priority for these rooms should be assigned according to a facility's healthcare-associated infection (HCAI) strategy.

4. Personal Protective Equipment (PPE)

PPE refers to a variety of barriers used either alone or in combination to protect healthcare workers from contact with transmissible pathogens (*See* Chapter 64).

5. Discontinuation of Isolation

In general, it would seem advisable to continue contact precautions for all patients who have been previously infected with, or are known to be colonised with the MDRO addressed in this document for the duration of their admission. On readmission rescreening is advised to facilitate an infection control risk assessment

6. Cleaning of the Environment and Patient Care Equipment

- Use of dedicated single-patient use non-critical medical equipment (blood pressure cuffs, thermometers, etc.).
- Assignment of dedicated cleaning staff to areas where patients with MDRO are being cared for

- Increased cleaning frequency and enhanced attention to frequently-touched surfaces, such as bed rails, bed side chairs and door handles.

7. Patient Movement and Transfer

When a patient colonised or infected with an MDRO is transferred to another hospital or healthcare facility, the clinical team responsible for the patient should inform the receiving clinical staff of the patient's MDRO carriage status.

8. Endoscopy

Special care should be taken to disinfect or protect delicate equipment used with endoscopes, such as cameras.

9. Education of Patients, Staff, Visitors and Carers

A patient who is found to be newly-colonised or infected with an MDRO should be informed about his colonisation/infection status by the clinical team with appropriate documentation in the patient's healthcare record. Visitors to the patient, as well as healthcare workers visiting the ward from other departments should be alerted to check with ward nursing staff for instructions prior to entering the room/cohort bed space.

10. Decolonisation

Currently there are no recommended regimens available for the routine decolonisation of patients harbouring MDRO other than MRSA.

11. Healthcare Workers and MDRO

If healthcare workers found to be colonised with MDRO adhere strictly to standard precautions (including hand hygiene) and contact precautions where indicated.

12. Intensified Interventions to Prevent MDRO Transmission

A decision to employ additional MDRO control measures may arise from surveillance data and assessments of the risk to patients in various settings.

13. MDRO Infection Prevention and Control Measures for Settings Outside of Hospitals

a. MDRO-colonised Patients in Long-term Care Facilities

Patients colonised with an MDRO may be encountered in healthcare facilities outside of the hospital setting, including long-term care facilities (LTCF), such as nursing homes and residential care centers. Alternatively, they may be cared for in their own home.

Before isolating a resident, a plan to review the need for ongoing contact precautions must be in place.

b. MDRO-colonised Patients in the Home

Standard precautions, hand hygiene and normal cleaning are sufficient as infection control measures in the home. Single-use patient care equipment should be used where possible.

KEY POINTS

- **Antimicrobial stewardship:** Antimicrobial stewardship (AMS) has been defined as "the optimal selection, dosage, and duration of antimicrobial treatment that results in the best clinical outcome for the treatment or prevention of infection, with minimal toxicity to the patient and minimal impact on subsequent resistance."
- **Multidrug-resistant organisms (MDRO):** Infections caused by bacterial organisms resistant to most available antibiotics, called multidrug resistant organisms (MDRO).
- **Methicillin-resistant staphylococci:** Methicillin-resistant *Staphylococcus aureus* (MRSA) and methicillin-resistant *Staphylococcus epidermidis* (MRSE), community associated methicillin-resistant *Staphylococcus aureus* (CAMRSA), healthcare-associated community-onset methicillin-resistant *Staphylococcus aureus* (HACO-MRSA).
- **Methicillin-resistant *Staphylococcus aureus* (MRSA)**
- **Infection control measures for the control of multidrug-resistant organisms (MDRO) in the healthcare setting:**
  1. Standard and contact precautions

2. Hand hygiene
3. Patient placement and priority for isolation
4. Personal protective equipment (PPE)
5. Discontinuation of isolation
6. Cleaning of the environment and patient care equipment
7. Patient movement and transfer
8. Endoscopy
9. Education of patients, staff, visitors and carers
10. Decolonisation
11. Healthcare workers and MDRO
12. Intensified interventions to prevent MDRO transmission
13. MDRO infection prevention and control measures for settings outside of hospitals MDRO-colonised patients in long-term care facilities.

IMPORTANT QUESTIONS

1. Write briefly on:
   a. Antibiotic stewardship
   b. Antimicrobial resistance (AMR)
   c. Prevention of methicillin-resistant *Staphylococcus aureus* (MRSA)
   d. Multidrug-resistant organisms (MDRO) in healthcare setting
   e. Infection control measures for multidrug-resistant organisms (MDRO) in the healthcare setting

MULTIPLE CHOICE QUESTIONS

1. **The major objectives of antimicrobial stewardship are:**
   a. To achieve best clinical outcomes related to antimicrobial use
   b. Minimizing toxicity and other adverse events
   c. Limiting the selective pressure on bacterial populations
   d. All of the above
2. **Intrinsic mechanisms of antimicrobial resistance can be caused by the following:**
   a. Lack of affinity of the drug for the bacterial target
   b. Inaccessibility of the drug into the bacterial cell
   c. Extrusion of the drug by chromosomally encoded efflux pumps;
   d. All of the above

ANSWERS

1. c   2. c

CHAPTER 70

Patient Safety Indicators

LEARNING OBJECTIVES

After reading and studying this chapter, you should be able to:
- Describe patient safety indicators (PSIS).
- Describe care of vulnerable patients.
- Describe prevention of iatrogenic injury.
- Describe the care of lines, drains and tubing's.
- Discuss restraint policy and care: Physical and chemical.
- Describe blood and blood transfusion policy.
- Describe prevention of IV complications.
- Describe fall prevention.
- Describe prevention of deep vein thrombosis (DVT).
- Discuss deep vein thrombosis (DVT) prevention.
- Discuss shifting and transporting of patients.
- Describe surgical safety.
- Describe medication reconciliation.
- Describe prevention of communication errors.
- Describe documentation.

INTRODUCTION

Patient safety is the absence of preventable harm to a patient during the process of health care and reduction of risk of unnecessary harm associated with health care to an acceptable minimum. The patient safety indicators (PSIs) are a set of measures that screen for adverse events that patients experience as a result of exposure to the health care system. These events are likely amenable to prevention by changes at the system or provider level. PSIs are defined on two levels: the provider level and the area level.

A. **Provider-level indicators** provide a measure of the potentially preventable complication for patients who received their initial care and the complication of care within the same hospitalization.

B. **Area-level indicators** capture all cases of the potentially preventable complication that occur in a given area (e.g., metropolitan area or county) either during hospitalization or resulting in subsequent hospitalization. Area-level indicators are specified to include principal diagnosis, as well as secondary diagnosis, for the complications of care.

CARE OF VULNERABLE PATIENTS

Vulnerable populations are defined as groups who are at increased risk of receiving a disparity in medical care on the basis of financial circumstances or social characteristics, such as age, race, gender, ethnicity, sexual orientation, spirituality, disability, or socioeconomic or insurance status. Hospitalists may play a significant role in influencing the health status, health care access, and health care delivery to vulnerable populations due to their higher rates of hospital utilization and lower access to outpatient care.

Vulnerability is the degree to which a population, individual or organization is unable to anticipate, cope with, resist and recover from the impacts of disasters. Children, pregnant women, elderly people, malnourished people, and people who are ill or immunocompromised are particularly vulnerable when a disaster strikes, and take a relatively high share of the disease burden associated with emergencies. Poverty and its common consequences, such as malnutrition, homelessness, poor housing and destitution is a major contributor to vulnerability (WHO). Hospitalists may serve as initial points of contact for the health care of these groups. Core competencies in communication, advocacy, and comprehension of the health care needs of vulnerable populations may influence health care expenditures, morbidity, and mortality. Hospitalists can lead initiatives that promote equity of health care provision.

A. Knowledge

Hospitalists should be able to:
- Explain key factors leading to disparities in health status among specific vulnerable populations.
- Explain disease processes.
- Describe key factors leading to disparities in the quality of care provided.
- List services in local healthcare system.
- Name local and institutional resources available to patients.
- Identify key elements of discharge planning for uninsured, underinsured, and disabled patients.

B. Skills

Hospitalists should be able to:
- Elicit elements of the history and physical examination
- Elicit a social history
- Tailor the therapeutic plan that takes into account discharge plan and outpatient resources.
- Identify vulnerable patients whose outpatient environment might benefit from additional community resources.
- Target vulnerable groups for indicated vaccinations and preventive care services or referrals.

C. Attitudes

Hospitalists should be able to:
- Utilize appropriate educational resources to inform vulnerable patients with low health literacy.
- Provide education and systems interventions
- Communicate openly to facilitate trust in patient-physician interactions.
- Actively involve patients and families in the design of care plans.
- Secure translators to assist with interviewing, physical examination, and medical decision making.
- Facilitate communication between vulnerable patient groups and consultants.
- Provide leadership to foster attitudes and systems improvements.
- Connect vulnerable patients with social services early in the hospital course.
- Coordinate adequate transitions of care from the inpatient to outpatient setting.
- Communicate with primary care physicians to facilitate transitions of care.

PREVENTION OF IATROGENIC INJURY

When medical or surgical treatment causes a new illness or injury, the result is considered to be iatrogenic. An iatrogenic event can either complicate existing medical condition or cause health issues unrelated to the illness sought treatment for in the first place.

Prevention of Iatrogenic Events

- Try to understand your treatments and ask as many questions as you need to ease your mind.
- After any procedures, remain aware of any potential adverse effects and contact a doctor immediately if you notice anything concerning.

- Try to bring a family member or trusted friend to your medical appointments.
- Communicate clearly and respectfully with your healthcare team.

CARE OF LINES, DRAINS AND TUBING'S

Step 1: When entering the room, wash your hands or use hand sanitizer. You will be in a hospital, so put on gloves before touching anything in the room. This process will significantly reduce the transmission of nosocomial infection.

Step 2: Upon entering the patient's room, introduce yourself and then observe and evaluate the different lines, tubes, and drains.

Step 3: Figure out what your plan of care is going to consist of, and what side of the bed you want to work from.

Step 4: Inform your patient what "the plan" is before making any adjustments to the room. Your patient will feel more comfortable with you if they know what you are doing.

Step 5: Prepare oxygen, by either attaching to bottle or remove oxygen from the equation (this will need nurses' approval).

Step 6: Move catheter to side of bed you are going to work from.

Step 7: Prepare intravenous (IV) lines for patient movement (lines will be tangled up). If there are several IV lines, ask the attending nurse if any can be disconnected for therapy. The nurse will do this for you if possible.

Note: If there are many medical devices needed to go with you out of the room, get help from a tech, a nurse's aid, or even family. Do not try to carry so much that you are not able to keep hands on your patient for safety.

Step 8: Before standing patient, put a gait belt on them, being conscious of abdominal incisions, tubes and drains. If there are abdominal interferences, put gait belt high on the chest–under the arms. Safety has to come first.

Step 9: Hook catheter to walker, have IV stand ready to go, if O_2 is necessary have enough hands to handle patient and equipment safely.

Note: If blood pressure is a concern, take vitals before and after therapy. If patient is on continuous O_2, check pulse-oximetry before and after treatment.

Step 10: Remember to be vigilant, patient, and kind. Take a deep breath, everything is going to be OK!

RESTRAINT POLICY AND CARE: PHYSICAL AND CHEMICAL

The forcible confinement or control of a subject, as of a confused, disoriented, psychotic, or irrational person.

Restraint of any kind is used only when the patient's behavior presents a danger to himself or herself or another person. It is never used for the convenience of staff or as a substitute for conscientious nursing care.

It may be either physical or chemical.

A. Physical Restraints

Physical restraints include restraining patient to prevent removal of drainage tubes, restraints of upper and lower limbs to limit mobility and prevent the patient from climbing out of bed or physically harming someone at the bedside, and waist and body restraints such as a **camisole** (**straitjacket**). Even though the patient might not fully understand the need for restraint, a brief explanation of why it is being done should be given.

Assessment of the need for physical restraint includes a systematic determination of the level of confusion or disorientation exhibited by the patient and objective observations of his behavior. If possible, the cause of the patient's behavior should be identified, e.g., trauma, drug or alcohol intoxication, electrolyte imbalance, elevated temperature, pain, fear, or mental exhaustion. Findings of the assessment should be well documented in specific terms for legal reasons as well as to inform other caretakers and provide continuity of care.

B. Chemical Restraint

It refers to the quieting of a violently psychotic or irrational person by means of medication. This medicine is not the regular medicines you may take every day for your medical or emotional problems.

What are the Safety Issues When Using Restraints?

The following safety things will be done if need restraints:
1. **Doctor's order:** Patient doctor must order restraints. The written order will tell the caregivers what type of restraint to use. The order also says how long they will be used and when they can be removed. Restraints should only be used for a short time. And, restraints are used only after other things have been tried to keep you safe.
2. **Family:** Family will be called, around the time patients are put into restraints. This is done only if patient and his/her family had both agreed to have patient family called.
3. **Safety checks:** Caregivers are especially trained in how to care for patients in restraints. Caregivers will check on patient often to make sure you are safe and all your needs are met.
   Since restraint of patients subjects them to the **hazards of immobility**, it is essential that they should be monitored closely, their vital signs should be checked regularly, and their position should be changed at least every 2 hours. The use of restraints is an active area of nursing research. The most appropriate and least restrictive type of restraint should always be the one chosen.
4. **Nursing intervention** defined as the application, monitoring, and removal of mechanical restraining devices or manual restraints which are used to limit the physical mobility of a patient.

BLOOD AND BLOOD TRANSFUSION POLICY

Blood transfusion service is a vital part of the health care service. In order to improve the standards of Blood Banks and the Blood Transfusion services in our country, National AIDS Control Organization through Technical Resource Group on Blood Safety, has formulated comprehensive standards to ensure better quality control system on collection, storage, testing and distribution of blood and its components.

For quality, safety and efficacy of blood and blood products, well-equipped blood centers with adequate infrastructure and trained manpower is an essential requirement. For effective clinical use of blood, it is necessary to train clinical staff. To attain maximum safety, the requirements of good laboratory practices (GLP), good manufacturing practices (GMP) and moving toward total quality management is vital for organization and management of Blood Transfusion Services.

The Blood Bank or Blood Transfusion Service should have its own constitution, which defines the responsibility and authority of the management. All blood banks should have their own quality policy and prepare a quality manual that addresses the systems in use. The blood banks and transfusion services should aim to accept blood from only voluntary nonremunerated safe blood donors and to do away with the high risk donors and blood sellers. They should gradually phase out replacement donors. (*Note:* Blood sellers have been banned as per Supreme Court directive).

The blood banks should establish and maintain a quality assurance system based on any current international standard. All blood banks should provide full time competent staff ensuring proper cadres for both medical and paramedical personnel. Accurate costing enables accurate planning and budgeting so that the department runs efficiently without shortage of supply in the middle of the year. It also enables planning for future expansion, evaluates cost effectiveness and helps in mobilization of resources.

PREVENTION OF INTRAVENOUS COMPLICATIONS

1. Infiltration

Infiltration occurs when intravenous (IV) fluid or medications leak into the surrounding tissue.

Prevention

- Select an appropriate IV site, avoiding areas of flexion.
- Use proper venipuncture technique.
- Follow your facility policy for securing the IV catheter.
- Observe the IV site frequently.
- Advise the patient to report any swelling or tenderness at the IV site.

2. Extravasation

Extravasation is the leaking of vesicant drugs into surrounding tissue.

Prevention

- Avoid veins that are small and/or fragile, veins in areas of flexion, veins in extremities with pre-existing edema, or veins in areas with known neurologic impairment.
- Be aware of vesicant medications, such as certain antineoplastic drugs (doxorubicin, vinblastine, and vincristine), and hydroxyzine, promethazine, digoxin, and dopamine.
- Follow your facility policy regarding vesicant administration via a peripheral IV; some institutions require that vesicants are administered via a central venous access device only.
- Give vesicants last when multiple drugs are ordered.
- Strictly adhere to proper administration techniques.

3. Phlebitis

Phlebitis is inflammation of a vein.

Prevention

- Use proper venipuncture technique.
- Use a trusted drug reference or consult with the pharmacist for instructions on drug dilution, when necessary.
- Monitor administration rates and inspect the IV site frequently.
- Change the infusion site according to your facility's policy.

4. Hypersensitivity

An immediate, severe hypersensitivity reaction can be life-threatening, so prompt recognition and treatment are imperative.

Prevention

- Ask the patient about personal and family history of allergies.
- For infants younger than 3 months, ask the mother about her allergy history because maternal antibodies may still be present.
- Stay with the patient for 5–10 minutes to detect early signs and symptoms of hypersensitivity.
- If the patient is receiving the drug for the first or second time, check him every 5–10 minutes or according to your facility's policy.

5. Infection

Local or systemic infection is another potential complication of IV therapy.

Prevention

- Perform hand hygiene, don gloves, and use aseptic technique during IV insertion.
- Clean the site with approved skin antiseptic before inserting IV catheter.
- Ensure careful hand hygiene before any contact with the infusion system or the patient.
- Clean injection ports before each use.
- Follow your institution's policy for dressing changes and changing of the solution and administration set.

FALL PREVENTION

Following are some things that can be done to make your room safe so you do not fall:
1. Chairs and the bed should be kept at the lowest height for you.
2. Use a night light at bedtime may help you know where you are.
3. Keep a clear path or area in your room so you do not trip.
4. Caregivers may put a commode chair beside your bed. Or, a raised seat may be put on the bathroom toilet.
5. Wear nonskid shoes or slippers that fit well.
6. Some hospitals have bed sensors that alarm at the nurses' station. The bed sensor alarms when weight is taken off the bed, such as when you try to get out of bed. Ask caregivers for more information on bed sensors.
7. Your mattress may be put right on the floor if falling out of bed is a problem.

PREVENTION OF DEEP VEIN THROMBOSIS

Deep vein thrombosis (DVT) is the formation or presence of a thrombus in the deep veins. DVT occurs mostly in the lower extremities and to a lesser extent in the upper extremities. Pulmonary embolism (PE) is an obstruction of the pulmonary artery or its branches by a thrombus (sometimes due to fat or air). The most likely source of thrombus in pulmonary arteries is an embolization from deep veins of the legs. Prevention of DVT thereby decreases the incidence of PE, a serious and life-threatening condition.

DVT prophylaxis methods target either venous stasis (mechanical methods) or hypercoagulability (pharmacological prophylaxis). DVT prophylaxis can be primary or secondary.
A. **Primary prophylaxis** is the preferred method with the use of medications and mechanical methods to prevent DVT.
B. **Secondary prophylaxis** includes early detection with screening methods and the treatment of subclinical DVT. It is a less commonly used method.

Deep Vein Thrombosis Prevention

1. **People with cancer:** In selected situations, people undergoing treatment for cancer who are at high risk for DVT (e.g., people with pancreatic cancer who are receiving chemotherapy), anticoagulants may be considered for use to prevent a DVT from occurring.
2. **During hospitalization:** Some people who are in the hospital, either for **surgery** (especially, bone or joint surgery and cancer surgery) or because of a **serious medical illness**, may be given anticoagulants to decrease the risk of blood clots. **Anticoagulants** may also be given to women at high risk for venous thrombosis during and after pregnancy.

   In people who are hospitalized and have a moderate to low risk of blood clots, other preventive measures may be used. For example, some people are fitted with **inflatable compression devices** after surgery. These devices are worn around the legs during and immediately after surgery and periodically fill with air. These devices apply gentle pressure to improve circulation and help prevent clots. **Compression stockings** may also be recommended.

   In all cases, walking as soon as possible after surgery can decrease the risk of a blood clot; it can also decrease the risk of chronic swelling in the legs from your DVT (also known as "post-thrombotic syndrome").
3. **Extended travel:** Prolonged travel (e.g., taking an airplane flight or car ride that lasts more than 5 hours) appears to increase the risk of developing blood clots, although the risk is very small. There are a few tips that may be of benefit during extended travel.

SHIFTING AND TRANSPORT OF PATIENTS

Transport of Patients

Movement and transportation of patients from the isolation room or area should be restricted to essential purposes only. This will reduce the possibility of transmission of microorganisms in other areas of the health care facility (HCF).

Appropriate precautions should be taken during transportation to reduce the risk of transmission of microorganisms to other patients, HCWs or the hospital environment (surfaces or equipment).

Infection Control Precautions During Transport of Patients

1. Place a surgical mask on the face of a patient with pulmonary tuberculosis during transit.
2. Care should be taken of drainage and shunts and IV lines as these are potential sources for contamination of the environment, trolleys, etc., during transportation, also a source of infection for the patient. Closed sterile drainage is to be maintained at all times. Shunts and IV lines should be covered with sterile dressing during transportation. A trolley should have the facility for hanging IV bottles, tying of urine bags below bladder level which helps in proper draining of urine and prevents stagnation of urine.
3. Change trolley cover between patients.
4. Spills of blood and body fluid should be taken care of immediately.
5. Routine cleaning schedules for trolleys and wheel-chairs should be maintained.

SURGICAL SAFETY

The Safe Surgery Saves Lives initiative was established by the World Alliance for Patient Safety as part of the World Health Organization's efforts to reduce the number of surgical deaths across the world. The aim of this initiative is to harness political commitment and clinical will to address important safety issues, including inadequate anesthetic safety practices, avoidable surgical infection and poor communication among team members. These have proved to be common, deadly and preventable problems in all countries and settings.

To assist operating teams in reducing the number of these events, the Alliance—in consultation with surgeons, anesthesiologists, nurses, patient safety experts and patients around the world-has identified a set of safety checks that could be performed in any operating room. The Checklist is not a regulatory device or a component of official policy; it is intended as a tool for use by clinicians interested in improving the safety of their operations and reducing unnecessary surgical deaths and complications (**Fig. 70.1**).

CARE COORDINATION EVENT RELATED TO MEDICATION RECONCILIATION AND ADMINISTRATION

Medication Reconciliation

Medication reconciliation is the process of comparing a patient's new medication orders with all the medications the patient had been taking prior to changing levels of care. These changes in levels of care occur as the patient moves through the health care system; from home to the emergency department (ED), from the ED to an inpatient bed, from a general medical-surgical unit to an intensive care unit (ICU) or vice versa, from the ICU to surgery, and from the hospital back to home or to an extended care facility. Care must be taken at each of these transitions to avoid drug-related errors (e.g., through omission, commission, duplication).

PREVENTION OF COMMUNICATION ERRORS

Medical errors arise in many situations, but can be broadly categorized into errors of proficiency, communication, execution, and judgment. **Errors of proficiency** arise when a physician does not have the required knowledge or current skill to perform a specific procedure or examination in a competent manner (e.g., a physician elects to perform a bronchoscopy although he/she is out of training for many years and has not done the procedure in years). **Communication errors** arise when crucial patient information is wrong, missing, misinterpreted, or not appreciated (e.g., a pulmonary angiogram is performed in a patient with an elevated creatinine level, but the radiologist is unaware that the patient has

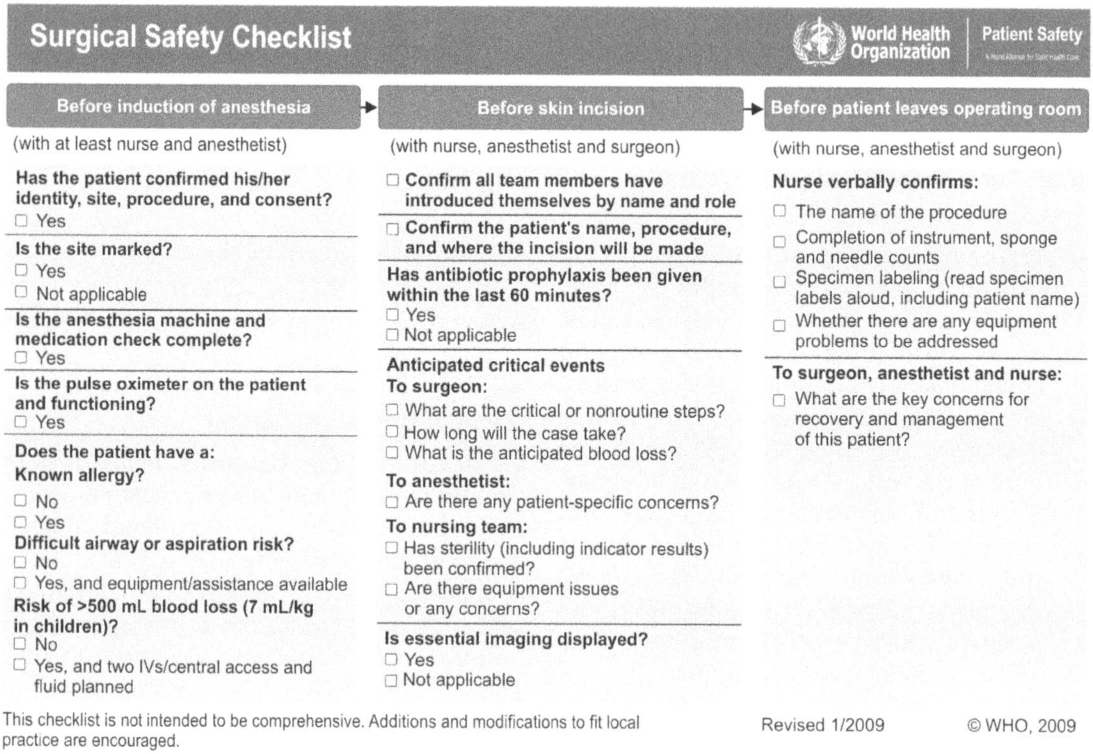

Surgical Safety Checklist

World Health Organization — Patient Safety

Before induction of anesthesia
(with at least nurse and anesthetist)

Has the patient confirmed his/her identity, site, procedure, and consent?
☐ Yes

Is the site marked?
☐ Yes
☐ Not applicable

Is the anesthesia machine and medication check complete?
☐ Yes

Is the pulse oximeter on the patient and functioning?
☐ Yes

Does the patient have a:
Known allergy?
☐ No
☐ Yes

Difficult airway or aspiration risk?
☐ No
☐ Yes, and equipment/assistance available

Risk of >500 mL blood loss (7 mL/kg in children)?
☐ No
☐ Yes, and two IVs/central access and fluid planned

Before skin incision
(with nurse, anesthetist and surgeon)

☐ Confirm all team members have introduced themselves by name and role
☐ Confirm the patient's name, procedure, and where the incision will be made

Has antibiotic prophylaxis been given within the last 60 minutes?
☐ Yes
☐ Not applicable

Anticipated critical events
To surgeon:
☐ What are the critical or nonroutine steps?
☐ How long will the case take?
☐ What is the anticipated blood loss?

To anesthetist:
☐ Are there any patient-specific concerns?

To nursing team:
☐ Has sterility (including indicator results) been confirmed?
☐ Are there equipment issues or any concerns?

Is essential imaging displayed?
☐ Yes
☐ Not applicable

Before patient leaves operating room
(with nurse, anesthetist and surgeon)

Nurse verbally confirms:
☐ The name of the procedure
☐ Completion of instrument, sponge and needle counts
☐ Specimen labeling (read specimen labels aloud, including patient name)
☐ Whether there are any equipment problems to be addressed

To surgeon, anesthetist and nurse:
☐ What are the key concerns for recovery and management of this patient?

This checklist is not intended to be comprehensive. Additions and modifications to fit local practice are encouraged.

Revised 1/2009 © WHO, 2009

Fig. 70.1: Surgical safety checklist.

---

renal failure). **Execution errors** occur when a physician is knowledgeable and skilled but makes a technical error even while following the correct procedures (e.g., a physician orders a wrong antibiotic dose for a patient with pneumococcal pneumonia). **Judgment errors** occur when a physician unnecessarily increases patient risk or willfully violates standards of care without a compelling reason.

Communication errors are considered the most common cause of medical errors and should be largely preventable by well-designed procedural policies and good execution. Professional communication among health care providers is a complex topic that is analogous to critical communications, as practiced by other high-risk professions. In addition, there are unique aspects to medical communication, including compassion, privacy, and the rich cultural heritage of medicine. Physicians can learn a lot from other high-risk professions with regard to good communication and avoidance of common communication pitfalls.

Errors in verbal communication are a common source of medical error.

Prevention of Verbal Communication Errors

1. Health care organizations should maintain policies that require printed prescriptions. If verbal orders are given, they should be read back orders and receive confirmation.
2. For critical test results and verbal or telephone orders, a "read-back" is required by the person receiving and recording the result or order, who must read back the order verbatim to the practitioner. The practitioner should verbally acknowledge the orders accuracy.
3. Clinicians should follow well-communicated protocols that guide care and communication.

4. Providers should listen to patient questions concerning how care is delivered.
5. To make patients active participants in avoiding medical errors, encourage patients to ask about unfamiliar tests, unplanned diagnostic tests, medications, and to verify the correct surgical site.

Written Errors

Using nonstandard abbreviations and illegible handwriting, failure to question inappropriately written orders, and failure to complete correct specimen labeling are common sources of written communication errors.

Prevention of Written Errors

1. Staff should never be reprimanded for questioning orders.
2. Healthcare professionals to use two or more patient identifiers when labeling, delivering and maintaining specimens.
3. Practitioners should always double-check that the patient's name is spelled correctly and their correct date of birth is present.

DOCUMENTATION

Documentation is a critical vehicle for conveying essential clinical information about each patient's diagnosis, treatment, and outcomes and for communication between clinicians and payers. Specifically in nursing, documentation helps to establish continuity of a patient's care, justify clinical reimbursement, safeguard providers from malpractice, and foster communication among rotating providers. One of the first and most important principles taught in nursing school is this: "If you did not document it, you did not do it." This rule is meant to protect both patients and providers. Nurses practice across settings at position levels from the bedside to the administrative office are responsible and accountable for the nursing documentation that is used throughout an organization.

For providers, patient records play an important role in the facility's ability to qualify for financial reimbursement from Medicare, Medicaid and other third-party payers. Additionally, health care facilities must meet stringent documentation standards. Meeting and exceeding charting standards also protect nurses providing care from possible ties to negligence or malpractice.

For patients, documentation ensures the delivery of safe, consistent, quality health care. Documentation is often the sole point of communication between nurses of changing shifts. This means that if no verbal conversation has taken place, the documented notes must be read by the incoming nurse in order to understand where in the care cycle the patient stands. In the case that a documentation error, or lack of documentation altogether, leads to a medical error that threatens a patient's life, the charting (or lack thereof) protects the patient in a court of law. Good health care providers should strive to improve their charting skills through ongoing continuing education opportunities. The health care arena is an ever-changing industry with many laws and regulations that have an impact on the documentation process.

Documentation of nurses' work is critical as well for effective communication with each other and with other disciplines. It is how nurses create a record of their services for use by payors, the legal system, government agencies, accrediting bodies, researchers, and other groups and individuals directly or indirectly involved with health care. It also provides a basis for demonstrating and understanding nursing's contributions both to patient care outcomes and to the viability and effectiveness of the organizations that provide and support quality patient care.

KEY POINTS

- **Patient safety indicators:** The patient safety indicators (PSIs) are a set of measures that screen for adverse events that patients experience as a result of exposure to the health care system.
- **Care of vulnerable patients:** Hospitalists may play a significant role in influencing the health status, health care access, and health care delivery to vulnerable populations due to their higher

rates of hospital utilization and lower access to outpatient care.
- **Prevention of iatrogenic injury:** Try to understand your treatments; after any procedures, remain aware of any potential adverse effects.
- **Care of lines, drains and tubing's:** It is done by various steps.
- **Restraint policy and care: physical and chemical**—The forcible confinement or control of a subject, as of a confused, disoriented, psychotic, or irrational person; it may be either physical or chemical.
- **Blood and blood transfusion policy:** For quality, safety and efficacy of blood and blood products, well-equipped blood centers with adequate infrastructure and trained manpower is an essential requirement. The Blood Bank or Blood Transfusion Service should have its own constitution, which defines the responsibility and authority of the management.
- **Prevention of IV complications:** (1) Infiltration; (2) Extravasation; (3) Phlebitis; (4) Hypersensitivity; (5) Infection
- **Fall prevention:** Some things that can be done to make your room safe so you do not fall.
- **Prevention of deep vein thrombosis (DVT):** DVT prophylaxis can be primary or secondary.
- **Transport of patients:** Appropriate precautions should be taken during transportation to reduce the risk of transmission of microorganisms to other patients, health care workers or the hospital environment (surfaces or equipment).
- **Surgical safety:** The Safe Surgery Saves Lives initiative aim is to harness political commitment and clinical will to address important safety issues, including inadequate anesthetic safety practices, avoidable surgical infection and poor communication among team members.
- **Medication reconciliation:** Medication reconciliation is the process of comparing a patient's new medication orders with all the medications the patient had been taking prior to changing levels of care.
- **Prevention of communication errors**—communication errors are considered the most common cause of medical errors and should be largely preventable by well-designed procedural policies and good execution. Errors in verbal communication are a common source of medical error.
- **Documentation:** Documentation is a critical vehicle for conveying essential clinical information about each patient's diagnosis, treatment, and outcomes and for communication between clinicians and payers.

IMPORTANT QUESTION

Write briefly on:
1. Patient Safety Indicators (PSIs)
2. Care of vulnerable patients
3. Prevention of iatrogenic injury
4. Prevention of communication errors
5. Care of lines, drains and tubing's
6. Restraint policy and care: Physical and chemical
7. Blood and blood transfusion policy
8. Prevention of IV complications
9. Fall prevention
10. Prevention of deep vein thrombosis (DVT)
11. Shifting and transporting of patients
12. Surgical safety
13. Medication reconciliation
14. Documentation

MULTIPLE CHOICE QUESTIONS

1. Patient safety indicators are defined on:
   a. Provider-level
   b. Area-level
   c. Provider-level and area-level
   d. None of the above
2. Restraint may be used as:
   a. Physical restraints
   b. Chemical restraints
   c. All of the above
   d. None of the above

ANSWERS

1. c   2. c

CHAPTER 71

Incidents and Adverse Events

LEARNING OBJECTIVES

After reading and studying this chapter, you should be able to:
- Describe capturing of incidents.
- Discuss root cause analysis.
- Describe report writing.

INTRODUCTION

Incident reporting is important for improving patient safety because it can lead to the identification of patient safety incidents (PSIs), defined by the World Health Organization as "event(s) or circumstance(s) that could have resulted, or did result, in unnecessary harm to a patient". PSI capture is a crucial step in patient safety improvement because it enables subsequent development and implementation of preventative measures.

The term "adverse event" describes harm to a patient as a result of medical care. Hospitals must track and analyze instances of patient harm as a condition of participation in the Medicare program. Incident reporting systems are a common means that hospitals use to meet this condition. Hospitals can demonstrate their compliance with this and all other conditions through a survey by a State Survey Agency or accreditation under an approved Medicare accreditation program. To standardize hospital event reporting, the Agency for Healthcare Research and Quality (AHRQ) developed a set of event definitions and incident reporting tools known as the Common Formats.

CAPTURING OF INCIDENTS

An incident report needs to include all the essential information about the accident or near-miss. The report-writing process begins with fact finding and ends with recommendations for preventing future accidents.

You may use a special incident reporting form, and it might be quite extensive. But writing any incident report involves four basic steps, and those are the focus of today's post.

1. Find the Facts

To prepare for writing an accident report, you have to gather and record all the facts. For example:
- Date, time, and specific location of incident
- Names, job titles, and department of employees involved and immediate supervisor(s)
- Names and accounts of witnesses
- Events leading up to incident
- Exactly what employee was doing at the moment of the accident
- Environmental conditions (e.g., slippery floor, inadequate lighting, noise, etc.)
- Circumstances (including tasks, equipment, tools, materials, PPE, etc.)

- Specific injuries (including part(s) of body injured and nature and extent of injuries)
- Type of treatment for injuries
- Damage to equipment, materials, etc.

2. Determine the Sequence

Based on the facts, you should be able to determine the sequence of events. In your report, describe this sequence in detail, including:

- **Events leading up to the incident:** Was the employee walking, running, bending over, squatting, climbing, lifting operating machinery, pushing a broom, turning a valve, using a tool, handling hazardous materials, etc.?
- **Events involved in the incident:** Was the employee struck by an object or caught in/on/between objects? Did the worker fall on the same level or from a height? Did the employee inhale hazardous vapors or get splashed with a hazardous chemical?
- **Events immediately following the incident:** What did the employee do: Grab a knee? Start limping? Hold his/her arm? Complain about back pain? Put a hand over a bleeding wound? Also, describe how other coworkers responded. Did they call for help, administer first aid, shutdown equipment, move the victim, etc.? The incident should be described on the report in sufficient detail that any reader can clearly picture what happened. You might consider creating a diagram to show, in a simple and visually effective manner, the sequence of events related to the incident and include this in your incident report. You might also wish to include photos of the accident scene, which may help readers follow the sequence of events.

3. Analyze

Your report should include an in-depth analysis of the causes of the accident. Causes include:

- Primary cause (e.g., a spill on the floor that caused a slip and fall)
- Secondary causes (e.g., employee not wearing appropriate work shoes or carrying a stack of material that blocked vision)
- Other contributing factors (e.g., burned out light bulb in the area).

4. Recommend

Recommendations for corrective action might include immediate corrective action as well as long-term corrective actions, such as:

- Employee training on safe work practices
- Preventive maintenance activities that keep equipment in good operating condition
- Evaluation of job procedures with a recommendation for changes
- Conducting a job on hazard analysis to evaluate the task for any other hazards and then train employees on these hazards
- Engineering changes that make the task safer or administrative changes that might include changing the way the task is performed

ROOT CAUSE ANALYSIS

Root cause analysis (RCA) is the process of discovering the root causes of problems in order to identify appropriate solutions. RCA assumes that it is much more effective to systematically prevent and solve for underlying issues rather than just treating ad hoc symptoms and putting out fires. Root cause analysis can be performed with a collection of principles, techniques, and methodologies that can all be leveraged to identify the root causes of an event or trend. Looking beyond superficial cause and effect, RCA can show where processes or systems failed or caused an issue in the first place.

Goals and benefits:
1. The first goal of root cause analysis is to discover the root cause of a problem or event.
2. The second goal is to fully understand how to fix, compensate, or learn from any underlying issues within the root cause.
3. The third goal is to apply what we learn from this analysis to systematically prevent future issues or to repeat successes.

Core Principles

There are a few core principles that guide effective root cause analysis, some of which should already be apparent. Not only will these help the analysis quality, these will also help the analyst to gain trust and buy-in from stakeholders, clients, or patients.

- Focus on correcting and remedying root causes rather than just symptoms.
- Do not ignore the importance of treating symptoms for short-term relief.
- Realize there can be, and often are, multiple root causes.
- Focus on HOW and WHY something happened, not WHO was responsible.
- Be methodical and find concrete cause-effect evidence to back up root cause claims.
- Provide enough information to inform a corrective course of action.
- Consider how a root cause can be prevented (or replicated) in the future.

As the above principles illustrate: When we analyze deep issues and causes, it is important to take a comprehensive and holistic approach. In addition, to discovering the root cause, we should strive to provide context and information that will result in an action or a decision. Remember: Good analysis is actionable analysis.

Tips for Performing Effective Root Cause Analysis

- Ask questions to clarify information and bring us closer to answers. The more we can drill down and interrogate every potential cause, the more likely we are to find a root cause. Once we believe we have identified the root cause of the problem (and not just another symptom), we can ask even more questions: Why are we certain this is the root cause instead of that? How can we fix this root cause to prevent the issue from happening again?
- Use simple questions, such as "Why?" "How?" and "so what does that mean here?" to carve a path toward understanding.

Work With a Team and Get Fresh Eyes

Whether it is just a partner or a whole team of colleagues, any extra eyes will help us figure out solutions faster and also serve as a check against bias. Getting input from others will also offer additional points of view, helping us to challenge our assumptions.

Plan for Future Root Cause Analysis

As we perform a root cause analysis, it is important to be aware of the process itself. Take notes. Ask questions about the analysis process itself. Find out if a certain technique or method works best for your specific business needs and environments.

Remember to Perform Root Cause Analysis for Successes Too

Root cause analysis is a great tool for figuring out where something went wrong. We typically use RCA as a way to diagnose problems but it can be equally as effective to find the root cause of a success. If we find the cause of a success or overachievement or early deadline, it is rarely a bad idea to find out the root cause of why things are going well. This kind of analysis can help to prioritize and pre-emptively protect key factors and we might be able to translate success in one area of business to success in another area.

REPORT WRITING

The Purpose of Reporting Adverse Events and Errors

- The primary purpose of patient safety reporting systems is to learn from experience. It is important to note that reporting in itself does not improve safety. It is the response to reports that leads to change. Within a health-care institution, reporting of a serious event or serious "near-miss" should trigger an in-depth investigation to identify underlying systems failures and lead to efforts to redesign the systems to prevent recurrence.
- In a state or national system, expert analyses of reports and dissemination of lessons learned are required if reports are to influence safety. Merely collecting data contributes little to patient safety advancement. Even monitoring for trends requires

considerable expert analysis and oversight of the reported data. The important point is that a reporting system must produce a visible, useful response by the receiver to justify the resources expended in reporting, or, for that matter, to stimulate individuals or institutions to report. The response system is more important than the reporting system.

- Adverse event reporting and learning systems should have as their main objective the improvement of patient safety through the identification of errors and hazards which may warrant further analysis and investigation in order to identify underlying systems factors report. The response system is more important than the reporting system.

Core Concepts

The four core principles underlying the guidelines are:
1. The fundamental role of patient safety reporting systems is to enhance patient safety by learning from failures of the healthcare system.
2. Reporting must be safe. Individuals who report incidents must not be punished or suffer other ill-effects from reporting.
3. Reporting is only of value if it leads to a constructive response. At a minimum, this entails feedback of findings from data analysis. Ideally, it also includes recommendations for changes in processes and systems of health care.
4. Meaningful analysis, learning, and dissemination of lessons learned requires expertise and other human and financial resources. The agency that receives reports must be capable of disseminating information, making recommendations for changes, and informing the development of solutions.

A successful reporting and learning system to enhance patient safety should have the following characteristics:
- Reporting is safe for the individuals who report;
- Reporting leads to a constructive response;
- Expertise and adequate financial resources are available to allow for meaningful analysis of reports; The reporting system must be capable of disseminating information on hazards and recommendations for changes.

KEY POINTS

- Incident reporting is important for improving patient safety because it can lead to the identification of patient safety incidents (PSIs), as "event (s) or circumstance (s) that could have resulted, or did result, in unnecessary harm to a patient".
- The term "adverse event" describes harm to a patient as a result of medical care.

Capturing of Incidents
- An incident report needs to include all the essential information about the accident or near-miss. The report-writing process begins with fact finding and ends with recommendations for preventing future accidents.
- Root cause analysis (RCA) is the process of discovering the root causes of problems in order to identify appropriate solutions.

Report Writing
The primary purpose of patient safety reporting systems is to learn from experience.

IMPORTANT QUESTION

Write short notes on:
1. Capturing of incidents.
2. Root cause analysis.
3. Report writing.

MULTIPLE CHOICE QUESTIONS

1. **Incident reporting is important:**
   a. For improving patient safety
   b. The identification of patient safety incidents
   c. All of the above
   d. None of the above
2. **Goals and benefits of root cause analysis:**
   a. To discover the root cause of a problem or event
   b. To fully understand how to fix, compensate, or learn from any underlying issues within the root cause
   c. To prevent future issues or to repeat successes
   d. All of the above

ANSWERS

1. c   2. d

CHAPTER 72
International Patient Safety Goals

LEARNING OBJECTIVES

After reading and studying this chapter, you should be able to:
- Describe International Patient Safety Goals (IPSG).
- Discuss applications of International Patient Safety Goals (IPSG) in the patient care system.

INTRODUCTION

These goals highlight problematic areas in health care. These promote specific improvements in patient safety, highlight problematic areas in health care and describe evidence- and expert-based consensus solutions to these problems.

INTERNATIONAL PATIENT SAFETY GOALS (IPSG)

1. Identify patients correctly
2. Improve effective communication
3. Improve the safety of high-alert medications
4. Ensure correct-site, correct-procedure, and correct patient surgery
5. Reduce the risk of healthcare-associated infections
6. Reduce the risk of patient harm resulting from falls

APPLICATIONS OF INTERNATIONAL PATIENT SAFETY GOALS (IPSG) IN THE PATIENT CARE SYSTEM

IPSG.1 Identify Patients Correctly

The hospital develops and implements a process to improve accuracy of patient identification.

Two-fold Intent

First: To identify the individual as the person for whom the service or treatment is intended.

Second: To match the service or treatment to that individual.

- Patients must be identified using **"two unique identifiers,"** i.e., Full Name and Medical Record Number (MRN)
- MUST NEVER use patient's room or location to identify patient.
- Patients are identified before providing treatments and procedures, e.g.,
  - Administering medications, blood, or blood products;
  - Serving a restricted diet tray;
  - Providing radiation therapy,
  - Taking blood and other specimens for clinical testing
  - Performing cardiac catheterization or diagnostic radiology procedure

IPSG. 2 Improve effective communication

The hospital develops and implements a process to improve the effectiveness of verbal and/or telephone communication among caregivers.

Verbal medication orders are reserved for code/emergency situations ONLY.
- When receiving a medication telephone order from a physician:
  - Nurse A writes the order in the physician order sheet.
  - Nurse B will read back the order written by Nurse A to the physician.
  - The prescriber will verify the order is correct to Nurse B.

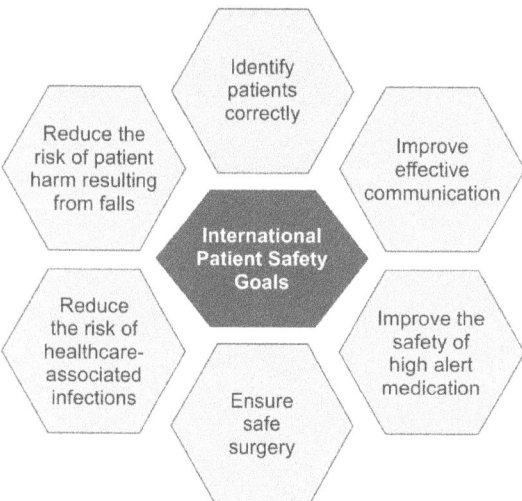

Fig. 72.1: Process for reporting critical results of diagnostic tests.

- Both nurse A and nurse B must document the date and time the order was received, badge number of the prescriber, and their own names, job title and badge numbers and both must sign the order sheet.

The hospital develops and implements a process for reporting critical results of diagnostic tests **(Fig. 72.1)**.

IPSG 2.1

- The technologist/reporter will provide the report to the Receiver (Requesting Physician/Ward Nurse).
- The receiver will document (hand-WRITE) the critical results.
- The receiver (or another person–could be another nurse) will READ BACK the information provided, including the patient's medical record number and name to the reporter.
- The technologists/reporter will verify the information is correct.
- Both the reporter and the receiver must document the READ BACK verification procedure was carried out; date and time the report was received, badge number of the person providing/receiving the report.

IPSG 2.2

The hospital develops and implements a process for handover communication.

IPSG. 3 Improve the Safety of High-Alert Medications

The hospital develops and implements a process to improve the safety of high-alert medications.

Look–alike, sound–alike and high-alert medications

High-Alert Medications

Medications that pose an increased risk of causing significant harm to patients if used in error.

Independent double checks in handling is one of the safety measures.

High-Alert Medications are:
- Medications involved in a high percentage of errors and/or sentinel events
- Medications that carry a higher risk for adverse outcomes
- Look-alike/sound-alike medications
  - Use TALL man Lettering labels for (Look-alike, sound-alike) LASA medications that are available via the Intranet, One Stop Resource.
  - Look-Alike, Sound-Alike medications without approved TALL Man Lettering will be labeled as "Name Alert".
  - Be aware of automated alerts/advisories for LASA medications that are in the HIS-CPR System.
  - Logistics and contracts management will consider the list of look-alike, sound-alike medications in the process of medication procurement.

IPSG.4 Ensure Correct-Site, Correct-Procedure, Correct-Patient Surgery

The hospital develops and implements a process for ensuring correct-site, correct-procedure, and correct-patient surgery.

Marking the surgical site should:
- Be made by the person performing the procedure with a permanent skin marker.

- Take place with the patient AWAKE and AWARE, if possible.
- Be done in all cases involving laterality (right, left), multiple structures (fingers, toes, lesions) or multiple levels or region (spine).
- Be done using an instantly recognizable mark (ARROW as per policy) that is consistent throughout the hospital.

TIME OUT–Pause with a purpose:
- Full verification that is performed immediately prior to the induction of anesthesia or the start of an invasive procedure
- **The entire care team actively and verbally presence and confirms:**
  - Patient's identity (two identifiers)
  - Procedure to be performed
  - Correct procedure side/site
  - Necessary imaging, equipment, implants or special requirements are present.

IPSG. 5 Reduce the Risk of Health Care-associated Infections

The hospital adopts and implements evidence-based hand-hygiene guidelines to reduce the risk of health care–associated infections.

Infection Control Manager (ICM)–II–04 Hand Hygiene

Reduce the risk of healthcare–associated infections:
- Wash hands with soap and water when hands are visibly soiled.
- Use alcohol-based hand rub when hands are not visibly soiled
- qABHR is ineffective—spore forming bacteria, e.g., *Clostridium difficile*.

Always remember: Wash your hands!!!!

IPSG.6 Reduce the Risk of Patient Harm Resulting from Falls

The hospital develops and implements a process to reduce the risk of patient harm resulting from falls.
- A process for assessing all inpatients and outpatients—identifies them as at high risk for falls.
- A process for the initial and ongoing assessment, reassessment, and interventions.
- Have measures implemented to reduce fall risk.
- Upon initial admission assessment, Physicians should screen Patient's Functional status which include "FALL RISK".
- Functional screening should be documented in the physicians history and physical form complimented by nurses' assessment.
- Communicate to nurses for implementation.

Multidisciplinary Team Effort
- Nurses
- Pharmacists
- Physiotherapist
- Physicians

KEY POINTS

International Patient Safety Goals (IPSG)
1. Identify patients correctly.
2. Improve effective communication.
3. Improve the safety of high-alert medications.
4. Ensure correct-site, correct-procedure, and correct patient surgery.
5. Reduce the risk of healthcare-associated infections.
6. Reduce the risk of patient harm resulting from falls.

IMPORTANT QUESTIONS

1. What are **International Patient Safety Goals (IPSG)**? Write briefly on them.
2. Write short notes on:
   a. Applications of International Patient Safety goals (IPSG) in the patient care system.

MULTIPLE CHOICE QUESTION

1. Applications of International Patient Safety Goals (IPSG) in the patient care system:
   a. Identify patients correctly
   b. Improve effective communication
   c. Improve the safety of high-alert medications
   d. All of the above.

ANSWER

1. d

CHAPTER 73

Safety Protocol

LEARNING OBJECTIVES

After reading and studying this chapter, you should be able to:
- Describe High 5s project.
- Discuss safe operating parameters.
- Describe the following: radiation safety; laser safety; fire safety; hazmat safety; spillage management; environmental safety; MSDS; environment health safety (EHS); audits; emergency codes; role of nurse in times of disaster.

HIGH 5s PROJECT

The High 5s project is a global patient safety initiative of the World Health Organization (WHO) to facilitate the development, implementation and evaluation of Standard Operating Protocols (SOPs) within a global learning community to achieve measurable, significant and sustainable reductions in challenging patient safety problems.

The objective of the High 5s initiative is to achieve a significant, sustained and measurable reduction in the occurrence of five patient safety problems, over 5 years, in at least seven countries, and to build an international collaborative learning network that fosters the sharing of knowledge and experience in implementing innovative standard operating protocols (SOPs). The project is best characterized as applying standardized patient care processes to improving patient safety and in evaluating the impact of these.

Working together, the High 5s partners achieve objectives that no single organization or patient safety agency could achieve individually. These include:

In action, the High 5s project draws on the specific strengths of its current and former partners. Since, the project's initiation the following types of organizations have contributed to its activities:

A written safety protocol, also known as a **"Standard Operating Procedure"**, is a document that includes the safety requirements developed in the risk assessment. It is used to ensure that everyone in the laboratory knows and understands the hazards, risks and protective measures needed to perform the procedure. There is no required format for this written protocol, but these Safety Protocol templates can be used and should become part of the research plan.

The information from your hazard and risk assessment is used to develop safe operating parameters. Developing safe operating parameters allows you to conduct research and change variables (i.e., substituting solvents, changing concentration or quantity, increasing temperature, etc.) without having to conduct a new hazard review and write a new safety protocol. These limits are critical when scaling up a procedure.

Safe Operating Parameters

The process limits need to be defined and included in the written procedures. This information must be conveyed to everyone working on procedure **(Box 73.1)**.

> **Box 73.1:** Information that needs to be included in the Safety Protocol.

1. List all Personal Protective Equipment (PPE) needed for the procedure. Be specific on type of gloves or eyewear needed.
2. List all chemicals (including concentration), biological materials and equipment needed for the procedure. Include chemical concentrations, catalog numbers, equipment names, model numbers, etc. Remember that liquid nitrogen, dry ice and compressed gases are hazardous materials.
3. List hazards of chemicals and biological material used in the procedure.
4. List any special emergency equipment needed (i.e., eyewash, spill kit, dry sand/Class D fire extinguisher, HF antidote, effective disinfectant).
5. List waste disposal requirements (chemical, biological waste, sharps containers).
6. Describe any anticipated problems that may occur while performing this procedure, the course of action to be taken, including the job title to consult/report to if problem occurs.

The written "safety protocol" must be made available to everyone working on the procedure. It can be used to train new researchers on the different protocols used in the laboratory. It ensures that everyone gets the information they need to conduct science safely.

RADIATION SAFETY

A radiation protection program (RPP) is one means of implementing occupational radiation protection by the adoption of appropriate management structures, policies, procedures and organizational arrangements. For medical staff in X-ray imaging, topics would include the need for local rules and procedures for personnel to follow, arrangements for the provision of personal protective equipment, a program for education and training in radiation protection, arrangements for individual monitoring, and methods for periodically reviewing and auditing the performance of the RPP.

The radiation protection measures should be designed, planned and implemented with the advice of the radiation protection officer and of the physician in charge of health surveillance, taking into account national regulations and the requirements of this code.

Preventive Measures

1. Inhalation, swallowing or direct contact with the skin should be avoided.
2. In case of X-rays, shielding should be used of such thickness and of such material as to reduce the exposure below allowable exposure.
3. The employee should be monitored at intervals not exceeding 6 months by the use of film badge or pocket electrometer devices.
4. Suitable protective clothing to prevent contact with harmful material should be used.
5. Adequate ventilation of work place is necessary to prevent inhalation of harmful gases and dusts
6. Replacement and periodic examination of workers should be done every 2 months. If harmful effects are found, the employee should be transferred to work not involving exposure to radiation.
7. Pregnant women should not be allowed to work in places where there is continuous exposure.

LASER SAFETY

1. **Wear laser safety glasses:** With the significant damage lasers can cause to your eyes, it is imperative that you are wearing the correct laser safety glasses. The wavelength range (in nanometers) and optical density measurements are imprinted on the glasses to help you match with your laser. Laser glasses should be worn throughout the entire procedure, taking them off during any laser application can lead to harmful effects.
2. **Utilize proper storage:** It is important to properly store laser glasses and equipment.

Protective eyewear should be stored in an individual case or protective unit to keep from scratches and contaminants. A comparable unit would be the Clearly Safe Acrylic Safety Eyeglass Dispenser, giving you the ability to store multiple pairs safely. When laser glasses are damaged it can compromise the protection level.

3. **Follow standards and regulations:** Healthcare facilities is to follow their laser safety standards and regulations.
4. **Work with trained personnel:** An individual working around high-powered lasers is required to have had proper training and education. Accidents can easily occur in laser procedures resulting in the loss or damage of vision. Well trained personnel will significantly reduce the risk of accidental laser exposure. A trained laser operator will know how to align the laser correctly, making sure to position the laser beam above or below the normal eye levels of seated and standing personnel. The initial machine alignment can take as little as 15 minutes but should be carefully done to ensure the highest safety measures.
5. **Use Warning Signs (Fig. 73.1):** Safety and warning signs can help your medical staff and patients be aware of caution areas in your facility. Throughout your controlled laser areas, easy-to-read signs should be posted in appropriate locations. (i.e., entrance of procedure rooms). You also will want to consider posting signs that indicate the type of reflective gear to avoid wearing during laser procedures. Some of these items include reflective identification badges, jewelry and tools.

Safety measures and policies should be enforced where all high-powered lasers are used. It is critical to keep physicians, staff and patients protected against harmful laser radiation.

FIRE SAFETY

Classes of Fires

Four classes of fires:
1. **Class A:** Ordinary solid combustibles, such as paper, wood, cloth and some plastics.
2. **Class B:** Flammable liquids, such as alcohol, ether, oil, gasoline and grease, which are best extinguished by smothering.
3. **Class C:** Electrical equipment, appliances and wiring in which the use or a nonconductive extinguishing agent prevents injury from electrical shock. Do not use water.
4. **Class D:** Certain flammable metallic substances such as sodium and potassium. These materials are normally not found in the Medical Center.

Fire Extinguishers

Portable extinguishers are useful for putting out small fires; however, they are not effective against large, spreading fires. In these situations, doors should be closed to contain the fire.

Types of Fire Extinguishers

Fire extinguishers are classified as types A, ABC, BC or K. It is important to use the right type of extinguisher on the specific class of fire to avoid personal injury or damage to property. The wrong type of extinguisher could cause electrical shock, explosion, or spread the fire.

Type A: Pressurized water to be used on Class A fire only. Do not use on Class B or C fires; may cause fire spread or electrical shock.

Type ABC: Dry chemical effective on all classes of fires.

Type BC: Carbon dioxide to be used on chemical or electrical fires.

Type K: Used in kitchens on grease fires.

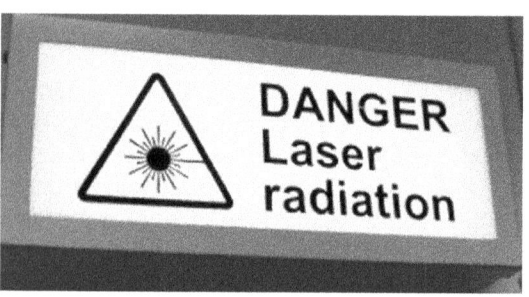

Fig. 73.1: Warning sign.

Locations

ABC fire extinguishers are located throughout the medical centers in corridors. Specialty areas, such as the operating rooms and kitchens have specific extinguishers.

Using a Fire Extinguisher

To use a fire extinguisher, follow the acronym **PASS**

Pull: Pull the pin on the extinguisher

Aim: Aim the nozzle at the base of the fire

Squeeze: Squeeze the trigger to release the product

Sweep: Sweep the nozzle from side to side (slowly)

General fire response procedures must be implemented immediately upon suspicion of a fire.

In the event of a SUSPECTED or CONFIRMED FIRE, remain calm and immediately do the following:

RACE: Remove, Alarm, Contain, and Extinguish

- **Remove** patients and personnel from the immediate fire area if safe to do so.
- Activate **Alarm** and notify others.
- Activate nearest audible fire alarm by pulling the handle down on alarm.
  - Report the fire to either the Medical Center Communications or the Police Department by dialing.
  - **Provide the following information:**
    - Location of event including building, floor and room number
    - Description of problem
    - Your name
  - Notify other staff members in the area and obtain assistance
- **Contain** the fire and the smoke by closing all doors leading into and surrounding the fire area. Do not lock them.
- **Extinguish** the fire if safe to do so or **Evacuate**—if the fire cannot be extinguished safely, evacuate the area horizontally to the next safest smoke compartment.

Do not open any door without first feeling it near the top. If it is hot, do not open the door.

If it is not safe to evacuate horizontally, evacuate vertically down a safe stairwell to the designated vertical evacuation staging floor/unit.

HAZMAT (HAZARDOUS MATERIALS) SAFETY

Hazardous materials (hazmat) are any material that has properties that may result in risk or injury to health and/or destruction of life or facilities. Many hazardous materials (hazmat) do not have a taste or an odor. Some can be detected because they cause physical reactions, such as watering eyes or nausea. Some hazardous materials exist beneath the surface of the ground and have an oil or foam-like appearance. The substance can be identified from placards, labels or markings on the transporters.

SPILL

A spill is defined as when used with reference to a pollutant, means a discharge:

- Into the natural environment
- From or out of a structure, vehicle or other container, and
- That is abnormal in quality or quantity in light of all the circumstances of the discharge.

Types of Spills

There are various types of spills that require attention. This list includes:

- Gas leak
- Oil spill
- Solid
- Liquid
- Biological
- Radioactive
- Mixed
- Unknown

Spillage Management

No matter what type of spill is present, the first step is always informing people in the surrounding area. If the spill is a major spill, contact Protection; they are responsible for securing the spill area and contacting the Office of Risk Management (ORM). For gas leaks, major oil spills and facility breakdowns, the ORM will work in conjunction with the Faculty of Science HSR and Facilities staff to address the issue.

For minor user generated solid or liquid spills, it is the responsibility of the user/researcher to clean the spill. If the user is unsure how to clean the spill or would like some advice on how to mitigate the spill, HSR can be contacted for information.

For a biological spill, please contact the Biosafety Office at the Office of Risk Management.

For a radioactive spill, contact the Radiation Safety Office at the Office of Risk Management.

Make every effort to identify a mixed or unknown spill. This information may greatly reduce the hazards involved in handling and classifying the material. Include the name of the research group, telephone number, type of research, storage method, approximate age of the container and all relevant information (i.e., organic, acid, air reactive, pH, oxidizer, etc.).

How to Clean a Spill—minor spills are to be cleaned by the user. The user must ensure that they are wearing the proper PPE and clean the spill.

MATERIAL SAFETY DATA SHEET (MSDS) OR SAFETY DATA SHEET (SDS)

Material Safety Data Sheet (MSDS) is a technical document which provides detailed and comprehensive information, such as the properties of each chemical; the physical, health, and environmental health hazards; protective measures; and safety precautions for handling, storing, and transporting the chemical.

It provides guidance for each specific chemical on things, such as:
- Personal protective equipment (PPE)
- First aid procedures
- Spill clean-up procedures

The data sheet may be written, printed or otherwise expressed, and must meet the availability, design and content requirements of legislation. The legislation provides for flexibility of design and wording but requires that a minimum number of categories of information be completed and that all hazardous ingredients meeting certain criteria be listed subject to exemptions granted under the Hazardous Materials Information Review Act.

Medical Access

Doctors and nurses can access withheld information however this information remains confidential.

ENVIRONMENT, HEALTH AND SAFETY (EHS)

Environment (E), health (H) and safety (S) (together **EHS**) is a discipline and specialty that studies and implements practical aspects of environmental protection and safety at work. In simple terms, it is what organizations must do to make sure that their activities do not cause harm to anyone.

From a **safety** standpoint, it involves creating organized efforts and procedures for identifying workplace hazards and reducing accidents and exposure to harmful situations and substances. It also includes training of personnel in accident prevention, accident response, emergency preparedness, and use of protective clothing and equipment.

Better **health** at its heart, should have the development of safe, high quality, and environmentally friendly processes, working practices and systemic activities that prevent or reduce the risk of harm to people in general, operators, or patients.

From an **environmental** standpoint, it involves creating a systematic approach to complying with environmental regulations, such as managing waste or air emissions all the way to helping site's reduce the company's carbon footprint.

Regulatory requirements play an important role in EHS discipline and EHS managers must identify and understand relevant EHS regulations, the implications of which must be communicated to executive management so the company can implement suitable measures.

Government is committed to regulate all economic activities for management of safety and health risks at workplaces and to provide measures so as to ensure safe and healthy working conditions for every working man and woman in the nation. The formulation of policy, priorities and strategies in occupational safety, health and environment at work places, is undertaken by national authorities in consultation with social partners for fulfilling such objectives. A critical role is played by the Government and the social partners, professional safety and health organizations in ensuring prevention and in also providing treatment, support and rehabilitation services. The policy seeks to bring the national objectives into focus as a step toward improvement in safety, health and environment at workplace.

What is EHS Risk Assessment?

An **EHS risk assessment** is a formal process to identify potential environmental, health and safety hazards related to your organization's operations. Conducting an EHS risk assessment can help you determine which risks pose the greatest threat to your operations, and identify controls to reduce the level of risk.

You should conduct a risk assessment any time a hazard is identified, or there's a change to your operations that could introduce new risks.

Since, there are so many different types of EHS risk, EHS risk assessments can vary widely in scope.

Steps to conduct an effective EHS risk assessment.

Review and monitor: In general, effective risk assessments follow this four-step process:
1. Identify hazards
2. Determine who might be harmed and how
3. Evaluate and prioritize
4. Implement controls

Aspect Impact Analysis

Environmental Aspects

In simple terms an environmental aspect is anything resulting from the organization's activities, products or services that has the potential to cause an environmental impact, even if it is presently controlled, or prevent such impact. The fact that the potential exists (if something goes wrong, for instance) makes it an environmental aspect. An environmental aspect can be either negative or positive. Negative aspects include emissions to the air or water, discharge of oil to the land or water, generation of hazardous waste, generation of solid waste, community impact, and the generation of dust and noise. Positive aspects include recycling of used materials, such as steel, aluminum, copper, glass bottles and paper, removal of pollutants from the air or water, and restoring land by removing decontaminated soil.

Environmental Impact

An environmental impact is any change to the environment, whether adverse or beneficial, wholly or partially resulting from the organization's activities, products or services. Essentially, the environmental impact is the result of the environmental aspect. For example, suppose a company is discharging wastewater to a nearby stream. A potential environmental impact of that activity is pollution to the water.

Examine Company Operations

Form a multidisciplinary team examining a company's operations helps one determine what environmental aspects/impacts it produces. One way to start this process is to form a team. Team members should bring different attributes to the group to allow for a holistic solution. Once the team is formed, it must select a method to document and track progress. Many different strategies exist for selecting which area to address first. One area to be addressed should be all permitted and regulatory areas to ensure that a company is operating legally.

Requirements

The Model Guidance document defines minimum standards for temperature and humidity monitoring and alarm systems and components, and for the operational management of these systems.

Temperature Monitoring Systems
Air temperature monitoring systems and devices should be installed in all temperature controlled rooms, cold rooms, freezer rooms, refrigerators and freezers used to store "time and temperature sensitive pharmaceutical product (TTSPP):TTSPPs". Electronic sensors should be accurate to $\pm$ 0.5°C or better 4. Sensors should be located in areas where the greatest variability in temperature is expected to occur within the qualified storage volume and they should be positioned so as to be minimally affected by transient events such as door opening.

Humidity Monitoring Systems
Humidity monitoring systems and devices should be used in temperature-controlled rooms that are used to store TTSPPs that require a humidity-controlled environment. Monitoring sensors should be accurate to $\pm$ 5% RH and located to monitor worst-case humidity levels within the qualified storage volume and they should be positioned so as to be minimally affected by transient events, such as door opening.

Alarm Systems
Temperature, and where necessary, humidity alarm systems should be linked to the monitoring system(s) with high and low alarm set points. There should be a visual alarm and also preferably an audible alarm, together with automatic telephone dial-up or SMS text warnings to key personnel.

Environment Health Safety (EHS) Audits

An EHS audit refers to relevant protocols and each of checklist items, reviews the client's existing EHS management system, regular operations and the procedures and records of such system and operations, and have interviews with the client's person in charge. The violation of laws and problems requiring improvements identified in the audit are summarized as findings, and propose measures to improve these individual findings.

EMERGENCY CODES

An emergency code is a notification of an event that requires immediate action. Preparing for the Unexpected emergencies can strike anywhere and at any time. In the spirit of proactivity, we encourage you to have your own emergency preparedness plan.

Hospital emergency codes are used in hospitals worldwide to alert staff to various emergencies. The use of codes is intended to convey essential information quickly and with minimal misunderstanding to staff, while preventing stress and panic among visitors to the hospital. These codes may be posted on placards throughout the hospital, or printed on employee identification badges for ready reference. Back of a hospital ID badge showing disaster codes. Hospital emergency codes may denote different events at different hospitals, including those in the same community. Because many physicians work at more than one facility, this may lead to confusion in emergencies, so uniform systems have been proposed.

Types of Codes (Fig. 73.2)
Some of the more widely used codes in hospitals include:
- **Code pink:** Infant or child abduction
- **Code orange:** Hazardous material or spill incident
- **Code silver:** Active shooter
- **Code violet:** Violent or combative individual
- **Code yellow:** Disaster
- **Code brown:** Severe weather
- **Code white:** Evacuation
- **Code green:** Emergency activation

How is an Emergency Code Called
The code should be called in a three-part statement to include alert category, specific code description, and location of emergency, for example, "Medical alert, cardiac arrest, Room 231." Additional information or instructions

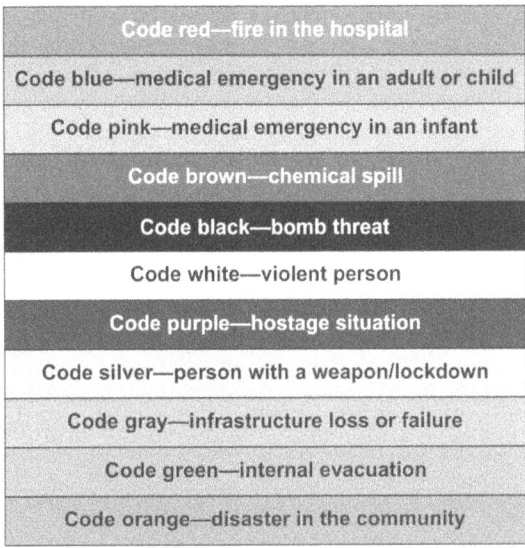

Fig. 73.2: Types of codes.

can be provided if known—for example, the description of a missing person.

Benefits to the Public

Hospital emergency codes are extremely important to the safety of people inside a hospital. Hospital employees, including doctors, undergo extensive training to respond to each of these events, allowing them to save lives. One of the primary benefits of a code system is that trained hospital employees know to respond to any given emergency without alarming those being treated and hospital visitors. Panicked bystanders can hinder the response efforts of emergency responders.

ROLE OF NURSE IN TIMES OF DISASTER

Disasters are catastrophic events that often result in extensive property damage and loss of life. Extreme devastation can occur from both man-made and natural disasters. Nurses play a major role in responding to disasters to help ensure the best possible outcomes. They usually have a desire to help, but they do not always know where to start. Nurses serve a critical role in emergency preparedness at the local, state, and national levels through planning, community and consumer education, and direct care provided during disasters. Nurses often facilitate communication and coordinate care among members of the health care team, patients, and their families during a disaster.

If inadequately prepared, a nurse can be more of a hindrance than a help in disaster relief efforts. The best time to prepare for a disaster is before it occurs. The unpredictable and chaotic events accompanying a disaster can leave people feeling helpless. A nurse can alleviate the helplessness by supporting those in need of care and empowering them with education. We cannot always predict when disaster will strike, but we can count on nurses to lend a helping hand. Extensive knowledge, adaptability, familiarity with a variety of settings, and a compassionate nature are only a few of the qualities that make nurses an essential resource for disaster response.

Nurses serve as an essential resource and can hold a wide range of responsibilities related to disaster preparedness and response including:

1. **Serving within their organization.** Developing an understanding of the disaster preparedness and response plans, operational protocols, and security measures can help nurses understand what their employers expect of them.
2. **Providing education.** Educating consumers and the community gives them the knowledge they need to make it safely through a disaster and help others. Knowledge can also do much to alleviate fear and anxiety.
3. **Volunteering.** Nurses who volunteer and become involved with an organized disaster response system are better prepared when disaster strikes. A few organizations that offer opportunities to assist with relief efforts include the American Red Cross, the Federal Emergency Management Agency (FEMA), and the United States Public Health Service (PHS).
4. **Assisting during a disaster.** A nurse may be assigned a variety of tasks during a disaster such as delivering first aid and medication,

assessing the state of victims, and monitoring mental health needs.
5. **Preparing self and family.** Some nurses have family members who rely on them. Personal preparation with an emergency plan and basic emergency supplies can help to ensure their families' safety while easing the nurse's worries. Other things to consider include arranging a meeting place if separated, ensuring reliable communication, and compiling important paperwork.

KEY POINTS

- The High 5s project is a global patient safety initiative of the World Health Organization (WHO) to facilitate the development, implementation and evaluation of Standard Operating Protocols (SOPs) within a global learning community to achieve measurable, significant and sustainable reductions in challenging patient safety problems.
- **Radiation safety:** A radiation protection program (RPP) is one means of implementing occupational radiation protection by the adoption of appropriate management structures, policies, procedures and organizational arrangements.
- **Laser safety:** 1. Wear laser safety glasses; 2. Utilize proper storage; 3. Follow standards and regulations; 4. Work with trained personnel; 5. Use warning signs.
- **Fire safety:** Four classes of fires—Class A; Class B; Class C; Class D.
  - Types of fire extinguishers: Type A; Type ABC; Type BC; Type K.
- **Hazmat (Hazardous materials) safety:** Hazardous materials (hazmat) are any material that has properties that may result in risk or injury to health and/or destruction of life or facilities.
- **Spill:** A spill is defined as when used with reference to a pollutant, means a discharge, (a) into the natural environment, (b) from or out of a structure, vehicle or other container, and (c) that is abnormal in quality or quantity in light of all the circumstances of the discharge.
- **Spillage management:** No matter what type of spill is present, the first step is always informing people in the surrounding area. If the spill is a major spill, contact protection. For minor user generated solid or liquid spills, it is the responsibility of the user/researcher to clean the spill.
- **How to clean a spill:** Minor spills are to be cleaned by the user. The user must ensure that they are wearing the proper PPE and clean the spill.
- **Material Safety Data Sheet (MSDS) or Safety Data Sheet (SDS):** Material Safety Data Sheet (MSDS) is a technical document which provides detailed and comprehensive information, such as the properties of each chemical; the physical, health, and environmental health hazards; protective measures; and safety precautions for handling, storing, and transporting the chemical.
- **Environment, health and safety (EHS):** Environment (E), health (H) and safety (S) (together EHS) is a discipline and specialty that studies and implements practical aspects of environmental protection and safety at work. In simple terms, it is what organizations must do to make sure that their activities do not cause harm to anyone.
- An **EHS risk assessment** is a formal process to identify potential environmental, health and safety hazards related to your organization's operations.
- **Environmental aspects:** In simple terms, an environmental aspect is anything resulting from the organization's activities, products or services that has the potential to cause an environmental impact, even if it is presently controlled, or prevent such impact.
- **Environmental impact:** An environmental impact is any change to the environment, whether adverse or beneficial, wholly or partially resulting from the organization's activities, products or services. Essentially, the environmental impact is the result of the environmental aspect.
- **Emergency codes:** Hospital emergency codes are used in hospitals worldwide to alert staff to various emergencies. The use of codes is intended to convey essential information quickly and with minimal misunderstanding to staff, while preventing stress and panic among visitors to the hospital. These codes may be posted on placards throughout the hospital, or printed on employee identification badges for ready reference. Back of a hospital ID badge showing disaster codes. Hospital emergency codes may denote different events at different hospitals, including those in the same community. Because many physicians work at more than one facility, this may lead to confusion in emergencies, so uniform systems have been proposed.
- **Types of codes:**
  1. **Code blue:** Cardiac arrest
  2. **Code red:** External disaster

3. **Code brown:** Internal disaster
4. **Code pink:** Baby disaster
5. **Code grey:** Security threats/workplace violence
6. **Code orange:** Medical emergency team (MET) codes shall be announced thrice over the PA system and shall be repeated every 30 seconds for 2 minutes. Mock drills at least every 6 months in all shifts and done areas specific especially in vulnerable areas, such as OT, ICUs, dialysis, etc.

- **Role of nurse in times of disaster:** Nurses play a major role in responding to disasters to help ensure the best possible outcomes. Nurses serve a critical role in emergency preparedness at the local, state, and national levels through planning, community and consumer education, and direct care provided during disasters. Nurses often facilitate communication and coordinate care among members of the healthcare team, patients, and their families during a disaster.

IMPORTANT QUESTION

Write briefly on:
1. 5S.
2. Radiation safety.
3. Laser safety.
4. Fire safety.
5. Types and classification of fire.
6. Fire alarms.
7. Firefighting equipment.
8. Hazmat safety.
9. Types of spill.
10. Spillage management.
11. MSDS.
12. Environmental safety:
    - Risk assessment
    - Aspect impact analysis
    - Maintenance of temperature and humidity (Department wise)
    - Audits
    - Emergency codes
13. Role of nurse in times of disaster.

MULTIPLE CHOICE QUESTIONS

1. **Information that needs to be included in the safety protocol:**
   a. List all personal protective equipment (PPE)
   b. List hazards of chemicals and biological material
   c. List any special emergency equipment needed
   d. All of the above.

2. **Classes of fires are:**
   a. Class A and B
   b. Class B and C
   c. Class A, B, and C
   d. Class A, B, C, D

3. **Hospital emergency codes are used in hospitals:**
   a. To alert staff to various emergencies
   b. For safety of hospital employees
   c. For safety of patients in the hospital
   d. None of the above

ANSWERS

1. d   2. d   3. a

Employee Safety Indicators

LEARNING OBJECTIVES

After reading and studying this chapter, you should be able to:
- Describe employee safety indicators.
- Discuss fall prevention.
- Describe annual health checkup.

EMPLOYEE SAFETY INDICATORS

One way to improve the effectiveness of your safety process is to change the way, it is measured. Measurement is an important part of any management process and forms the basis for continuous improvement. Measuring safety performance is not different and effectively doing so will compound the success of your improvement efforts.

Finding the perfect measure of safety is a difficult task. What you want is to measure both the bottom-line results of safety as well as how well your facility is doing at preventing accidents and incidents. To do this, you will use a combination of lagging and leading indicators of safety performance.

1. Leading Indicators

Leading indicators, one type of accident precursor, are conditions, events or measures that precede an undesirable event and that have some value in predicting the arrival of the event, whether it is an accident, incident, near miss, or undesirable safety state. Leading indicators are associated with proactive activities that identify hazards and assess, eliminate, minimize, and control risk. Leading indicators are focused on future safety performance and continuous improvement. These measures are proactive in nature and report what employees are doing on a regular basis to prevent injuries.

2. Lagging Indicators

Lagging indicators, in contrast, are measures of a system that are taken after events, which measure outcomes and occurrences. These are the traditional safety metrics used to indicate progress toward compliance with safety rules. These are the bottom-line numbers that evaluate the overall effectiveness of safety at your facility. They tell you how many people got hurt and how badly.

FALL PREVENTION

Although, fall prevention in hospitals typically focuses on patients, it is important to recognize the impact on workers, visitors, and others as well. Multiple factors place patients at risk for falls while in healthcare facilities, including compromised cognitive and physical status, disorientation, effects of medication, age, and balance and mobility issues. Falls cause physical harm and psychological distress, and fall-related injuries can impair rehabilitation, increase length of stay, and escalate the cost of care.

Interventions to Prevent Falls

Specific interventions to prevent falls include the following:

1. **Keep floors clean and dry. Contaminants on walking surfaces, such as water, grease,

and soap are common risk factors in healthcare facilities.
- Promote prompt reporting of observed hazards (such as spills and obstructions) by patients and visitors, as well as staff.
- Encourage workers to clean or cover spills promptly.
- Install spill clean-up materials, such as wall mounted spill pads or paper towel dispensers throughout the facility and near drinking fountains for quick and easy access.
- Make floor signs readily available to warn of wet or slippery floors.
- Place umbrella sleeves/bags available near building entrances.
- Place water-absorbent mats with beveled edges as wide as the entrance area. Ideally, mats should be of sufficient size to remove all water, ice, and snow from the soles of shoes, so that no tracks are on the flooring surface beyond the last mat.
- Prominently, post and disseminate housekeeping contact information (telephone or beeper numbers) as part of a general awareness campaign.

2. **Prevent entry to wet areas**
   - Use barriers and special signage to block access to wet areas.
   - Block off areas where floor wax is being stripped or applied and use a doorstop to prevent wax overflow to adjacent areas.
   - Promptly remove (within 10 minutes) "wet floor" signs when flooring is dry.

3. **Housekeeping**
   - Keep walkways clear of objects and reduce clutter.
   - Address the risk from electrical and equipment cords in the following ways:
     – Secure loose cords and wires with cord organizers in patient rooms, operating rooms, computer stations, and other high-traffic areas.
     – Use retractable cord holders for phones in patient rooms and nursing stations.
     – Cover cords on floor with a beveled protective cover.
     – Organize operating rooms to minimize equipment cords across walkways.

4. **Ice and snow removal**
   - Prominently, post and disseminate contact information (telephone or beeper numbers) for snow removal staff.
   - Encourage home health and maintenance workers to use ice cleats.
   - Conveniently, place bins of ice-melting chemicals near outdoor stairs and heavily traveled walkways so that any employee can apply them if they notice icy patches.

ANNUAL HEALTH CHECKUP

An annual health checkup is a yearly visit to an individual's healthcare provider wherein the general condition of one's health is assessed. It is also known as a **routine physical examination, preventive health check, or master health checkup**. The benefits of undergoing an annual master health checkup have been under debate for quite some time, specifically in terms of its necessity when it comes to healthy individuals.

Benefits of Health Checkups

There are several advantages of regular health checkup with a doctor. One of the most important benefits is the **prevention of disease**. Preventive health checks are important especially, for individuals with risk factors for different health conditions. A master health checkup can also aid in the early detection and treatment of a health problem, which is valuable especially in cases of cancer. The examinations and laboratory tests that will be done during a health checkup vary depending on an individual's age, sex, family history, and lifestyle. Health checkups also promote **better patient-doctor relationships** and allow the doctor to promote healthy habits through patient education.

No need for yearly preventive health check for healthy individuals

Although medical experts used to advocate undergoing an annual health examination for all individuals, a lot of medical professionals have moved away from conducting yearly health checkups depending on the health condition of the individual.

Instead of an annual checkup, several medical groups now advocate Periodic Health Assessments which is done every 5 years for adults over 18 years of age until he/she reaches the age of 40 years, after which the individual should have a checkup at every 1–3 years. For individuals taking prescription medications, there may be a need for more frequent health evaluations.

Things to Expect During a Periodic Health Assessment

During a health checkup, there are several things you can expect that will be done. The doctor will ask about your health history which includes family history, past immunizations, medical history, lifestyle, and habits. A physical examination will also be conducted, the extent of which depends on age, sex, and findings from the health history. Screening tests will also be done.

A health checkup can be useful in detecting various health conditions so that these can be promptly treated. Annual checkups are not actually a necessity for healthy individuals and tend to be inefficient in terms of cost. Each individual is different and a personalized approach to health checkups can prove to be more valuable in health maintenance.

KEY POINTS

- Combination of lagging and leading indicators of safety performance are used.
- Fall prevention: Specific interventions to prevent falls include:
  1. Keep floors clean and dry.
  2. Prevent entry to wet areas.
  3. Housekeeping.
  4. Ice and snow removal.
- An annual health checkup is a yearly visit to an individual's healthcare provider wherein the general condition of one's health is assessed. It is also known as a routine physical examination, preventive health checkup, or master health checkup.

IMPORTANT QUESTIONS

1. Describe Employee safety indicators.
2. Write briefly on:
   a. Fall prevention
   b. Radiation safety
   c. Annual health checkup

MULTIPLE CHOICE QUESTIONS

1. **Employee safety indicators use:**
   a. Lagging indicators of safety performance
   b. Leading indicators of safety performance
   c. Lagging and leading indicators of safety performance
   d. All of the above
2. **All statements of annual health check-up are true, *except*:**
   a. It is also known as a routine physical examination
   b. There are several advantages of regular health check-up with a doctor
   c. Health check-ups also promote better patient-doctor relationships
   d. Need for yearly preventive health check-up for healthy individuals

ANSWERS

1. c   2. a

Healthcare Worker Immunization and Management of Occupational Exposure

CHAPTER 75

LEARNING OBJECTIVES

After reading and studying this chapter, you should be able to:
- Describe occupational health program.
- Discuss vaccines for healthcare workers.
- Discuss needle stick injuries (NSI).
- Describe postexposure prophylaxis (PEP)

OCCUPATIONAL HEALTH AND SAFETY (OHS) LEGISLATION IN INDIA

Like most other countries, India tries to reinforce occupational health and safety (OHS) by implementing laws which regulate the measures that companies have to take. In order to guarantee, a sufficient level of OHS throughout the country, these Acts lay down very basic minimum requirements. In this way, the differences between states in the administration of the Act can be minimized. Another intention of these detailed provisions is to streamline the work of inspectors who have to examine the conditions of work in factories, thereby implying that inspectors have expert knowledge of the subject.

The main objectives of OHS-related legislation are:
1. Providing a statutory framework including the enactment of a general enabling legislation on OHS in respect of all sectors of economic activities, and designing suitable control systems of compliance, enforcement and incentives for better compliance.
2. Providing administrative and technical support services.
3. Providing a system of incentives to employers and employees so that they achieve higher health and safety standards.
4. Establishing and developing research and development capabilities in emerging areas of risk and effective control measures.
5. Reducing the incidence of work related injuries, fatalities and diseases.
6. Reducing the cost of workplace injuries and diseases.
7. Increasing community awareness regarding areas related to OHS.

OCCUPATIONAL HEALTH PROGRAM

An occupational health program is essential for an effective infection, prevention, and control (IPC) program and has implications for patient safety. The components of such a program are:
- Evaluation for general health of employees including infectious diseases at entry, periodically as required.
- Screening for vaccination for childhood communicable diseases (measles, rubella, chickenpox, diphtheria, pertussis, tetanus).
- Hepatitis B status and immunization
- Influenza vaccine, TST status
- Screening for tuberculosis
- **Surveillance and management of exposure risk:** Hazard identification, risk assessment and control, postexposure management
- Education and training

Occupational Vaccination Program

- A vaccination policy (also for contractual staff)
- Maintenance of vaccination records
- Providing information about vaccine-preventable diseases and offering vaccination for the same.
- Modification of duties if a healthcare worker (HCW) has an infection that has a risk of transmission during exposure-prone procedures.
- Explaining the consequences of vaccine refusal.
- Vaccine refusal, contraindication to vaccination and vaccine nonresponse may be managed by ensuring appropriate work placements, work adjustments, and work restrictions. This should be documented.

Vaccines for Healthcare Workers

Healthcare workers (HCWs) are at risk for exposure to serious, and sometimes deadly, diseases. If you work directly with patients or handle material that could spread infection, you should get appropriate vaccines to reduce the chance that you will get or spread vaccine-preventable diseases. Protect yourself, your patients, and your family members. Make sure you are up-to-date with recommended vaccines **(Table 75.1)**. Healthcare workers include physicians, nurses, emergency medical personnel, dental professionals and students, medical and nursing students, laboratory technicians, pharmacists, hospital volunteers, and administrative staff.

Needle Stick Injuries (NSI)

Needle stick injuries are known to occur frequently in healthcare settings and can be serious. Awareness of needle stick injuries started to develop soon after the identification of human immunodeficiency virus (HIV) in the early 1980s. However, today the major

Table 75.1: Recommended vaccines for healthcare workers.

Vaccines	Recommendations in brief
Hepatitis B	If you do not have documented evidence of a complete hepatitis B vaccine series, or if you do not have an up-to-date blood test that shows you are immune to hepatitis B (i.e., no serologic evidence of immunity or prior vaccination) then you should • Get a 3-dose series of Recombivax HB or Engerix-B (dose #1 now, #2 in 1 month, #3 approximately 5 months after #2) or a 2-dose series of Heplisav-B, with the doses separated by at least 4 weeks • Get an anti-HBs serologic test 1–2 months after the final dose.
Flu (Influenza)	Get 1 dose of influenza vaccine annually
MMR (Measles, Mumps, and Rubella)	If you were born in 1957, or later and have not had the MMR vaccine, or if you do not have an up-to-date blood test that shows you are immune to measles or mumps (i.e., no serologic evidence of immunity or prior vaccination), get 2 doses of MMR (1 dose now and the 2nd dose at least 28 days later). If you were born in 1957, or later and have not had the MMR vaccine, or if you do not have an up-to-date blood test that shows you are immune to rubella, only 1 dose of MMR is recommended. However, you may end up receiving 2 doses, because the rubella component is in the combination vaccine with measles and mumps. For HCWs born before 1957, *see* the MMR ACIP vaccine recommendations
Varicella (Chickenpox)	If you have not had chickenpox (varicella), if you have not had varicella vaccine, or if you do not have an up-to-date blood test that shows you are immune to varicella (i.e., no serologic evidence of immunity or prior vaccination) get 2 doses of varicella vaccine, 4 weeks apart
Tdap (Tetanus, Diphtheria, Pertussis)	Get a one-time dose of Tdap as soon as possible if you have not received Tdap previously (regardless of when previous dose of Td was received) Get Td boosters every 10 years thereafter Pregnant HCWs need to get a dose of Tdap during each pregnancy
Meningococcal	Those who are routinely exposed to isolates of *N. meningitidis* should get one dose

(ACIP: Advisory Committee on Immunization Practices; HCW: healthcare worker)

concern after a needle stick injury is not HIV but hepatitis B or hepatitis C. Guidelines have been established to help healthcare institutions manage needle stick injuries and when to initiate postexposure HIV prophylaxis. Healthcare professionals at the highest risk for needle stick injuries are surgeons, emergency room workers, laboratory room professionals, and nurses.

Postexposure Prophylaxis (PEP)

"Postexposure prophylaxis" (PEP) refers to the comprehensive management given to minimize the risk of infection following potential exposure to blood-borne pathogens (HIV, HBV, HCV). This includes counseling, risk assessment, relevant laboratory investigations based on informed consent of the source and exposed person, first aid and depending on the risk assessment, the provision of short-term (4 weeks) of antiretroviral drugs, with follow-up and support.

If an accidental exposure occurs, any wound should be washed with soap and water, or mucous membranes flushed with water. The accident must be reported so that, if necessary, prophylaxis can be started as soon as possible. Knowledge of the status of the source patient is essential.

Postexposure Prophylaxis (PEP) for HIV

Eligibility for PEP

- PEP should be offered, and initiated as early as possible, to all individuals with exposure that has the potential for HIV transmission, and ideally, within 2 hours (but certainly within the first 72 hours) of exposure and the risk evaluated as soon as possible.
- Exposures that may warrant occupational PEP include:
  - Parenteral or mucous membrane exposure (splashes to the eye, nose or oral cavity)
  - The following bodily fluids may pose a risk of HIV infection: blood, blood-stained saliva, breast-milk, genital secretions and cerebrospinal, amniotic, rectal, peritoneal, synovial, pericardial or pleural fluids

Postexposure Prophylaxis Regimen for HIV

In contrast to the earlier recommendation of two antiretroviral drugs, recent guidelines including World Health Organization (WHO) 2014c, WHO 2018d, Department of Health and Human Services (DHHS) 2013e, BHIVAf and NACOg prefer three antiretroviral drugs for PEP, irrespective of the degree of exposure (irrespective of percutaneous or mucous membrane exposure and irrespective of mild, moderate or severe exposure).

This change was aimed at simplification of the recommendation to improve uptake and completion rates for PEP. This shift toward recommending a three-drug regimen for everyone was based on the availability of less toxic and better-tolerated medications, the difficulty in evaluating the risk of drug resistance and need to simplify prescribing **(Table 75.2)**.

Postexposure Prophylaxis for HBV

- **If the source is HBV-positive:** Appropriate and timely prophylaxis can prevent HBV infection and subsequent development of chronic infection or liver disease. The mainstay of PEP is hepatitis B vaccine, but in certain circumstances, hepatitis B immune globulin is recommended in addition to vaccine for added protection.
- **If the source is known or shown to be positive for HBsAg**, the level of anti-HBs antibodies in the HCW is important. If the injured HCW is immunized (anti-HBs antibodies >10 IU/mL)—whether from vaccination or past infection they are protected, and there is no need for hepatitis B immunoglobulin after a potential or confirmed exposure to hepatitis B.
- **When a source patient is unknown**, the exposed HCW should be managed as if the source patient were HBsAg-positive.
- **When indicated, immune prophylaxis** should be initiated as soon as possible, preferably within 24 hours.
- **If the HCW is unimmunized or a nonresponder** (did not seroconvert to the vaccine)

Table 75.2: Postexposure prophylaxis (PEP) for HIV.

Recommendations

A regimen for postexposure prophylaxis for HIV with two antiretroviral drugs (ARV) drugs is effective, but three drugs are preferred.

Postexposure prophylaxis ARV regimens–adults and adolescents

TDF + 3TC (or FTC) is recommended as the preferred backbone regimen for HIV postexposure prophylaxis for adults and adolescents.

LPV/r or ATV/r is recommended as the preferred third drug for HIV postexposure prophylaxis for adults and adolescents. Where available RAL, DRV/r or EFV can be considered as alternative options.

Postexposure prophylaxis ARV regimens–children (≤10 years old)

AZT + 3TC is recommended as the preferred backbone regimen for HIV postexposure prophylaxis for children 10 years and younger.

ABC + 3TC or TDF + 3TC (or FTC) can be considered as alternative regimens.

LPV/r is recommended as the preferred third drug for HIV postexposure prophylaxis for children younger than 10 years. An age-appropriate alternative regimen can be identified among ATV/r, RAL, DRV, EFV and NVP. **Prescribing frequency**

A 28-day prescription of antiretroviral drugs should be provided for HIV postexposure prophylaxis following initial risk assessment

Adherence strategies

Enhanced adherence counseling is suggested for individuals initiating HIV postexposure prophylaxis.

(TDF: tenofovir disoproxil fumarate; 3TC: lamivudine; FTC: emtricitabine; LPV/r: lopinavir/ritonavir; ATV/r: atazanavir/ritonavir; RAL: raltegravir; DRV/r: darunavir + ritonavir; EFV: efavirenz; AZT: azidothymidine; HIV: human immunodeficiency virus)

---

or has antibody levels to HBsAg <10 IU/mL), and sustains a needle-stick injury from a patient with evidence of chronic HBV (HBsAg-positive), they should be given HBIG (hepatitis B hyperimmune globulin) 0.06 mL/kg as soon as possible, preferably within 24 hours and should simultaneously start/reinitiate the course of HBV immunization with three doses of hepatitis B vaccine at a different site for unimmunized/previously unfinished second hepatitis B series. The second and third doses should be separated by at least 2 months' interval.

- **If the HCW has had two series of the HBV vaccine and was still a nonresponder**, they should receive a second dose of HBIG, 1 month after the first dose.
- Following completion of three-dose vaccination series, the level of immunity (antibodies to surface antigen, i.e., anti-HBs titers) should be checked 1–2 months later. Those whose anti-HBs titers are <10 mIU/mL should complete a second three-dose vaccine series or be evaluated for HBsAg positivity. If HBsAg is positive after exposure, the person should be counseled regarding the modes of prevention of HBV transmission to others and to seek treatment for HBV.

Exposure to Hepatitis C (HCV) Virus

1. If the source patient tests positive for HCV, the employee will receive a baseline test.
2. At 4 weeks after exposure, the employee is to be offered a HCV-RNA test to determine if the employee contracted HCV.
3. If positive, the employee is started on treatment. (There is no prophylactic treatment for HCV after exposure).
4. Early treatment for infection has the potential to prevent chronic infections.

Prevention of Needle Stick Injuries (NSI)

It is necessary for employees to be aware of the consequence of needle stick and what can be done to prevent them. Today most hospitals have instituted policies and protocols to prevent needle stick injuries by advocating the following:

- Used needles must not be recapped by hand; if necessary, use the single hand "scoop" method.
- Used needles should not be bent or broken after use.
- Avoid recapping needles
- Before beginning any procedure using needles, plan for safe handling and proper disposal. Minimize the use of needles where possible.
- Help your employer select and evaluate devices with safety features.
- Encourage use of needles with safety features
- Alters any dangerous work practice on the floor and in the operating room.
- Report all needle stick and other sharps-related injuries.
- Dispose of used needles in appropriate sharps disposal containers.
- Inform your employer of hazards from needles that you observe at work.
- Participate in bloodborne pathogen training and follow recommended infection prevention practices, including hepatitis B vaccination.

KEY POINTS

- **Occupational health and safety (OHS) Legislation in India:** Like most other countries, India tries to reinforce occupational health and safety (OHS) by implementing laws which regulate the measures that companies have to take.
- **Vaccines for healthcare workers:** Healthcare workers (HCWs) are at risk for exposure to serious, and sometimes deadly, diseases. If you work directly with patients or handle material that could spread infection, you should get appropriate vaccines to reduce the chance that you will get or spread vaccine-preventable diseases.
- **Needle stick injuries (NSI):** Needle stick injuries are known to occur frequently in healthcare settings and can be serious. Guidelines have been established to help healthcare institutions manage needle stick injuries and when to initiate postexposure HIV prophylaxis.

- **Postexposure prophylaxis (PEP):** If an accidental exposure occurs, any wound should be washed with soap and water, or mucous membranes flushed with water. The accident must be reported so that, if necessary, prophylaxis can be started as soon as possible. Knowledge of the status of the source patient is essential.
- **Prevention of needle stick injuries (NSI):** It is necessary for employees to be aware of the consequence of needle stick and what can be done to prevent them. Today most hospitals have instituted policies and protocols to prevent needle stick injuries.

IMPORTANT QUESTIONS

1. Discuss vaccines for healthcare workers.
2. Discuss prevention of needle stick injuries (NSI).
3. Describe postexposure prophylaxis (PEP).
   Write briefly on:
   a. Occupational health program.
   b. Annual health checkup.

MULTIPLE CHOICE QUESTIONS

1. Occupational vaccination program include:
   a. A vaccination policy (also for contractual staff)
   b. Maintenance of vaccination records
   c. Explaining the consequences of vaccine refusal
   d. All of the above.
2. Postexposure prophylaxis for Hepatitis B virus (HBV) is initiated:
   a. If the source is HBV-positive
   b. If the source is known or shown to be positive for HBsAg
   c. When a source patient is unknown
   d. All of the above

ANSWERS

1. d 2. d

Index

Page numbers followed by *f* refer to figure and *t* refer to table.

A

Abscess 103, 391
  amebic 282
  deeper 340
  intra-abdominal 105
Accidental inoculation 187
Acetone 40
Acid
  alcohol decolorizer 42
  fast 136
    bacilli 41, 142
    organisms 42
    stain 39, 41
Acidic dyes 38
Acidic protoplasm 39
Acinetobacter 206
  baumannii 206, 352
Acquired immunodeficiency syndrome 145, 147, 251, 252, 271, 348
Acridine dyes 383
Acriflavine 383
Actinomadura 146
Actinomycetes 146, 343
Actinomycosis 146, 343
  treatment for 147
Active immunization 224 225, 332
Acute human immunodeficiency virus infection 252
Acyclovir 229
Adenocarcinoma 171
Adenosatellovirus 226
Adenovirus 226, 231, 315, 317, 318
Adrenals 282
Adult T-cell leukemia 348

Adult worm 294, 295, 298*f*, 301*f*, 303, 306, 308, 310
  detection of 307
Aedes aegypti 247
Aeromonas hydrophila 318
African sleeping sickness 345
Agalactia 104
Agar dilution method 321, 322
Agglutinable vibrios 167
Agglutination 316
  reaction 67
    applications of 67
Agranulocytosis 85
Air removal 379
Air-borne transmission 351, 352
Alarm systems 432
Albert's stain 42, 43*f*, 117
Alcaligenes faecalis 18, 205, 206, 343
Alcohol 40, 42, 377, 381, 382, 387
Aldehyde 377, 381, 383
  test 288
Algae 3, 259
Algid malaria 292
Alkaline
  bile salt agar 166
  peptone water 27, 166
Allantoic cavity 221
Allergens 83
Allergic reactions 56
Alpha-hemolytic streptococci 100, 325
Alphavirus 247
Amebiasis 281
Amebic dysentery, acute 282
Aminacrine 383
Aminoglycosides 328

Amniotic sac 221
Amoxicillin 172
Ampholytic compounds 382
Amphoteric compounds 382
Ampicillin 132, 200
Anaerobic culture methods 29
Anal canal 115
Anaphylaxis 83
  localized 84
  mechanism of 83
  primary mediators of 84
  secondary mediators of 84
Anchovy sauce pus 282
Ancylostoma duodenale 303, 345
Anemia, hemolytic 85
Angular cheilitis 271
Angular stomatitis 271
Aniline dyes 383
Animal anatomical waste 394
Animal inoculation 124, 138, 196, 198, 220, 263, 287
  test 272
Animal oncoviruses 348
Animal rabies 245
Anopheles 288
Anthracoid bacilli 124, 125*t*
Anthrax 5
  bacilli 123*f*
  causal agents of 6
  cutaneous 124
Antibacterial drug, mechanisms of action of 327, 328*t*
Antibacterial therapy 168
Antibiotic 6, 327, 329
  antibacterial 219
  disks 321
  prophylaxis 130

rational use of 403
resistance 403
  causes of 404
sensitivity test 97, 110, 135, 151, 174, 183, 321
susceptibility test 154
therapy 342, 403
Antibody 53
  demonstration of 162, 234
  dependent cell 84, 85
  detection 253
  excess, zone of 63, 63f
  generator 51
  production of 79
  reactions 63
  structure 53
  synthesis of 78
Anticoagulants 414
Anti-deoxyribonuclease 104b
Antigen 51, 66, 83
  antibody
    binding 58
    interaction 62
    reactions 62
  binding site 53
  biological classes of 52
  detection 104, 176, 183, 231, 253, 297, 316
    techniques 202
  excess, zone of 63f
  group-specific 191
  internal 243
  nonspecific 191
  processing and presentation 79
  specific 191
  types of 51, 63
Antigenic
  classification 112, 243
  determinant sites 51
  drift 243
  shift 243
  structure 53, 108, 114, 150, 153, 156, 160, 166, 191, 236, 243
Antiglobulin test 67
  principle of 67
Antimicrobial
  agent 327
  chemotherapy 327
  drugs 329
  policy 402
  resistance 404
    mechanism of 404

stewardship 401, 407
  goal of 401
  program 401, 402
  team 401
  therapy, laboratory control of 321
Antimony test 288
Antirabic vaccines 246
Antiretroviral treatment 255
  highly active 255
Antiseptic 327, 376
  surgery, system of 6
Antisera 6, 335
Antisheep-red cell antibody 68
Anti-streptolysin O test 104
Antitetanus serum 131
Antitoxin 121
Antral gastritis 171
Arboviruses 247, 315
Arenaviridae 347, 348
Arsphenamine 6
Arthritis 341
Arthropod-borne
  diseases 32
  infection 196
  viruses 247
Arthrospores formation 268f
Arthus reaction 85
Asbestos filters 380
Ascariasis 345
Ascaris lumbricoides 301, 301f, 318, 345
  eggs of 301f
  life cycle of 302f
Ascaris pneumonia 302
Asepsis 386
Aseptic meningitis 198, 242, 315, 315t, 317
Aspergilloma 273
Aspergillosis 252, 261, 273, 275, 344
  bronchopulmonary 273
  colonizing 273
Aspergillus
  fumigatus 261, 273, 344
  niger 273
Asphyxia 341
Asthma, allergic 273
Astrovirus 318
Atopic reactions, clinical expression of 84
Atopy, mechanism of 84
Attitudes 410

Auramine
  phenol 138
  rhodamine fluorescent dyes 138
Australia antigen 236
Autoclave tapes 379
Autoimmune diseases 61
  classification of 88
Autoimmunity 88
  mechanisms of 88
Axoneme 286
Azidothymidine 255

B

B cell 75, 228
  activation 79
  lymphoma 252
  maturation 75
Bacillary dysentery 157, 282
Bacillus 14, 17, 123, 174
  anthracis 6, 17, 123, 125, 341
  cereus 123, 125, 318
  identification of 160
  isolation of 132
  stearothermophilus 20
Bacitracin 328
Bacteremia 105, 109, 160, 174, 341
Bacteria 3, 6, 13, 14, 72, 219, 259, 318, 337
  aerobic 23
  anaerobic 23, 28, 134
  arrangement of 15f
  cultures of 6
  microscopy of 11
  miscellaneous 204
  morphology of 11, 13, 14
  physiology of 22
  shape of 14, 14f
  size of 14
  study of 14
Bacterial antigens, detection of 186
Bacterial cell
  anatomy of 14, 15f, 20
  arrangement of 14
  components 15
  wall synthesis 327, 328
Bacterial culture 67
  methods of 28
Bacterial cytoplasmic membrane
  function, inhibition of 328

Bacterial endotoxin,
    demonstration of 316
Bacterial growth
    curve 22, 22f
    phases of 22
    principles of 22
Bacterial nucleic acid synthesis,
    inhibition of 328
Bacterial parasites 213
Bacterial protein 382
    synthesis, inhibition of 328, 329
Bacterial spore 19, 19f, 379
Bacterial vaccines 49, 331
Bacterial vaginosis 343
Bactericidal drugs 139
Bacteriological index 143
Bacteriophage 34
    typing 96, 97
Bacteristatic drug 139
Bacterium anitratum 206
Bacteriuria, significant 151
Bacteroides 315
Balanitis 271
Balantidial dysentery 345
Balantidium coli 318, 345
Bamboo-stick appearance 123
Bancroftian filariasis 345
Barber's itch 344
Bartonella 211
Bartonellaceae 208
Basophilic intranuclear inclusion
    body 230
Basophils 76
Bedsores 174
Beef tape worm 294, 345
Bell's palsy 228
Benzyl penicillin 97
Betadine 382
Beta-hemolytic streptococci 101
Beta-lactam
    agents 327
    antibiotics 328
    production of 97
Beta-propiolactone 383
    vaccine 246
Bile
    culture of 162
    solubility test 108
Biliary tract infection 105, 319
Binary fission 22, 219
Biochemical
    reactions 102, 108, 112, 124, 128, 151, 124, 152, 157, 159, 162, 168, 176, 179, 182, 185
    tests 237, 316
Biological control 378, 379
Biomedical waste 393, 400
    categories of 393, 393b, 394t
    handlers 399
    management 393, 399
Biopsy 147
    urease test 172
Bipolar metachromatic staining 185
Bipolaris 261, 344
Bisphenols 381
Black death 4
Black piedra 261, 344
Blackwater fever 292
Bladder worm 296
Blastomyces dermatitidis 261, 266, 266f, 344
Blastomycosis 261, 266, 269, 344
    cutaneous 267
Bleaching powder 382
Blood 188f, 198, 252
    agar 26, 28, 102, 108, 112, 118, 119, 124, 130, 150, 153, 156, 159, 165, 173, 174, 178
    plate 96, 129
    and blood transfusion policy 412, 418
    and tissues, antibacterial substances in 48
    borne infections 352
    count 288, 293
    culture 110, 113, 129, 160, 161, 183, 287, 316
        Castaneda's method of 161, 188
    examination 283, 300, 303, 305
    flukes 310, 345
    products 252
    trematodes 310
Bloodstream infection 103, 352, 353, 355, 356, 391
Bone marrow 188
    biopsy 287
    culture 162
Bordetella pertussis 185, 317, 342
Bordet-Gengou medium 185
Borrelia
    burgdorferi 196, 343
    isolation of 197
    recurrentis 198, 343

    vincentii 196
Botulinum toxin 131
Botulism 131, 132, 341
Brain 282
    CT scan of 297
Brazilian purpuric feve 183, 342
Breakbone fever 248
Bronchial washings 137
Bronchiolitis 244
Bronchitis, chronic 109
Bronchopneumonia 96, 109
Bronchopulmonary disease 147
Broth dilution method 321, 322
Browne's tubes 378
Brucella 78, 187
    infections 189
    melitensis 342
Brucellin skin test 188
Brucellosis 188, 319, 337, 342
Bubonic plague 179
Buccal capsule 303
Buffalopox 227
Bullous impetigo 96
Bunyaviridae 347, 348
Burkholderia
    cepacia 174, 342
    mallei 175, 342
    pseudomallei 175, 342
Butzler's selective medium 170

C

Calicivirus 318
Calymmatobacterium granulomatis 205, 206, 319, 343
Campylobacter 170, 171
    coli 170
    jejuni 170, 318
Campylobacteriaceae 170
Candida albicans 261, 270, 270f, 317, 319, 344, 352
Candidiasis 252, 270, 271
    bronchopulmonary 271
Capsid 220, 241
Capsomers 220
Capsular antigens 108, 150, 152, 182
Capsule
    composition of 17
    demonstration of 17
    functions of 18
    staining of 43

swelling
   reaction 17
   tests 109
Carbapenems 328
Carbohydrate
   assimilation tests 272
   fermentation 272
   group specific 102f
Carbol fuchsin 39
Carbon dioxide 23
Carcinoma, hepatocellular 348
Cardiobacterium hominis 343
Carpet culture 29
Carrom coin appearance 108
Cary-Blair medium 166
Casoni reaction 300
Castaneda's method 188f
Castaneda's stain 208
Catalyst 29
Cefixime 115
Ceftriaxone 115
Cell
   count 112, 315
   culture 208, 220, 221
      vaccine 246, 247
      primary 221, 222
   envelope 16
   membrane 286, 381, 382, 387
   surface proteins 94
   virus 230
   wall 15, 16, 41
      defective organisms 20
      integrity 40
      structure 39
Cellular organization 219
Cellulitis 182
Central nervous system 272, 391
Cephalic tetanus 130
Cephalosporin 110, 132, 328
Cerebral malaria 292
Cerebrospinal fluid 36, 111f, 260, 316, 317, 392
Cervical alae 306
Cervicitis 341
Cervix cell line, human carcinoma of 222
Cestodes 294, 318
Cetrimide 382
   agar 173, 174
Chaga's disease 337, 345
Chancre 191
Chancroid 184, 319, 342
Charcot-Leyden crystals 283

Chemical
   agents 377, 381, 387
   composition 13
   control 379
   disinfection 398
   food preservatives 377
   indicator 378
   liquid waste 395
   nature 51
   sterilization 377, 384
   waste 395
Chemoprophylaxis 113, 225
Chemotaxis 61
Chemotherapeutic agents 327, 329
Chemotherapy 6
Chick embryo fibroblast cell culture 222
Chickenpox 229, 440
Chigger-borne typhus 209
Chikungunya virus 247
Chinese liver fluke 345
Chlamydia 213, 214t, 215, 344
   growth cycle 214f
   infections, laboratory diagnosis of 215
   pneumonia 214
   psittaci 214, 344
   trachomatis 214, 215, 319, 325, 344
Chlamydophila 213, 215, 344
   pneumoniae 215, 344
   psittaci 215
Chlamydospores 272
Chloramines 382
Chloramphenicol 110, 196, 328, 329
Chlorhexidine 382, 387
Chlorine 382, 387
   dioxide 384
Chloroxylenol 382, 387
Chocolate agar 26, 112, 114, 171, 172, 181
Cholera 6, 337
   classical 167t
   red reaction 166
   toxin 167
   vibrio 165, 165f
   serotypes of 167t
Chorioallantoic membrane 221, 226
Chromobacterium violaceum 205, 343

Chromoblastomycosis 261, 263, 344
Chromomycosis 263
Chronic persistent infection 238
Ciliophora 345
Ciprofloxacin 113, 115
Circumoral candidal dermatitis 271
Cirrhosis 238, 348
Clindamycin 132
Clonorchis sinensis 345
Clostridial endometritis 129
Clostridium
   botulinum 131, 318, 341
   difficile 132, 341, 385
      diarrhea 352
   perfringens 127-129, 318, 341
      colitis 129
   tetani 23, 129, 130, 341
   welchii 127
Clot culture 161
   advantage of 161
Coagulase test 95, 97
Coccidioides immitis 261, 267, 268f, 344
Coccidioidomycosis 252, 267, 269, 344
Codes, types of 433
Cold
   agglutination test 202
   chain 332
   equipment 332
   sterilization 380
Colistin 112, 114
Colitis, hemorrhagic 150
Colony-stimulating factors 80
Colorado tick fever virus 348
Complement fixation test 63, 68, 69f 244, 288
Conjugate vaccines 183
Conjunctiva 48
   normal flora of 324
Conjunctival swab 115
Conjunctivitis 214, 271, 341
   follicular 228, 231, 346
Contact dermatitis 86
Cooked meat broth 135
Coombs' serum 67
Corneal infections 342
Corneal test 245
Corneal ulcers 228
Corneybacterium 117
Coronavirus 348

Corynebacterium 324
 diphtheria 42, 117, 117f, 118, 121, 317
 type of 118t
 xerosis 324
Cotton plugs 378
Cough plate method 186
COVID-19 352
Cowpox 227
Coxiella 208
 burnetii 211, 221
Coxsackievirus 315, 317, 346
C-reactive protein 109
Creutzfeldt-Jakob disease 223
Cryptococcal meningitis 272
Cryptococcosis 252, 261, 272, 344
Cryptococcus neoformans 260, 261, 272, 272f, 317, 344
Cryptosporidiosis 252
Cryptosporidium parvum 318
Crystal violet 39
 blood agar 102, 104
 iodine complex 40
Cuneiform arrangement 117
Cycloheximide 187
Cycloserine 328
Cyst 280, 284
Cysticercosis, diagnosis of 297
Cysticercus
 bovis 296, 310
 cellulosae 296, 297, 297f, 310
Cystosome 285
Cytokines 80, 84
Cytolytic toxins 95
Cytomegalovirus 72, 226, 228, 230, 232, 252, 319, 337, 346
Cytoplasm 13, 15, 19, 102, 280, 286
Cytoplasmic membrane 15, 17, 18, 94, 102f
Cytotoxic reaction 84
 drug-induced 84
Cytotoxicity 85
Cytotoxin 79, 132

D

Dane particle 236
Dapsone 328
Dasypus novemcinctus 141
Deep vein thrombosis 414
 prevention of 414, 418
Delta hepatitis virion 238f

Dengue 247
 fever, classic 247
 hemorrhagic fever 248, 249
 shock syndrome 248, 249
Densovirus 226
Dental caries 105
Deoxycholate citrate agar 27, 156, 159
Deoxyribonucleic acid
 probes 230
 vaccines 332
 viruses 226
Dependovirus 346
Dermatophytosis 261, 344
Diaminapyrimidines 329
Diarrhea 150, 152, 231, 317, 341, 346
 acute 337
 antibiotic-associated 341
 chronic recurrent 285
 infantile 342
 infective 318t
 laboratory diagnosis of 150
Dienes phenomenon 153
Dilution methods 321, 322
Dimorphic fungi 260
Diphtheria 186
 bacilli 65
 pertussis-tetanus vaccine 121
Diphtheroids 121
Diphyllobothriasis 345
Diphyllobothrium latum 345
Diplococcus 107
 intracellularis meningitidis 111
 pneumomiae 107
Diploid cell strains 222
Dip-stick assay 198
Direct fluorescent antibody test 124
Dirofilaria immitis 345
Disinfection 376, 380
 guidelines 383
 methods of 376, 377b
 procedures 384
Diverticulitis 105
Doderlien's bacilli 326
Dog tapeworm 345
Domestic livestock 211
Donovan bodies 206
Donovania granulomatis 205, 343
Donovanosis 319
Dot blot assays 253
Drumstick appearance 129

Dry heat 376, 377
 sterilization 376
Duck embryo vaccine 246
Duodenal aspiration 285
Duodenal ulcer disease 171
Dwarf tapeworm 345
Dysentery 318, 318t
 amebic 281, 282, 282t, 345

E

Ear, infection of 154, 392
Earthware filters 380
Ebola virus 348
Echinococcus granulosus 298f, 310, 345
 egg of 298f
 life cycle of 299f
Echoviruses 315, 346
Ecthyma gangrenosum 342
Eczema herpeticum 228
Edwardsiella tarda 152
Ehrlichia 208
 sennetsu 210
Eikenella corrodens 343
Electron microscopy 222, 224, 229
Elek's gel precipitation test 65, 120, 120f
Elephantiasis 345
Embryos 308
Empirical therapy 403
Employee safety indicators 436
Empyema 96, 109
Encephalitis virus 247
Endemic syphilis 194
Endocarditis 105, 271, 273, 341-343
 infective 105, 319
Endoscopy 407
Endospore 19, 20
Endotoxin 17, 33, 33t
Enrichment media 26, 159, 166
Entamoeba histolytica 72, 280, 280f, 281, 293, 318, 319, 345
 life cycle of 281f
Enteric fever 159, 160, 319
 phases of 161t
Enteritis necroticans 129
Enterobacter 153, 317, 352
Enterobacteriaceae 149, 149t
 classification of 149
Enterobius vermicularis 306, 345
 egg of 306f
 life cycle of 307f

Enterococcus 100, 105
　faecium 352
Enterotoxin 95, 129, 132, 150
Enteroviruses 315
Enzyme 3, 34, 95, 102, 103
　detection of 222
　drug-inactivating 329
　immunoassay 194, 202, 229
Enzyme-linked immunosorbent
　　assay 70, 171, 188, 260, 283
　indirect 70
　sandwich 71
　tests 239, 253
　types of 70, 71*f*
　uses of 72
Eosinophil 76
　chemotactic factor 84
Eosinophilia 297
Epidemic viral gastroenteritis 348
Epidermolytic toxins 95
Epidermophyton 262
　floccosum 261, 344
Epididymo-orchitis 244
Epiglottitis 182
Episomes 19
Epithelial cells 228
Epitome 51
Epitopes 51
Epstein-Barr virus 226, 228, 230,
　　232, 252, 317, 319, 346
　infection 319
Erysipeloid 343
Erysipelothrix rhusiopathiae 205,
　　206, 343
Erythema multiforme 228
Erythrocytic schizogony 288
Erythrogenic toxins 103
Erythromycin 110, 121, 194, 196
Erythrovirus 346
Escherichia coli 40, 149, 151, 154,
　　315, 317, 318, 341, 352, 353
　enterohemorrhagic 318
　enteroinvasive 318
Eskape' pathogens 352
Ethanol 382
Ethyl alcohol 382
Ethylene oxide 383, 384
Ethylenediamine tetra acetic acid
　124
Euflavine 383
Eukaryotes 14
Eukaryotic cell 13, 13*t*
Exfoliative diseases 96

Exophiala 261, 344
Exotoxin 33, 33*t*, 150, 156
Exserohilum 261, 344
Eye 363
　infections 174, 231, 346
　lens antigen of 88

F

Facial protection 363, 366
Famciclovir 229
Fasciola 310
　hepatica 310, 345
Fascioliasis 345
Fecal antigen test 172
Feces 157, 390
　culture 161, 161*f*
Fernandez reaction 142
Fever of unknown origin 319
Fever
　glandular 230
　hemorrhagic 348
Fibrinolysin 103
Filamentous fungi 270*f*
Filariasis 309, 319, 345
Filoviridae 348
Fimbria 18
　antigen 150
　demonstration of 18
Fire extinguishers 428
　types of 428
Fire safety 428, 434
Fish tapeworm 345
Fit test 361
Flagella 18
　arrangement of 18*f*
　demonstration of 18
Flageller antigen 166
Flagellin 18
Flagellum 286
Flavivirus 247
Flavobacterium meningosepticum
　205, 343
Flocculation tests 63, 193
　types of 63
Flu 440
Fluorescent 69, 173
　antibody 229
　technique 229
　dyes 69
　isothiocyanate 69
　microscopy 224
　treponemal antibody test 194

Fluorometric microparticle
　　technologies 253
Foamy cells 141
Fonecaea pedrosoi 261, 344
Fontana's method 190
Food poisoning 96, 129, 160, 163,
　　318, 337
　causative agents of 318*t*
Formaldehyde gas 383
Formol gel test 288
Formol toxoid 131
Foscarnet 230
Fosfomycin 328
Francisella tularensis 342
Frei test 215
Fresh clotted rabbit blood 183
Fried egg appearance 201, 202
Fumigation 338
Fungal
　antibodies 260
　disease, classification of 344*t*
Fungi 3, 259, 315, 317
　beneficial effects of 259
　classification of 259
　general properties of 259
　laboratory diagnosis of 259
　study of 259
Fungus 317
　infections 260
Furazolidone 329
Fusidic acid 328
Fusion protein 244
Fusobacterium fusiforme 196
Fusospirochetosis 196

G

Gaffkya tetragena 15*f*
Gamma herpes virinae 228
Ganciclovir 230
Gardnerella vaginalis 206, 317,
　　319, 325, 343
Gas gangrene 129
Gas-Pak system 135
Gastric
　adenocarcinoma 342
　lavage 137
　malignancies 171
　ulcers 171
Gastritis 342
Gastroenteritis 160, 342
　infantile 343
　septicemia 159

Gastrointestinal disease 231
Gastrointestinal tract 47, 390
  normal flora of 325
Gel diffusion precipitation 283
Gelatin stab culture 124, 166
Gell and Coombs classification 82
Genital
  cells 308f
  disease 228
  infections 214, 228, 391
  lesions 226
  mycoplasmas 201
  tract 391
  warts 319
Genitourinary infections 343
Genitourinary tract 48
  normal flora of 325
Genome 241, 242, 245, 251
Germ
  theory 5
  tube test 272
German measles 248
Giardia intestinalis 284, 345
Giardia lamblia 284, 293, 318, 319, 345
  cyst of 284
Giardiasis 345
Giemsa stain 124, 196, 206, 208
Gingivostomatitis, acute 228
Glomerulonephritis, acute 103, 340
Glottis 390
Glutaraldehyde 383
Glycopeptides 98, 328
Gonococcal disease, disseminated 114
Gonorrhea 114, 319
  acute 115
  diagnosis of 115
  uncomplicated 115
Gram stain 17, 20, 39, 40f, 104, 115, 260
  mechanism 39
  interpretation of 39
Gram's iodine 39
Gram's method 124
Gramicidin 328
Gram-negative bacteria, cell walls of 16, 16f, 17t
Gram-positive bacteria cell wall 16, 17t, 33, 41t
Granular lymphocytes, large 75
Granuloma inguinale 343

Ground itch 305
Growth media, phases of 25
Guillain-Barre syndrome 228, 342
Guinea pig skin, fixing to 54

H

Haemophilus
  ducreyi 183, 319, 342
  influenzae 17, 68, 72, 181-183, 315, 317, 342
Hair, infection of 262
Halogens 381, 382, 387
Halophilic vibrios 169
Hand hygiene 358, 362, 364, 368, 373, 406
  essential 368b
  implementation of 369
Hand rub 369, 371f
Hand wash 369, 370f
Handwashing techniques 372f
Hanging drop
  method 6
  preparation 36, 36f, 37, 37f
Hansen's disease 136
Haptens 51
Hard chancre 191
Hazardous waste 393
Healthcare worker 364, 368, 407, 439, 440
  vaccines for 440, 443
Healthcare-associated infections, types of 352, 356
Heart muscle antigens 88
Heartworm 345
Heated blood agar 112, 129, 181
Heat-labile enterotoxin 170
Heavy metals 381, 382, 387
Helical nucleocapsid 244
Helicobacter pylori 171, 342
Helminthic parasites, immunity against 56
Helminths 3
Helper T-cells, activity of 88
Hemadsorption 222
Hemagglutination 283
  inhibition tests 68, 244
Hemagglutinin 243, 243f
Hemolysins 102, 130, 150
Hemolytic uremic syndrome 150
Hepadnaviridae 235
Heparin 84
Hepatic amebiasis 319
  diagnosis of 283

Hepatic trematodes 310
Hepatitis 193, 225, 228
  A 225, 332
    exclusion of 239
    vaccine 235
    virus 234, 235f, 337, 346, 352
    acute 238, 348
    amebic 282
  B 337, 346, 440
    core antigen 236
    exclusion of 239
    immune globulin 237
    surface antigen 236
    vaccine, plasma-derived 237
    virus 226, 232, 234, 235, 236f, 319, 332, 346, 389
  BE antigen 236
  C 238
    virus 234, 238, 319, 352, 442
  chronic 348
  E virus 239, 348
  G virus 239
  infectious 234
  virus 234, 235t
    antigens 72
Herpes
  febrilis 228
  genitalis 319
  gladiatorum 228
  lymphotropic virus 228
  simplex 226, 228, 315
  virus 227, 345
    infections 227
    typical structure of 227f
Herpetic stomatitis 228
Heterophile antigens 52
Hexachlorophane 382, 387
Histamine 84
Histocompatibility complex, major 76
Histoplasma capsulatum 261, 344
Histoplasmin skin test 268
Histoplasmosis 252, 261, 267, 269, 344
Hookworm 303f, 318, 345
  disease 345
  egg of 304f
  infection, clinical features of 305
  life cycle of 304f
Horse anti-rabies serum 247
Horse blood agar 131

Hortaea werneckii 261, 344
Hospital associated infection
   control of 353, 356
   diagnosis of 353, 356
   prevention of 354, 356
Hot air oven 377
   uses of 378
Hot-stain procedure 138
Human amnion cell culture 222
Human anatomical waste 394
Human antitetanus
   immunoglobulin 131
Human body, normal microbial
   flora of 324
Human diploid cell vaccine 246
Human embryonic lung cell strain 222
Human epithelioma 222
Human erythrocytes antigens 51
Human herpes virus 226, 228, 232, 252
   classification of 228*t*
Human immunodeficiency virus 251, 319, 348, 389, 440
   infection 271, 319
      clinical features of 252
   structure of 251*f*
Human leukocyte antigen
   complex 76
Human life, microorganisms on 3
Human papilloma virus 319, 332
Human plague, forms of 179
Human rabies 245
   immune globulin 247
Human serum immunoglobulins 55*t*
Human synovial carcinoma cell line 222
Human T-cell
   leukemia virus 348
   lymphotropic viruses 337
Humidity monitoring systems 432
Humoral response
   primary 79
   secondary 79
Hyaluronic acid capsule 102*f*
Hyaluronidase 103
Hybrid virus vaccine 238, 332
Hydatid cyst 298*f*
   pathogenesis of 300
Hydatid disease 310
Hydrogen peroxide 382, 383, 385, 387

Hydrogen sulfide 112
Hydrolyze urea 201
Hymenolepasis 345
Hymenolepis nana 318, 345
Hypersensitivity 82-85, 85*f*, 86, 413
   cell-mediated 86*f*
   delayed 85
   reactions 61, 82, 131
      classification of 82
      types of 83*t*
   test 188
   types of 82*t*, 86
Hypochlorite solution 382
Hypochlorites 382, 387

I

Iatrogenic injury, prevention of 410, 418
Idoxuridine 229
Immune complex 85
   mediated disease, models of 85
Immune elimination 131
Immune reaction, cell-mediated 80
Immune response 78
   cell-mediated 80
   primary 78*f*
   theories of 80
   types of 74, 78
Immune system 47
   functions of 74
   organs of 74
   structure of 74
   tissues of 74
Immunity 6, 47, 229, 292
   acquired 48
   active 48, 48*t*, 121, 131, 183
   antibody-mediated 62, 74, 78
   artificial
      active 49
      passive 49
   cell-mediated 74, 78, 80
   classification 47
   herd 50
   humoral 78
   innate 47, 48
   natural 47, 49
   nonspecific 47
   passive 48*t*, 49
   premunition 292

   specific 47
   types of 48
Immunization 6, 235, 237, 239, 242, 332
   schedule 242, 333
Immunochromatographic tests 72
Immunodiffusion test 120
   types of 64
Immunoelectroblot techniques 72
Immunoelectron microscopy 224, 239
Immunoelectrophoresis 65, 66*f*
Immunoenzyme test 72
Immunoferritin test 72
Immunofluorescence 69, 183, 222, 229
   indirect 70
   methods 190
   test 254
   types of 69
Immunoglobulin 53
   A 54
   classes 54
      role of 57
   D 56
   E 56
   G 54
   M 56
Immunological tests 254
Immunoprophylaxis 113, 131, 331
In vitro
   method 119
   test 120
In vivo
   method 119
   test 120
Incinerator
   disadvantages of 398
   types of 397
Indirect fluorescent antibody test 288
Indole 112
Inducer cell 75
Industrial eye injuries 342
Infection 31, 204, 413
   chronic 115
   community-associated 351
   control 5
      and safety 349
      committee 354 356
      nurse 354
      policy 354, 356
      team 4, 354, 356

cutaneous 95, 97, 148, 227, 340
deep 96
diagnosis of 4
healthcare-associated 351, 352, 356
iatrogenic 32
laboratory 32
mode of 32, 124
nature of 4
neonatal 104, 204
primary 137
route of 34
sources of 32, 351
treatment of 4
types of 238
Infectious diseases
anemia due to 85
types of 34
Infestation 338
Inflammation 48
Influenza 225, 332, 440
immunization 50
virus 242, 243f
Inner membrane 19
Interleukin 80
Intertriginous infection 271
Intestinal
amebiasis 281, 282
anthrax 124
candidosis 271
entamoebae 283t
flagellates 283, 284
flukes 310
parasitic infestation 337
trematodes 310
Intestine 222
Intracutaneous test 120
Intradermal test 120, 283
Intraperitoneal injection 109
Inulin fermentation 108
Invasive aspergillosis 273
Iodine 382, 387
Iodophors povidone-iodine 382
Ionizing radiation 377, 380
Isolation
discontinuation of 406
technique 358
Isoniazid 328
Isopropyl alcohol 382
Isospora belli 318
Isosporiasis 252
Ixodid ticks 211

J

Jacuzzi rash 342
Japanese encephalitis 225, 247, 249
Jarisch-Herxheimer reaction 194
Jaundice 348

K

K antigen 150
Kahn test 64, 193
Kaposi's sarcoma 228, 252
Karyosome 280
Keratitis 271
amebic 345
dendritic 228
Keratoconjunctivitis
epidemic 231, 346
severe 228
Kidney 222
infections 271
Kirby-Bauer disk diffusion method 321, 321f
Kissing disease 230
Klebsiella 17, 149, 152, 154
granulomatis 205
pneumoniae 152, 154, 341, 352
Koch's phenomenon 6, 139
Koch's postulates 6, 7b
Koplik's spots 244
Kovacs' method 112
Kyasanur forest disease 248

L

Lactophenol cotton 44
blue preparation 273
Lag phase 23
Lancefield
grouping 101
technique 104
Lanceolate appearance 107
Larva migrans, cutaneous 305, 306
Laryngeal swabs 137
Larynx cell line 222
Laser safety 427, 434
Lassa fever virus 348
Latex agglutination 229, 283
test 68
Lattice hypothesis 63
Lawn culture 29

Legionella 176
pneumophila 176, 342
Legionellaceae 176
Legionnaire's disease 176, 342
Leishman stain 196
Leishmania donovani 286, 286f
life cycle of 287f
pathogenicity of 287
Leishmaniasis 319
Leishmanin skin test 288
Lepra-cell 142
Lepromatous leprosy 142
Lepromin reaction, uses of 142
Lepromin test 142, 143
Leprosy 193
lesions of 142
Leptospira 191, 195, 197, 199
demonstration of 198
interrogans 197
Leptospirosis 343
Leptotrichia buccalis 196, 317
Lesion
localized 174
mild superficial 97
primary 195
Leukocytes 75, 178f
Leukotrienes 84
Levaditi's method 190
Lid 379
Light microscope, use of 12
Lincosamides 328
Lipooligosaccharide 114
Lipopolysaccharide 16, 17
Lipoprotein 16
bullet-shaped 245
envelope 251
Liquid culture 28
Liquid media 108, 137, 187
types of 27t
Listeria 206
monocytogenes 204, 315, 343
Litmus milk medium 128
Live attenuated anthrax vaccine 5
Live oral vaccine 169
Live vaccines 331
Live virus 331
Liver 222
abscess, amebic 283
biopsy 188, 283
flukes 310
Living bacteria, examination of 36
Living leptospira, appearance of 197f

Local immune complex disease 85
Local immunity 50, 56
Loeffler's serum slope 26, 118, 119
Loeffler's syndrome 302
Lophotrichous 18
Louse-borne 196
  relapsing fever 196
Low egg passage vaccine 246
Lowenstein-Jensen medium 136, 317
Lower respiratory tract 390
  infections 201
Ludlam's medium 94
Lung 319
  fluke 345
  trematodes 310
Lyme disease 196, 343
Lymphadenopathy 228, 248, 287
Lymphocytes 74, 75, 228
Lymphocytic choriomeningitis virus 348
Lymphogranuloma
  inguinale 215
  venereum 215, 319
Lymphoid cells 74, 75
Lymphoid tissue, mucosa associated 171
Lymphokine 80, 137
  activated killer cells 76
Lymphoma 171, 348
Lymphoreticular cells 74
Lymphoreticular system, cells of 75

M

MacConkey
  agar 27, 28, 94, 151, 156, 157, 159, 165, 174
  medium 150, 168, 180
Macrogametocyte 289
Macrolides 328
Macrophages 74
  functions of 76
Madurella mycetomatis 261, 344
Magic bullet 6
Malaria 193, 293, 319, 337
  clinical features of 292
  hemoglobinuria 292
  parasite 288, 291f
    life history of 289f
  relapses of 292
Malta fever 188

Mancini method 65
Mannitol salt agar 94
Mantoux test 139
Marburg virus 348
Mast cell 83f
Mastigophora 345
Matrix protein 243-245
McFadyean's method 124
McIntosh and Filde's anaerobic jar 29, 29f
Measles 225, 244, 315
  mumps, and rubella 440
  vaccine 248
Medical asepsis 386
Medical microbiology 3
Medusa head appearance 123
Membrane attack complex 59
  formation of 59
Membrane filters 380
Membrane protein 243f, 245
Memory cells 75, 79
Meningitis 109, 112, 174, 182, 271, 315, 316t, 341, 342
  acute pyogenic 315, 316
Meningococcal
  infections, stages of 112
  polysaccharide antigen 113
  septicemia 112
Meningococcemia 112
Meningococcus 111
Meningoencephalitis 341
Mercury drops 185
Mesenteric adenitis 231, 346
Mesosomes 15
  functions of 19
Metabolic antagonism 328, 329
Metabolic inhibition 222
Metachromatic granules 117, 117f
Metacystic trophozoites 281
Metallic body implants 396
Methicillin-resistant
  Staphylococcus
    aureus 97, 405-407
    epidermidis 407
Methylene blue 39, 41, 42
  counterstain 42
  reduced 29
Microaerophilic organisms 23
Microbial antagonisms 48
Microbial antigen, detecting 71
Microbial pathogenicity 32
Microbiology 3, 4
  branches of 7

development of 5
historical development of 3
research in 7
Micrococcus luteus 98
Microencephalitis 345
Microfilaria
  bancrofti, morphology of 308f
  detection of 310
Microorganisms
  discovery of 5
  first observation of 5
  relevance of 3
Microscope 11
  parts of 11
Microscopic agglutination test 198
Microscopic appearance 283
Microscopic examination 272, 273
Microscopy 142
  and antigen detection 109
  dark
    field 192
    ground 196
  direct 135
Microsporidiosis 252
Microsporum 262
Microwave irradiation 398
Midstream urine specimen 151
Milk
  agar 94
  pasteurization of 378
Milker's node 227
Millionaire molecule 56
Mima polymorpha 206
Minimum bactericidal concentration 322
Minocycline 113
Mites 209
Mitsuda reaction 142
Modern surgery 6
Molecular diagnostic methods 143
Molecular mimicry 88
Molecular techniques 183
Molluscum contagiosum virus 227, 319
Monkeypox 227
Monobactams 328
Monoclonal antibody 79
  uses of 80
Monocyte 228
Monokines 80
Mononuclear cells 76

Mononucleosis, infectious 193, 230, 337
Monotrichous 18
Monsur's gelatin taurocholate trypticase tellurite agar 166
Monsur's medium 168
Monsur's taurocholate tellurite peptone water 166
Moraxella 111
   catarrhalis 325
   lacunata 324
Morganella 153, 154
Morphological index 143
Morphology 226, 244, 267, 270
Mosquito-borne group 247
Mother to fetus, transfer from 54
Mother yaw 195
Motile gram negative bacilli 38
Motility, true 37
Mouse
   bioassay 132
   inoculation 245
Mouth 363
   cavity 47
   normal flora of 324
Mucocutaneous lesions 271
Mucoepithelial cells 228
Mucomycosis 344
Mucopolysaccharide 48
Mucormycosis 261, 273
Mucosa 267
   candidiasis of 261, 344
Mucous
   diarrhea 285
   membrane 47
Mueller-Hinton agar 114, 322
Multibacillary disease 142
Multidrug resistant
   Mycobacterium tuberculosis 140
   organisms 406, 407
Mumps 225, 315
   virus 244
Mupirocins 328
Mycelium 259
Mycetoma 261, 263, 264, 344
Mycobacteria, atypical 42, 343
Mycobacterial disease, types of opportunist 145, 145t
Mycobacterium 136, 342
   bovis 42
   leprae 42, 78, 136, 141, 343
   smegmatis 325
   tuberculosis 78, 136, 252, 317, 352
Mycolic acid 41
Mycoplasma 14, 200-202, 219, 343
   antigens 202
   genitalium 319
   hominis 201, 319
   pneumoniae 201, 202, 343
Mycosis 260, 261, 344
   classification of 260
   cutaneous 262
   superficial 262
   type of 261, 344
Mycotic infections 344
Myelography 297
Myeloma 79

N

Naegleria fowleri 345
Nagler's reaction 128
Nail
   bed, infection of 342
   candidiasis of 261, 344
   infections 271
Nalidixic acid 329
Napkin
   dermatitis 271
   rash 227
Nasal
   mucosa 152
   scrapings 142
Nasopharyngeal
   infection 112
   swabs 390
Nasopharynx 324
   cell line, human carcinoma of 222
Natural killer cell 75, 80
Necator americanus 305, 345
Neck 296, 298
Necrotic enteritis 129
Necrotizing fasciitis 103
Necrotizing jejunitis 129
Needle stick injuries 440, 443
   prevention of 363, 442, 443
Needle-mount method 44
Negler reaction 129f
Negri bodies 245
Neill-Mooser reaction 209
Neisseria 111, 112
   catarrhalis 15f
   gonorrhoeae 113, 317, 319, 341
   meningitidis 17, 68, 111, 315, 332, 341
   species 115
Nematoda 345
Nematodes 301, 318
Neoantigens 88
Neuraminidase 243
Neuron 228
Neurotoxin 130
Neutralization tests 69
Neutrophil 76
   chemotactic factors 84
Niacin test 137
Nichol's strain 190
Nicotinamideadenine dinucleotidase 103
Nitrate reduction
   positive 162
   test 137
Nitrofurans 328, 329
Nitrofurantoin 329
Nitrogen fixers 3
Nitroimidazoles 328, 329
Nocardia 146, 147
   asteroids 42
   braziliensis 42
Nocardiosis 147
Nonagglutinable vibrios 167
Noncholera vibrios 167
Nongonococcal urethritis 319
Nonhemolytic streptococci 101
Non-Hodgkin's lymphoma 252
Noninvasive disease 182
Noninvasive tests 172
Nonmotile gram negative bacteria 38
Non-neural vaccines 246
Nonparalytic poliomyelitis 242
Nonpathogenic treponemes 195
Nonphotochromogens 144
Nonsporing anaerobes 134
   classification of 134b
Nontreponemal tests 192, 193
Nontuberculous mycobacteria 144, 144t
Nontypable strains 182
Nonvenereal treponematoses 194
Norwalk virus 318, 348
Nose 363
   normal flora of 324
Nosocomial infections 154, 343
Novobiocin 328, 329
Nuclear membrane 280

Nucleic acid 381, 382
  detection of 245
  synthesis, inhibitors of 328
  technology 138
Nucleocapsid 220, 251
Nucleus 13, 280, 285, 286
Null cells 75
Nursing intervention 412
Nutrient
  agar 25, 93, 123, 124, 150, 153, 156, 159, 165, 173, 178
  broth 25
  media 153
Nutritional factors, based on 25
Nystatin 112, 114

O

O antigen 17, 150, 166
O polysaccharide 17
O serogroups 167
Oakley-Fulthorpe procedure 64, 64f
Obligate aerobes 23
Obligate anaerobes 23
Oculogenital serotypes 214
Ofloxacin 115
Onychomycosis 271
Ophthalmia neonatorum 114
Opportunist pathogens 31
Opportunistic fungi 270, 343
Opportunistic mycobacteria 144
Opportunistic mycoses 270
Opportunistic pulmonary disease 147
Optical instrument 11
Optical system 11
Optimum temperature 23
Optochin sensitivity 108
Oral
  cavity 47, 390
  infection 228
  lesions 226
  manifestations 268, 271
  polio vaccine 242
  rehydration therapy 168
  thrush 271
  vaccine 163, 169
Organ specificity 52
Organic acids 381
Organisms, observing motility of 37
Orientia
  species 208, 209t
  tsutsugamushi 209
Ornithodoros 196
Ornithosis 344
Oropharyngitis 196
Orthomyxoviridae 242, 249, 347, 348
Osmotic effect 24
Osteomyelitis 96
Otitis
  externa 342
  media 341
Ouchterlony technique 65, 65f
Outer membrane 16, 17
Oxidase test 112
Oxidizing agents 381, 382, 387
Oxygen 23

P

Pain, epigastric 285
Painful genital ulcers 319
Palladinized alumina 29
Papillomavirus 226, 232, 346
Papovaviruses 232, 346
Paracoccidioides brasiliensis 261, 267, 267f
Paracoccidioidomycosis 261, 267, 344
Paraffin baiting 147
Paragonimiasis 345
Paragonimus westermani 310, 345
Parainfluenza viruses 244
Paramyxoviruses 244
Paranasal granuloma 273
Paranasal sinuses 390
Parasite 31, 72, 279, 337
  classification of 279
Paratyphoid fever 160
Paravaccinia 227
Parrot fever 215
Particle agglutination 253
Parvovirus 226, 232, 346
Passive agglutination 68
  reversed 68
  test 67
Passive immunity, natural 49
Passive immunization 224, 225, 230, 237, 247, 332, 335
  indications of 49
  preparations for 335
Pasteurella 178
  multocida 342
Pasteurization 5
Pathogenic microorganisms 4
Pathogenicity 184
Pathogens 31
  types of 31
Patient safety indicators 409, 417
Patient's serum 68
  test 194
Paucibacillary disease 142
Paul-Bunnell test 231
Pediculus humanus corporis 196
Pelvic inflammatory disease 341
Pemphigus neonatorum 96
Penicillin 110, 113, 121, 147, 194, 196, 197, 200, 328
  destroying enzymes, production of 328
Penicillinase 97, 329
  producing gonococci 115
Penicilliosis 261, 273, 344
Penicillium 275f
  marneffei 261, 344
  notatum 6
Peptic ulcers 342
Peptide subunit vaccines 332
Peptidoglycan 16, 94, 102f
  smaller amount of 40
Peptone water 166
Peracetic acid 385
Periostitis 96
Peripheral blood 287
Peritonitis 105
Peritrichous 18
Pernasal swab 186, 390
Pernicious malaria 292
Peroxyacetic acid 385
Peroxygens 381
Personal protective equipment 358, 362, 364, 366, 399, 406, 430
Pertussis vaccine 121
Petechial lesions 113
Petroff's method 138
pH 24
Phaeohyphomycosis 261, 344
Phagocytic cells 74, 76
Phagocytosis 56, 76
Pharyngitis 96, 228, 231, 341, 346
Pharyngoconjunctival fever 231, 346
Pharynx 119
Phenol 41, 377, 381, 382
  derivatives 382

Phenolphthalein phosphate agar 94
Phenyl pyruvic acid test 153
Phialophora verrucosa 261, 344
Phlebitis 413
Phlebotomus argentipes 287
Phosphatase test 94
Phosphonoformic acid 230
Photochromogens 144
Phthirus pubis 319
Physicochemical structure 53
Picornaviridae 241*b*, 346, 348
Picornaviruses 241
Piedraia hortae 261, 344
Pigment production 173
Pilins 18
Pilli 18, 114
    functions of 18
Pinta 194, 195
Pinworm 345
    feotalism 345
Pityriasis versicolor 261, 344
Plague 4
Plain toxoid 131
Plasma
    cell 74, 75, 79
    tumor 79
    membrane 15, 17
Plasmids 19, 34
    function of 19
Plasmodium
    falciparum 288, 291*f*, 293
    malariae 288, 291*f*, 293
    ovale 288, 291*f*, 293
    vivax 288, 291*f*, 293
Platelet activating factor 84
Plating media 166
Platyhelminthes 345
Pleomorphism 178
Plesiomonas shigelloides 318
Pleuropneumonia 200
Pleuropulmonary amebiasis 282
Pneumexystis
    carinii 274
    jiroveci 274
Pneumococci 107*f*, 110*t*
Pneumococcus 17, 107, 108
Pneumocystis 286
    carinii 270
        pneumonia 252, 274
Pneumocystosis 274
Pneumonia 109, 152, 154, 174, 182, 201, 202, 231, 244, 319, 341, 344, 346

    chronic 267
    infant 214
    primary atypical 201, 343
    ventilator-associated 352, 353, 355, 356
Pneumonic plague 179
Pneumonitis 228
Polar bodies 117
Polio 332, 346
    vaccine, inactivated 225, 242
Poliomyelitis 225, 337
    abortive 242
    immunization 50
Poliovirus 241, 249, 315, 346
    types of 241
Pollution, cleaning up 4
Polyclonal B-cell activation 88
Polymerase chain reaction 113, 120, 172, 186, 210, 229-232, 237, 239, 248, 260, 273
Polymorphonuclear leukocytes 74
Polymorphonuclear microphages 76
Polymyxin 200, 328
Polyomavirus 232, 346
Polysaccharide antigen, group-specific 102
Pomona 197
Pontiac fever 176
Pork tapeworm 295, 345
Postdiphtheritic paralysis 341
Post-exposure prophylaxis 246 255, 441, 443
Post-kala-azar dermal leishmaniasis 286
Postnasal swab 186, 390
Potassium hydroxide 260, 271
    preparation 43, 260
Potassium tellurite 118
    medium 27
Potato-blood-glycerol agar 185
Pour-plate culture 28
Poxvirus 226
    diseases 227
Precipitation reaction 63
    applications of 63
Pre-erythrocytic schizogony 288
Pressure filtration 380
Prevotella melaninogenica 135
Primitive communities 124
Proctitis 341, 342
Proflavine 383
Prokaryotes 14
Prokaryotic cell 13, 13*t*

Promote health 4
Prophylaxis 4, 113, 121, 129, 130, 132, 139, 162, 168, 188, 237, 238, 242, 245, 248, 254, 298
    pre-exposure 247
    vaccination 186
Propionibacterium 324
Prostaglandin 84
Prostate per rectum, massage of 391
Prostatitis 391
Protein 245, 381, 382
    A 94
    abnormal 109
    acute phase 48
    derivative, purified 139
    lipoteichoic acid fimbria 102*f*
Proteinase 103
Proteus 149, 153
    bacilli 153, 154
    mirabilis 317
    vulgaris 171
Proton pump inhibitor 172
Protoplasm 39
Protozoa 3, 279, 315, 318
    vaginitis 345
Providencia 153, 154
Prozone 63
    phenomenon 67
Pseudallescheria boydii 261, 344
Pseudo anthrax 124
Pseudomembrane 119
    candidiasis 271
    formation 317
Pseudomembranous colitis 132, 341
Pseudomonas 95, 173, 315
    aeruginosa 135, 173-175, 317, 324, 342, 352
Pseudo-reaction 121
Psittacosis 344
Puberty 326
Public health, contribution to 3
Puerperal sepsis 103
Pulmonary anthrax 124
Pulmonary aspergillosis 273
Pulmonary infection 267
Pulmonary tuberculosis 137, 342
Purified chick embryo cell vaccine 246
Purulent meningitis 315
Pus 107*f*
    smear of 93*f*
Pustule, malignant 124

Pyelonephritis 319
Pyemia 103
Pyocyanin 173
Pyogenes 197
Pyogenic cutaneous infections 340
Pyogenic infections 105, 150, 151, 341
Pyomelanin 173
Pyorubrin 173
Pyoverdine 173
Pyrexia 287
  of unknown origin 319
Pyrogenic exotoxins 102
Pyrrolidonyl naphthylamine, hydrolysis of 102

Q

Q fever 211
Quality of life 3
Quellung reaction 17, 183
Quinolones 328

R

Rabbit-blood agar 183
Rabies 225, 332
  antigens 245
  vaccine 246b
    developed 5
  virus 245, 348
    antigen 245
    isolation of 245
Radial immunodiffusion 65, 65f
Radiation 377, 380
  safety 427, 434
Radioimmunoassay 70
Rail road track 183
Rapid diagnostic tests 293
Rapid dipstick assay 188
Rapid plasma regain test 193
Rapid slide agglutination test 231
Rash 248
Rat
  bite fever 206, 343
  fleas 179, 338
Rattus rattus 338
Raveler's diarrhea 150
Reaction
  localized 83
  negative 120
  positive 121
  types of 120

Rectal swabs 157
Red blood cell 69, 178f
Regional lymph nodes 191
Regulatory T cells 75
Relapsing fever 193, 196, 198
Reservoir hosts 32
Respiratory diphtheria 119
Respiratory diseases 231, 346
  acute 231, 346
Respiratory hygiene 358, 362
Respiratory infection 103, 340
Respiratory syncytial virus 72, 244, 249
Respiratory syndrome, severe acute 358
Respiratory tract 103
  disease 201
  infection 154
Retroviruses 251
Reverse camp test 128f
Reynolds-Braude phenomenon 272
Rhabdoviruses 245
Rhesus
  embryo cell strain 222
  monkey kidney cell culture 222
Rheumatic fever 340
  acute 103
Rheumatoid arthritis 88
Rhinosporidiosis 263, 264, 264f
Rhinosporidium 264
  seeberi 264
Rhinovirus 346
Rhizopoda 345
Rhodamine 69, 69b
Ribonucleoprotein 243
Ribosomes 15, 19, 219
Riboviruses 222
Rickettsia 208, 209t, 211
  antigens 210
  diseases 210t
  isolation of 210
  rickettsiae 344
Rifampin 113
Rifamycins 328, 329
Ring test 63
Ritter's disease 96
Robertson's cooked meat
  broth 127
  medium 96, 127
Rocky mountain spotted fever 344

Rose Bengal plate test 188
Rose-Waaler test 68
Rotavirus 248, 249, 318, 348
Roundworm 345
Rubella 225, 248
  congenital 248
  vaccine 248
Runyon classification 144t

S

Sabin live polio vaccine 242
Sabouraud's dextrose agar 260, 271, 273
Sacral autonomic dysfunction 228
Safety-pin appearance 178
Safranin counterstain 39
Salmonella 28, 67, 78, 159, 162
  dublin 318
  enteritidis 318
  gastroenteritis 160, 163
  heidelberg 318
  indiana 318
  newport 318
  typhi 332
  typhimurium 318
Salpingitis 341
Salt milk agar 94, 96
San Joaquin valley fever 267
Saprophytes 31
Sarcina 15f
Sarcoptes scabei 319
Satellitism 181, 182f
Scalded skin syndrome 340
Scarlatinal toxin 102
Scarlet fever 340
Schick test 120
Schistosoma mansoni 318
Schistosomiasis 345
Schultz-Charlton reaction 103
Scistosoma
  haematobium 310
  japonicum 310
  mansoni 310
Scolex 294, 296, 298
Scotochromogens 144
Screw-feed technology 398
Scrub typhus 209
Seitz filter 380
Semisynthetic media 197
Sensitivity testing 138
Sepsis 342
Septicemia 96, 103, 150, 152, 154, 271, 319, 342, 343

plague 179
Septicemic
  illnesses 343
  malaria 292
Sequestrated antigens 52
Serogroup-specific tests 198
Serological methods 17
Serological reactions 62
Serological screening 194
Serological test 97, 143, 162, 188, 192, 249, 260, 268, 272, 273, 283, 293, 300, 303
  nonspecific 202
Serology 176, 229, 230, 232, 244, 245, 247, 248, 263, 297
Serotherapy 6
Serotinin 84
Serotypes, host-adapted 160
Serratia 153
Serum
  dextrose 188
  dextrose agar 187
  hepatitis 235, 346
  opacity factor 103
  potato infusion agar 187
  sickness 85
Sexually transmitted disease 252, 319, 319t, 342, 343
Shake culture 28
Shanghai fever 342
Sheep liver fluke 345
Shiga toxin 156, 157
Shigella 27, 28, 67, 156, 157
  boydii 318
  dysenteriae 149, 318, 341
  fiexneri 318
  organisms 157
  sonnei 318
Shock 248
  anaphylactic 83
  endotoxic 61
Shwartzman reaction 86
Sinusitis 96, 341
Skin 47, 103, 267
  candidiasis of 261, 344
  disinfectant 382
  infection 103, 262, 271
  lesions, secondary 195
  normal flora of 324
  smears 142
  test 215, 263, 272, 273, 303
Skirrow's campylobacter 171
Skull, X-ray of 297

Slide
  agglutination 67, 157, 168
    test 162
  coagulase test 95
  flocculation test 64
  test 64
Slim disease 252
Slit and scrape method 142
Small intestine 47
Smallpox 225, 345
  classical 226
  virus 345
Smear 38
  preparation 38
Soft chancres 184
Soft sore 184, 342
Soft tissue
  infection 103, 129
  X-ray of 297
Soiled waste 394
Somatic antigen 109, 150, 152, 182
Somatic cells 308
Sonic stresses 24
Sore mouth 227
Sore throat 103, 317
  causative agents of 317t
Spaulding's classification 386, 387t
Specimens, collection of 315, 390, 391
Sperm antigens 88
Spermine 48
Spill 429, 434
  clean-up procedures 430
  types of 429
Spillage management 429, 434
Spinal fluid 272f
Spiral bacteria 315
Spirilla 14
Spirillum minus 206
Spirochetes 14, 190, 191f, 191t, 343
Spleen 282
  punctures 287
Splenic enlargement 287
Spoliative action 303
Spontaneous abortion 342
Sporadic encephalitis 228
Sporangia 264
Spore 386
  coat 19
  septum 19

staining of 43
  types of 20f
  uses of 20
Sporothrix schenckii 261, 263, 264, 264f, 344
Sporotrichosis 261, 263, 264, 344
Sporozoa 288
Spotted fever group 209
Sputum 137, 390
  culture 183
Stab culture 28
Stain 38
  differential 39
  methods 36, 38
  negative 38
  preparations 14, 38
  simple 39
  smear for 38
  special 43
  techniques 6
  types of 38
Standard agglutination test 188
Standard loop method 151
Staphylococcal cell wall, structure of 94f
Staphylococci 98t
  species of 93
Staphylococcus 13, 93, 93f, 98t
  aureus 13, 68, 93-95, 97, 315, 318, 340, 352, 353, 385, 405
  epidermidis 97, 315, 324, 326
  saprophyticus 97, 317
Steam sterilizers, types of 379
Stenotrophomonas 173
  maltophilia 173, 174
Sterile technique 386
Sterilization 376
  control 20, 378, 379
  methods of 376, 377b
Stokes disk diffusion method 321, 322, 322f
Stomach aspiration 391
Stool 168
  examination of 282, 283, 297, 305
Stormy clot reaction 128
Stormy fermentation 128
Streak culture 28, 28f
Streptobacillus moniliformis 206, 343
Streptococcal
  gangrene 103
  pharyngitis 340

pyrogenic exotoxin 102
toxic shock syndrome 103, 340
Streptococci 100f
  classification of 101
  group B 315, 319
  pathogenic 104
Streptococcus 100, 107
  agalactiae 104
  pneumoniae 17, 68, 107f, 110, 315, 332, 341
  pyogenes 101, 103, 317, 340
Streptogramins 328
Streptokinase 103
Streptolysin
  O 102
  S 102
String test 166
Stroke culture 28
Strongyloides stercoralis 318, 345
Strongyloidiasis 345
Stuart's transport medium 28
Subcutaneous mycoses 262-264
Subcutaneous test 120
Sucking disk 284
Suckling mice 247
Sugar
  fermentation 94, 112, 166
  utilization tests 113
Sulfonamide 148, 328
Sulfur granules 146, 147f
Sulfuric acid 42
  decolorizer 42
Sun-ray appearance 147
Superkingdoms system 13
Suppurative complications 103
Suppurative streptococcal disease 103
Suprapubic stab 151
Surface antigens 243
Surgical asepsis 386
Surgical hand scrub 369
Surgical prophylaxis 130
Surgical safety 415, 418
Surgical site infections 352, 353, 356
Swarming appearance 153
Synthetic peptide vaccines 238
Syphilis 64, 319, 337, 343
  congenital 192, 194
  diagnosis of 70
  diagnostic tests for 192t
  late 192
  secondary 191

serological tests in untreated 194t
standard tests for 192
tertiary 192
Systemic anaphylaxis 83
Systemic aspergillosis 273
Systemic bacteriology 91
Systemic candidiasis 261, 271, 344
Systemic disease, severe 198
Systemic immune complex disease 85
Systemic mycoses 266
Systemic phycomycosis 273
Systemic reactions 83

T

T cell 74, 75
  activation 79
  cytotoxic 75, 79
  dependent 52
  independent antigens 52
  suppressor 75, 88
T lymphocytes 75
Tacaribe virus complex 348
Taenia
  saginata 294, 295t, 345
  solium 295, 295t, 345
  eggs of 295f
Taeniasis 345
Tanapox 227
Tapeworm 294
  general cycle of 296f
  infection, laboratory diagnosis of 297
Teichoic acids 16, 94
Teicoplanin 98
Tellurite blood agar 118, 119
Tetanolysin 130
Tetanospasmin 130
Tetanus
  diphtheria, pertussis 440
  generalized 130
  neonatorum 130
  toxin 130
  toxoid 131
Tetracycline 147, 194, 196, 328, 329
Tetramethylparaphenylene-diamine-dihydrochloride 112
Tetranucleate amoeba 281
Tetrathionate broth 27

Thallophyta 259
Thayer-Martin medium 114
Thicker peptidoglycan cell wall 40
Thioglycollate broth 135
Thiosulfate-citrate-bile-sucrose agar 166
Threadworm 345
Throat 390
Thrombocytopenic purpura 84
Thumb print appearance 185
Tick-borne 196
  relapsing fever 196
Tinea nigra 261, 344
Tissue enzymes, susceptibility to 51
Togaviridae 347, 348
Toluidine
  blue 42
  red unheated serum test 193
Tonsillitis 96, 228
Tonsils 119
Tooth decay 105
Toxic epidermal necrolysis 96
Toxic shock syndrome 95, 96, 340
Toxigenicity 33, 65
  test 130
Toxin 95, 102, 119, 128, 132, 150, 157
  consists 119
  demonstration of 132
  induced diseases 340
  major 129
  mediated diseases 96
  properties of 119
  standardization of 64
Toxocara canis 306
Toxocara cati 306
Toxoid 331
  standardization of 64
Toxoplasma 72
Toxoplasmosis 252, 319
Tracheobronchitis 201, 228
Trachoma 214, 344
Transcription-polymerase chain reaction, reverse 245
Transformation 222
Transmembrane pedicle glycoprotein 251f
Transport media 28
Trematodes 310, 318
  classification of 310
Treponema 190, 191, 195
  antigen, species-specific 191

pallidum 190, 191, 191f, 198, 319, 343, 391
   agglutination test 193
   hemagglutination 68
   immune adherence test 193
   tests 192, 193
   vincentii 196, 317
Tribe proteae 153
Tric agents 214
Trichinaworm 345
Trichinella spiralis 345
Trichinosis 345
Trichomonas 285
   hominis 285
   tenax 285
   vaginalis 285, 285f, 293, 319, 345
Trichomoniasis 319
Trichophyton 262
Trichuriasis 345
Trichuris trichiura 318, 345
Trimethoprim 328
Trophozoite 280, 284, 284f
Tropical bubo 215
Tropical eosinophilia 193
Trypanosoma
   brucei 345
   cruzi 337, 345
Trypanosomes 78
Trypanosomiasis 319, 337
Trypticase soy agar 187
Tryptose agar 187
Tsugamushi 209
Tsutsugamushi disease 209
Tube agglutination 67
   uses of 67
Tube coagulase test 95
Tubercle bacilli 136, 144
   constituents of 137
Tuberculate macroconidia 268
Tuberculin
   test 138, 139
   type 86
Tuberculosis 6, 319, 342
   extrapulmonary 138
Tuberculous meningitis 316, 317
Tumor necrosis factor 76
Tunica reaction 209
Tyndallization 378
Typhoid fever 160, 337
   diagnosis of 161f
   vaccines 162, 163

Typhus fever group 209
Tyrocidine 328
Tzanck smear 229

U

Ulcerative gingivostomatitis 196
Ulcers, flask-shaped 281
Undulant fever 188
Unilocular echinococcosis 310
Universal Immunization Program 333
Upper respiratory tract 47, 119
   normal flora of 325
Urea
   breath test 172
   hydrolysis 153
Ureaplasma 200, 202, 343
   urealyticum 201, 202, 319, 325
Urethra 115
   discharge 319, 391
   pus 114f
Urethritis 341
   acute 114
Urinary tract infection 105, 150, 151, 174, 271, 317, 319, 341, 343, 353, 391
   catheter-associated 352, 353, 355, 356
   causes of 317t
Urine 151, 198
   culture 162
   microscopy of 151
   normal flow of 48
   specimen 115

V

Vaccines 3, 331, 440
   types of 331
Vaccinia virus 226, 227
Vacuole 286
Vaginal discharge 319
Vaginal swab, high 391
Vaginitis 319
Valaciclovir 229
Valley fever 267
Vancomycin 98, 112, 328
Vancomycin-resistant
   Staphylococcus aureus 406
Varicella 225, 229, 440
Varicella-zoster
   immunoglobulin 230

   virus 226, 228, 229, 232 252, 345
Varicose ulcers 342
Variola
   major 226
   minor 227
   virus 226
VDRL-ELISA test 193
Venereal disease research laboratory 193
Venkatraman-Ramakrishnan medium 166
Vesicle formation 228
Vesicular stomatitis virus 348
Vibrio 14, 165
   cholerae 165, 169, 318, 342
   parahaemolyticus 318
Vincent's angina 119, 196, 198
Violet dye 39
Viral
   envelope 220
   hepatitis 234
   infections, laboratory diagnosis of 224
   markers, detection of 237
   meningitis 316
   proteins, detection of 224
   vaccines 49, 225t, 332
Viral diseases
   chemotherapy of 224
   immunoprophylaxis of 224
   laboratory diagnosis of 224
   prophylaxis of 224
Viral nucleic acid 220
   detection of 253
Virchow's lepra cells 141
Viridans streptococci 105, 108, 110t
Virulence 33
   determinants of 33
   tests 119
Virus 3, 72, 219, 234, 242, 249, 315, 317, 318, 337, 345
   antigen 229, 243
   capsid antigen 231
   classification of 222
   cultivation of 220
   detection 248
   direct demonstration of 231
   direct detection of 224
   discovery of 6
   diseases, chemotherapy of 225
   general properties of 219

growth, detection of 222
isolation 224, 229-231, 235, 244, 245, 247-249, 253, 380
morphology of 219
shape of 220, 221f
sizes of 221f
structure 235
Visceral larva migrans 306
Vitamins 3
Volutin containing organisms, staining of 42
Volutin granules 117
Vulvovaginal candidiasis 319
Vulvovaginitis 114, 271

W

Walking pneumonia 201
Warning sign 428
Waste
 disposal 363
 infectious 393
 management program 399
 segregation 394, 400
 treatment 394
 type of 394, 395, 396
Waterhouse-Friderichsen syndrome 112
Wear laser safety glasses 427
Weil's disease 198
Weil-Felix reaction 210, 210t
Western blot 72
 assay 239
 test 253
Wet coverslip preparation 36
Wet thermal treatment 398
Whipworm 345
Whirlpool rash 342
White cell count 231
Whittaker's system 13
Whole cell agglutination 260
Whooping cough 186, 342
Widal agglutination 161f
Widal test 161, 162
Wilson and Blair medium 27
Wolinella 170
Wool-Sorter's disease 124
Wound 391
 botulism 132
 infection 105, 154, 174, 390
 local treatment of 246
Wright's stain 206
Wuchereria bancrofti 307, 310, 345
 life cycle of 309f

X

Xenopsylla cheopis 179
Xylose lysine deoxycholate agar 156, 159

Y

Yaws 194, 195
Yeast 259, 260, 270
 like fungi 260, 270
Yellow fever 225, 247
Yersinia 17, 178
 enterocolitica 180, 318
 pestis 17, 178, 342
 pseudotuberculosis 179
Yersiniosis 179
Yolk sac 208, 221

Z

Ziehl-Neelsen
 carbol fuchsin 42
 method 136
 reagents 42
 stain 41, 41f, 141, 145, 147, 316, 317
 modified 20
 technique 138
Zinc 48
Zone phenomenon 63
Zoonosis 32, 211
Zoonotic
 bacterial disease 198
 disease 179
 infection 342
Zygomycosis 261, 273, 344

EU GSPR Authorised Reprsentative
Logos Europe, 9 rue Nicolas Poussin
1700, La Rochelle, France
Phone: +33 (0) 6 67 93 73 78
E-mail: contact@logoseurope.eu

www.ingramcontent.com/pod-product-compliance
Ingram Content Group UK Ltd.
Pitfield, Milton Keynes, MK11 3LW, UK
UKHW050456150426
5217IPUK00025B/1706